Handbook of Cardiovascular Immunology

Handbook of Cardiovascular Immunology

Editor: Rebbeca Atwell

AMERICAN
MEDICAL PUBLISHERS
www.americanmedicalpublishers.com

AMERICAN
MEDICAL PUBLISHERS
www.americanmedicalpublishers.com

Cataloging-in-Publication Data

Handbook of cardiovascular immunology / edited by Rebbeca Atwell.
p. cm.
Includes bibliographical references and index.
ISBN 978-1-63927-964-7
1. Cardiovascular system--Diseases--Immunological aspects. 2. Cardiovascular system--Diseases.
3. Immunology. I. Atwell, Rebbeca.
RC669 .H36 2023
616.1--dc23

American Medical Publishers,
41 Flatbush Avenue,
1st Floor, New York,
NY 11217, USA

ISBN 978-1-63927-964-7 (Hardback)

Contents

Preface

It is often said that books are a boon to mankind. They document every progress and pass on the knowledge from one generation to the other. They play a crucial role in our lives. Thus I was both excited and nervous while editing this book. I was pleased by the thought of being able to make a mark but I was also nervous to do it right because the future of students depends upon it. Hence, I took a few months to research further into the discipline, revise my knowledge and also explore some more aspects. Post this process, I begun with the editing of this book.

Cardiovascular immunology involves the interaction of immune cells with cardiomyocytes, cardiac stromal cells and endothelial cells, which adjust their metabolism for supporting the continuing inflammatory process. The immune system has a crucial role in cardiac homeostasis and illness. If atherothrombotic occlusion disturbs oxygen transport, the downstream hypoxic tissues and cells begin to die within minutes. In case this condition remains untreated, the organism can succumb to stroke or myocardial infarction (MI). The immune system plays a significant role in cardiac growth, composition and function. The immune cells infiltrate the heart during gestation and remain in the myocardium where they perform vital housekeeping functions. A large numbers of immune cells are employed by the heart after a myocardial infarction, or in reaction to infection for promoting recovery, eliminating dying tissue and scavenging pathogens. Immune cells might cause irreparable harm in some cases which leads to heart failure. This book is a compilation of chapters that discuss the most vital aspects in the field of cardiovascular immunology. Through it, we attempt to further enlighten the readers about the new aspects in this field.

I thank my publisher with all my heart for considering me worthy of this unparalleled opportunity and for showing unwavering faith in my skills. I would also like to thank the editorial team who worked closely with me at every step and contributed immensely towards the successful completion of this book. Last but not the least, I wish to thank my friends and colleagues for their support.

Editor

1

Cardioprotection of Ginkgolide B on Myocardial Ischemia/Reperfusion-Induced Inflammatory Injury via Regulation of A20-NF-κB Pathway

*Rui Zhang [1], Lin Xu [2], Dong Zhang [3], Bo Hu [4], Qi Luo [1], Dan Han [5], Jiangbing Li [6] and Chengwu Shen [1]**

[1] Department of Pharmacy, Shandong Provincial Hospital Affiliated to Shandong University, Jinan, China, [2] Department of Thoracic Surgery, Shandong Provincial Hospital Affiliated to Shandong University, Jinan, China, [3] Department of Urology, Shandong Provincial Hospital Affiliated to Shandong University, Jinan, China, [4] Minimally Invasive Urology Center, Shandong Provincial Hospital Affiliated to Shandong University, Jinan, China, [5] Department of Pharmacy, Nanjing Drum Tower Hospital, The Affiliated Hospital of Nanjing University Medical School, Nanjing, China, [6] Department of Cardiology, Shandong Provincial Hospital Affiliated to Shandong University, Jinan, China

***Correspondence:**
Chengwu Shen
525500290@qq.com

Inflammation urges most of the characteristics of plaques involved in the pathogenesis of myocardial ischemia/reperfusion injury (MI/RI). In addition, inflammatory signaling pathways not only mediate the properties of plaques that precipitate ischemia/reperfusion (I/R) but also influence the clinical consequences of the post-infarction remodeling and heart failure. Here, we studied whether Ginkgolide B (GB), an effective anti-inflammatory monomer, improved MI/RI via suppression of inflammation. Left anterior descending (LAD) coronary artery induced ischemia/reperfusion (I/R) of rats or A20 silencing mice, as well as hypoxia/reoxygenation (H/R) induced damages of primary cultured rat neonatal ventricular myocytes or A20 silencing ventricular myocytes, respectively, served as MI/RI model *in vivo* and *in vitro* to discuss the anti-I/R injury properties of GB. We found that GB significantly alleviated the symptoms of MI/RI evidently by reducing infarct size, preventing ultrastructural changes of myocardium, depressing Polymorphonuclears (PMNs) infiltration, lessening histopathological damage and suppressing the excessive inflammation. Further study demonstrated that GB remarkably inhibited NF-κB p65 subunit translocation, IκB-α phosphorylation, IKK-β activity, as well as the downstream inflammatory cytokines and proteins expressions via zinc finger protein A20. In conclusion, GB could alleviate MI/RI-induced inflammatory response through A20-NF-κB signal pathway, which may give us new insights into the preventive strategies for MI/RI disease.

Keywords: Ginkgolide B, Myocardial ischemia/reperfusion injury, Inflammation, A20, NF-κB

INTRODUCTION

Myocardial ischemia/reperfusion injury (MI/RI) with high morbidity and mortality rates has become one of the decisive factors for the events of cardiovascular diseases (1, 2). The mechanisms of MI/RI refer to a series of complicated pathological processes, including inflammatory response, calcium overload, complement activation, cell autophagy, and apoptosis (3). And, it has repeatedly been shown that the earliest phases of ischemia/reperfusion (I/R) are dominated by an acute inflammatory response. Presently, the mechanisms driving this acute and robust inflammatory response are still unknown. However, over the last decades, it has become increasingly clear that Zinc finger protein A20 is considered to be a pivotal link to the inflammation throughout the whole pathological process of myocardial ischemia/reperfusion induced tissue injury (4).

Zinc finger protein A20, also described as the TNF-α-induced protein 3 (TNFAIP3), is a widely expressed cytoplasmic signaling protein, commonly deemed as an anti-inflammatory, nuclear factor-kappa B (NF-κB) inhibitory, and anti-apoptotic molecule (5, 6). A20 was one key part of the mechanisms involved in multiple autoimmune and inflammatory diseases, such as coronary artery disease, psoriasis, systemic sclerosis, coeliac disease, type 1 diabetes, inflammatory bowel disease, and rheumatoid arthritis. A20 comprehensively results in alterations to the signaling pathways leading to inflammatory changes, and in consequence, regulates the intensity and duration of signaling by several critical factors mainly dependent on NF-κB pathway (7). And, we have also reported that up-regulating A20 could protect blood brain barrier against ischemic stroke superimposed on systemic inflammatory challenges (8). However, no data have been published focused on the role of A20 in pathogenesis of MI/RI.

Moreover, an increasing body of evidence suggested that I/R could elevate the activation of NF-κB, whereas inflammatory response was inhibited after NF-κB deactivation, and cardiac function restored. IκB-α, regarded as an inhibitor, binds to NF-κB p65/p50 heterodimer in cytoplasm (9–11). Phosphorylation and subsequent degradation of IκB-α caused by IKK-β activation lead to the release of NF-κB and then translocation to nucleus. Ultimately, that will stimulate the production of various inflammatory cytokines, such as interleukin (IL)-1β, tumor necrosis factor (TNF)-α, IL-6 and cell adhesion molecules which acts directly or indirectly to depress cardiac function (12). Meanwhile, PMNs infiltration also remarkably influences the post-ischemic perfused myocardium and various metabolites into the myocardial cells as well. Therefore, suppressing PMNs infiltration and NF-κB activation can obviously alleviate MI/RI induced damages and consequently offer myocardial protection (13, 14).

Ginkgolide B (GB, **Figure 1**), an effective flavonoid monomer, was extracted from Ginkgo biloba leaves with multiple modulatory or protective functions and has been used in the treatment of cardio-cerebral vascular system damage for years (15–17). Most recently, researchers have discovered that GB could exert modulatory or protective functions against inflammatory reactions induced cascade effect to subsequently alleviate ischemia reperfusion diseases (18, 19). Moreover, there has been reported that GB could protect against IR-induced myocardial dysfunction and degradation of the membrane phospholipids (20). However, there has been no research reported on the relations between A20 and GB, meanwhile the specific mechanism of its anti-inflammatory effects is still limited and need an in-depth elucidation.

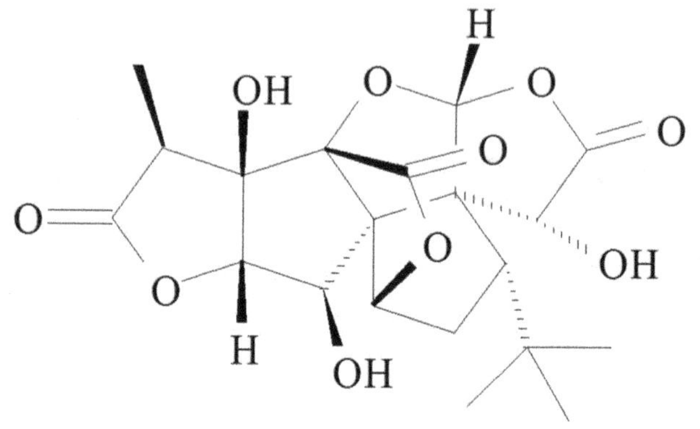

FIGURE 1 | Chemical structure of GB.

Thus, in this study, we investigated the role of GB in the protection of inflammation induced by MI/RI *in vivo*. We also made positive efforts to elucidate the role of A20-NF-κB signal pathway in the protection of ventricular myocytes exposed to H/R *in vitro*.

MATERIALS AND METHODS

Materials and Reagents

GB (PubChem CID: 65243), 2, 3, 5-Triphenyltetrazolium chloride (TTC) was purchased from Sigma (St. Louis, MO, United States). DMEM medium (high glucose) and newborn calf serum were purchased from Gibco (Grand Island, NY, United States). TNF-α, IL-1β, and IL-6 ELISA kits were products of Sigma (St. Louis, MO, United States). Anti-A20, anti-ICAM-1, anti-VCAM-1, anti-iNOS, anti-NF-κB p65, anti-p-IκB-α, anti-IKK-β, anti-Histone, anti-β-actin, goat anti-rabbit and anti-mouse IgG antibodies were products of Santa Cruz (Santa Cruz, CA, United States). Enhanced chemiluminescence (ECL) plus kit was product of Keygen Biotech.

Animals

Male Sprague-Dawley rats (250–300 g, Experimental Animal Center of Shandong University) were used for the current study. A20 gene silencing male mouse strains were provided by Beijing Biocytogen Co., Ltd. Rats and mice were housed in a temperature-controlled environment (18–22°C) with a 12 h light-dark cycle and allowed free access to food and water before the experiment. All the experiments were approved by the ethics committee of the Shandong Provincial Hospital affiliated to Shandong University (NSFC: No. 2018-019).

In vivo I/R Procedure to Induce MI/RI in Rats

I/R surgery was exactly carried out in accordance with the procedure in **Figure 2A**. The rats were anesthetized with 300 mg/kg chloral hydrate (i.p.). Electrocardiograph was continuously applied to monitor the changes of S-T segment so as to determine the success of surgery. After a left thoracotomy, the left anterior descending (LAD) coronary artery was twined with a plastic tube by a 6-0 silk suture for reversible LAD occlusion. Reperfusion for 120 min was initiated by releasing the suture and removing the tension after transient regional myocardial ischemia for 40 min according to the procedure. Before the rats were sacrificed, the blood samples were collected.

Randomly selected rats were divided into 5 groups as follows ($n = 8$ per group): (1) Control group, rats did not receive I/R, saline was administered; (2) I/R group, I/R rats administered with saline; (3) 8 mg/kg GB group, I/R rats received 8 mg/kg of GB; (4) 16 mg/kg GB group, I/R rats received 16 mg/kg of GB; (5) 32 mg/kg GB group, I/R rats received 32 mg/kg of GB. Saline and

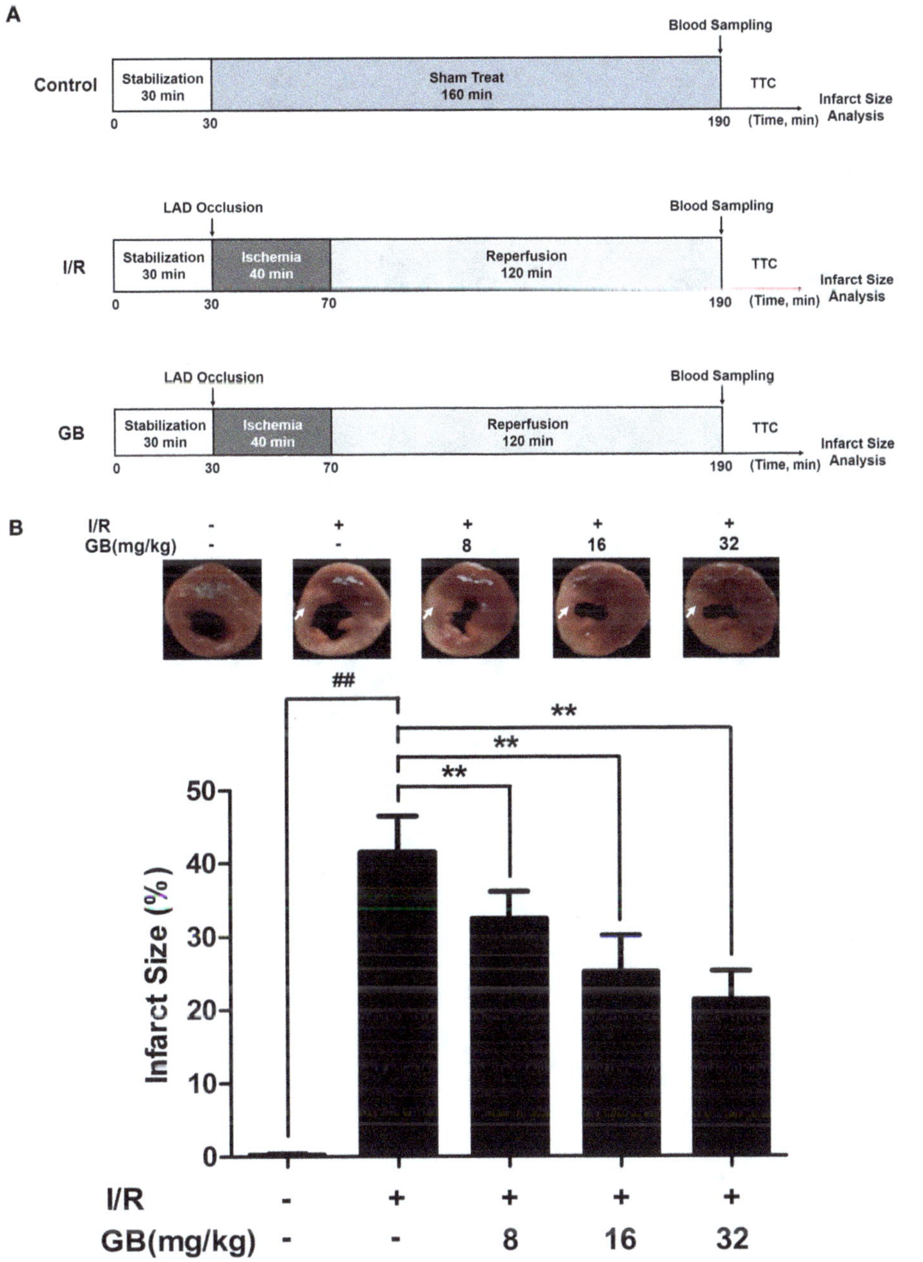

FIGURE 2 | Effects of GB on infarct size in MI/RI rats model. **(A)** The experimental procedures of *in vivo* MI/RI rats model. **(B)** Treatment with GB significantly reduced the infarct size in MI/RI rats model. Data were expressed as mean ± S.D. ($n = 8$). ##$P < 0.01$, I/R group vs. control group; *$P < 0.05$, **$P < 0.01$, 8, 16, 32 mg/kg GB groups vs. I/R group.

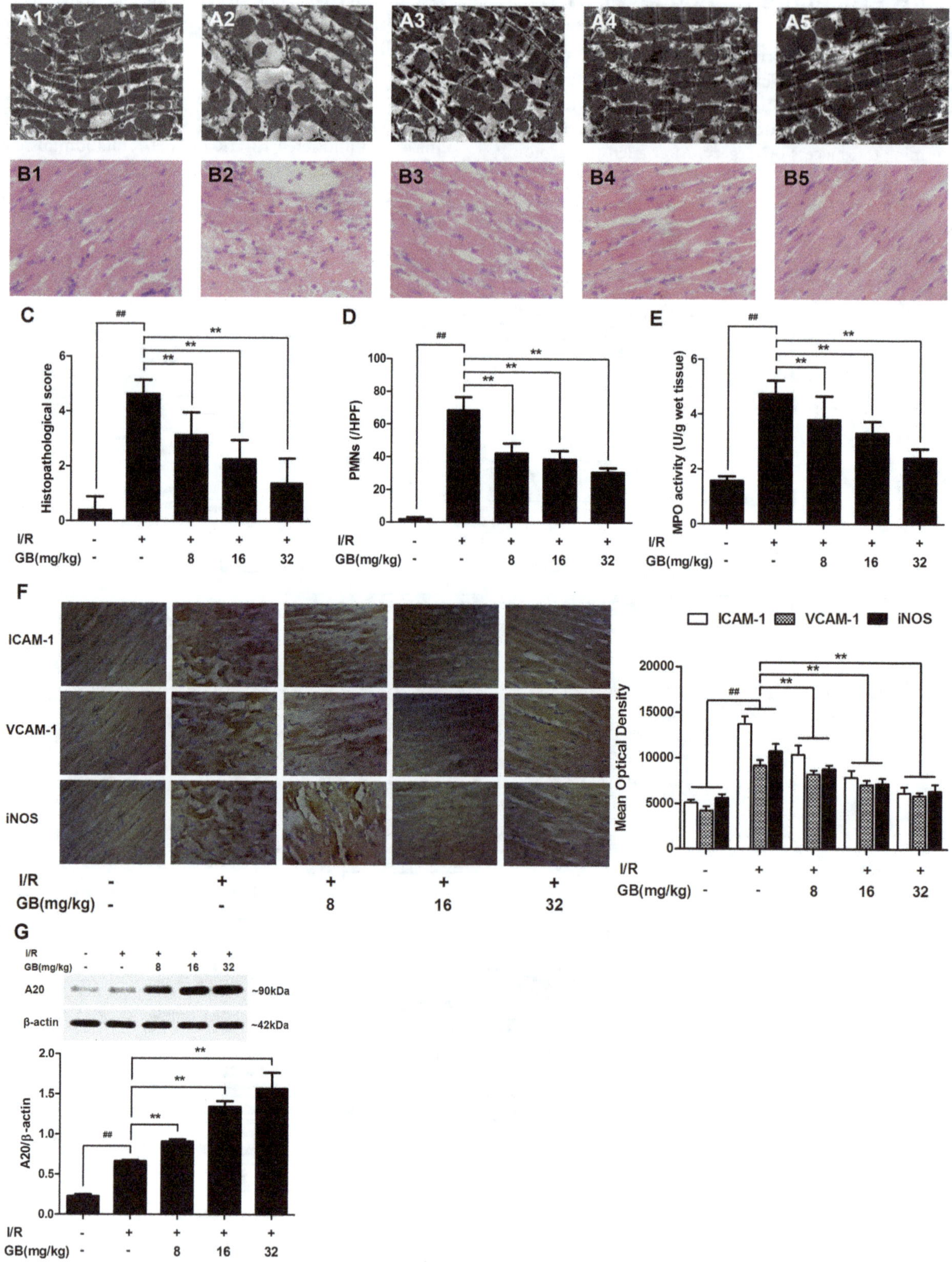

FIGURE 3 | Effects of GB on the ultrastructure of myocardial tissue, histopathological changes, histopathological scores, PMNs counting, MPO activity and ICAM-1, VCAM-1, iNOS expressions in MI/RI rats model. **(A1–5)** Representative transmission electron microscopy (TEM) observation of myocardial tissue injury for control group **(A1)**, I/R group **(A2)**, I/R + 8 mg/kg GB group **(A3)**, I/R + 16 mg/kg GB group **(A4)**, I/R + 32 mg/kg GB group **(A5)**. **(B1-5)** Representative light microscopic *(Continued)*

FIGURE 3 | appearance of rat myocardial histopathological morphology (HE staining; original magnification × 200) for control group **(B1)**, I/R group **(B2)**, I/R + 8 mg/kg GB group **(B3)**, I/R + 16 mg/kg GB group **(B4)**, I/R + 32 mg/kg GB group **(B5)**. **(C)** Effect of GB on histopathological scores, **(D)** effect of GB on myocardial PMNs counting, **(E)** effect of GB on MPO activity, effect of GB on expressions of ICAM-1, VCAM-1, iNOS **(F)** and effect of GB on expression of A20 **(G)**. The location of the histological images were taken in three random fields of infarcted area. Data were expressed as mean ± S.D. ($n = 8$). ##$P < 0.01$, I/R group vs. control group; *$P < 0.05$, **$P < 0.01$, 8, 16, 32 mg/kg GB groups vs. I/R group.

GB were, respectively administered intraperitoneally for 7 days before cardiac I/R operation.

In vivo I/R Procedure to Induce MI/RI in A20 Gene Silencing Mice

I/R surgery was exactly carried out in accordance with the procedure in **Figure 5A**. The mice were anesthetized with 60 mg/kg 3% sodium pentobarbital (i.p.). Electrocardiograph was continuously applied to monitor the changes of S-T segment so as to determine the success of surgery. A longitudinal incision was made at the left margin of the sternum 2~3 mm and between the second and third costal points. The intercostal artery was ligatured and the thymus and pericardium were separated to expose the heart. After a left thoracotomy, the LAD coronary artery was tied in a slipknot using a 7-0 silk suture. In sham operated mice, silk sutures were placed around LAD but were not ligated. After transient regional myocardial ischemia for 30 min, unlock slipknot, the blood flow of the coronary artery was recovered for 90 min. Before the rats were sacrificed, the blood samples were collected.

Randomly selected mice were divided into 5 groups as follows ($n = 8$ per group): (1) Control group, A20 gene silencing mice did not receive I/R, saline was administered; (2) I/R group, I/R A20 gene silencing mice administered with saline; (3) 12 mg/kg GB group, I/R A20 gene silencing mice received 12 mg/kg of GB; (4) 24 mg/kg GB group, I/R A20 gene silencing mice received 24 mg/kg of GB; (5) 48 mg/kg GB group, I/R A20 gene silencing mice received 48 mg/kg of GB. Saline and GB were, respectively administered intraperitoneally for 7 days before cardiac I/R operation.

Measurement of Infarct Size

Infarct size was determined by TTC staining technique. After I/R procedure, the hearts were excised and frozen at −80°C for 4 h. The left ventricle area of heart was cut into five 2-3 mm-thick slices from the apex to the base. After incubation in 2% TTC in PBS (pH 7.4) solution for 15 min (37°C), the third slice was immersed in formalin (4%) for another 30 min. Then, the area of the infarcted tissues was photographed with a digital camera and measured by Image-Pro Plus software (version 6.0, Media Cybernetic, United States) according to computerized planimetry. Infarct size was expressed as the percentage of infarcted area to the risk region × 100%.

Transmission Electron Microscopy

The third heart slice was fixed in 3.0%, pH 7.2 glutaraldehyde buffered fixative for 2-3 days. Then the specimens were embedded in Polybed 812 before being rinsed in PBS. 60-80 nm-thick specimens were analyzed with a transmission electron microscope (JEM-2000EX) in three random fields.

Histopathological Examination and Analysis of PMNS Infiltration Intensity

The third heart slice was stained with hematoxylin-eosin (H&E) and analyzed by light microscopy in three random fields. The intensity of histopathological damage was evaluated via pathological scores in accordance with the criteria reported by the previous study (21): (1) score 0: no damage; (2) score 1: mild damage; (3) score 2: moderate damage; (4) score 3: severe damage; (5) score 4: highly severe damage. The mean of the absolute number of PMNs was also recorded in three random high-power fields (HPF).

Immunohistochemistry

Immunohistochemistry was applied to evaluate the expressions of ICAM-1, VCAM-1, and iNOS. The third heart slice was frozen and blocked by 10% normal serum. And, anti-ICAM-1, anti-VCAM-1 and anti-iNOS antibodies were incubated overnight at 4°C after being. Then, the heart slice was incubated with anti-rabbit IgG primary antibody for 30 min. Immunohisochemical staining protocol was used for further immunohistological analysis under the fluorescence microscope in three random fields. Image-Pro Plus software (version 6.0) was applied to quantify the optical density of positive staining area, as described previously (22). The results were expressed as mean optical density mean ± S.D.

MPO Activity Assay

The ischemic tissue samples were homogenized and sonicated to release the MPO into the supernatant. Then, the activity of MPO was measured using kits according to the manufacture instructions (AmyJet Scientific Inc., Wuhan, China).

In vitro H/R Procedure to Induce H/R Injury in Ventricular Myocytes

Rat ventricular myocytes were separated from the hearts of 1–4-day-old Sprague-Dawley rats according to trypsin enzymic digestion and differential attachment methods as described previously (21). Three days later, the cells were finally purified at a density of 1×10^5/mL in DMEM medium supplemented with 10% fetal calf serum in 95% air/5% CO_2 at 37°C.

H/R treatment procedure (**Figure 4A**). The cells were incubated in 95% N_2/5% CO_2 for 2 h (hypoxia) and then in 95% air/5% CO_2 for 2 h (reoxygenation). Randomly selected cells were divided into five groups as follows ($n = 8$ per group): (1) Control group, cells did not receive H/R and were cultured in DMEM medium; (2) H/R group, cells receive H/R; (3) 1 μM GB group, H/R cells were pre-incubated with 1 μM GB for 24 h; (4) 10 μM GB group, H/R cells were pre-incubated with 10 μM GB for 24 h; (5) 100 μM GB group, H/R cells were pre-incubated with 100 μM GB for 24 h.

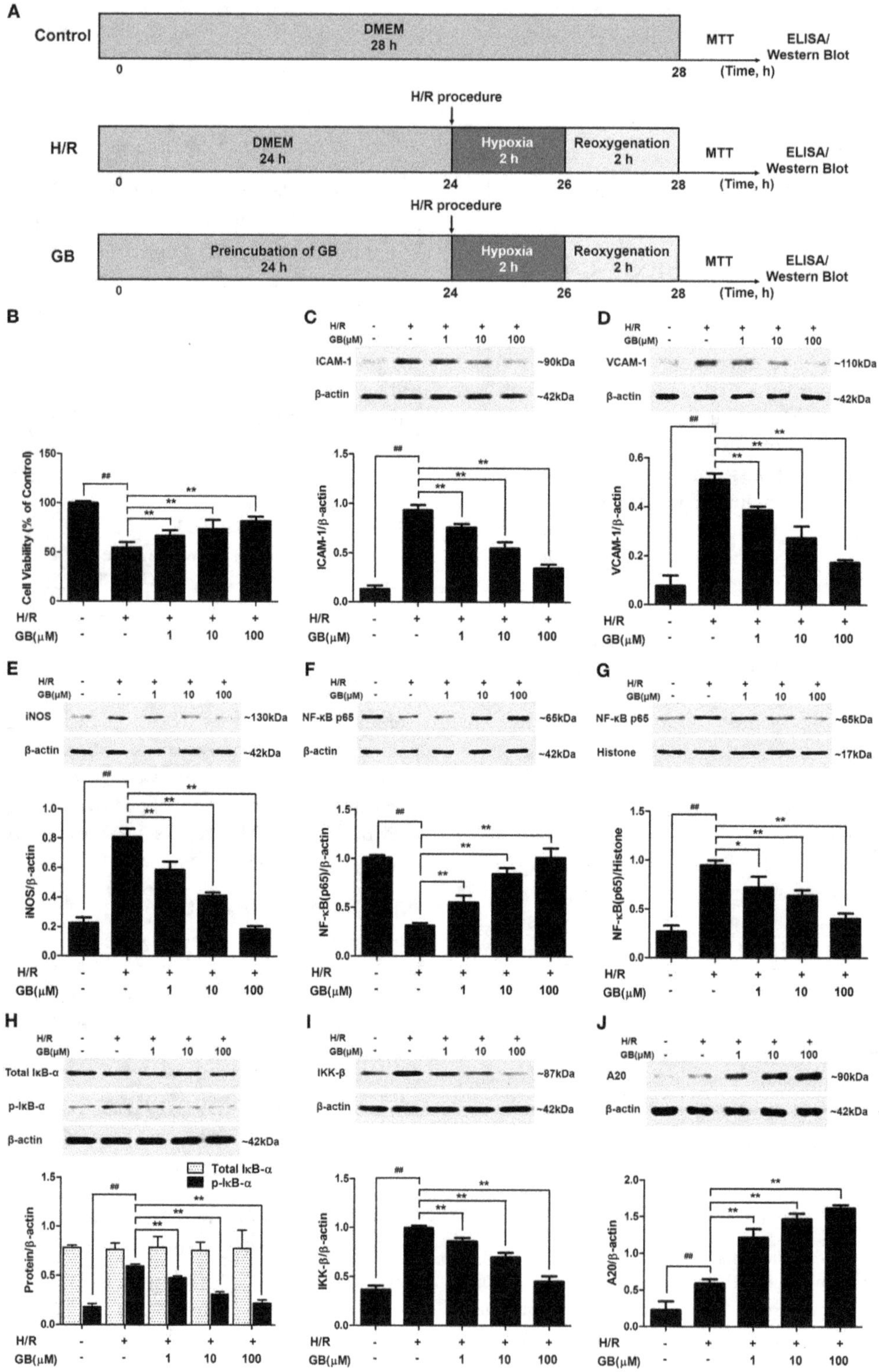

FIGURE 4 | Effects of GB on cell viability and the expressions of ICAM-1, VCAM-1, iNOS, NF-κB p65, p-IκB-α, IKK-β by Western blot in H/R ventricular myocytes model. **(A)** The experimental procedures of *in vitro* H/R ventricular myocytes model. **(B)** GB significantly increased the cell viability after H/R procedure. **(C)** GB decreased the expression of ICAM-1. **(D)** GB decreased the expression of VCAM-1. **(E)** GB decreased the expression of iNOS. GB blocked the translocation of NF-κB p65 from cytosolic **(F)** to nuclear **(G)**. **(H)** GB down-regulated the expression of p-IκB-α. **(I)** GB decreased the expression of IKK-β. **(J)** GB increased the expression of A20. The NF-κB p65 protein levels were assayed separately in cytosolic **(F)** and nuclear **(G)** extracts. Results were expressed as Protein/reference protein ratio. Data were expressed as mean ± S.D. of three independent experiments. ##$P < 0.01$ H/R group vs. control group; *$P < 0.05$, **$P < 0.01$, 1, 10, 100 μM GB groups vs. I/R group.

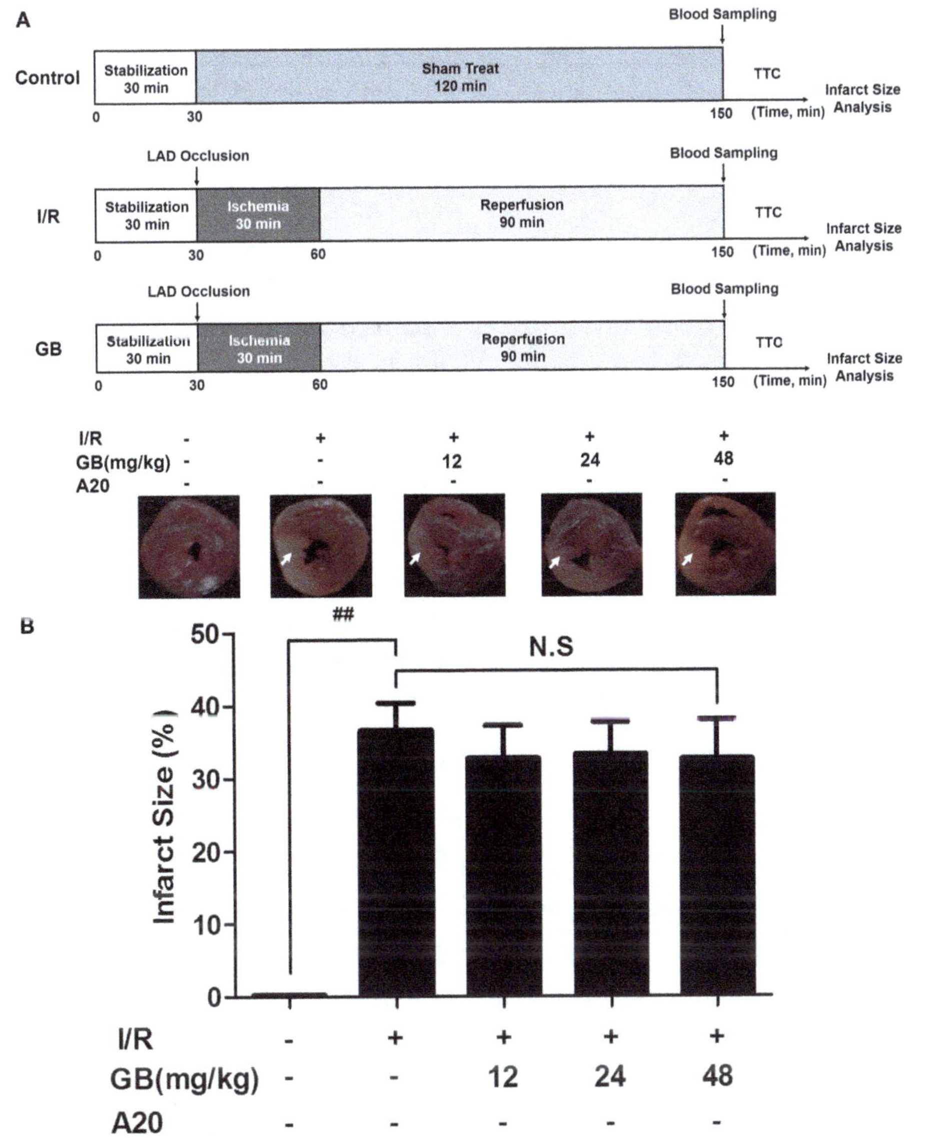

FIGURE 5 | Effects of GB on infarct size in A20 gene silencing MI/RI mice model. **(A)** The experimental procedures of *in vivo* A20 gene silencing MI/RI mice model. **(B)** Treatment with GB significantly reduced the infarct size in A20 gene silencing MI/RI mice model. Data were expressed as mean ± S.D. ($n = 8$). ##$P < 0.01$, I/R group vs. control group; *$P < 0.05$, **$P < 0.01$, 12, 24, 48 mg/kg GB groups vs. I/R group.

Reconstruction of A20 Gene Silencing Ventricular Myocytes

After the density of ventricular myocytes reached 1×10^5/mL, the cells were transfected with pGPU6/Hygro in control group while pGPU6/Hygro-A20 in other groups for 24 h using the GenePharma Transfection Reagent. After the transfection, cells were treated with H/R.

In vitro H/R Procedure to Induce H/R Injury in A20 Gene Silencing Ventricular Myocytes

The A20 gene silencing cells were incubated in 95% N_2/5% CO_2 for 2 h (hypoxia) and then in 95% air/5% CO_2 for 2 h (reoxygenation). Randomly selected cells were divided into 5 groups as follows ($n = 8$ per group): (1) Control group, cells did not receive H/R and were cultured in DMEM medium; (2) H/R group, A20 gene silencing cells receive H/R; (3) 1 μM GB group, H/R A20 gene silencing cells were pre-incubated with 1 μM GB for 24 h; (4) 10 μM GB group, H/R A20 gene silencing cells were pre-incubated with 10 μM GB for 24 h; (5) 100 μM GB group, H/R A20 gene silencing cells were preincubated with 100 μM GB for 24 h.

Analysis of Cell Vitality

Cell viability of ventricular myocytes was quantified with 3-(4,5-dimethylthiazol-2-yl)-2,5-diphenyl tetrazolium bromide (MTT) colorimetric assay. At the end of H/R procedure, cells were

TABLE 1 | Effects of GB on serum inflammatory cytokines in MI/RI rats model.

Group	Dose (mg/kg)	TNF-α (pg/mL)	IL-1β (pg/mL)	IL-6 (pg/mL)
Control		13.63 ± 3.61	56.41 ± 12.19	31.94 ± 8.34
I/R		86.34 ± 15.40##	239.56 ± 17.38##	103.78 ± 10.45##
I/R+GB	8	66.34 ± 10.98**	185.65 ± 21.76**	90.13 ± 14.53*
	16	48.54 ± 8.07**	133.49 ± 23.68**	62.34 ± 8.31**
	32	27.39 ± 6.31**	85.68 ± 9.78**	50.49 ± 3.98**

Values were expressed as mean ± SD (n = 8).
*##P < 0.01 I/R group vs. control group; *P < 0.05, **P < 0.01, 8, 16, 32 mg/kg GB groups vs. I/R group.*

TABLE 2 | Effects of GB on supernatant inflammatory cytokines in H/R ventricular myocytes model.

Group	Concentration (μM)	TNF-α (pg/mL)	IL-1β (pg/mL)	IL-6 (pg/mL)
Control		5.21 ± 2.16	87.29 ± 6.89	23.10 ± 3.15
H/R		62.17 ± 5.96##	875.09 ± 47.10##	681.34 ± 29.32##
H/R+GB	1	43.26 ± 10.11**	529.21 ± 43.43**	501.21 ± 22.31**
	10	32.18 ± 2.98**	329.11 ± 20.98**	209.34 ± 13.34**
	100	16.88 ± 2.16**	192.10 ± 40.19**	102.09 ± 21.08**

Values were expressed as mean ± SD (n = 8).
*##P < 0.01 H/R group vs. control group; *P < 0.05, **P < 0.01, 1, 10, 100 μM GB groups vs. I/R group.*

incubated with 5 mg/mL MTT for 4 h at 37°C and the insoluble formazan crystals were dissolved in 100 μl of DMSO for 15 min. Results were expressed as percentage of the optical density (OD) at 490 nm measured in control cells.

Measurement of TNF-α, Il-1β, and Il-6

Before rats and mice were sacrificed, the blood samples were obtained. After H/R procedure, the cell supernatant was collected from medium. The expressions of TNF-α, IL-1β, and IL-6 were determined via ELISA kits both in blood samples and cell supernatant.

Extraction of Myocardial Tissues Protein

RIPA Lysis Buffer (Beyotime Inc., China) and 1% phenylmethanesulfonyl fluoride (PMSF) were used to extract the proteins in myocardial tissue. Then, the myocardial tissues were homogenized and ultrasonically ground to no precipitation. Finally, the samples were centrifuged at 12,000 × g at 4°C for 30 min and the total protein was collected from the supernatant. All the steps above were carried out on the ice in order to avoid protein denaturation.

Western Blot Analysis

Nuclear and Cytoplasmic Protein Extraction Kit (Beyotime Biotechnology, Beijing, China) was applied to extract the cytoplasmic and nuclear proteins from cells according to the manufacturer's instruction as described previously (21). The protein concentrations were determined by BCA assay.

Protein samples (50 μg) was loaded to SDS-PAGE gel, and then transferred to a PVDF membrane at 20 V and 100 mA overnight. The membranes were blocked with 5% skim milk, and then incubated with primary antibodies (1:800) against CD40, ICAM-1, VCAM-1, iNOS, NF-κB p65, p-IκB-α, and IKK-β proteins for 4 h at 37°C. The horseradish peroxidase-conjugated secondary antibody (1:1,000) was added and detected using an ECL plus kit. Protein expression levels were determined by quantitating protein band densities of images taken by Gel Imaging System using Quantity One software.

Statistical Analysis

The results were expressed as the mean ± S.E.M. Significance of difference between groups were compared using one-way analysis of variance (ANOVA) followed by Bonferroni correction for multiple comparisons. A probability value of $P < 0.05$ was considered to be statistically significant. All statistical figures were performed using Graph Pad Prism software (Version 5.0).

RESULTS

Effect of GB on MI/R-Induced Inflammatory Injury IN MI/RI Rats Model

GB Reduced Infarct Size in MI/RI Rats

As the results shown in **Figure 2B**, infarct size in the I/R group was 41.5 ± 4.9% ($P < 0.01$ vs. control group), whereas 8, 16, 32 mg/kg GB decreased infarct size to 32.4 ± 3.7%, 25.2 ± 5.0% and 21.3 ± 4.0% ($P < 0.01$), respectively, compared with the I/R group.

GB Improved Cardiac Ultrastructural Characterization, Alleviated Pmns Infiltration, Decreased the Amount of Serum Inflammatory Cytokines and Inhibited Overexpressions of Myocardial Tissue ICAM-1, VCAM-1, and iNOS in MI/RI Rats

In the control group, mitochondria containing cristae with high electron density are elongated and tightly aligned between myofibrils (**Figure 3A1**). However, in I/R group, the cardiac myofibers were disconnected and damaged, nuclear stained deeper, and the mitochondria became swelling and degeneration (**Figure 3A2**). In 8 mg/kg GB group, there were still some breaks and loss of mitochondrial cristae associated with loss of the mitochondrial matrix (**Figure 3A3**). In 16 mg/kg GB group, the damaged mitochondria showed mild loss of cristae, swelling, myelin figures and membrane disruption (**Figure 3A4**). In 32 mg/kg GB group, only a few swollen mitochondria was observed (**Figure 3A5**).

In the control group, the myocytes arranged regularly and no inflammatory cells were observed in the myocardial interstitium. After I/R procedure, the myocytes arranged irregularly, the tissue became necrotic, and a large number of inflammatory cells were observed in the myocardial interstitium accompanied by the formation of fibrotic scars. But GB could significantly improve the histological injury, characterized by regularly arranged myocytes and alleviative inflammatory infiltration (**Figures 3B1–5**). As demonstrated in **Figure 3C**, 8, 16, 32 mg/kg

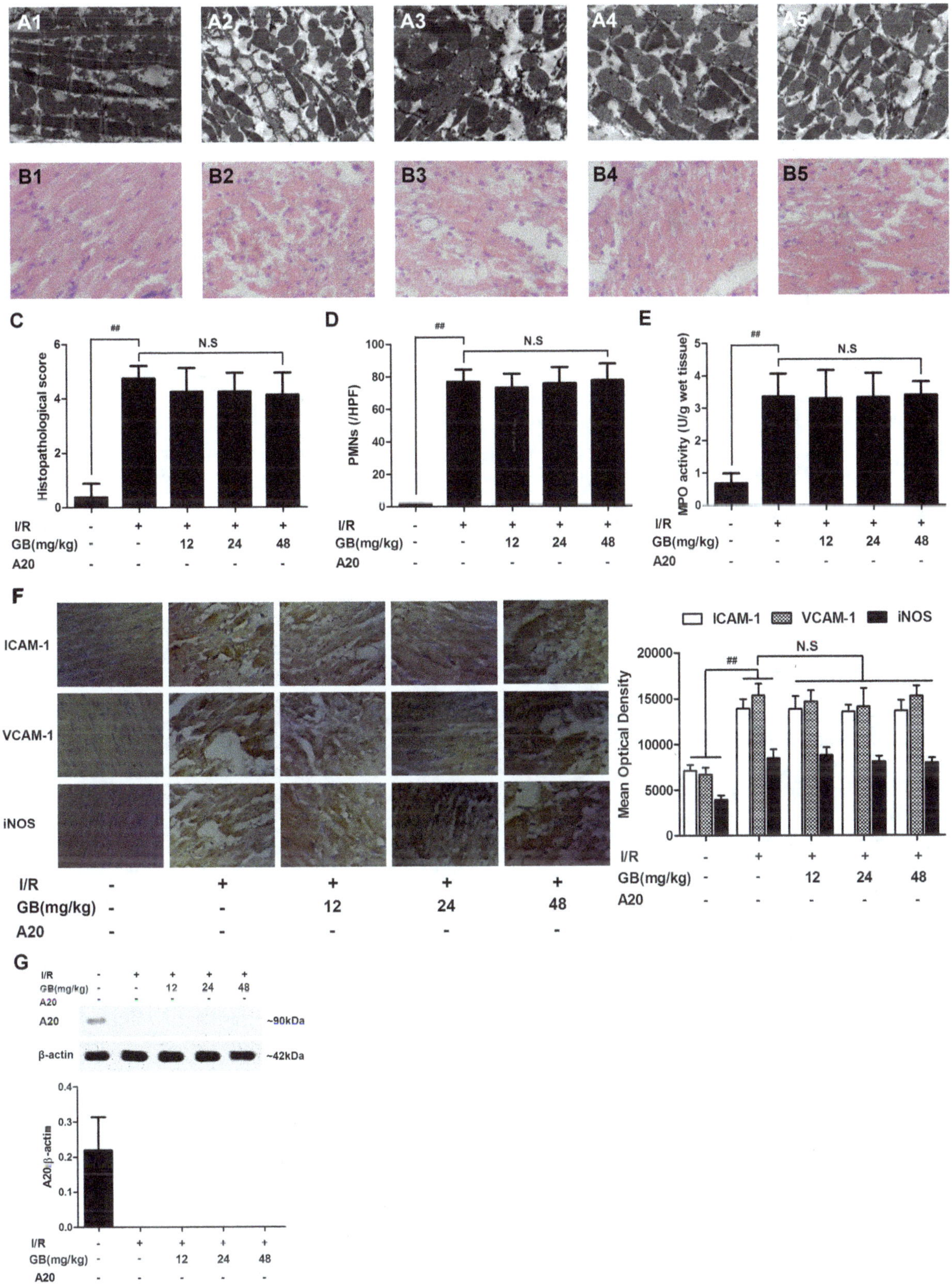

FIGURE 6 | Effects of GB on the ultrastructure of myocardial tissue, histopathological changes, histopathological scores, PMNs counting, MPO activity and ICAM-1, VCAM-1, iNOS expressions in A20 gene silencing MI/RI mice model. **(A1-5)** Representative transmission electron microscopy (TEM) observation of myocardial tissue injury for control group **(A1)**, I/R group **(A2)**, I/R + 12 mg/kg GB group **(A3)**, I/R + 24 mg/kg GB group **(A4)**, I/R + 48 mg/kg GB group **(A5)**. **(B1-5)** Representative

(Continued)

FIGURE 6 | light microscopic appearance of rat myocardial histopathological morphology (HE staining; original magnification × 200) for control group **(B1)**, I/R group **(B2)**, I/R + 12 mg/kg GB group **(B3)**, I/R + 24 mg/kg GB group **(B4)**, I/R + 48 mg/kg GB group **(B5)**. **(C)** Effect of GB on histopathological scores, **(D)** effect of GB on myocardial PMNs counting, **(E)** effect of GB on MPO activity, effect of GB on expressions of ICAM-1, VCAM-1, iNOS **(F)** and effect of GB on expression of A20 **(G)**. The location of the histological images were taken in three random fields of infarcted area. Data were expressed as mean ± S.D. (n = 8). ##P < 0.01 I/R group vs. control group; *P < 0.05, **P < 0.01, 12, 24, 48 mg/kg GB groups vs. I/R group.

GB markedly decrease the histopathological scores compared with I/R group ($P < 0.01$). Meanwhile, all GB groups remarkably decreased the total numbers of infiltrated and adherent PMNs compared with I/R group (**Figure 3D**).

Then, MPO activity was measured to evaluate the level of neutrophilic infiltration. In control group, the MPO activity was very low at 1.57 ± 0.16 U/g protein (**Figure 3E**). However, the MPO activity was significantly elevated in I/R group (4.72 ± 0.51 U/g protein) ($P < 0.01$ vs. control group). Interestingly, the current study indicated that pretreatment with GB 8 mg/kg (3.79 ± 0.86 U/g protein, $P < 0.05$), 16 mg/kg (3.30 ± 0.43 U/g protein, $P < 0.01$) and 32 mg/kg (2.40 ± 0.33 U/g protein, $P < 0.01$) could inhibit MPO activity in myocardial tissue compared with I/R group.

As shown in **Table 1**, the levels of TNF-α, IL-1β, and IL-6 were increased by 6.33-fold, 4.25-fold, and by 3.25-fold ($P < 0.01$), respectively, compared with control group. 8, 16, 32 mg/kg GB could dose-dependently decrease the levels of TNF-α by 23.2% ($P < 0.05$), 43.8% ($P < 0.01$) and 68.3% ($P < 0.01$), respectively, IL-1β by 22.5, 44.3, and 64.2% ($P < 0.01$), respectively, and IL-6 by 13.2% ($P < 0.05$), 39.9% ($P < 0.01$) and 51.3% ($P < 0.01$), respectively, compared with I/R group.

As shown in **Figure 3F**, the expressions of ICAM-1, VCAM-1, and iNOS in I/R group were significantly elevated compared with control group. However, 8, 16, 32 mg/kg GB could effectively reduce the expressions of ICAM-1, VCAM-1 and iNOS compared with I/R group. The original pictures were put in the **Supplementary Material**.

Gb Increased Expression of A20 in MI/RI Rats

As shown in **Figure 3G**, the level of A20 in I/R group was obviously higher in contrast with control group ($P < 0.01$). But 8, 16, 32 mg/kg GB remarkably increased the level of A20 in response to I/R injury ($P < 0.01$ vs. I/R group).

Effect of GB on H/R-Induced Injury in H/R Ventricular Myocytes Model

GB Increased Cell Viability Against H/R Injury in Ventricular Myocytes

As shown in **Figure 4B**, the cell viability in H/R group was markedly reduced to 54.5 ± 5.6% ($P < 0.01$ vs. control group). 1, 10, 100 μM GB could significantly increase the viability of cells received H/R injury (66.6 ± 5.8, 73.6 ± 9.3, 81.8 ± 4.7%, $P < 0.01$ vs. H/R group).

GB Inhibited Overproduction of Inflammatory Cytokines in H/R Ventricular Myocytes

The productions of TNF-α, IL-1β, and IL-6 in H/R group were markedly increased by 11.93-, 10.03-, and 29.50-fold, respectively, compared with control group ($P < 0.01$) in **Table 2**. Pretreatment with 1, 10, 100 μM GB could significantly reduce the levels of TNF-α by 30.4, 48.2, and 72.8% ($P < 0.01$), IL-1β by 39.5, 62.4, and 78.0% ($P < 0.01$), IL-6 by 26.4, 69.3, and 85.0% ($P < 0.01$), respectively, compared with H/R group.

GB Prevented Overexpressions of ICAM-1, VCAM-1 and iNOS, Translocation of NF-κB p65, Phosphorylation of IκB-α, Activity of IKK-β and Increased Expression of A20 in H/R Ventricular Myocytes

Compared with control group, the expressions of ICAM-1, VCAM-1, and iNOS markedly increased to about 7.18-, 6.65-, and 3.56-fold ($P < 0.01$) after H/R procedure (**Figures 4C–E**). While pretreatment with 1, 10, 100 μM GB reduced the expressions of ICAM-1 by 18.6, 41.4, and 63.2% ($P < 0.01$), VCAM-1 by 24.2, 46.4, and 66.0% ($P < 0.01$) and iNOS by 27.3, 48.8, and 76.9% ($P < 0.01$) compared with H/R group.

As shown in **Figures 4F,G**, the levels of NF-κB p65 were relatively high in the cytoplasm of cells but low in nucleus in control group. However, an evident translocation of p65 from the cytosol into nucleus showed in H/R group. Pretreatment with 1, 10, 100 μM GB could inhibit such nuclear translocation in a concentration-dependent manner.

As shown in **Figure 4H**, the total IκB-α in each group was not different. Then we checked the level of p-IκB-α in each group. Compared with control group, the level of p-IκB-α in H/R group significantly increased by 3.25-fold ($P < 0.01$). However, 1, 10, 100 μM GB all showed a notably inhibitory effect on phosphorylation of IκB-α by 19.6, 47.5, and 62.6% ($P < 0.01$) compared with H/R group.

And, we furtherly checked whether GB had an influence on IKK-β activity. The results in **Figure 4I** showed that the level of IKK-β significantly increased by 2.72-fold in H/R group ($P < 0.01$ vs. control group). In contrast, 1, 10, 100 μM GB could reduce the expressions of IKK-β by 13.7, 29.8, and 54.5% ($P < 0.01$) compared with H/R group.

As shown in **Figure 4J**, there was a small increased expression of A20 after H/R procedure ($P < 0.01$ vs. control group). While pre-incubation of GB (1, 10, 100 μM) all significantly enhanced the expressions of A20 in response to H/R injury ($P < 0.01$ vs. H/R group).

Effect of GB on MI/R-Induced Inflammatory Injury in A20 Gene Silencing MI/RI Mice Model

In I/R group, it was found that I/R procedure could markedly increase infarct size (**Figure 5B**), destroy cardiac ultrastructural

TABLE 3 | Effects of GB on serum inflammatory cytokines in A20 gene silencing MI/RI mice model.

Group	Dose (mg/kg)	TNF-α (pg/mL)	IL-1β (pg/mL)	IL-6 (pg/mL)
Control		34.21 ± 6.44	39.53 ± 10.98	18.39 ± 3.14
I/R		134.31 ± 10.98##	193.53 ± 23.67##	76.55 ± 6.98##
I/R+GB	12	119.82 ± 14.33*	153.12 ± 17.09**	68.05 ± 3.29*
	24	87.09 ± 5.09**	89.31 ± 14.13**	52.12 ± 6.99**
	48	40.01 ± 13.32**	58.39 ± 4.56**	48.15 ± 6.11**

Values were expressed as mean ± SD (n = 8).
*##P < 0.01, I/R group vs. control group; *P < 0.05, **P < 0.01, 12, 24, 48 mg/kg GB groups vs. I/R group.*

characterization (**Figures 6A1–5**), aggravate pathological changes (**Figures 6B1–5C**), trigger PMNs infiltration (**Figure 6D**), cause inflammatory cytokines overproduction (**Table 3**) and upregulate expressions of ICAM-1, VCAM-1, iNOS (**Figure 6F**). As shown in **Figure 6G**, there showed successful and stable A20 gene silencing in mice except the control group. It was interesting that, after A20 gene was silenced, 12, 24, 48 mg/kg GB all failed to improve the outcomes induced by MI/RI (**Figure 6** and **Table 3**).

Effect of GB on H/R-Induced Injury in A20 Gene Silencing H/R Ventricular Myocytes Model

GB Could Not Increase Cell Viability After A20 Gene Silencing

The cell viabilities in H/R + A20 silencing group (**Figure 7A**) were significantly reduced ($P < 0.01$ vs. control group). After A20 gene silencing, GB could not elevate the cell viability against to H/R injury.

GB Could Not Inhibit the Expression of Inflammatory Factors, Translocation of NF-κB p65, Phosphorylation of IκB-α and Activity of IKK-β After A20 Gene Silencing

Compared with control group, the expressions of TNF-α, IL-1β, IL 6, ICAM 1, VCAM-1, and iNOS in H/R + A20 silencing group were obviously increased (**Table 4** and **Figures 7B–D**). Whereas, after A20 gene silencing, GB could not influence the expressions of TNF-α, IL-1β, IL-6, ICAM-1, VCAM-1, and iNOS.

The levels of NF-κB translocation, IκB-α phosphorylation and IKK-β activity were significantly affected in H/R + A20 silence group (**Figures 7E–H**). Nevertheless, after A20 gene silencing, all GB groups had no impact on NF-κB p65 translocation, IκB-α phosphorylation and IKK-β activity compared with H/R + A20 silence group.

Stable A20 Gene Silencing in Ventricular Myocytes

As shown in **Figure 7I**, there was little A20 expressed after transfection by preincubation with pGPU6/Hygro in control group. In addition, the ventricular myocytes in other groups were preincubated with pGPU6/Hygro-A20 and no A20 expressed after transfection.

DISCUSSION

This is the first investigation studied on MI/RI both *in vivo* and *in vitro* to examine whether GB played a vital role in the whole pathological process of MI/RI, whether GB regulated the expression of A20 in response to H/R injury, and whether NF-κB signal pathway was heavily involved in the whole pathogenesis.

Inflammation is responsible for the development of many cardiovascular or cerebrovascular diseases, such as atherosclerosis, myocardial infarction, stroke, hyperlipidemia, and neurodegeneration (23, 24). And, it is an important form of cardiomyocyte death in the early stage of MI/RI, which further leads to severe complications such as arrhythmia and heart failure. It was traditionally believed that the process of I/R gradually provokes severe inflammatory response and subsequent cardiac rupture, ventricular aneurysm formation, and exacerbation of left ventricular (LV) remodeling (25). However, not only the pathogenesis of I/R may lead to the inflammatory response, but inflammation itself may aggravate the I/R injury. But so far, the information of molecular mechanisms underlying the proinflammatory process of MI/RI is far from certain. Therefore, study on inflammation participating in MI/RI is quite meaningful for preventive therapy.

Recently, herbal treatment of cardiovascular and cerebrovascular diseases has gained much attention. GB, a major monomer of extracts from leaves of *Ginkgo biloba* traditionally used in Chinese herbal medicine, displays a wide range of biological activities, including anti-inflammatory and anti-oxidant effects (26). It has been reported that GB could exert neuroprotective effects against cerebral ischemia/reperfusion injury (CI/RI) via suppressing inflammatory response and scavenging oxygen free radical (27, 28). Both MI/RI and CI/RI are hypoxic and anoxic diseases, which have similar characteristics in pathogenesis and treatment, suggesting that GB may possess a potential value in the treatment strategy of MI/RI. Meanwhile, we have just proved that Ginkgolide C (GC) which possessed the similarity chemical structure to GB could exert a protective effect against MI/RI via inhibiting inflammation which might involve in blocking CD40-NF-κB signal pathway (21). However, it has not been illuminated whether GB has the similar effect of improving MI/RI yet. Consequently, in this study we investigated whether the strong anti-inflammatory property of GB constituted a part of molecular mechanisms of MI/RI protective effect.

It is well established that infarct size is a very important indicator reflecting therapeutic effect of MI/RI. One of the most effective strategy for reducing the size followed by acute myocardial infarction is the early and successful myocardial reperfusion which can improve the clinical outcome to a great degree (29). In this study, we found that pretreatment of GB for 7 days could remarkably protect against the I/R insult through significant reduction of infarct size. In addition, we found that GB largely improves myocardium damage as evidenced by restoration of myocardial ultrastructure and suppression of myofibrillar degeneration.

PMNs, which are involved in multiple non-infectious inflammatory processes including the response to MI/RI, serves

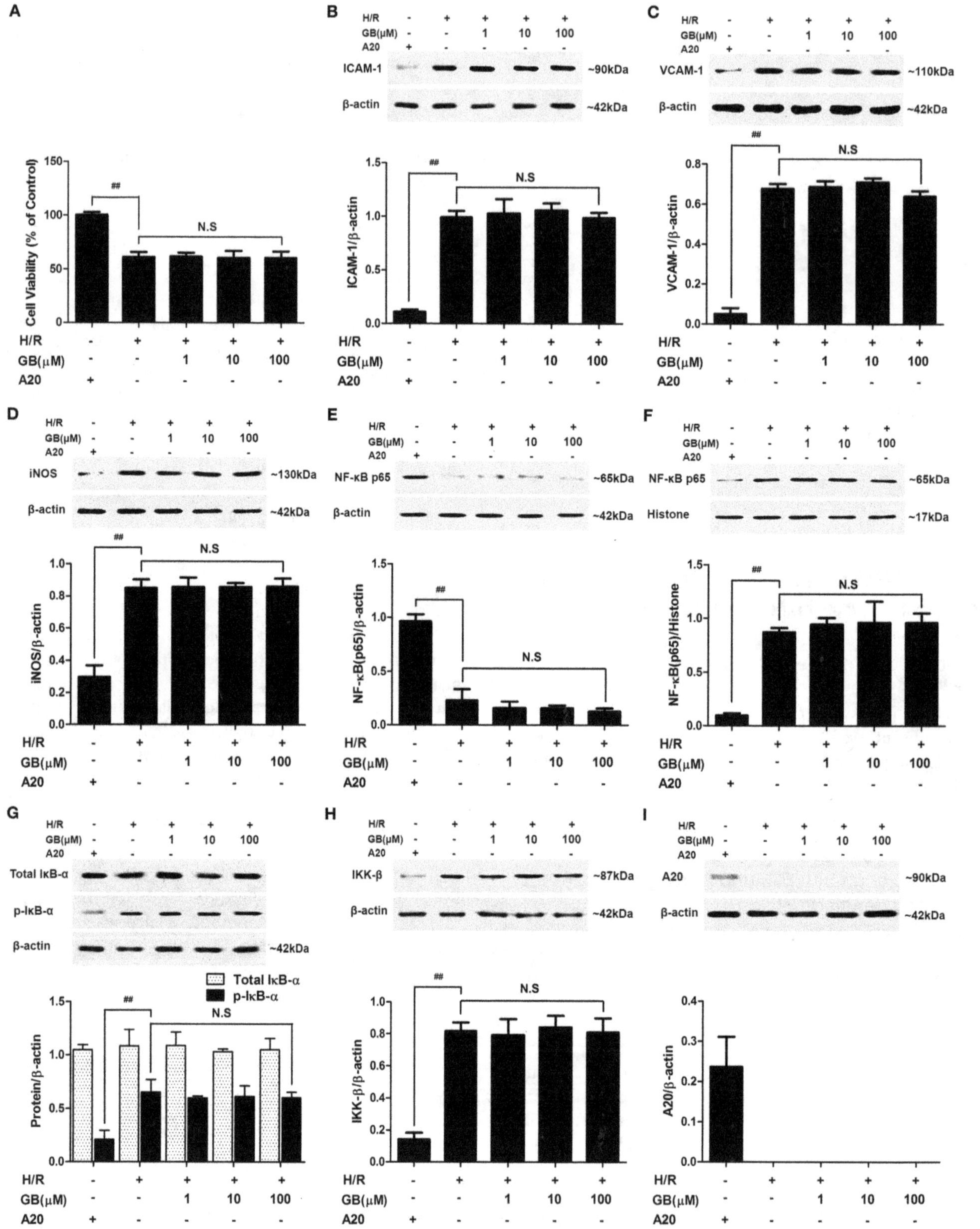

FIGURE 7 | Effects of GB on cell viability **(A)** and the expressions of **(B)** ICAM-1, **(C)** VCAM-1, **(D)** iNOS, **(E)** cytoplasm NF-κB p65, **(F)** nucleus NF-κB p65, **(G)** p-IκB-α, **(H)** IKK-β and **(I)** A20 by Western blot in A20 gene silence H/R ventricular myocytes model. Results were expressed as Protein/reference protein ratio. Data were expressed as mean ± S.D. of three independent experiments. ##$P < 0.01$, H/R group vs. control group; *$P < 0.05$, **$P < 0.01$, 1, 10, 100 μM GB groups vs. I/R group.

TABLE 4 | Effects of GB on supernatant inflammatory cytokines in A20 gene silence H/R ventricular myocytes model.

Group	Concentration (μM)	TNF-α (pg/mL)	IL-1β (pg/mL)	IL-6 (pg/mL)
Control		4.13 ± 0.18	69.33 ± 18.25	16.19 ± 2.26
H/R+A20⁻		72.19 ± 6.59##	906.10 ± 73.20##	729.35 ± 81.00##
H/R+GB+A20⁻	1	68.33 ± 10.31	872.12 ± 67.34	681.98 ± 69.21
	10	62.18 ± 5.68	912.33 ± 89.76	633.10 ± 58.22
	100	65.33 ± 8.32	890.65 ± 76.38	637.39 ± 58.31

Values were expressed as mean ± SD (n = 8).
*##P < 0.01, H/R group vs. control group; *P < 0.05, **P < 0.01, 1, 10, 100 μM GB groups vs. I/R group.*

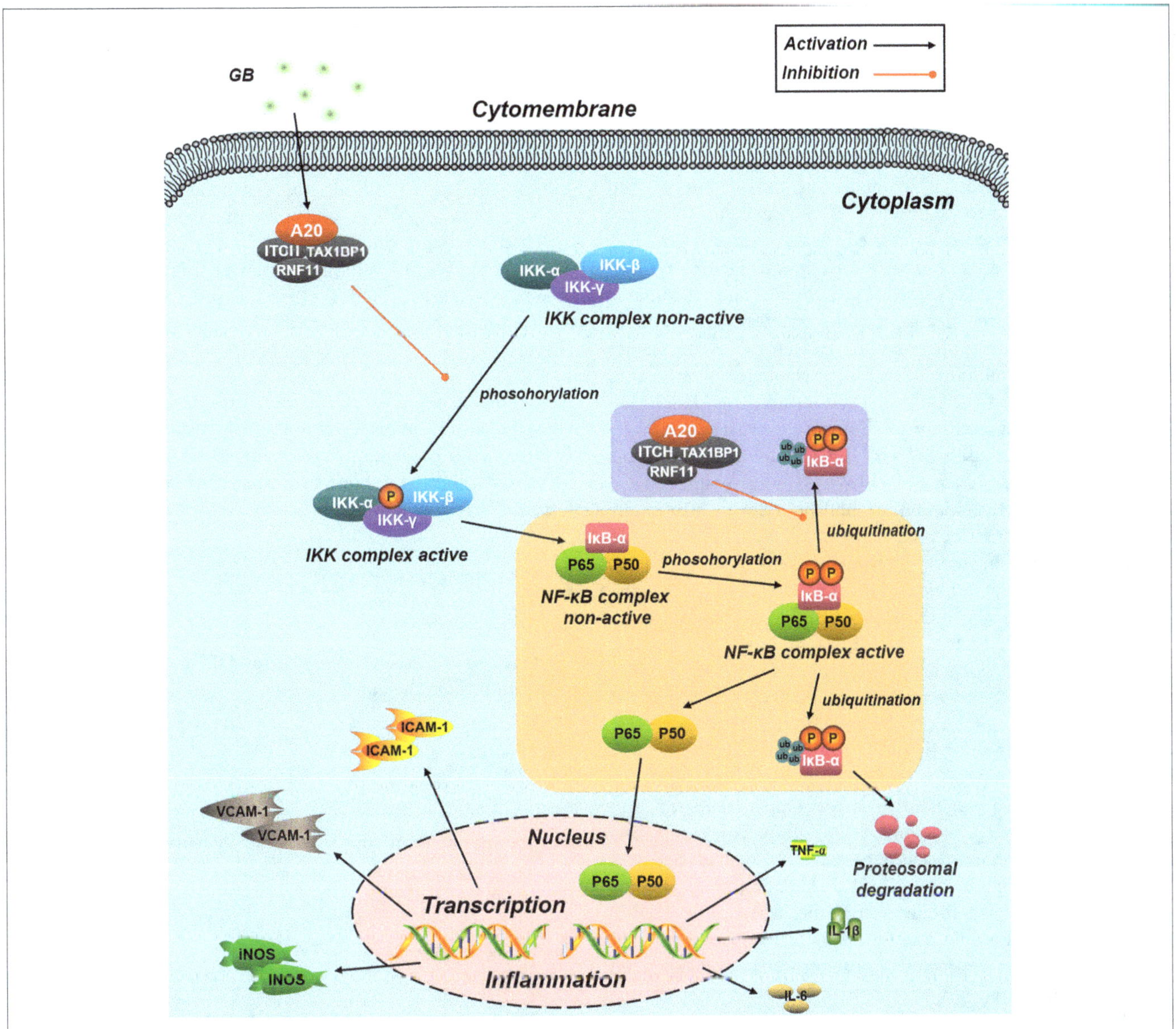

FIGURE 8 | Schematic diagram describing the mechanism in the inhibitory effect of GB on H/R induced ventricular myocytes inflammatory injury. GB could alleviate MI/RI-induced inflammatory injury via up-regulating A20 and inhibiting IKK/IκB/NF-κB signal pathway.

as a key effector in the innate immune system (30). Following MI/RI, a large increase in the number of circulating PMNs occurred, which could predict the major adverse cardiac events in MI/RI patients with larger infarct size and worse cardiac function (31). Therefore, suppression of PMNs infiltration is a main resource of relieving the damage of MI/RI. In this study, a convincing show of histopathological damage was found in *in vivo* I/R groups which suggested that there was a definite relationship between MI/RI and PMNs infiltration. Nevertheless, pretreatment with GB could significantly attenuate PMNs infiltration, as determined by histopathological scores and the counting of PMNs. MPO, regarded as a precise marker of MI/RI and a risk factor for long-term mortality, is secreted by PMNs. Similarly, the elevated level of MPO in I/R groups was decreased after pretreatment with GB. These findings provide a potential link between GB's MI/RI protective effect and PMNs infiltration inhibitory property.

Moreover, *in vitro* H/R-treated ventricular myocytes were applied to imitate the pathological process of *in vivo* I/R injury, which helped to thoroughly validate the cardioprotective property of GB. Interestingly, we found for the first time that GB could significantly increase the cell viability after I/R-like insult which indicated that GB could exert anti-MI/RI effect via promoting viability and tolerance of cells injured by H/R-induced inflammation.

So far, observed data implicate that NF-κB is deemed as one of the key players in pathogenesis of I/R injury. And they have also shown that active NF-κB-mediated signaling significantly increased I/R-induced heart damage (32, 33). NF-κB functions as a crucial transcription factor in both inflammatory cells and myocardial cells, linking the coordinated inflammatory and cell death signaling pathways proposed in the concept of necroinflammation. However, lots of studies indicated that inhibition of NF-κB signal pathways could remarkably suppress the inflammation induced by MI/RI (34–36). Under normal conditions, NF-κB proteins were bound by members of the inhibitor of κB (IκB) family as components of inactive cytoplasmic complexes (37, 38). After ubiquitylation and proteasomal degradation of phosphorylated IκB family members, nuclear translocation of NF-κB family members would be released (39). In the present work, the level of NF-κB p65 translocation was obviously elevated after H/R procedure. Whereas, our results indicated that GB could effectively reverse this activated effect. In addition, pretreatment with GB could significantly block the notable phosphorylation of IκB-α triggered by H/R procedure. These results suggest that the reduction in phosphorylation of IκB-α and translocation of NF-κB p65 is at least one of the targets of GB for inhibiting I/R-induced inflammation.

Genetic evidence suggests that IKK complex (IKK-α, β, and γ), a supporting role in activating the NF-κB pathway, is pivotal for activating phosphorylation-dependent IκB degradation and NF-κB nuclear translocation (40). Therefore, we detected whether GB had an influence on the activity of IKK-β. Unsurprisingly, GB could also inhibit IKK-β activation in H/R injured ventricular myocytes. Consequently, we determined that IKK-β/IκB-α/NF-κB signal pathway was one of the anti-inflammatory targets of GB.

Numerous data have proved that there was a positive feedback between NF-κB activation and its downstream inflammatory cytokines, such as TNF-α, IL-1β, and IL-6; cell adhesion molecules, such as ICAM-1 and VCAM-1; and nitric oxide synthase (NOS) (41–43). Therefore, this study has also checked this point. It implies that, blockade of NF-κB pathway by GB has shown positive efficacy in the management of MI/RI induced inflammation.

NF-κB signal pathway is mediated by several regulatory mechanisms to keep the homeostasis of tissue. Zinc finger protein A20, serves as a tumor suppressor gene and susceptibility gene/biomarker of disease, involved in various inflammatory diseases, especially MI/RI (44, 45). Previous studies have verified that A20 was a central and inducible negative regulator of NF-κB which regulates multiple inflammatory signaling cascades. Silencing of A20 can significantly promote the translocation of NF-κB p65, finally leading to a pro-inflammatory state (46). Our present study showed that the level of A20 is low under normal conditions. However, A20 was significantly up-regulated by all GB-treated groups and the consequences were severe inhibition of NF-κB signal pathway. According to the fact, we concluded that the MI/RI protective effect of GB might partly attribute to NF-κB inhibition mediated by upregulation of A20. Furthermore, we silence the A20 gene both *in vivo* and *in vitro* to verify our hypothesis. After A20 was silenced, GB failed to reduce infarct size, improve cardiac ultrastructural characterization, inhibit PMNs infiltration and downregulate expressions of inflammatory cytokines and proteins *in vivo*. In addition, GB had no effect on cell viability and inflammatory factors at all (**Data Sheet 1** in **Supplementary Material**). Therefore, it was obvious that GB exerted the protective effect against MI/RI through inhibiting NF-κB signal pathway via A20 (**Figure 8**).

In conclusion, this is the first time to find out that GB alleviated MI/RI-induced inflammatory insult both *in vivo* and *in vitro* via up-regulating A20 dependent NF-κB signal pathway. Thus, GB could be applied as a preventive and valuable agent against MI/RI.

AUTHOR CONTRIBUTIONS

RZ, LX, DZ, BH, and QL performed the research. RZ, DH, JL, and CS designed the research study. RZ and CS analyzed the data. RZ wrote and edited the paper.

FUNDING

This study was supported by grants from the Natural Science Foundation of Shandong Province (Program No. ZR2018PH037), National Natural Science Foundation of China (Program No. 81602226, 81572534), China Postdoctoral Science Foundation (No. 2016M590641) and Health Foundation of Shandong Province (No. 2017WS292).

SUPPLEMENTARY MATERIAL

Supplementary Figure 1 | The LPS experimental procedure *in vitro*.

Supplementary Figure 2 | Effects of GB on cell viability and the expressions of A20, ICAM-1, VCAM-1, iNOS, NF-κB p65, p-IκB-α, IKK-β after LPS procedure.

Supplementary Figure 3 | Effects of GB on cell viability and the expressions of A20, ICAM-1, VCAM-1, iNOS, NF-κB p65, p-IκB-α, IKK-β after A20 silencing.

REFERENCES

1. Ibanez B, Heusch G, Ovize M, Van de Werf F. Evolving therapies for myocardial ischemia/reperfusion injury. *J Am Coll Cardiol.* (2015) 65:1454–71. doi: 10.1016/j.jacc.2015.02.032
2. Costa MA, Paiva AE, Andreotti JP, Cardoso MV, Cardoso CD, Mintz A, et al. Pericytes constrict blood vessels after myocardial ischemia. *J Mol Cell Cardiol.* (2018) 116:1–4. doi: 10.1016/j.yjmcc.2018.01.014
3. Thind GS, Agrawal PR, Hirsh B, Saravolatz L, Chen-Scarabelli C, Narula J, et al. Mechanisms of myocardial ischemia-reperfusion injury and the cytoprotective role of minocycline: scope and limitations. *Fut Cardiol.* (2015) 11:61–76. doi: 10.2217/fca.14.76
4. Enesa K, Evans P. The biology of A20-like molecules. *Adv Exp Med Biol.* (2014) 809:33–48.
5. Wertz IE, Newton K, Seshasayee D, Kusam S, Lam C, Zhang J, et al. Phosphorylation and linear ubiquitin direct A20 inhibition of inflammation. *Nature* (2015) 528:370–5. doi: 10.1038/nature16165
6. Lawless D, Pathak S, Scambler TE, Ouboussad L, Anwar R, Savic S. A Case of Adult-Onset still's disease caused by a novel splicing mutation in TNFAIP3 successfully treated with tocilizumab. *Front Immunol.* (2018) 9:1527. doi: 10.3389/fimmu.2018.01527
7. Osorio J. Inflammation: A20-NEMO interaction prevents autoinflammation. *Nat Rev Rheumatol.* (2016) 12:134. doi: 10.1038/nrrheum.2016.19
8. Han D, Fang W, Zhang R, Wei J, Kodithuwakku ND, Sha L, et al. Clematichinenoside protects blood brain barrier against ischemic stroke superimposed on systemic inflammatory challenges through up-regulating A20. *Brain Behav Immun.* (2016) 51:56–69. doi: 10.1016/j.bbi.2015.07.025.
9. Lee GJ, Lee HM, Kim TS, Kim JK, Sohn KM, Jo EK. Mycobacterium fortuitum induces A20 expression that impairs macrophage inflammatory responses. *Pathog Dis.* (2016) 74:ftw015. doi: 10.1093/femspd/ftw015
10. Zilberman-Rudenko J, Shawver LM, Wessel AW, Luo Y, Pelletier M, Tsai WL, et al. Recruitment of A20 by the C-terminal domain of NEMO suppresses NF-kappaB activation and autoinflammatory disease. *Proc Natl Acad Sci USA.* (2016) 113:1612–7. doi: 10.1073/pnas.1518163113
11. Aksentijevich I, Zhou Q. NF-kappaB pathway in autoinflammatory diseases: dysregulation of protein modifications by ubiquitin defines a new category of autoinflammatory diseases. *Front Immunol.* (2017) 8:399. doi: 10.3389/fimmu.2017.00399
12. Gray CB, Suetomi T, Xiang S, Mishra S, Blackwood EA, Glembotski CC, et al. CaMKIIdelta subtypes differentially regulate infarct formation following *ex vivo* myocardial ischemia/reperfusion through NF-kappaB and TNF-alpha. *J Mol Cell Cardiol.* (2017) 103:48–55. doi: 10.1016/j.yjmcc.2017.01.002
13. de Aquino PE, Magalhaes TR, Nicolau LA, Leal LK, de Aquino NC, Dos Santos SM, et al. The anti-inflammatory effects of N-methyl-(2S,4R)-trans-4-hydroxy-l-proline from Syderoxylon obtusifolium are related to its inhibition of TNF-alpha and inflammatory enzymes. *Phytomedicine* (2017) 24:14–23. doi: 10.1016/j.phymed.2016.11.010
14. Hall CHT, Campbell EL, Colgan SP. Neutrophils as components of mucosal homeostasis. *Cell Mol Gastroenterol Hepatol.* (2017) 4:329–37. doi: 10.1016/j.jcmgh.2017.07.001
15. Wan F, Zang S, Yu G, Xiao H, Wang J, Tang J. Ginkgolide B suppresses methamphetamine-induced microglial activation through TLR4-NF-kappaB signaling pathway in BV2 cells. *Neurochem Res.* (2017) 42:2881–91. doi: 10.1007/s11064-017-2309-6
16. Hu H, Li Y, Xin Z, Zhanga X. Ginkgolide B exerts anti-inflammatory and chondroprotective activity in LPS-induced chondrocytes. *Adv Clin Exp Med.* (2018) 27:913–20. doi: 10.17219/acem/70414
17. Zhang M, Sun J, Chen B, Zhao Y, Gong H, You Y, et al. Ginkgolide B inhibits platelet and monocyte adhesion in TNFalpha-treated HUVECs under laminar shear stress. *BMC Complement Altern Med.* (2018) 18:220. doi: 10.1186/s12906-018-2284-8
18. Chen A, Xu Y, Yuan J. Ginkgolide B ameliorates NLRP3 inflammasome activation after hypoxic-ischemic brain injury in the neonatal male rat. *Int J Dev Neurosci.* (2018) 69:106–11. doi: 10.1016/j.ijdevneu.2018.07.004
19. Zheng PD, Mungur R, Zhou HJ, Hassan M, Jiang SN, Zheng JS. Ginkgolide B promotes the proliferation and differentiation of neural stem cells following cerebral ischemia/reperfusion injury, both *in vivo* and *in vitro*. *Neural Regen Res.* (2018) 13:1204–11. doi: 10.4103/1673-5374.232476
20. Pei HX, Hua R, Guan CX, Fang X. Ginkgolide B reduces the degradation of membrane phospholipids to prevent ischemia/reperfusion myocardial injury in Rats. *Pharmacology* (2015) 96:233–9. doi: 10.1159/000438945
21. Zhang R, Han D, Li Z, Shen C, Zhang Y, Li J, et al. Ginkgolide C alleviates myocardial ischemia/reperfusion-induced inflammatory injury via inhibition of CD40-NF-kappab pathway. *Front Pharmacol.* (2018b) 9:109. doi: 10.3389/fphar.2018.00109
22. Mukaino M, Nakamura M, Yamada O, Okada S, Morikawa S, Renault-Mihara F, et al. Anti-IL-6-receptor antibody promotes repair of spinal cord injury by inducing microglia-dominant inflammation. *Exp Neurol.* (2010) 224:403–14. doi: 10.1016/j.expneurol.2010.04.020
23. Agita A, Alsagaff MT. Inflammation, Immunity, and Hypertension. *Acta Med Indones* (2017) 49:158–65.
24. Messer JS. The cellular autophagy/apoptosis checkpoint during inflammation. *Cell Mol Life Sci.* (2017) 74:1281–96. doi: 10.1007/s00018-016-2403-y
25. Arfvidsson J, Ahlin F, Vargas KG, Thaler B, Wojta J, Huber K. Monocyte subsets in myocardial infarction: a review. *Int J Cardiol.* (2017) 231:47–53. doi: 10.1016/j.ijcard.2016.12.182
26. Lv Z, Yang Y, Wang J, Chen J, Li J, Di L. Optimization of the preparation conditions of borneol-modified ginkgolide liposomes by response surface methodology and study of their blood brain barrier permeability. *Molecules* (2018) 23:E303. doi: 10.3390/molecules23020303
27. Chang J, Xue X, Song C, Liu B, Gao L. Ginkgolide B promotes cell growth in endothelial progenitor cells through miR-126 and the Akt signaling pathway. *Mol Med Rep.* (2017) 16:5627–32. doi: 10.3892/mmr.2017.7254
28. Gill I, Kaur S, Kaur N, Dhiman M, Mantha AK. Phytochemical ginkgolide B attenuates amyloid-beta1-42 induced oxidative damage and altered cellular responses in human neuroblastoma SH-SY5Y Cells. *J Alzheimers Dis.* (2017) 60:S25–40. doi: 10.3233/jad-161086
29. van Hout GP, Bosch L, Ellenbroek GH, de Haan JJ, van Solinge WW, Cooper MA, et al. The selective NLRP3-inflammasome inhibitor MCC950 reduces infarct size and preserves cardiac function in a pig model of myocardial infarction. *Eur Heart J.* (2017) 38:828–36. doi: 10.1093/eurheartj/ehw247
30. Gao W, Zhao B, Liu L, Yuan Q, Wu X, Xia Z. Myocardial ischemic post-conditioning protects the lung against myocardial ischemia/reperfusion-induced damage by activating GSK-3beta. *Acta Cir Bras.* (2017) 32:376–87. doi: 10.1590/s0102-865020170050000007
31. Butler T. The Jarisch-herxheimer reaction after antibiotic treatment of spirochetal infections: a review of recent cases and our understanding of pathogenesis. *Am J Trop Med Hyg.* (2017) 96:46–52. doi: 10.4269/ajtmh.16-0434
32. Yue Y, Yang X, Feng K, Wang L, Hou J, Mei B, et al. M2b macrophages reduce early reperfusion injury after myocardial ischemia in mice: a predominant role of inhibiting apoptosis via A20. *Int J Cardiol.* (2017) 245:228–35. doi: 10.1016/j.ijcard.2017.07.085
33. Hoshino M, Yonetsu T, Murai T, Kanaji Y, Usui E, Yamaguchi M, et al. Multimodality coronary imaging to predict periprocedural myocardial necrosis after an elective percutaneous coronary intervention. *Coron Artery Dis.* (2018) 29:237–45. doi: 10.1097/mca.0000000000000595
34. EMP, Mopuri R, Pulaganti M, Kareem MA, Islam MS, KRDG, et al. Molecular assessment of protective effect of Vitex negundo in ISO induced myocardial infarction in rats. *Biomed Pharmacother.* (2017) 92:249–53. doi: 10.1016/j.biopha.2017.05.078
35. Erikson JM, Valente AJ, Mummidi S, Kandikattu HK, DeMarco VG, Bender SB, et al. Targeting TRAF3IP2 by genetic and interventional approaches inhibits ischemia/reperfusion-induced myocardial injury and adverse remodeling. *J Biol Chem.* (2017) 292:2345–58. doi: 10.1074/jbc.M116.764522
36. Yu B, Wang W. cardioprotective effects of morroniside in rats following acute myocardial infarction. *Inflammation* (2018) 41:432–6. doi: 10.1007/s10753-017-0699-x
37. Kljucevic N, Milat AM, Grga M, Mudnic I, Boban M, Grkovic I. White wine consumption influences inflammatory phase of repair after myocardial infarction in rats. *J Cardiovasc Pharmacol.* (2017) 70:293–9. doi: 10.1097/fjc.0000000000000519
38. Mongue-Din H, Patel AS, Looi YH, Grieve DJ, Anilkumar N, Sirker A, et al. NADPH Oxidase-4 driven cardiac macrophage polarization protects against

myocardial infarction-induced remodeling. *JACC Basic Transl Sci.* (2017) 2:688–98. doi: 10.1016/j.jacbts.2017.06.006

39. Rothschild DE, McDaniel DK, Ringel-Scaia VM, Allen IC. Modulating inflammation through the negative regulation of NF-kappaB signaling. *J Leukoc Biol.* (2018) 103:1131–50. doi: 10.1002/jlb.3mir0817-346rrr
40. Samidurai M, Ramasamy VS, Jo J. beta-amyloid inhibits hippocampal LTP through TNFR/IKK/NF-kappaB pathway. *Neurol Res.* (2018) 40:268–76. doi: 10.1080/01616412.2018.1436872
41. Catrysse L, van Loo G. Inflammation and the metabolic syndrome: the tissue-specific functions of NF-kappaB. *Trends Cell Biol.* (2017) 27:417–29. doi: 10.1016/j.tcb.2017.01.006
42. Durand JK, Baldwin AS. Targeting IKK and NF-kappaB for therapy. *Adv Protein Chem Struct Biol.* (2017) 107:77–115. doi: 10.1016/bs.apcsb,.2016.11.006
43. Kondylis V, Kumari S, Vlantis K, Pasparakis M. The interplay of IKK, NF-kappaB and RIPK1 signaling in the regulation of cell death, tissue homeostasis and inflammation. *Immunol Rev.* (2017) 277:113–27. doi: 10.1111/imr.12550
44. Lee HR, Choi J, Lee SH, Cho ML, Jue DM. Intracelluar delivery of A20 protein inhibits TNFalpha-induced NF-kappaB activation. *Protein Expr Purif.* (2018) 143:14–9. doi: 10.1016/j.pep.2017.10.005
45. Van Quickelberghe E, Martens A, Goeminne LJE, Clement L, van Loo G, Gevaert K. Identification of Immune-Responsive Gene 1 (IRG1) as a Target of A20. *J Proteome Res.* (2018) 17:2182–91. doi: 10.1021/acs.jproteome.8b00139
46. Jarosz M, Olbert M, Wyszogrodzka G, Mlyniec K, Librowski T. Antioxidant and anti-inflammatory effects of zinc. Zinc-dependent NF-kappaB signaling *Inflammopharmacology* (2017) 25:11–24. doi: 10.1007/s10787-017-0309-4

2

C-Reactive Protein and N-Terminal Pro-Brain Natriuretic Peptide Levels Correlate with Impaired Cardiorespiratory Fitness in Patients with Heart Failure Across a Wide Range of Ejection Fraction

Jessie van Wezenbeek[1†], Justin M. Canada[1†], Krishna Ravindra[1†], Salvatore Carbone[1], Cory R. Trankle[1], Dinesh Kadariya[1], Leo F. Buckley[1], Marco Del Buono[1], Hayley Billingsley[1], Michele Viscusi[1], George F. Wohlford[2], Ross Arena[3], Benjamin Van Tassell[2] and Antonio Abbate[1]*

[1] VCU Pauley Heart Center, Virginia Commonwealth University, Richmond, VA, United States, [2] Department of Pharmacotherapy and Outcome Sciences, Virginia Commonwealth University, Richmond, VA, United States, [3] Department of Physical Therapy, College of Applied Health Sciences, University of Illinois, Chicago, IL, United States

Correspondence:
Antonio Abbate
antonio.abbate@vcuhealth.org

[†] These authors have contributed equally to this work

Background: Impaired cardiorespiratory fitness (CRF) is a hallmark of heart failure (HF). Serum levels of C-reactive protein (CRP), a systemic inflammatory marker, and of N-terminal pro-brain natriuretic peptide (NT-proBNP), a biomarker of myocardial strain, independently predict adverse outcomes in HF patients. Whether CRP and/or NT-proBNP also predict the degree of CRF impairment in HF patients across a wide range of ejection fraction is not yet established.

Methods: Using retrospective analysis, 200 patients with symptomatic HF who completed one or more treadmill cardiopulmonary exercise tests (CPX) using a symptom-limited ramp protocol and had paired measurements of serum high-sensitivity CRP and NT-proBNP on the same day were evaluated. Univariate and multivariate correlations were evaluated with linear regression after logarithmic transformation of CRP ($\log_{10}$) and NT-proBNP ($\log_N$).

Results: Mean age of patients was 57 ± 10 years and 55% were male. Median CRP levels were 3.7 [1.5–9.0] mg/L, and NT-proBNP levels were 377 [106–1,464] pg/ml, respectively. Mean peak oxygen consumption (peak VO_2) was 16 ± 4 $mlO_2 \bullet kg^{-1} \bullet min^{-1}$. CRP levels significantly correlated with peakVO_2 in all patients ($R = -0.350$, $p < 0.001$) and also separately in the subgroup of patients with reduced left ventricular ejection fraction (LVEF) (HFrEF, $N = 109$) ($R = -0.282$, $p < 0.001$) and in those with preserved EF (HFpEF, $N = 57$) ($R = -0.459$, $p < 0.001$). NT-proBNP levels also significantly correlated with peak VO_2 in all patients ($R = -0.330$, $p < 0.001$) and separately in patients with HFrEF ($R = -0.342$, $p < 0.001$) and HFpEF ($R = -0.275$, $p = 0.032$). CRP and NT-proBNP did not correlate with each other ($R = 0.05$, $p = 0.426$), but independently predicted peak VO_2 ($R = 0.421$, $p < 0.001$ and $p < 0.001$, respectively).

Conclusions: Biomarkers of inflammation and myocardial strain independently predict peak VO_2 in HF patients. Anti-inflammatory therapies and therapies alleviating myocardial strain may independently improve CRF in HF patients across a large spectrum of LVEF.

Keywords: heart failure, biomarker, systemic inflammation, myocardial strain, cardiorespiratory fitness, cardiopulmonary exercise testing

INTRODUCTION

Heart failure (HF) is a syndrome that presents clinically with dyspnea, fatigue, and/or edema caused by structural or functional cardiac defects that lead to reduced cardiac output and/or increased cardiac pressure at rest or during stress. Impaired cardiorespiratory fitness (CRF) is a hallmark of heart failure (HF) (1). CRF is defined as the ability of the circulatory, respiratory, and muscular systems to supply oxygen during sustained physical activity (2). CRF is expressed in metabolic equivalents (METs) and measured by peak oxygen uptake (peak VO_2) using exercise tests (3). CRF is both an objective measure of habitual physical activity, as well as a prognostic indicator in HF.

C-reactive protein (CRP), a marker for systemic inflammation, is produced by the hepatocytes upon inflammation, infection, or tissue injury (4). Patients with HF show signs of chronic systemic inflammation, as shown by elevated serum levels of CRP (5). Increased levels of CRP are associated with an increased risk for CVD events and for mortality (6, 7). Higher CRP levels are also associated with worse cardiopulmonary exercise performance in patients with ischemic heart disease and systolic HF (8, 9).

Natriuretic peptides are peptide hormones that function as counter-regulatory mechanisms for the Renin-Angiotensin-Aldosterone-system (RAAS), and therefore cause a decrease in arterial pressure, central venous pressure, pulmonary capillary wedge pressure, cardiac output, and total blood volume through natriuresis and diuresis (10). Brain natriuretic peptide (BNP) is produced by the ventricles in response to an increase in myocardial stretch, damage, or ischemia (10). N-terminal pro-brain natriuretic peptide (NT-proBNP) is the biologically inactive peptide that is cleaved off the pro-hormone, proBNP (11). The diagnostic and prognostic power of both BNP and NT-proBNP is similar, however, NT-proBNP is less sensitive to breakdown than BNP is, which results in a more accurate measurement and reproducibility (11). Plasma levels of NT-proBNP have shown to relate to a low peak oxygen uptake (peak VO_2) in HF patients (12).

Serum levels of CRP and NT-proBNP have shown to predict adverse outcomes in patients with HF, both in HF with reduced ejection fraction (HFrEF, LVEF <50%) and in HF with preserved ejection fraction (HFpEF, LVEF >50%). Although CRP and NT-proBNP provide independent and complementary insight into CRF, whether CRP and/or NT-proBNP also independently predict the degree of CRF impairment in HF patients is not yet established. We hypothesize that two biomarkers, CRP, and NT-proBNP, by acting as surrogates for different pathophysiologic mechanisms, inflammation and myocardial strain, respectively, will independently predict the degree of CRF impairment in patients with HF across the spectrum of LVEF including both HFrEF and HFpEF. The objective of this study was to investigate whether CRP and/or NT-proBNP can independently predict CRF impairment, defined as reduced peak VO_2 in patients with HF across a wide range of ejection fraction.

MATERIALS AND METHODS

Study Design

We retrospectively queried a database of de-identified data that was prospectively collected data from patients with symptomatic HF who completed one or more cardiopulmonary exercise tests (CPX) using a symptom-limited ramp protocol on a treadmill and had paired measurements of serum high-sensitivity CRP and NT-proBNP on the same day. All members of the research team have completed training on the ethical conduct of research on human subjects. The VCU Institutional Review Board approved of the study, which was conducted according to the International Conference on Harmonization Good Clinical Practice Guidelines and the Declaration of Helsinki.

Cardiopulmonary Exercise Testing

All patients underwent maximal CPX with a certified exercise physiologist under the supervision of a physician with a metabolic cart connected to a treadmill (Vmax Encore, Viasys, Yora Linda, CA) using a ramp protocol, as described before (13). Oxygen and carbon dioxide sensors were calibrated before the test with known oxygen, nitrogen, and carbon dioxide concentrations and the flow sensor was calibrated using a 3-L syringe. Subjects were asked to exercise to maximal fatigue. Twelve-lead ECG measurements were done at baseline,

Abbreviations: CRF, Cardiorespiratory Fitness; HF, Heart Failure; HFrEF, Heart Failure with Reduced Ejection Fraction; HFpEF, Heart Failure with Preserved Ejection Fraction; METs, Metabolic Equivalents; VO_2, Oxygen Consumption; CRP, C-Reactive Protein; NT-proBNP, N-Terminal Pro-Brain Natriuretic Peptide; WBC, White Blood Cell; NLR, Neutrophil to Leukocyte Ratio; ANP, Atrial Natriuretic Peptide; CVD, Cardiovascular Disease; CVP, Central Venous Pressure; RAAS, Renin Angiotensin Aldosterone System; LVEF, Left Ventricular Ejection Fraction; LVEDV, Left Ventricular End Diastolic Volume; LVESV, Left Ventricular End Systolic Volume; CPX, Cardiopulmonary Exercise Test; TET, Treadmill Exercise Time; Peak VO_2, Peak Oxygen Consumption; VE/VCO_2, Ventilatory Efficiency; ACS, Acute Coronary Syndrome; MI, Myocardial Infarction; ARNI, Angiotensin Receptor-Neprilysin Inhibitor; ACEI, Angiotensin-Converting-Enzyme Inhibitor; PARADIGM-HF, Prospective Comparison of ARNI with ACEI to Determine Impact on Global; Mortality and Morbidity in Heart Failure; CANTOS, Canakinumab Antiinflammatory Thrombosis Outcome Study; ROC, Receiver Operating Characteristic; AUC, Area Under the Curve.

throughout the test, and during recovery. Every 2 min blood pressure was measured using an automated exercise compatible device (Tango, SunTech Medical). Expired gases were sampled during exercise with a mouthpiece-mounted sensor and were analyzed continuously to measure oxygen consumption (VO_2), carbon dioxide production (VCO_2), and minute ventilation (VE). The peak VO_2 ($mlO_2{\bullet}kg^{-1}{\bullet}min^{-1}$) during exercise was defined as the highest 10-s average value for VO_2 during the last 30 s of the exercise. Peak VO_2 measured during exercise is the most objective variable for assessment of functional capacity as is an important prognostic indicator (3). American Heart Association/American College of Cardiology guidelines for exercise testing contraindications and termination criteria were followed.

Doppler Echocardiography

Subjects underwent transthoracic Doppler echocardiogram. Echocardiography was performed according to the American Society of Echocardiography measurement guidelines and provides information on both cardiac dimensions and function (14). LV end-diastolic and end-systolic volumes (LVEDV, LVESV), EF, and early transmitral E wave velocities were obtained. Early mitral annulus (e′) velocities obtained by tissue Doppler were averaged between lateral and septal e′ and tricuspid annulus plane systolic excursion. The E/e′ ratio provides information on diastolic function and was calculated to estimate LV filling pressures (15, 16).

Biomarker Analysis

We analyzed differential comprehensive metabolic profile and plasma levels of biomarkers including high-sensitivity CRP and NT-proBNP. CRP, a marker for systemic inflammation, is increased in HF and has shown to relate to poor exercise performance (8, 9). CRP values <3.0 mg/L were considered within normal range. CRP values >3.0 mg/L have shown to be associated with an increased risk of cardiovascular disease (6). N-terminal pro-brain natriuretic peptide (NT-proBNP), a biomarker of myocardial strain, correlates with exercise capacity in HF (12). NT-proBNP values <300 ng/ml were considered within normal range (17). Both CRP and NT-proBNP independently predict adverse outcomes in patients with HF (7, 18, 19). Furthermore, we analyzed White Blood Cell (WBC) count, absolute neutrophils, and leukocyte count. Neutrophil to leukocyte ratio (NLR) is a measure for systemic inflammation (20). A NLR >4 has prognostic value in cardiovascular disease (21).

Data Analysis

For the data analysis, each of the tests were considered as a separate measurement for data analysis. We assessed the correlation between different clinical parameters and peak oxygen consumption (peak VO_2), as the preferred measures of CRF obtained during effort-limited maximal cardiopulmonary exercise testing (CPX). This was done for the entire HF group and then analyzed separately for 2 groups of patients stratified according to LVEF <50% (HFrEF) or ≥50% (HFpEF). According to the Fick principle, peak VO_2 is determined by stroke volume, heart rate, and arterial-venous oxygen difference and therefore reflects both cardiac, vascular, and peripheral skeletal muscle components. The cause of exercise intolerance has been proposed to be different in HFrEF and HFpEF patients, therefore we stratified according to LVEF (22).

Statistical Analysis

Data was tested for deviation from Gaussian distribution using the Kolmogorov–Smirnov test, and due to a lack of deviation, is presented as mean and standard deviation. Data that deviated from Gaussian distribution is presented as median and interquartile range. For normally distributed continuous variables, differences between groups were evaluated using independent-samples *t*-test, and for not normally distributed variables with the Mann–Whitney *U*-test. Correlations between continuous variables were assessed using linear regression. Multivariate analysis using stepwise linear regression was used to assess predictors of CRF with available clinical parameters. A ROC curve analysis was performed to evaluate whether the biomarkers had discriminative value for reduced CRF defined as peak VO_2 <10 $mlO_2{\bullet}kg^{-1}{\bullet}min^{-1}$ and peak VO_2 <14 $mlO_2{\bullet}kg^{-1}{\bullet}min^{-1}$. SPSS Statistics 24.0 (IBM, Armonk, NY) statistical software package was used for all analyses. No missing data imputation method used. A p-value < 0.05 was considered statistically significant.

TABLE 1 | Clinical characteristics in all patients.

Patient characteristics (*N* = 200)	
Age, y	57 (10)
Male sex, *n* (%)	110 (55%)
BMI, kg/m^2	35 (8)
BIOMARKERS	
CRP, mg/L	7.1 (8.9) 3.7 [1.5–9.0]
WBC, ×10^9/L	7.2 (2.4)
Absolute Neutrophils, ×10^9/L	4.0 [3.1–5.2]
Absolute Lymphocytes, ×10^9/L	1.9 (0.6)
Neutrophil-to-Lymphocyte ratio	2.3 [1.6–3.1]
NT-proBNP, ng/ml	1306 (3092) 377 [106–1464]
DOPPLER ECHOCARDIOGRAPHY PARAMETERS	
LVEF, %	44 (14)
E/e′	15 (8)
CARDIOPULMONARY EXERCISE PARAMETERS	
Treadmill exercise time, min	8.7 (2.8)
Peak VO_2, $mlO_2{\bullet}kg^{-1}{\bullet}min^{-1}$	16 (4)
Peak VO_2 % of predicted	54 (16)
VE/VCO_2 slope	33 (7)
DASI score	30 (16)
MLWHF score	46 (26)

BMI, Body Mass Index; WBC, White Blood Cell Count; NLR, Neutrophil to Leukocyte Ratio; DASI, Duke Activity Status Index; MLWHF, Minnesota Living With Heart Failure; LVEF, Left Ventricular Ejection Fraction; VO_2, Oxygen uptake; VE, Minute Ventilation; VCO_2, Carbon Dioxide output. Data shown as mean and (standard deviation) or median and [interquartile range].

RESULTS

We evaluated a total of 366 CPX from 200 different patients (2.0 ± 1.3 studies per patient) of which the clinical characteristics are shown in **Table 1** for all patients. Clinical characteristics are shown separately for patients with HF with reduced LVEF (LVEF <50%) and for patients with HF with preserved LVEF HFpEF (LVEF ≥50%) in **Table 2**. Mean age of patients was 57 ± 10 years and 110 (55%) were male. Mean LVEF was 44 ± 14% (HFrEF, $N = 109$ and HFpEF, $N = 57$) (**Figure 1**), with a mean LVEF of 36 ± 11% in HFrEF, and 58 ± 6% in HFpEF. Median high-sensitivity CRP levels were 3.7 [1.5–9.0] mg/L, respectively and median NT-proBNP levels were 377 [106–1,464] pg/ml, respectively. In HFrEF, median CRP levels were 4.2 [1.9–9.2] mg/L, and median NT-proBNP levels were 1,029 [280–2,263] pg/ml. In HFpEF, median CRP levels were 3.7 [0.6–10.8] mg/L and median NT-proBNP levels were 102 [46–183] pg/ml, respectively ($P < 0.001$ for NT-proBNP, $P = 0.03$ for CRP between HFpEF and HFrEF). The distribution of LVEF, CRP, and NT-proBNP is shown in **Figure 1**. Mean White Blood Cell (WBC) count and median Neutrophil to Leukocyte Ratio (NLR) was 7.2 (2.4) × 10^9/L and 2.3 [1.6–3.1], with a mean WBC count and median NLR of 7.4 (2.6) × 10^9/L and 2.0 [1.5–2.7] in HFpEF, and 6.9 (2.1) × 10^9/L and 2.3 [1.6–3.2] in HFrEF, respectively, ($P = 0.198$ for WBC count, $P = 0.07$ for NLR). Mean peak oxygen consumption (peak VO_2) was 16 ± 4 $mlO_2 \bullet kg^{-1} \bullet min^{-1}$and mean treadmill exercise time (TET) was 8.7 ± 2.8 min.

CRP as a Predictor of CRF

CRP levels significantly and inversely correlated with peak VO_2 ($R = -0.350$, $p < 0.001$, $N = 316$), and with TET ($R = -0.342$, $p < 0.001$, $N = 314$) as shown in **Figure 2**. The association between CRP and peak VO_2 and between CRP and TET remained significant when the analysis was limited to HFrEF patients ($R = -0.282$, $p < 0.001$, $N = 192$ for peak VO_2 and $R = 0.336$, $p < 0.001$, $N = 190$ for TET) and to HFpEF patients ($R = -0.459$, $p < 0.001$, $N = 90$ for peak VO_2 and $R = -0.345$, $p < 0.01$, $N = 90$ for TET).

NT-proBNP as a Predictor of CRF

NT-proBNP levels significantly and inversely correlated with peak VO_2 ($R = -0.330$, $p < 0.001$, $N = 258$) and with TET ($R = -0.412$, $p < 0.001$, $N = 256$) as shown in **Figure 3**. The association between NT-proBNP and peak VO_2 and between NT-proBNP and TET remained significant when the analysis was limited to HFrEF patients ($R = -0.354$, $p < 0.001$, $N = 168$ for peak VO_2 and $R = -0.437$, $p < 0.001$, $N = 166$ for TET) as well as in HFpEF patients ($R = -0.275$, $p = 0.032$, $N = 61$ for peak VO_2 and $R = -0.459$, $p < 0.001$, $N = 61$ for TET).

Multivariate Analysis

Multivariate analysis including CRP and NT-proBNP showed that both CRP and NT-proBNP independently predicted peak VO_2 ($R = 0.421$, $p < 0.001$ and $p < 0.001$, respectively), and TET ($R = 0.478$, $p < 0.001$, and $p < 0.001$, respectively). CRP and NT-proBNP did not exhibit collinearity ($R = +0.05$,

TABLE 2 | Clinical characteristics in HFpEF and HFrEF patients.

	HFpEF ($N = 57$)	HFrEF ($N = 109$)	
Age, y	53 (9)	57 (10)	$P = 0.03$
Male sex, n (%)	19 (33%)	78 (72%)	$P < 0.001$
BMI, kg/m^2	40 (8)	34 (8)	$P < 0.001$
BIOMARKERS			
CRP, mg/L	6.4 (7.1) 3.7 [0.6–10.8]	7.7 (9.7) 4.2 [1.9–9.2]	$P = 0.03$
NT-proBNP, ng/ml	172 (266) 102 [46-183]	1906 (3693) 1029 [280–2263]	$P < 0.001$
HgB, g/dl	13.1 (1.8)	13.2 (1.7)	$P = 0.75$
HBA1c, %	7.7 (1.9)	6.8 (1.4)	$P < 0.001$
WBC, ×10^9/L	7.4 (2.6)	6.9 (2.1)	$P = 0.198$
Absolute Neutrophils, ×10^9/L	4.1 [3.0–5.4]	4.0 [3.1–5.2]	$P = 0.71$
Absolute Lymphocytes, ×10^9/L	2.1 (0.6)	1.8 (0.6)	$P = 0.002$
Neutrophil-to-Lymphocyte ratio	2.0 [1.5–2.7]	2.3 [1.6–3.2]	$P = 0.07$
DOPPLER ECHOCARDIOGRAPHY PARAMETERS			
LVEF, %	58 (6)	36 (11)	$P < 0.001$
LVEDV, ml	110 (32)	172 (62)	$P < 0.001$
LVESV, ml	47 (19)	115 (55)	$P < 0.001$
E′	8.1 (2.4)	6.5 (3.6)	$P = 0.01$
E/e′	11.3 (4.7)	17.2 (8.3)	$P < 0.001$
CARDIOPULMONARY EXERCISE PARAMETERS			
Treadmill exercise time, min	9.4 (2.6)	8.4 (2.8)	$P = 0.005$
Peak VO_2, $mlO_2 \bullet kg^{-1} \bullet min^{-1}$	16.5 (4.6)	15.4 (4.3)	$P = 0.04$
Peak VO_2 % of predicted	55 (17)	52 (14)	$P = 0.356$
VE/VCO_2 slope	30 (5)	33 (7)	$P < 0.001$

BMI, Body Mass Index; HgB, Hemoglobin; HBA1c, Hemoglobin A1c; WBC, White Blood Cell Count; NLR, Neutrophil to Leukocyte Ratio; LVEF, Left Ventricular Ejection Fraction; LVEDV, Left Ventricular End Diastolic Volume; LVESV, Left Ventricular End Systolic Volume; VO_2, Oxygen uptake; VE, Minute Ventilation; VCO_2, Carbon Dioxide output. Data shown as mean and (standard deviation) or median and [interquartile range].

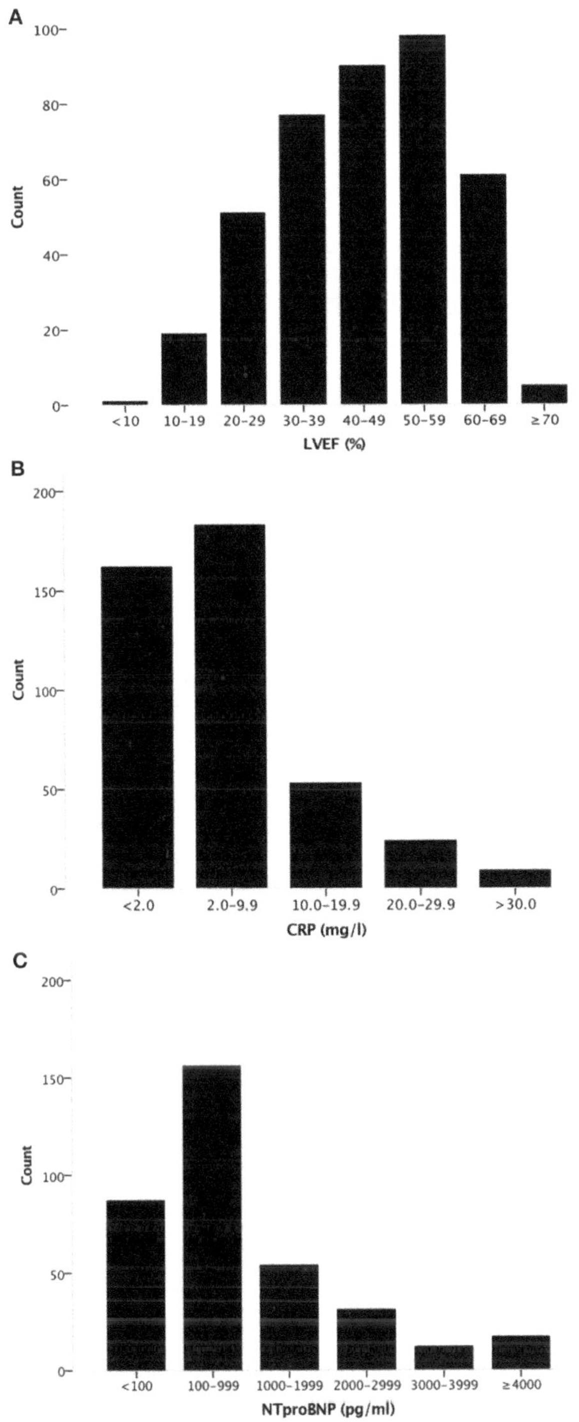

FIGURE 1 | Distribution of LVEF, CRP, and NT-proBNP levels in the population. Histogram showing the distribution of **(A)** LVEF, **(B)** CRP levels, and **(C)** NT-proBNP levels in the population. LVEF, Left Ventricular Ejection Fraction.

$p = 0.426$, $N = 255$). When the analysis was limited to HFrEF patients, CRP and NT-proBNP predicted peak VO_2 ($R = 0.432$, $p < 0.001$, $p < 0.001$, respectively) and TET ($R = 0.496$, $p < 0.001$, $p < 0.001$, respectively). When the analysis was limited to HFpEF patients, NT-proBNP predicted peak VO_2 independent from CRP ($R = 0.287$, $p = 0.5$ for CRP, $p = 0.04$ for NT-proBNP) and TET ($R = 0.459$, $p = 0.988$ for CRP, $p < 0.001$ for NT-proBNP). Furthermore, multivariate analysis including NT-proBNP, BMI, age, and sex significantly predicted peak VO_2 ($R = 0.631$, $p < 0.001$, $p < 0.001$, $p = 0.04$, respectively, with a trend for sex ($p = 0.08$). NT-proBNP, CRP, BMI, age, and sex significantly predicted TET ($R = 0.651$, $p < 0.001$, $p = 0.006$, $p < 0.001$, $p < 0.001$, $p = 0.029$, respectively). When the analysis was limited to HFrEF patients, BMI, age, sex, NT-proBNP, and CRP predicted Peak VO_2 ($R = 0.669$, $p < 0.001$, $p < 0.001$, $p < 0.001$, $p < 0.001$, $p = 0.03$, respectively) and TET ($R = 0.716$, $p < 0.001$, $p < 0.001$, $p < 0.001$, $p < 0.001$, $p = 0.002$, respectively). When the analysis was limited to HFpEF patients, BMI, and age significantly predicted peak VO_2 ($R = 0.669$, $p < 0.001$, and $p < 0.001$, respectively) and BMI, age, and NT-proBNP predicted TET ($R = 0.680$ $p < 0.001$, $p = 0.017$, $p = 0.03$, respectively).

ROC Curve Analysis

A ROC curve analysis was performed to evaluate whether CRP and NT-proBNP have discriminative value for reduced CRF, defined as peak VO_2 <10 $mlO_2 \bullet kg^{-1} \bullet min^{-1}$and peak VO_2 <14 $mlO_2 \bullet kg^{-1} \bullet min^{-1}$(**Figure 4**). For peak VO_2 < 10 $mlO_2 \bullet kg^{-1} \bullet min^{-1}$, the area under the curve (AUC) = 0.660 95% CI [0.544–0.776], $P = 0.014$ for CRP and AUC = 0.749 95% CI [0.669–0.829], $P < 0.001$ for NT-proBNP. For peak VO_2 <14 $mlO_2 \bullet kg^{-1} \bullet min^{-1}$, AUC = 0.658 95% CI [0.597–0.718], $P < 0.001$ for CRP and AUC = 0.608 95% CI [0.537–0.678] $P = 0.003$ for NT-proBNP.

DISCUSSION

CRF is an important determinant of quality of life and prognostic indicator in patients with HF (23, 24). In the current study, we show that systemic inflammation, as measured by elevated CRP levels, and myocardial strain, as indicated by elevated NT-proBNP levels, independently predict impaired CRF in patients with HF, reflected in reduced peak VO_2. Both CRP and NT-proBNP show a high discriminative value for reduced CRF as defined by peak VO_2 <10 $mlO_2 \bullet kg^{-1} \bullet min^{-1}$and peak VO_2 <14 $mlO_2 \bullet kg^{-1} \bullet min^{-1}$.

Systemic Inflammation in Heart Failure

HF is characterized by systemic inflammation, as shown by elevated circulating levels of inflammatory biomarkers in patients that increase with progression of the disease (25). For one, systemic inflammation may be the result of HF by means of tissue hypoperfusion and neurohormonal activation (26), or inflammation may play a pathophysiologic role in HF (27, 28). It is suggested that the pro-inflammatory state contributes to the development and progression of HF, not only by impairing myocardial function but also by affecting other organs and tissues and thereby adding to other aspects of the HF syndrome including cachexia and anemia (25).

The preferred inflammatory biomarker in cardiovascular disease is CRP (29, 30). HF patients have elevated CRP levels and such levels tend to increase with clinical decompensation and predict worse outcomes (5, 31, 32). Elevated CRP levels reflect inflammatory and immune deregulation in HF (31, 33). Elevated CRP levels also correlate with worse cardiac function (34, 35), and worse functional capacity in patients with ischemic heart disease and systolic HF (8, 9). The association between elevated CRP levels and HF is however complex and likely only incompletely understood. CRP is produced in the liver in response to cytokines such as Interleukin-6 (IL-6) (36). IL-6 is considered a secondary cytokine produced by myeloid cells in response to Interleukin-1 (IL-1) and Tumor Necrosis Factor-α (TNF-α) (36). Elevated IL-1 and TNF-α levels have been reported in patients with HF (33, 37). Moreover, IL-1 and TNF-α are also known as soluble cardiodepressant factors in patients with sepsis (38). More recently enhanced IL-1 activity has been described in patients with acute decompensated HF (31). IL-1 induces a reversible left ventricular systolic dysfunction in the mouse that is characterized by β-adrenergic receptor desensitization and impaired contractile reserve (39). This data points to an active role of IL-1 in the pathophysiology of HF.

Myocardial Strain

Elevated NT-proBNP levels reflect myocardial strain due to increased pressure, however, levels may also increase in response to other insults such as ischemia or inflammatory cytokines. NT-proBNP has shown to predict adverse outcomes in HF patients (10). Although BNP exerts protective effects on the heart during HF, the circulating levels of BNP or NT-proBNP reflect worse hemodynamics (elevated filling pressures) and neurohormonal activation (40). A lack of endogenous BNP response facilitates the onset of HF in animal experimental models (41), whereas potentiation of the BNP effects using recombinant BNP or neprylisin inhibitors help prevent HF (42).

Limitations

The retrospective nature of the study limited the power of our analyses, specifically in the HFpEF cohort for which the sample size was smaller than for HFrEF patients. Another limitation of our study is that every visit in the data analysis was used as separate data point, which results in some patients being represented more than once in the database. Having patients represented more than once can alter the representation of the patient population, as a single patient could have provided more than one data entry leading to an over-representation of their specific clinical characteristics. Lastly, we were not able to address the role of other biomarkers for inflammation in HF in our study.

Potential Implications for Diagnosis, Risk Stratification, and Treatment

According to our findings, both elevated CRP and NT-proBNP levels are independently predictive of impaired CRF in HF and predictive of moderately or severe reduction in peak VO_2. A scoring system that would include both biomarkers is therefore likely to yield a better discrimination than only one of the markers. In non-ST elevation ACS, CRP, and BNP in combination with troponin I were predictive of mortality, MI and CHF. Further, a combination of the biomarkers provided additional prognostic value (43). These observations were validated in a cohort of 1,635 patients in the TACTICS-TIMI 18 study, and after adjustment for known clinical predictors, the number of elevated biomarkers remained predictive of the composite end point. Specifically, patients with one, two, and three elevated biomarkers had a 2.1, 3.1, and 3.7-fold increase in the risk of death, MI, or development of CHF after 6 months (43). A scoring system that could utilize the prognostic power of both CRP and NT-proBNP would allow for risk stratification beyond that solely provided by each of the markers used separately to predict CRF in patients with HF across a wide range of LVEF.

Inhibiting systemic inflammation with anti-inflammatory therapies and alleviating myocardial strain may represent two independent therapeutic strategies to improve CRF in patients with HF. Phase II studies have started exploring the effects of Interleukin-1 blockers in HF. A pilot feasibility study in 7 patients was conducted to test the efficacy of Anakinra on CP exercise performance in patients with HF and evidence of CRP. CRP levels were greatly reduced and peak VO_2 significantly improved (31). In the REDHART sub study, 60 patients with HFrEF and elevated CRP were randomly assigned to daily subcutaneous injections of Anakinra 100 mg for weeks, 12 weeks, or placebo (44). Treatment with Anakinra did not affect peak VO_2 or VE/VCO_2 slope at 2 weeks; however, patients showed improvement in peak VO_2 when assigned to the 12-week group. Further, the incidence of death or rehospitalization for HF at 24 weeks was 6, 31, and 30% for the Anakinra 12-week, Anakinra 2-week, and placebo groups, respectively. In the D-HART pilot study, the effects of IL-1 blockade with Anakinra on aerobic exercise capacity and CRP in patients with HFpEF were examined (45). Anakinra led to a statistically significant improvement in peak VO_2 consumption and a significant reduction in plasma CRP levels.

In a follow up study, the Diastolic Heart Failure Anakinra Response Trial-2 (DHART-2), patients with stable symptomatic HFpEF were treated with Anakinra to confirm the effects on peak VO_2 and CRP and observe its effects on serum NT-proBNP (46). Twenty-eight patients completed two visits or more and Anakinra was found to significantly reduce CRP as well as NT-proBNP levels. After 12 weeks of IL-1 blockade with Anakinra, NT-proBNP was reduced at a magnitude that correlated with CRP reduction. Anakinra however failed to increase peak VO_2 in the DHART2 study. The potential benefits of IL-1 blockade in patients with heart disease is further supported by the results of the phase III Canakinumab Antiinflammatory Thrombosis Outcome Study (CANTOS) (47), in which patients with prior acute myocardial infarction were randomized to canakinumab, IL-1β blocker, or placebo, and showed a significant reduction in major adverse cardiac events. A small single-center sub-study of the CANTOS trial showed a significant improvement in peak VO_2 in canakinumab-treated patients at 3 and 12 months (46).

Neprilysin inhibitors have also provided a novel therapeutic strategy to combat HF symptoms and promote CRF. Another

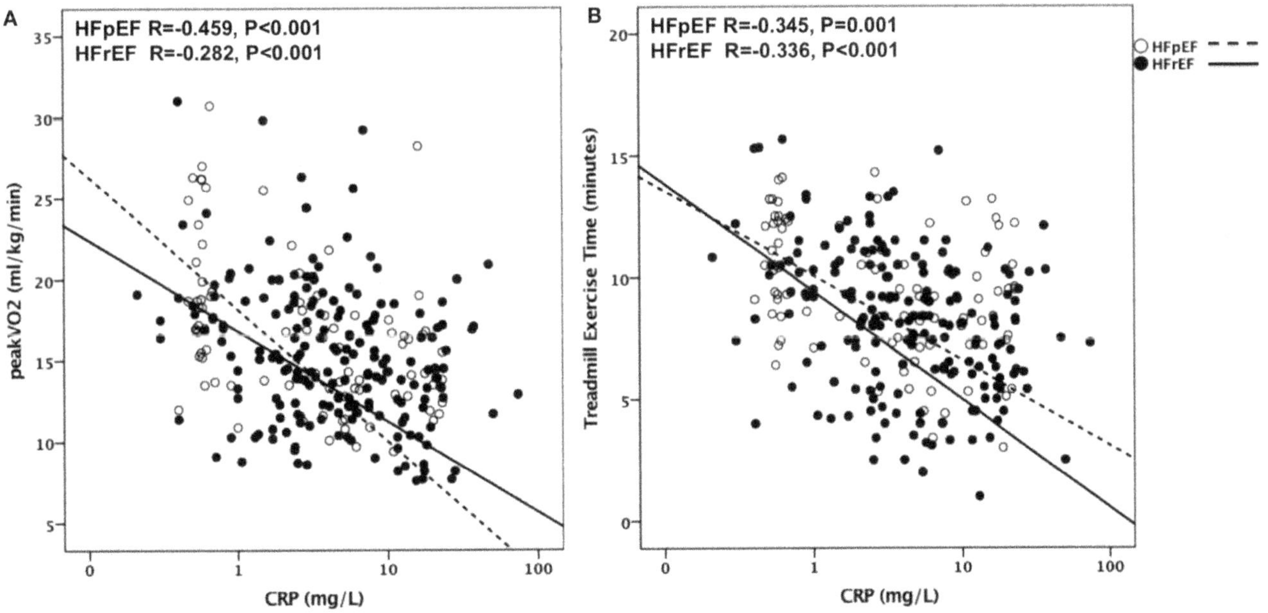

FIGURE 2 | CRP as predictor of CRF in HFrEF and HFpEF. Correlations are shown in **(A)** between CRP and Peak VO_2 in patients with HFpEF ($R = -0.459$, $P < 0.001$) and with HFrEF ($R = -0.282$, $P < 0.001$) and in **(B)** between CRP and TET in patients with HFpEF ($R = -0.345$, $P < 0.001$) and with HFrEF ($R = -0.336$, $P < 0.001$). VO_2, Oxygen uptake; HFpEF, Heart Failure with preserved Ejection Fraction; HFrEF, Heart Failure with reduced Ejection Fraction; TET, Treadmill Exercise Time.

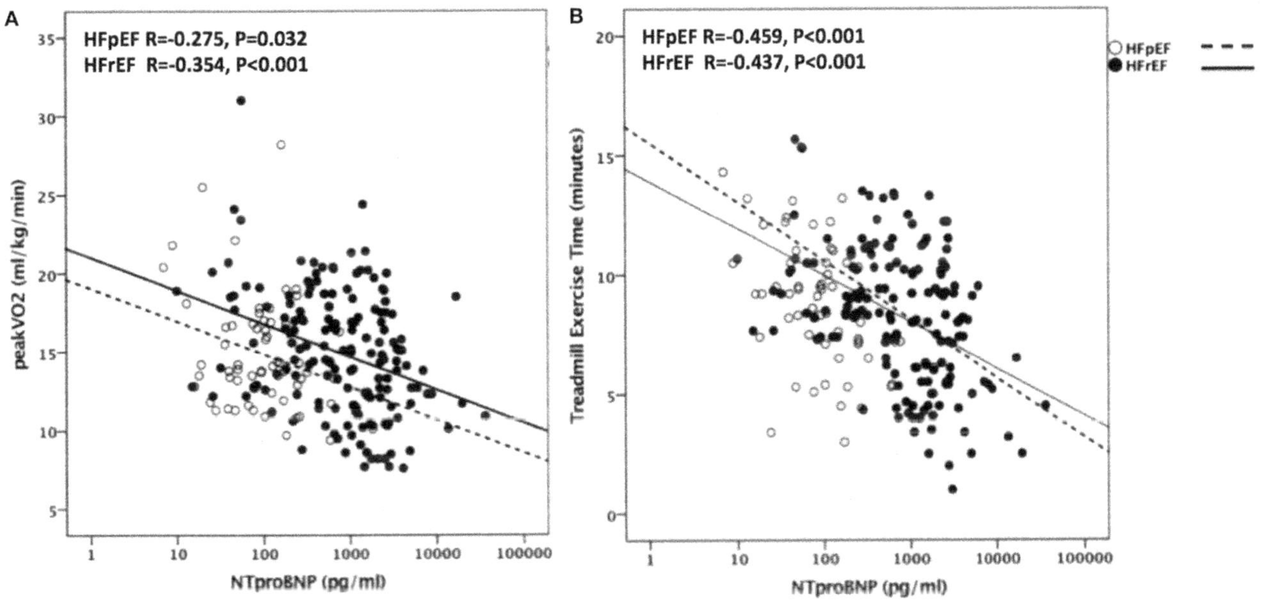

FIGURE 3 | NT-proBNP as predictor of CRF in HFrEF and HFpEF. Correlations are shown in **(A)** between NT-proBNP and Peak VO_2 in patients with HFpEF ($R = -0.275$, $P = 0.032$) and with HFrEF ($R = -0.354$, $P < 0.001$) and in **(B)** between NT-proBNP and TET in patients with HFpEF ($R = -0.459$, $P < 0.001$) and with HFrEF ($R = -0.437$, $P < 0.001$). VO_2, oxygen uptake; HFpEF, Heart Failure with preserved Ejection Fraction; HFrEF, Heart Failure with reduced Ejection Fraction; TET, Treadmill Exercise Time.

study was completed to compare the effects of Candoxatril (novel neutral endopeptidase inhibitor) with those of Furosemide in the treatment of patients with mild HF (37). Male patients with mild HF were randomly assigned to treatment with 20 mg of Furosemide twice a day, 200 mg of Candoxatril twice a day, or 400 mg of Candoxatril twice a day, for 9 days. For patients

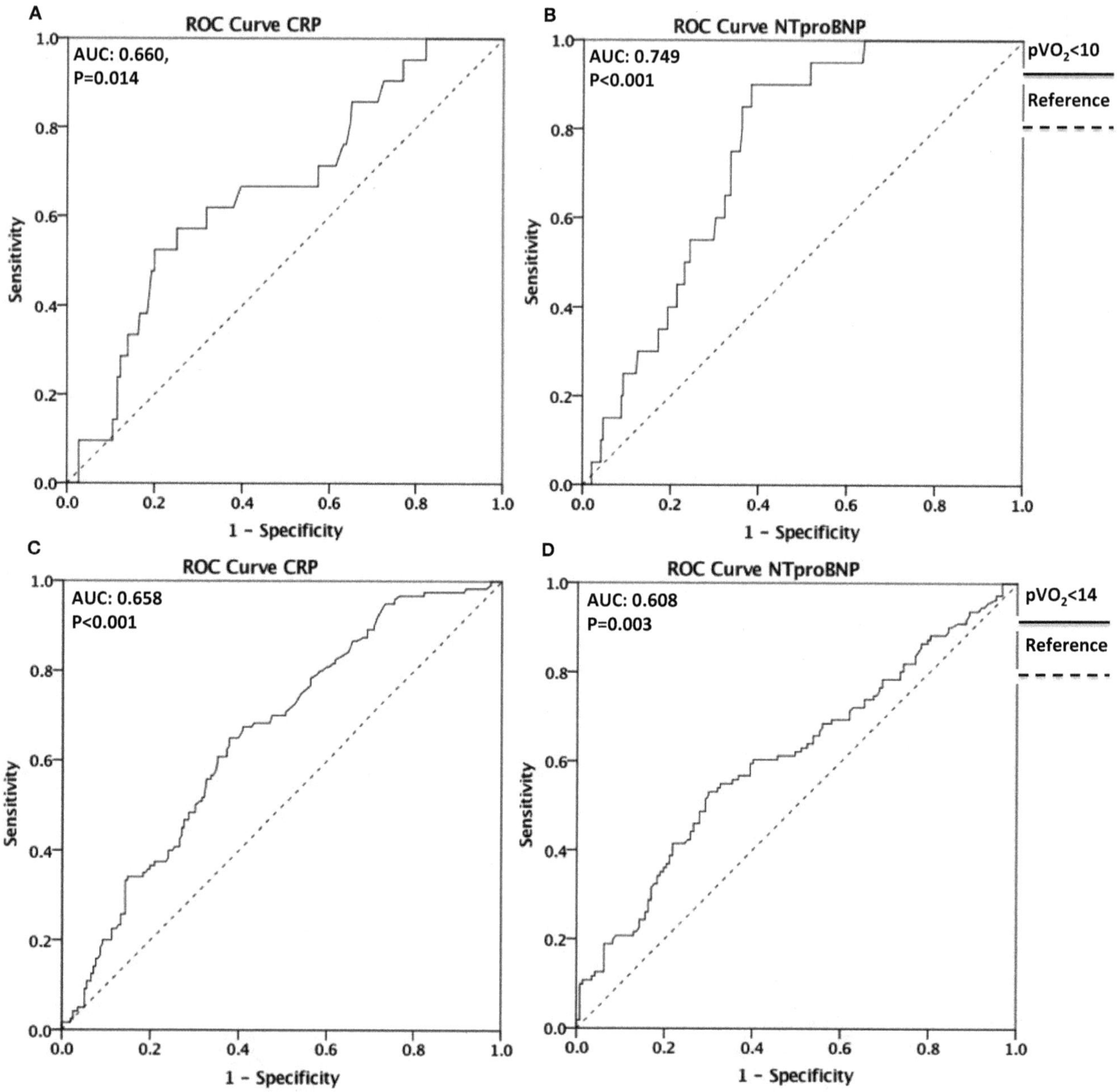

FIGURE 4 | Discriminative value of CRP and NT-proBNP for reduced CRF. ROC curves depicting the discriminative value of CRP in **(A)** and of NT-proBNP in **(B)** for reduced CRF defined as Peak $VO_2 < 10$ $mlO_2 \bullet kg^{-1} \bullet min^{-1}$ (AUC = 0.660, $P = 0.014$ for CRP and AUC = 0.749, $P < 0.001$ for NT-proBNP). ROC curves depicting the discriminative value of CRP in **(C)** and NT-proBNP in **(D)** for reduced CRF defined as Peak $VO_2 < 14$ $mlO_2 \bullet kg^{-1} \bullet min^{-1}$ (AUC = 0.658, $P < 0.001$ for CRP and AUC = 0.608, $P = 0.003$ for NT-proBNP). ROC, Receiver operating characteristic; CRF, Cardiorespiratory Fitness; VO_2, oxygen uptake; AUC. Area Under the Curve.

assigned to Furosemide, treadmill exercise capacity decreased by 30 ± 26 s compared to an increase of 12 ± 35 and of 35 ± 31 s for 200 mg of Candoxatril twice a day and 400 mg of Candoxatril twice a day, respectively (37). A pilot study was completed to evaluate the short-term effects of sacubitril/valsartan on maximal exercise capacity evaluated by peak VO_2 in stable patients with symptomatic HFrEF, with a secondary end point looking at changes in the VE/VCO_2 slope. When compared with baseline peak VO_2, patients experienced a significant increase in peak VO_2 at 30 days ($+0.92$ $mlO_2 \bullet kg^{-1} \bullet min^{-1}$), which corresponded to a 7.9% increase (38). These beneficial effects on CRF, fit well with the overall favorable effects of sacubitril/valsartan on major adverse cardiovascular events and cardiac death in the Prospective Comparison of ARNI (Angiotensin Receptor-Neprilysin Inhibitor) with ACEI (Angiotensin-Converting-Enzyme Inhibitor) to Determine Impact on Global Mortality and Morbidity in Heart Failure (PARADIGM-HF) trial (48).

CONCLUSION

Biomarkers of inflammation and myocardial strain independently predict reduced peak VO_2 in HF patients. Anti-inflammatory therapies and therapies alleviating myocardial strain may independently improve CRF in HF patients across a large spectrum of LVEF.

ETHICS STATEMENT

The study was completed with a de-identified database available at VCU. The research was considered exempt from Institutional Review Board review as per VCU IRB guidelines.

AUTHOR CONTRIBUTIONS

JC, SC, CT, DK, LB, HB, GW, BV, and AA clinical data collection. JW, KR, and AA database analysis, drafting of the manuscript. LB, MB, MV, and RA critical revision of the manuscript.

ACKNOWLEDGMENTS

AA and BV are supported by the United States of America National Heart & Lung Institute award (1R61HL139943). AA has served as a consultant to Novartis, Swedish Orphan Biovitrum, Janssen, Merck, and Olatec. BV has served as consultant to Novartis.

REFERENCES

1. Kondamudi N, Haykowsky M, Forman DE, Berry JD, Pandey A. Exercise training for prevention and treatment of heart failure. *Prog Cardiovasc Dis.* (2017) 60:115–20. doi: 10.1016/j.pcad.2017.07.001
2. Lavie CJ, Arena R, Swift DL, Johannsen NM, Sui X, Lee DC, et al. Exercise and the cardiovascular system: clinical science and cardiovascular outcomes. *Circ Res.* (2015) 117:207–19. doi: 10.1161/CIRCRESAHA.117.305205
3. Balady GJ, Arena R, Sietsema K, Myers J, Coke L, Fletcher GF, et al. Clinician's guide to cardiopulmonary exercise testing in adults: a scientific statement from the American heart association. *Circulation* (2010) 122:191–225. doi: 10.1161/CIR.0b013e3181e52e69
4. Libby P, Ridker PM, Maseri A. Inflammation and atherosclerosis. *Circulation* (2002) 105:1135–43. doi: 10.1161/hc0902.104353
5. Van Tassell BW, Abouzaki NA, Oddi Erdle C, Carbone S, Trankle CR, Melchior RD, et al. Interleukin-1 blockade in acute decompensated heart failure: a randomized, double-blinded, placebo-controlled pilot study. *J Cardiovasc Pharmacol.* (2016) 67:544–51. doi: 10.1097/FJC.0000000000000378
6. Emerging Risk Factors Collaboration, Kaptoge S, Di Angelantonio E, Lowe G, Pepys MB, Thompson SG, et al. C-reactive protein concentration and risk of coronary heart disease, stroke, and mortality: an individual participant meta-analysis. *Lancet* (2010) 375:132–40. doi: 10.1016/S0140-6736(09)61717-7
7. Ridker PM, MacFadyen JG, Everett BM, Libby P, Thuren T, Glynn RJ, et al. Relationship of C-reactive protein reduction to cardiovascular event reduction following treatment with canakinumab: a secondary analysis from the CANTOS randomised controlled trial. *Lancet* (2017) 391:319–28. doi: 10.1016/S0140-6736(17)32814-3
8. Canada JM, Fronk DT, Cei LF, Carbone S, Erdle CO, Abouzaki NA, et al. Usefulness of C-reactive protein plasma levels to predict exercise intolerance in patients with chronic systolic heart failure. *Am J Cardiol.* (2016) 117:116 20. doi: 10.1016/j.amjcard.2015.10.020
9. Rahimi K, Secknus MA, Adam M, Hayerizadeh BF, Fiedler M, Thiery J, et al. Correlation of exercise capacity with high-sensitive C-reactive protein in patients with stable coronary artery disease. *Am Heart J.* (2005) 150:1282–9. doi: 10.1016/j.ahj.2005.01.006
10. de Lemos JA, McGuire DK, Drazner MH. B-type natriuretic peptide in cardiovascular disease. *Lancet* (2003) 362:316–22. doi: 10.1016/S0140-6736(03)13976-1
11. Pan Y, Li D, Ma J, Shan L, Wei M. NT-proBNP test with improved accuracy for the diagnosis of chronic heart failure. *Medicine* (2017) 96:e9181. doi: 10.1097/MD.0000000000009181
12. Felker GM, Whellan D, Kraus WE, Clare R, Zannad F, Donahue M, et al. N-terminal pro-brain natriuretic peptide and exercise capacity in chronic heart failure: data from the heart failure and a controlled trial investigating outcomes of exercise training (HF-ACTION) study. *Am Heart J.* (2009) 158(4 Suppl.):S37–44. doi: 10.1016/j.ahj.2009.07.011
13. Arena R, Humphrey R, Peberdy MA, Madigan M. Predicting peak oxygen consumption during a conservative ramping protocol implications for the heart failure population. *J Cardiopulm Rehabil.* (2003) 23:183–9. doi: 10.1097/00008483-200305000-00004
14. Porter TR, Shillcutt SK, Adams MS, Desjardins G, Glas KE, Olson JJ, et al. Guidelines for the use of echocardiography as a monitor for therapeutic intervention in adults: a report from the american society of echocardiography. *J Am Soc Echocardiogr.* (2015) 28:40–56. doi: 10.1016/j.echo.2014.09.009
15. Barmeyer A, Müllerleile K, Mortensen K, Meinertz T. Diastolic dysfunction in exercise and its role for exercise capacity. *Heart Fail Rev.* (2009) 14:125–34. doi: 10.1007/s10741-008-9105-y
16. Terzi S, Sayar N, Bilsel T, Enc Y, Yildirim A, Ciloglu F, et al. Tissue doppler imaging adds incremental value in predicting exercise capacity in patients with congestive heart failure. *Heart Vessels* (2007) 22:237–44. doi: 10.1007/s00380-006-0961-x
17. van Kimmenade RR, Pinto YM, Bayes-Genis A, Lainchbury JG, Richards AM, Januzzi JL. Usefulness of intermediate amino-terminal pro-brain natriuretic peptide concentrations for diagnosis and prognosis of acute heart failure. *Am J Cardiol.* (2006) 98:386–90. doi: 10.1016/j.amjcard.2006.02.043
18. Yin WH, Chen JW, Jen HL, Chiang MC, Huang WP, Feng AN, et al. Independent prognostic value of elevated high-sensitivity C-reactive protein in chronic heart failure. *Am Heart J.* (2004) 147:931–8. doi: 10.1016/j.ahj.2003.11.021
19. Park JJ, Choi DJ, Yoon CH, Oh IY, Jeon ES, Kim JJ, et al. Prognostic value of C-reactive protein as an inflammatory and n-terminal probrain natriuretic peptide as a neurohumoral marker in acute heart failure (from the Korean heart failure registry). *Am J Cardiol.* (2014) 113:511–7. doi: 10.1016/j.amjcard.2013.10.022
20. Ackland GL, Minto G, Clark M, Whittle J, Stephens RCM, Owen T, et al. Autonomic regulation of systemic inflammation in humans: a multi-center, blinded observational cohort study. *Brain Behav Immun.* (2018) 67:47–53. doi: 10.1016/j.bbi.2017.08.010
21. Uthamalingam S, Patvardhan EA, Subramanian S, Ahmed W, Martin W, Daley M, et al. Utility of the neutrophil to lymphocyte ratio in predicting long-term outcomes in acute decompensated heart failure. *Am J Cardiol.* (2011) 107:433–8. doi: 10.1016/j.amjcard.2010.09.039
22. Dhakal BP, Malhotra R, Murphy RM, Pappagianopoulos PP, Baggish AL, Weiner RB, et al. Mechanisms of exercise intolerance in heart failure with preserved ejection fraction: the role of abnormal peripheral oxygen extraction. *Circ Hear Fail.* (2015) 8:286–94. doi: 10.1161/CIRCHEARTFAILURE.114.001825
23. Kupsky DF, Ahmed AM, Sakr S, Qureshi WT, Brawner CA, Blaha MJ, et al. Cardiorespiratory fitness and incident heart failure: the henry ford exercise testing (FIT) project. *Am Heart J.* (2017) 185:35–42. doi: 10.1016/j.ahj.2016.12.006
24. Szlachcic J, Massie BM, Kramer BL, Topic N, Tubau J. Correlates and prognostic implication of exercise capacity in chronic congestive heart failure. *Am J Cardiol.* (1985) 55:1037–42. doi: 10.1016/0002-9149(85)90742-8
25. Yndestad A, Damås JK, Oie E, Ueland T, Gullestad L, Aukrust P. Systemic inflammation in heart failure - the whys and

wherefores. *Heart Fail Rev.* (2006) 11:83–92. doi: 10.1007/s10741-006-9196-2

26. Van Linthout S, Tschöpe C. Inflammation—cause or consequence of heart failure or both? *Curr Heart Fail Rep.* (2017) 14:251–65. doi: 10.1007/s11897-017-0337-9
27. Buckley LF, Abbate A. Interleukin-1 blockade in cardiovascular diseases: a clinical update. *Eur Heart J.* (2018) 39:2063–9. doi: 10.1093/eurheartj/ehy128
28. Buckley LF, Abbate A. Interleukin-1 blockade in cardiovascular diseases: from bench to bedside. *BioDrugs* (2018) 32:111–8. doi: 10.1007/s40259-018-0274-5
29. Pearson TA, Mensah GA, Wayne R, Anderson JL, CannonIII RO, Criqui M, et al. Markers of inflammation and cardiovascular disease. *Circulation* (2003) 107:499–511. doi: 10.1161/01.cir.0000052939.59093.45.
30. Ridker PM. Clinical application of C-reactive protein for cardiovascular disease detection and prevention. *Circulation* (2003) 107:363–9. doi: 10.1161/01.CIR.0000053730.47739.3C
31. Van Tassell BW, Arena RA, Toldo S, Mezzaroma E, Azam T, Seropian IM, et al. Enhanced interleukin-1 activity contributes to exercise intolerance in patients with systolic heart failure. *PLoS ONE* (2012) 7:e33438. doi: 10.1371/journal.pone.0033438
32. Elster SK, Braunwald E, Wood HF. A study of C-reactive protein in the serum of patients with congestive heart failure. *Am Heart J.* (1956) 51:533–41. doi: 10.1016/0002-8703(56)90099-0
33. Testa M, Yeh M, Lee P, Fanelli R, Loperfido F, Berman JW, et al. Circulating levels of cytokines and their endogenous modulators in patients with mild to severe congestive heart failure due to coronary artery disease or hypertension. *J Am Coll Cardiol.* (1996) 28:964–71. doi: 10.1016/S0735-1097(96)00268-9
34. Shah SJ, Marcus GM, Gerber IL, McKeown BH, Vessey JC, Jordan MV, et al. High-sensitivity C-reactive protein and parameters of left ventricular dysfunction. *J Card Fail.* (2006) 12:61–5. doi: 10.1016/j.cardfail.2005.08.003
35. Tang WH, Shrestha K, Van Lente F, Troughton RW, Martin MG, Borowski AG, et al. Usefulness of C-reactive protein and left ventricular diastolic performance for prognosis in patients with left ventricular systolic heart failure. *Am J Cardiol.* (2008) 101:370–3. doi: 10.1016/j.amjcard.2007.08.038
36. Ridker PM. C-Reactive protein: Eighty eighty years from discovery to emergence as a major risk marker for cardiovascular disease. *Clin Chem.* (2009) 55:209–15. doi: 10.1373/clinchem.2008.119214
37. Vasan RS, Sullivan LM, Roubenoff R, Dinarello CA, Harris T, Benjamin EJ, et al. Inflammatory markers and risk of heart failure in elderly subjects without prior myocardial infarction: the framingham heart study. *Circulation* (2003) 107:1486–91. doi: 10.1161/01.CIR.0000057810.48709.F6
38. Kumar A, Thota V, Dee L, Olson J, Uretz E, Parrillo JE. Tumor necrosis factor alpha and interleukin 1 beta are responsible for in vitro myocardial cell depression induced by human septic shock serum. *J Exp Med.* (1996) 183:949–58. doi: 10.1084/jem.183.3.949
39. Van Tassell BW, Seropian IM, Toldo S, Mezzaroma E, Abbate A. Interleukin-1β induces a reversible cardiomyopathy in the mouse. *Inflamm Res.* (2013) 62:637–40. doi: 10.1007/s00011-013-0625-0
40. Díez J. Chronic heart failure as a state of reduced effectiveness of the natriuretic peptide system: implications for therapy. *Eur J Heart Fail.* (2017) 19:167–76. doi: 10.1002/ejhf.656
41. Tamura N, Ogawa Y, Chusho H, Nakamura K, Nakao K, Suda M, et al. Cardiac fibrosis in mice lacking brain natriuretic peptide. *Proc Natl Acad Sci U.S.A.* (2000) 97:4239–44. doi: 10.1073/pnas.070371497
42. Gong X, Mou Z, Shao L, Zou Y, Gu Y, Sun S. Human recombinant-B-type natriuretic peptide protect ventricular function and structure in ST-elevation myocardial infarction. *Int J Clin Exp Pathol.* (2015) 8:11622–8.
43. Sabatine MS, Morrow DA, de Lemos JA, Gibson CM, Murphy SA, Rifai N, et al. Multimarker approach to risk stratification in non-ST elevation acute coronary syndromes. *Circulation* (2002) 105:1760–3. doi: 10.1161/01.CIR.0000015464.18023.0A
44. Van Tassell BW, Canada J, Carbone S, Trankle C, Buckley L, Oddi Erdle C, et al. Interleukin-1 blockade in recently decompensated systolic heart failure: Results from REDHART (Recently Decompensated Heart Failure Anakinra Response Trial). *Circ Hear Fail.* (2017) 10:e004373.doi: 10.1161/CIRCHEARTFAILURE.117.004373
45. Van Tassell BW, Arena R, Biondi-Zoccai G, Canada JM, Oddi C, Abouzaki NA, et al. Effects of interleukin-1 blockade with anakinra on aerobic exercise capacity in patients with heart failure and preserved ejection fraction (from the D-HART Pilot Study). *Am J Cardiol.* (2014) 113:321–7. doi: 10.1016/j.amjcard.2013.08.047
46. Trankle C, Canada J, Carbone S, Buckley LF, Del Buono MG, Christopher S, et al. Interleukin-1 blockade reduces Nt-probnp serum levels in patients with stable heart failure with preserved ejection fraction. *J Am Coll Cardiol.* (2018) 71:A869. doi: 10.1016/S0735-1097(18)31410-4
47. Ridker PM, Everett BM, Thuren T, MacFadyen JG, Chang WH, Ballantyne C, et al. Antiinflammatory therapy with canakinumab for atherosclerotic disease. *N Engl J Med.* (2017) 377:1119–31. doi: 10.1056/NEJMoa1707914
48. McMurray JJ, Packer M, Desai AS, Gong J, Lefkowitz MP, Rizkala AR, et al. Angiotensin–neprilysin inhibition versus enalapril in heart failure. *N Engl J Med.* (2014) 371:993–1004. doi: 10.1056/NEJMoa1409077

3

Cardiac Complications in Immune Checkpoint Inhibition Therapy

Kazuko Tajiri and Masaki Ieda*

Department of Cardiology, Faculty of Medicine, University of Tsukuba, Tsukuba, Japan

***Correspondence:**
Kazuko Tajiri
ktajiri@md.tsukuba.ac.jp

Immune checkpoint inhibitors (ICIs) have changed the treatment landscape of advanced cancers. Unfortunately, these agents can induce a wide spectrum of immune-related adverse events (irAEs) through activation of immune responses in non-target organs, including the heart. As the clinical use of ICI therapy increases rapidly, management of irAEs is becoming extremely important. The most commonly presented cardiac irAE is myocarditis. Histopathologically, T-cell (with a predominance of $CD8^+$ cells) and macrophage infiltration in the myocardium is typically observed in ICI-associated myocarditis. Other presentations of cardiac irAEs include congestive heart failure, Takotsubo cardiomyopathy, pericardial disease, arrhythmias, and conduction disease. Although cardiac irAEs are relatively rare, they can be life-threatening. Hence, cardiologists and oncologists should be vigilant for these presentations.

Keywords: immune checkpoint inhibitors, myocarditis, cardiotoxicity, programmed cell death protein 1, cytotoxic T-lymphocyte antigen 4, immune-related adverse events, immune checkpoint, autoimmunity

INTRODUCTION

Immune checkpoint inhibitors (ICIs), including monoclonal antibodies (mAbs) against cytotoxic T-lymphocyte-associated antigen 4 (CTLA-4), programmed cell death protein 1 (PD-1), and programmed cell death ligand 1 (PD-L1), are being routinely used in clinical settings and have shown unprecedented efficacy in treating multiple cancers (1–6). Unfortunately, these agents can induce a wide spectrum of immune-related adverse events (irAEs) (7–9) through activation of immune responses in non-target organs, including the heart. In recent years, several cases of cardiotoxicity have been reported in cancer patients treated with ICIs (10–17). Although its frequency is lower than that for other irAEs, cardiotoxicity can become life-threatening, making it an important consideration for cardiologists, oncologists, and immunologists.

In this review, we describe the mechanisms and summarize the reported clinical scenarios of cardiotoxicities associated with ICIs. Evidence available for diagnosis, management, and prognosis are considered.

PHYSIOLOGICAL ROLES OF IMMUNE CHECKPOINTS

T lymphocytes play a pivotal role as modulators and effectors of the immune system. Naïve T cells are activated after recognizing a cognate peptide presented by antigen-presenting cells (APCs) via interaction between the major histocompatibility complex (MHC) on the APCs and the T cell receptor (TCR), but further co-stimulatory signals are required for activation. CD28 is a stimulatory co-receptor expressed on T cells. Binding of CD80 (also known as B7-1) or CD86 (also known as B7-2) molecules on APCs with CD28 molecules provides an essential signal for T cell activation. However, to prevent destructive immune activation, these signals are finely regulated by immune checkpoints (e.g., CTLA-4 and PD-1) (18).

CTLA-4

CTLA-4 is an inhibitory co-receptor expressed on activated T cells. CTLA-4 inhibits T cell functions by competing with CD28 for binding with B7 ligands, CD80, and CD86. CTLA-4 is homologous to CD28 but has much higher binding affinity and avidity for B7 ligands. In resting naïve T cells, unlike CD28, which is constitutively expressed on the cell surface, CTLA-4 is localized primarily in intracellular vesicles (19). CTLA-4 is upregulated on the cell surface in response to TCR activation and the signal is enhanced by co-stimulation through CD28 and/or interleukin-2 (20). Of note, the stronger the TCR signal, the greater the CTLA-4 translocation to the cell surface, thereby preventing harmful T cell activation (19–21).

PD-1:PD-L1/2 Pathway

PD-1 is another inhibitory receptor and plays a pivotal role in regulating the effector phase of T cell responses through binding with its ligands PD-L1 and programmed death ligand 2 (PD-L2) (21). PD-L1 is expressed constitutively on hematopoietic cells and a wide range of non-hematopoietic cells, including hepatocytes, astrocytes, epithelial cells, muscle cells including cardiomyocytes, vascular endothelial cells, and pancreatic cells (22, 23). PD-L1 is also expressed on numerous tumors, and its expression is reported to be associated with poor prognosis in several cancers (24–26). In contrast to PD-L1, PD-L2 is expressed primarily on APCs and certain B cell lymphomas (20, 21). Similar to CTLA-4 signaling, PD-1 signaling abrogates T cell proliferation and cytokine production and reduces T cell survival (23). PD-1 exhibits minimal expression on resting immune cells. However, upon activation, PD-1 expression is induced on the surface of T cells, B cells, natural killer cells, natural killer T cells, dendritic cells, and macrophages (23).

IMPLICATIONS OF BLOCKING THE CTLA-4 AND PD-1 PATHWAYS IN CANCER

To date, six ICIs have been approved by the United States Food and Drug Administration: ipilimumab (anti-CTLA-4 mAb); nivolumab and pembrolizumab (anti-PD-1 mAbs); and atezolizumab, avelumab, and durvalumab (anti-PD-L1 mAbs) (**Table 1**). Antibody therapies against the CTLA-4 and PD-1/PD-L1 axes have revolutionized the treatment of cancer (**Figure 1**).

Cancer is characterized by genetic mutations that can lead to the expression of various tumor-associated antigens. APCs present these antigens via MHC molecules expressed on their surface, which interact with TCRs. Thus, T cells can recognize tumor-associated antigens as "non-self" and attack tumor cells expressing these antigens (27). However, CTLA-4 inhibits T cell activation and clonal expansion. In the tumor immunotherapy setting, CTLA-4-targeting mAbs support the activation and proliferation of effector T cells, resulting in broad activation of immune responses against tumor cells (28). In contrast, CTLA-4 blockade inhibits regulatory T cell-mediated immunosuppression (28). These are thought to be the main mechanisms of action of CTLA-4 blockade.

PD-1 is expressed on tumor-infiltrating lymphocytes in many cancers. Chronic or high exposure to tumor antigens can induce persistent PD-1 expression, which leads to a state of exhaustion or anergy (lack of response). PD-1 blockade may reverse anergy of tumor-specific T cells. PD-1 is upregulated on the cell surface of many different tumor types. Tumor PD-L1 expression indicates an active tumor immune microenvironment and is strongly associated with efficacious responses to PD-1- and PD-L1-targeting mAbs (29). It is commonly accepted that PD-L1 expression on tumors and immune cells can inhibit the T-cell antitumor response and facilitate cancer development. However, the role of PD-L2 in antitumor immunity remains controversial (30, 31).

irAEs

Due to the central role played by immune checkpoints in the maintenance of self-tolerance, immune checkpoint blockade can induce a spectrum of adverse events, called irAEs (32). Remarkably, irAEs can affect almost any organ system (**Figure 2**) and have been reported at a substantially high frequency. irAEs occur in up to 90% of patients (10–15% grade 3/4) treated with ipilimumab (1) and 79% of patients (13% grade 3/4) treated with pembrolizumab (3). In a meta-analysis, the incidence was reported to be 75% in patients treated with CTLA-4-targeting mAbs and 30% for PD-1- and/or PD-L1-blocking mAbs (33). The frequency of grade 3/4 irAEs was substantially higher in patients treated with a combination of ipilimumab and nivolumab (54%) than in those receiving ipilimumab monotherapy (20%) (34).

irAEs are generally managed with corticosteroids, and less commonly, with other immunomodulatory agents (35). There are no prospective studies that have investigated management strategies for irAEs. According to the various organs involved, grade 1–2 events mainly affect the gut and skin, whereas grade 3–4 events are mainly restricted to the digestive tract. Cardiac, neurologic, renal, ocular, and hematologic irAEs are uncommon (35).

CARDIOTOXICITY ASSOCIATED WITH IMMUNE CHECKPOINT INHIBITION

Insights From Animal Studies

During the establishment of central tolerance in the thymus, most autoreactive T cells are deleted; however, some autoreactive T cells are released into the periphery (36, 37). In healthy individuals, peripheral tolerance mechanisms regulate the numbers of these cells. CTLA-4 competes with CD28 to downregulate T cell activation, resulting in immunotolerance and prevention of pathologic immune responses to cardiac antigens

Abbreviations: α-MHC, myosin heavy chain α isoform; APC, antigen-presenting cells; CTLA-4, cytotoxic T-lymphocyte-associated antigen 4; ICI, immune checkpoint inhibitor; irAE, immune-related adverse event; mAb, monoclonal antibody; PD-1, programmed cell death protein 1; PD-L1, programmed cell death ligand 1; TCR, T cell receptor.

TABLE 1 | FDA-approved ICIs for cancer therapy.

Target	Drug	Indication
CTLA-4	Ipilimumab	Melanoma
PD-1	Nivolumab	Melanoma, NSCLC, SCLC, RCC, HCC, Hodgkin lymphoma, head and neck cancer, urothelial carcinoma, microsatellite instability-high, or mismatch repair-deficient metastatic colorectal cancer
PD-1	Pembrolizumab	Melanoma, NSCLC, head and neck squamous cell carcinoma, Hodgkin lymphoma, urothelial carcinoma, microsatellite instability-high cancer, gastric cancer, cervical cancer, primary mediastinal large B-cell lymphoma
PD-L1	Atezolizumab	NSCLC, urothelial carcinoma
PD-L1	Durvalumab	NSCLC, urothelial carcinoma
PD-L1	Avelumab	Urothelial carcinoma, Merkel cell carcinoma
CTLA-4 and PD-1 in combination	Ipilimumab and nivolumab	Melanoma, RCC, microsatellite instability-high, or mismatch repair-deficient metastatic colorectal cancer

CTLA-4, cytotoxic T lymphocyte-associated antigen 4; FDA, Food and Drug Administration; HCC, hepatocellular carcinoma; ICI, immune checkpoint inhibitor; NSCLC, non-small cell lung cancer; PD-1, programmed cell death protein 1; PD-L1, programmed cell death ligand 1; RCC, renal cell carcinoma; SCLC, small cell lung cancer.

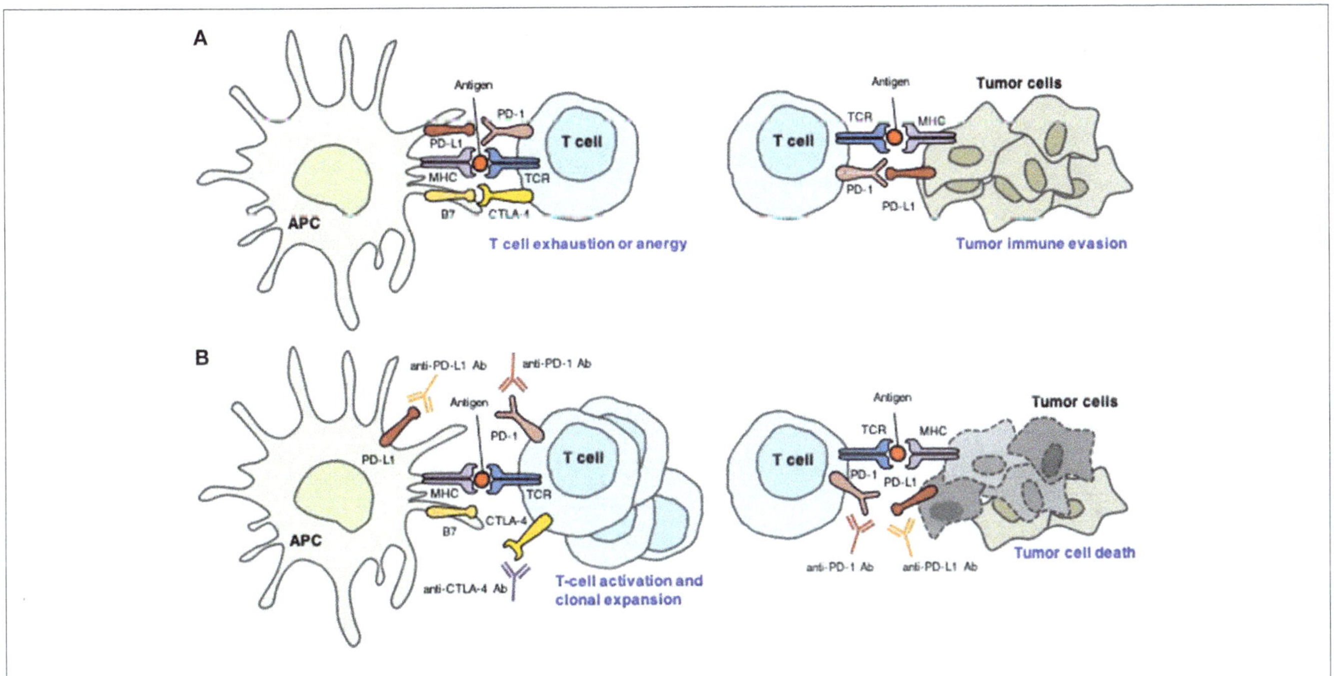

FIGURE 1 | Distinct roles of CTLA-4 and PD-1/PD-L1 in the regulation of antitumor immune responses. **(A)** Interactions between CTLA-4/B7 and PD-1/PD-L1 inhibit T cell-mediated tumor cell killing. **(B)** Blockade of CTLA-4, PD-1, and PD-L1 results in T cell activation and proliferation, which reactivates T cell-mediated tumor cell killing.

(38). Interactions between PD-1 and its ligands also maintain cardiac-reactive T cells in an anergic state (38) (**Figure 3**).

Mice deficient in CTLA-4 develop severe myocarditis with massive T cell infiltration (39). The cardiac presentation of PD-1-deficient mice is dependent on their background; mice on the BALB/c background develop autoimmune dilated cardiomyopathy (40), but PD-1-deficient autoimmune-prone MRL mice show lymphocytic myocarditis with massive infiltration of $CD4^+$ and $CD8^+$ T cells (41). PD-L1 is significantly upregulated on the surface of cardiac endothelial cells during myocarditis. PD-L1 deficiency in MRL mice induces similar severe myocarditis (42).

Cardiac irAEs of ICIs in Patients With Cancer

Incidence

There are contrasting reports on the rates of cardiac irAEs associated with ICI therapies. For example, no incidence of myocarditis was identified after a pooled analysis of 448 patients treated with nivolumab and ipilimumab combination therapy (43). In contrast, a pharmacovigilance study identified myocarditis in 18 of 20,594 patients (0.09%) treated with nivolumab alone or in combination with ipilimumab (13), and a cohort study of 964 patients from a multicenter registry reported a prevalence of 1.14%, which increased to as high as

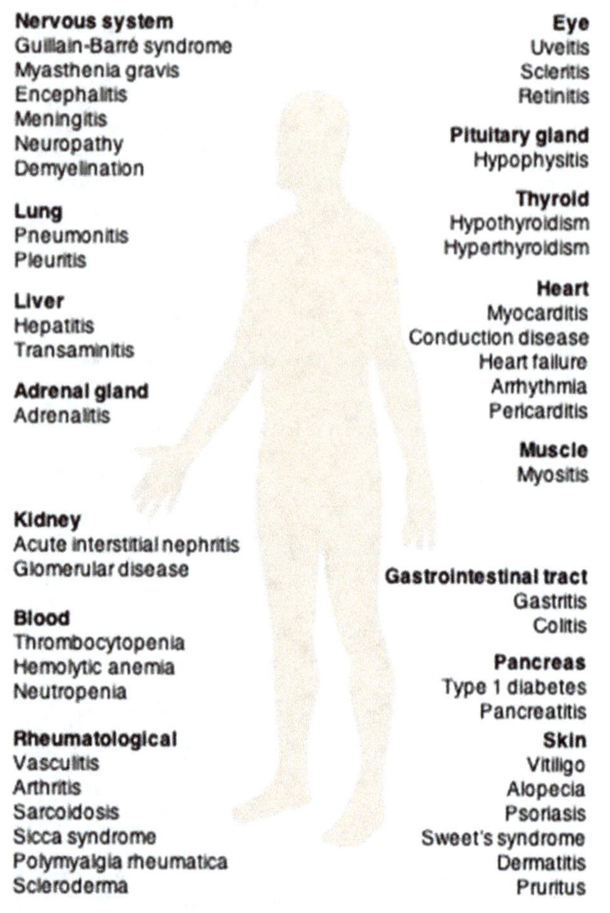

FIGURE 2 | The clinical spectrum of irAEs associated with immune checkpoint inhibitors. irAEs, immune-related adverse events.

2.4% for combination therapy with anti-PD-1/anti-CTLA-4 (44). According to the latter report, ICI-associated myocarditis can no longer be considered a "rare" adverse effect. So far, ICI-associated myocarditis appears to be a class effect, and the incidence seems to be higher when patients are treated with a combination of ICIs (13, 44).

Clinical Presentation and Management

The most common cardiac irAE is myocarditis (45). Histopathologically, T cell (with a predominance of $CD8^+$ cells) and macrophage infiltration in the myocardium are typically observed in ICI-related myocarditis (10, 12–15, 46). This myocarditis sometimes involves the cardiac conduction system, leading to conduction block. Other presentations of cardiac irAEs include congestive heart failure, Takotsubo cardiomyopathy, pericardial disease, arrhythmias, and conduction disease (47).

The time to onset of myocarditis is variable. An analysis of VigiBase, the World Health Organization's database of individual case safety reports that includes 101 cases of severe myocarditis, revealed that myocarditis was diagnosed at a median of 27 days (range, 5–155 days) after the initiation of ICI therapy, with 76% of the cases occurring in the first 6 weeks of treatment (48). A medical record review of 30 ICI-related cardiotoxicity patients from two cardio-oncology units revealed that the median onset of cardiotoxicity was 65 days (range, 2–454 days) and it occurred after a median of three (range, 1–33) infusions (49). In a multicenter cohort including 35 myocarditis patients, the median time to onset was 34 days and 81% of the patients developed cardiac irAE within 3 months (44). Notably, fatal myocarditis can develop after only a single treatment with an ICI (11, 13). Unfortunately, there is insufficient information regarding the time of onset of cardiac irAEs relating to specific treatment regimes. In general, most irAEs were reported to occur within 3–6 months of the initiation of anti-CTLA-4- or anti-PD-1-targeting therapy (47, 50). While the risk of severe irAEs appears to be dose-dependent with anti-CTLA-4 antibodies, toxicities with anti-PD-1/anti-PD-L1 antibodies are reported to be dose-independent (47, 50).

Cardiac signs and symptoms of ICI-related cardiotoxicity vary from asymptomatic to sudden death (10–17, 51) and lack specificity. Sometimes cardiac irAE is accompanied by other organ irAEs, especially those in skeletal muscles (11, 13).

Currently, patients who are likely to develop cardiac irAEs cannot be identified before ICI therapy. Therefore, early detection of ICI-related myocarditis is thought to be important for improved management. Mahmood et al. (44) showed that measuring troponin levels at baseline and at each cycle of ICI treatment may be useful for surveillance because this parameter was abnormal in 94% of ICI-myocarditis patients at clinical presentation. In contrast, Sarocchi et al. (52) measured troponin levels at each nivolumab administration in 59 patients and found an elevation in only six patients, none of whom developed overt cardiac irAEs. These researchers mentioned possible reasons for a "false positive" elevation of troponin, including it being a consequence of myocardial oxygen demand-supply mismatch due to aggravation of the clinical status or the presence of subclinical ICI-induced myocarditis. An elevation of troponin indicates the presence of, but not the underlying reason for, myocardial injury. Therefore, myocarditis or other myocardial damage should be considered in cases presenting with elevated troponin, and these patients should be referred immediately to cardiologists/onco-cardiologists for further evaluation (44). Mahmood et al. (44) also reported abnormal electrocardiograms in 89% of ICI-related myocarditis patients. In contrast, NT-ProBNP was abnormal in 66%, and the left ventricular ejection fraction (LVEF) was abnormal in only 49% of these patients. Thus, NT-proBNP or LVEF may be less useful for early diagnosis of cardiac irAEs than troponin or ECG. Information on the utility of hsCRP as an early biomarker of cardiac irAEs is lacking.

Pharmacovigilance data show that the mortality of ICI-associated myocarditis exceeded 60% in patients receiving ipilimumab-nivolumab combination therapy (13). Mahmood et al. (44) reported that nearly half of all myocarditis cases developed a major adverse cardiac event (a combination of cardiovascular death, cardiac arrest, cardiogenic shock, and hemodynamically significant complete heart block). Escudier et al. (49) reported after a medical record review of 30 ICI-related cardiotoxicity patients that eight (27%) died of cardiovascular

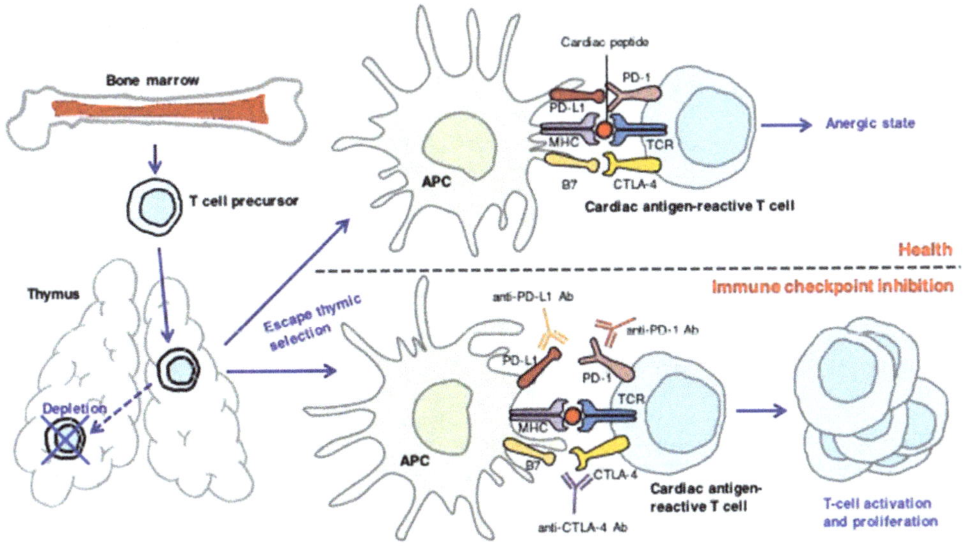

FIGURE 3 | The role of immune checkpoints in establishing peripheral tolerance to the heart. During the establishment of central tolerance in the thymus, most autoreactive T cells are deleted, however, some autoreactive T cells are released into the periphery. In health, peripheral tolerance mechanisms keep these cells in check. CTLA-4 competes with CD28 to downregulate T-cell activation, resulting in immunotolerance and prevention of pathologic immune responses to cardiac-antigens. PD-1-PD-1 ligand interactions also maintain the cardiac-reactive T cells in an anergic state. Antibodies against CTLA-4, PD-1, or PD-L1 may activate cardiac antigen-reactive T cells that escape central tolerance. These T cells can clonally expand and attack the heart.

complications. They also reported that cardiovascular mortality was significantly associated with conduction abnormalities and ipilimumab-nivolumab combination therapy (49).

Currently, there are no guidelines for the treatment of cardiac irAEs. Steroids have been used to treat cardiac irAEs in most cases (11, 13–16, 44, 45). For steroid non-responders, other immunosuppressive agents, high-dose intravenous immunoglobulin therapy, plasmapheresis, and immunoadsorption therapy have been used (45, 53).

CONCLUSIONS

ICI therapies have changed the treatment landscape of advanced cancer. As the clinical use of ICI therapy rapidly increases, management of irAEs is extremely important. Cardiac irAEs are relatively rare but can be life-threatening. Large scale, prospective, and longitudinal cohort studies are needed to clarify predisposing risk factors and long-term consequences of ICI-induced cardiac irAEs. In addition to clinical studies, basic studies are crucially needed to provide insights into underlying mechanisms and to find biomarkers to identify high risk patients and minimize the risk of ICI-associated cardiac irAEs.

AUTHOR CONTRIBUTIONS

KT has written the main manuscript text and prepared the figures. MI participated to the redaction of the manuscript and its extensive revision.

FUNDING

This study was supported in part by Grant-in-Aid for Scientific Research (Japan Society for the Promotion of Science KAKENHI Grant Number 17K09567) to KT and a grant from Japan Cardiovascular Research Foundation (The Bayer Scholarship for Cardiovascular Research) to KT.

ACKNOWLEDGMENTS

We would like to thank Editage (www.editage.jp) for English language editing.

REFERENCES

1. Hodi FS, O'Day SJ, McDermott DF, Weber RW, Sosman JA, Haanen JB, et al. Improved survival with ipilimumab in patients with metastatic melanoma. *N Engl J Med.* (2010) 363:711–23. doi: 10.1056/NEJMoa1003466
2. Robert C, Long GV, Brady B, Dutriaux C, Maio M, Mortier L, et al. Nivolumab in previously untreated melanoma without BRAF mutation. *N Engl J Med.* (2015) 372:320–30. doi: 10.1056/NEJMoa1412082
3. Hamid O, Robert C, Daud A, Hodi FS, Hwu WJ, Kefford R, et al. Safety and tumor responses with lambrolizumab (Anti–PD-1) in melanoma. *N Engl J Med.* (2013) 369:134–44. doi: 10.1056/NEJMoa1305133
4. Brahmer J, Reckamp KL, Baas P, Crinò L, Eberhardt WEE, Poddubskaya E, et al. Nivolumab versus docetaxel in advanced squamous-cell non–small-cell lung cancer. *N Engl J Med.* (2015) 373:123–35. doi: 10.1056/NEJMoa1504627

5. Borghaei H, Paz-Ares L, Horn L, Spigel DR, Steins M, Ready NE, et al. Nivolumab versus docetaxel in advanced nonsquamous non–small-cell lung cancer. *N Engl J Med.* (2015) 373:1627–39. doi: 10.1056/NEJMoa1507643
6. Motzer RJ, Escudier B, McDermott DF, George S, Hammers HJ, Srinivas S, et al. Nivolumab versus everolimus in advanced renal-cell carcinoma. *N Engl J Med.* (2015) 373:1803–13. doi: 10.1056/NEJMoa1510665
7. Chen TW, Razak AR, Bedard PL, Siu LL, Hansen AR. A systematic review of immune-related adverse event reporting in clinical trials of immune checkpoint inhibitors. *Ann Oncol Off J Eur Soc Med Oncol.* (2015) 26:1824–9. doi: 10.1093/annonc/mdv182
8. Boutros C, Tarhini A, Routier E, Lambotte O, Ladurie FL, Carbonnel F, et al. Safety profiles of anti-CTLA-4 and anti-PD-1 antibodies alone and in combination. *Nat Rev Clin Oncol.* (2016) 13:473–86. doi: 10.1038/nrclinonc.2016.58
9. Champiat S, Lambotte O, Barreau E, Belkhir R, Berdelou A, Carbonnel F, et al. Management of immune checkpoint blockade dysimmune toxicities: a collaborative position paper. *Ann Oncol.* (2016) 27:559–74. doi: 10.1093/annonc/mdv623
10. Koelzer VH, Rothschild SI, Zihler D, Wicki A, Willi B, Willi N, et al. Systemic inflammation in a melanoma patient treated with immune checkpoint inhibitors—an autopsy study. *J Immunother Cancer* (2016) 4:13. doi: 10.1186/s40425-016-0117-1
11. Kimura T, Fukushima S, Miyashita A, Aoi J, Jinnin M, Kosaka T, et al. Myasthenic crisis and polymyositis induced by one dose of nivolumab. *Cancer Sci.* (2016) 107:1055–8. doi: 10.1111/cas.12961
12. Läubli H, Balmelli C, Bossard M, Pfister O, Glatz K, Zippelius A, et al. Acute heart failure due to autoimmune myocarditis under pembrolizumab treatment for metastatic melanoma. *J Immunother Cancer* (2015) 3:11. doi: 10.1186/s40425-015-0057-1
13. Johnson DB, Balko JM, Compton ML, Chalkias S, Gorham J, Xu Y, et al. Fulminant myocarditis with combination immune checkpoint blockade. *N Engl J Med.* (2016) 375:1749–55. doi: 10.1056/NEJMoa1609214
14. Tadokoro T, Keshino E, Makiyama A, Sasaguri T, Ohshima K, Katano H, et al. Acute lymphocytic myocarditis with anti-PD-1 antibody nivolumab. *Circ Heart Fail.* (2016) 9:e003514. doi: 10.1161/CIRCHEARTFAILURE.116.003514
15. Heinzerling L, Ott PA, Hodi FS, Husain AN, Tajmir-Riahi A, Tawbi H, et al. Cardiotoxicity associated with CTLA4 and PD1 blocking immunotherapy. *J Immunother Cancer* (2016) 4:50. doi: 10.1186/s40425-016-0152-y
16. Semper H, Muehlberg F, Schulz-Menger J, Allewelt M, Grohé C. Drug-induced myocarditis after nivolumab treatment in a patient with PDL1-negative squamous cell carcinoma of the lung. *Lung Cancer* (2016) 99:117–9. doi: 10.1016/j.lungcan.2016.06.025
17. Gibson R, Delaune J, Szady A, Markham M. Suspected autoimmune myocarditis and cardiac conduction abnormalities with nivolumab therapy for non-small cell lung cancer. *BMJ Case Rep.* (2016) 2016:bcr2016216228. doi: 10.1136/bcr-2016-216228
18. Chen L, Flies DB. Molecular mechanisms of T cell co-stimulation and co-inhibition. *Nat Rev Immunol.* (2013) 13:227–42. doi: 10.1038/nri3405
19. Walker LSK, Sansom DM. Confusing signals: recent progress in CTLA-4 biology. *Trends Immunol.* (2015) 36:63–70. doi: 10.1016/j.it.2014.12.001
20. Intlekofer AM, Thompson CB. At the bench: preclinical rationale for CTLA-4 and PD-1 blockade as cancer immunotherapy. *J Leukoc Biol.* (2013) 94:25–39. doi: 10.1189/jlb.1212621
21. Buchbinder EI, Desai A. CTLA-4 and PD-1 pathways: similarities, differences, and implications of their inhibition. *Am J Clin Oncol.* (2016) 39:98–106. doi: 10.1097/COC.0000000000000239
22. Gianchecchi E, Delfino DV, Fierabracci A. Recent insights into the role of the PD-1/PD-L1 pathway in immunological tolerance and autoimmunity. *Autoimmun Rev.* (2013) 12:1091–100. doi: 10.1016/j.autrev.2013.05.003
23. Keir ME, Butte MJ, Freeman GJ, Sharpe AH. PD-1 and its ligands in tolerance and immunity. *Annu Rev Immunol.* (2008) 26:677–704. doi: 10.1146/annurev.immunol.26.021607.090331
24. Hino R, Kabashima K, Kato Y, Yagi H, Nakamura M, Honjo T, et al. Tumor cell expression of programmed cell death-1 ligand 1 is a prognostic factor for malignant melanoma. *Cancer* (2010) 116:1757–66. doi: 10.1002/cncr.24899
25. Thompson RH, Gillett MD, Cheville JC, Lohse CM, Dong H, Webster WS, et al. Costimulatory B7-H1 in renal cell carcinoma patients: Indicator of tumor aggressiveness and potential therapeutic target. *Proc Natl Acad Sci USA.* (2004) 101:17174–9. doi: 10.1073/pnas.0406351101
26. Mu CY, Huang JA, Chen Y, Chen C, Zhang XG. High expression of PD-L1 in lung cancer may contribute to poor prognosis and tumor cells immune escape through suppressing tumor infiltrating dendritic cells maturation. *Med Oncol.* (2011) 28:682–8. doi: 10.1007/s12032-010-9515-2
27. Chen DS, Mellman I. Oncology meets immunology: the cancer-immunity cycle. *Immunity* (2013) 39:1–10. doi: 10.1016/j.immuni.2013.07.012
28. Pardoll DM. The blockade of immune checkpoints in cancer immunotherapy. *Nat Rev Cancer* (2012) 12:252–64. doi: 10.1038/nrc3239
29. Pitt JM, Vétizou M, Daillère R, Roberti MP, Yamazaki T, Routy B, et al. Resistance mechanisms to immune-checkpoint blockade in cancer: tumor-intrinsic and -extrinsic factors. *Immunity* (2016) 44:1255–69. doi: 10.1016/j.immuni.2016.06.001
30. Umezu D, Okada N, Sakoda Y, Adachi K, Ojima T, Yamaue H, et al. Inhibitory functions of PD-L1 and PD-L2 in the regulation of anti-tumor immunity in murine tumor microenvironment. *Cancer Immunol Immunother.* (2018) doi: 10.1007/s00262-018-2263-4. [Epub ahead of print].
31. Wang H, Yao H, Li C, Liang L, Zhang Y, Shi H, et al. PD-L2 expression in colorectal cancer: Independent prognostic effect and targetability by deglycosylation. *Oncoimmunology* (2017) 6:e1327494. doi: 10.1080/2162402X.2017.1327494
32. Postow MA, Sidlow R, Hellmann MD. Immune-related adverse events associated with immune checkpoint blockade. *N Engl J Med.* (2018) 378:158–68. doi: 10.1056/NEJMra1703481
33. Bertrand A, Kostine M, Barnetche T, Truchetet ME, Schaeverbeke T. Immune related adverse events associated with anti-CTLA-4 antibodies: systematic review and meta-analysis. *BMC Med.* (2015) 13:211. doi: 10.1186/s12916-015-0455-8
34. Hodi FS, Chesney J, Pavlick AC, Robert C, Grossmann KF, McDermott DF, et al. Combined nivolumab and ipilimumab versus ipilimumab alone in patients with advanced melanoma: 2-year overall survival outcomes in a multicentre, randomised, controlled, phase 2 trial. *Lancet Oncol.* (2016) 17:1558–68. doi: 10.1016/S1470-2045(16)30366-7
35. Palmieri DJ, Carlino MS. Immune checkpoint inhibitor toxicity. *Curr Oncol Rep.* (2018) 20:72. doi: 10.1007/s11912-018-0718-6
36. Lv H, Lipes MA. Role of impaired central tolerance to α-myosin in inflammatory heart disease. *Trends Cardiovasc Med.* (2012) 22:113–7. doi: 10.1016/j.tcm.2012.07.005
37. Strasser A, Puthalakath H, O'Reilly LA, Bouillet P. What do we know about the mechanisms of elimination of autoreactive T and B cells and what challenges remain. *Immunol Cell Biol.* (2008) 86:57–66. doi: 10.1038/sj.icb.7100141
38. Mueller DL. Mechanisms maintaining peripheral tolerance. *Nat Immunol.* (2010) 11:21–7. doi: 10.1038/ni.1817
39. Waterhouse P, Penninger JM, Timms E, Wakeham A, Shahinian A, Lee KP, et al. Lymphoproliferative disorders with early lethality in mice deficient in Ctla-4. *Science* (1995) 270:985–8.
40. Nishimura H, Okazaki T, Tanaka Y, Nakatani K, Hara M, Matsumori A, et al. Autoimmune dilated cardiomyopathy in PD-1 receptor-deficient mice. *Science* (2001) 291:319–22. doi: 10.1126/science.291.5502.319
41. Wang J, Okazaki IM, Yoshida T, Chikuma S, Kato Y, Nakaki F, et al. PD-1 deficiency results in the development of fatal myocarditis in MRL mice. *Int Immunol.* (2010) 22:443–52. doi: 10.1093/intimm/dxq026
42. Lucas JA, Menke J, Rabacal WA, Schoen FJ, Sharpe AH, Kelley VR. Programmed death ligand 1 regulates a critical checkpoint for autoimmune myocarditis and pneumonitis in MRL mice. *J Immunol.* (2008) 181:2513–21. doi: 10.4049/jimmunol.181.4.2513
43. Sznol M, Ferrucci PF, Hogg D, Atkins MB, Wolter P, Guidoboni M, et al. Pooled analysis safety profile of nivolumab and ipilimumab combination therapy in patients with advanced melanoma. *J Clin Oncol.* (2017) 35:3815–22. doi: 10.1200/JCO.2016.72.1167
44. Mahmood SS, Fradley MG, Cohen JV, Nohria A, Reynolds KL, Heinzerling LM, et al. Myocarditis in patients treated with immune checkpoint inhibitors. *J Am Coll Cardiol.* (2018) 71:1755–64. doi: 10.1016/j.jacc.2018.02.037
45. Mir H, Alhussein M, Alrashidi S, Alzayer H, Alshatti A, Valettas N, et al. Cardiac complications associated with checkpoint inhibition: a systematic review of the literature in an important emerging area. *Can J Cardiol.* (2018) 34:1059–68. doi: 10.1016/j.cjca.2018.03.012

46. Tajiri K, Aonuma K, Sekine I. Immune checkpoint inhibitor-related myocarditis. *Jpn J Clin Oncol.* (2018) 48:7-12. doi: 10.1093/jjco/hyx154
47. Kumar V, Chaudhary N, Garg M, Floudas CS, Soni P, Chandra AB. Current diagnosis and management of immune related adverse events (irAEs) induced by immune checkpoint inhibitor therapy. *Front Pharmacol.* (2017) 8:49. doi: 10.3389/fphar.2017.00049
48. Moslehi JJ, Salem JE, Sosman JA, Lebrun-Vignes B, Johnson DB. Increased reporting of fatal immune checkpoint inhibitor-associated myocarditis. *Lancet* (2018) 391:933. doi: 10.1016/S0140-6736(18)30533-6
49. Escudier M, Cautela J, Malissen N, Ancedy Y, Orabona M, Pinto J, et al. Clinical features, management, and outcomes of immune checkpoint inhibitor-related cardiotoxicity. *Circulation* (2017) 136:2085-7. doi: 10.1161/CIRCULATIONAHA.117.030571
50. Michot JM, Bigenwald C, Champiat S, Collins M, Carbonnel F, Postel-Vinay S, et al. Immune-related adverse events with immune checkpoint blockade: a comprehensive review. *Eur J Cancer* (2016) 54:139-48. doi: 10.1016/j.ejca.2015.11.016
51. Thibault C, Vano Y, Soulat G, Mirabel M. Immune checkpoint inhibitors myocarditis: not all cases are clinically patent. *Eur Heart J.* (2018) 39:3553. doi: 10.1093/eurheartj/ehy485
52. Sarocchi M, Grossi F, Arboscello E, Bellodi A, Genova C, Dal Bello MG, et al. Serial troponin for early detection of nivolumab cardiotoxicity in advanced non-small cell lung cancer patients. *Oncologist* (2018) 23:936-42. doi: 10.1634/theoncologist.2017-0452
53. Caforio ALP, Pankuweit S, Arbustini E, Basso C, Gimeno-Blanes J, Felix SB, et al. Current state of knowledge on aetiology, diagnosis, management, and therapy of myocarditis: a position statement of the European Society of Cardiology Working Group on Myocardial and Pericardial Diseases. *Eur Heart J.* (2013) 34:2636-48. doi: 10.1093/eurheartj/eht210

4

First Report of the Italian Registry on Immune-Mediated Congenital Heart Block (Lu.Ne Registry)

Micaela Fredi [1], Laura Andreoli [1], Beatrice Bacco [2], Tiziana Bertero [2], Alessandra Bortoluzzi [3], Silvia Breda [4], Veronica Cappa [5], Fulvia Ceccarelli [6], Rolando Cimaz [7], Salvatore De Vita [8], Emma Di Poi [8], Elena Elefante [9], Franco Franceschini [1], Maria Gerosa [10], Marcello Govoni [3], Ariela Hoxha [11], Andrea Lojacono [12], Luca Marozio [13], Alessandro Mathieu [14], Pier Luigi Meroni [15], Antonina Minniti [6], Marta Mosca [9], Marina Muscarà [16], Melissa Padovan [3], Matteo Piga [14], Roberta Priori [6], Véronique Ramoni [17], Amelia Ruffatti [11], Chiara Tani [9], Marta Tonello [11], Laura Trespidi [18], Sonia Zatti [12], Stefano Calza [5], Angela Tincani [1] and Antonio Brucato [4,19]*

[1] Rheumatology and Clinical Immunology Unit, Department of Clinical and Experimental Science, ASST Spedali Civili, University of Brescia, Brescia, Italy, [2] S.S.d.D.U. Immunologia, Allergologia, A.O. Ordine Maurziano di Torino, Torino, Italy, [3] UO e Sezione di Reumatologia, Dipartimento di Scienze Mediche, Universita' degli Studi di Ferrara, Cona, Italy, [4] Struttura Complessa Medicina Interna, ASST Papa Giovanni XXIII, Bergamo, Italy, [5] Unit of Biostatistics, Biomathematics, and Bioinformatics, Department of Molecular and Translational Medicine, University of Brescia, Brescia, Italy, [6] UO Complessa Reumatologia, Policlinico Umberto I- University La Sapienza, Rome, Italy, [7] Anna Meyer Children's Hospital, University of Firenze, Firenze, Italy, [8] Clinica di Reumatologia, Azienda Sanitaria Universitaria Integrata di Udine, Udine, Italy, [9] UO Reumatologia, Dipartimento di Medicina Clinica e Sperimentale, Universita' di Pisa, Pisa, Italy, [10] Istituto Ortopedico Gaetano Pini, University of Milan, Milan, Italy, [11] Unità di Reumatologia, Dipartimento di Medicina, Università di Padova, Padova, Italy, [12] Department of Obstetrics and Gynecology, ASST Spedali Civili and University, Brescia, Italy, [13] Ginecologia e Ostetricia 1, Dipartimento di Scienze Chirurgiche, Università di Torino, Turin, Italy, [14] Cattedra e Struttura Complessa di Reumatologia, Universita' degli Studi e AOU di Cagliari, Cagliari, Italy, [15] Immunorheumatology Research Laboratory, Istituto Auxologico Italiano, Milan, Italy, [16] UO Reumatologia, ASST Ospedale Niguarda, Milan, Italy, [17] Rheumatology, IRCCS Policlinico San Matteo Foundation, University of Pavia, Padova, Italy, [18] Dipartimento per la Salute della Donna, Bambino e Neonato, Fondazione Ospedale Maggiore, Milan, Italy, [19] Dipartimento di Scienze Biomediche e Cliniche "Sacco", Università degli Studi di Milano, Milan, Italy

Correspondence:
Micaela Fredi
fredi.micaela@gmail.com

Objective: Neonatal Lupus (NL) is a rare syndrome caused by placental transfer of maternal anti-SSA/Ro and anti-La/SSB autoantibodies to the fetus. The rarity of this condition requires the establishment of multidisciplinary registries in order to improve our knowledge.

Method: Inclusion criteria in this retrospective study were the maternal confirmed positivity for anti-SSA/Ro and/or anti-SSB/La antibodies, and the presence of II or III degree congenital heart block (CHB) *in utero* or neonatal period (up to 27 days after birth).

Result: Eighty-nine cases of CHB were observed in 85 women with 88 pregnancies that occurred between 1969 and 2017. CHB was mostly detected *in utero* (84 cases, 94.2%), while five cases were observed in the neonatal period. A permanent pacemaker was implanted in 51 of 73 children born alive (69.8), whereas global mortality rate was 25.8% (23 cases): 16 *in utero*, five perinatal, and two during childhood. By univariate analysis, factors associated with fetal death were pleural effusion ($p = 0.005$, OR > 100; CI 95% 2.88->100 and hydrops ($p = 0.003$, $OR = 14.09$; CI 95% 2.01–122). Fluorinated steroids (FS) were administered in 71.4% pregnancies, and its use was not associated with better survival. Some centers treated all cases with fluorinated steroids and some centers did not treat any case. CHB was initially incomplete in 24 fetuses, and of them five cases of II degree block reverted to a lower degree block after treatments. Recurrence rate in subsequent pregnancies was 17.6% (3 out of 17). A prophylactic treatment was introduced in 10 of these 16 subsequent (58.8%) pregnancies, mostly with FS or high dose intravenous immunoglobulins.

Conclusion: This is the first report from the Italian Registry of neonatal lupus/CHB. The live birth rate was nearly 80%, with nearly two thirds of the children requiring the implantation of a pacemaker. The management of fetuses diagnosed with CHB was heterogeneous across Italian Centers. The registry at present is mainly rheumatological, but involvement of pediatric cardiologists and gynecologists is planned.

Keywords: pregnancy, congenital heart block, neonatal lupus, outcome, risk factors, therapy

INTRODUCTION

Neonatal lupus (NL) is a rare disorder mainly caused by the transplacental passage of maternal autoantibodies anti-SSA/Ro and/or anti-SSB/La (1, 2), usually during the second trimester of gestation (3, 4); these antibodies can reach the fetal heart, inducing inflammation (macrophage infiltration and giant cell formation), calcification, and fibrosis, which lead to aberrant signal conduction at the atrio-ventricular node. The most common manifestations are cutaneous or cardiac, while liver damage or cytopenia are less frequent. NL can occur in the offspring of mothers with a diagnosis of connective tissue disease (CTD), mostly Sjögren Syndrome (SS), or Systemic Lupus Erythematosus (SLE), but most cases are reported in asymptomatic women.

Cardiac involvement is usually irreversible and represents the most feared manifestation. It is characterized by advanced congenital heart block (CHB) (II or III degree) in an otherwise structurally normal heart.

Anti-SSA/Ro autoantibodies are found in ~85–90% of mothers of children with CHB (1), and prospective studies of pregnancies in anti-SSA/Ro positive patients estimated the risk of CHB to be 1–2% (5, 6). Recurrence rate in subsequent pregnancies is about 12–19% (1, 7, 8).

Several groups addressed the morbidity and mortality associated with CHB in different countries (9–13). Mortality ranges from 16 to 29%, whereas the rates of children receiving pacemaker vary from 50 to 79%, frequently within the first year of life. Studies are heterogeneous, also including cases not associated with maternal antibodies (9–14) (**Table 1**). The Italian Registry of Neonatal Lupus (Lu.Ne registry) was created to collect data also in Italy, supported by a grant from the Italian Society of Rheumatology. The aim was to determine the mortality and morbidity associated with CHB in an Italian cohort enrolling women with a confirmed positivity for anti-SSA/Ro and/or anti-SSB/La antibodies.

PATIENTS AND METHODS

Study Cohort

The Lu.Ne registry was created in 2016, partially funded by the Italian Society of Rheumatology, after approval of the Institutional Review Board of the Coordinating Center in Brescia. Inclusion criteria were the maternal confirmed positivity for anti-SSA/Ro and/or anti-SSB/La antibodies and the presence of II or III degree CHB *in utero* or within the neonatal period (0–27 days after birth) (15) documented by electrocardiography and/or fetal echocardiography. For this study cases enrolled in the registry up to May 2018 were included. Medical records of pregnant women attending 11 Italian referral centers (mainly Rheumatology or Internal Medicine Departments, whose ethical committees approved the study) from 1969 to 2017 were retrospectively evaluated. In cases of variability of CHB grade, the most severe degree of CHB ever reached was considered for statistical analysis. This study was performed according to the principles of the Declaration of Helsinki with written informed consent from all subjects and was approved by the Ethic Committee of the Coordinating Center (approval number 2,417) and the participating centers.

Data Collection and Definitions

Data were collected through an online electronic data sheet prepared in a Research Electronic Data Capture (REDCap) platform. Data obtained from medical files included: maternal age at birth, ethnicity, obstetrical history, the presence of a systemic connective tissue disease (CTD), an organ autoimmune disease or other known obstetrical risk factors.

The following data were collected about the fetus/child: the time of occurrence of CHB, the lowest prenatal ventricular and atrial heart rate, the presence of endocardial fibroelastosis (EFE), pericardial effusion, hydrops, dilated cardiomyopathy (DCM), valvulopathy or other anomalies (including ventricular and atrial-septal defects, intraauricular communication), treatment for CHB (dose and duration), maternal, and fetal outcomes. For

TABLE 1 | Outcome of infants with CHB in the present study and in five large international series of cases (9–13).

	Lopes et al. (9)	Eliasson et al. (10)	Izmirly et al. (11)	Levesque et al. (12)	Van der Berg et al. (13)	Present study
N. of fetuses	57 with normal cardiac anatomy	175	325	202 *in utero* +12 in the neonatal period	56	84 *in utero* +5 in the neonatal period
Total mortality	13 (23%)	27 (15%)	57 (17.5%)	49 (23%)	9 (16%)	23 (25.8%)
Mortality *in utero*	6 (10%)	16 (9%)	18 (6%)	27 (13%)	8 (14.2%) (five additional cases of termination of pregnancies for various reasons	16 (17.9%)
Perinatal mortality	7 (14%)	10 (6.2%)	39 (12.7%) considered as 1 year after birth	8 (4%)	1 (2.3)	5 (5.6%)
PM cumulative prevalence	29 (56.7%)	102 (64%)	70% (the cumulative probability)	148 (79%)	30 (70%)	51 (69.8%)
Late onset cardiomiopathy	3 (5.6%)	8 (5.8%)	Four cases of heart transplantation	35 (18%)	6 (14%)	2 (2.2%)
Treated with FS	6 (10%)	67 (38%)	152 (47.8%)	79 (39%)	14 (27%)	60 (71.4%%)
Effects of FS	None	None on mortality; possibly reversal on II CHB	Possibly reversal on II CHB	None	None	None on mortality; possibly reversal on II CHB
Reversal of II degree CHB after FS	None	In 3/7 fetuses treated vs. 0/8 untreated	In 4/13 fetuses treated vs. 1/8 untreated	In 1/13 treated vs. 1/11 untreated	In 2/14 treated vs. 1/42	Five cases, all treated; see footnote*
Variables associated with death	Atrial rate <120 bpm, ventricular rate <55 bpm, hydrops,	Detection <20 gw, ventricular rate <50 bpm, hydrops, impaired left ventricular function	Earlier gestational age, lower ventricular rate, hydrops, EFE	Hydrops, prematurity (<37 weeks gestation)	Not analyzed	Hydrops, pleural effusion
Survival rate at 10 years for a child born alive	NA	NA	86%	88%	NA	90%
Maternal anti-SSA/Ro antibodies	72%	80% of 162 pregnancies with documented antibody status	100%	99.5 %	89%	100%

1 case regressed from II degree to variable CHB (alternating between I and II degree), 2 from II to I degree and 2 regression from II degree to no CHB. Three out of the five fetuses were treated with a combined protocol composed by fluorinated steroids plus plasmapheresis plus IVIg, one received dexametasone plus plasmapheresis and one only dexametasone. NA, not available; CHB, congenital heart block; EFE, endocardial fybroelastosis; DCM, dilated cardiomyopathy; FS, fluorinated steroids; bpm, beats per minute.

children, we collected information on pacemaker implantation (PM), postnatal DCM, death, and other complications.

Fetal complications were defined according to common definitions (10–13). Atrioventricular block (AVB)-II° was defined as the intermittent mechanical dissociation of atrial and ventricular activation diagnosed by M-mode echocardiography and AVB-III° as the complete mechanical dissociation of atrial and ventricular activation diagnosed by M-mode (10, 13). AVB-I° was assessed only in the recent years, using pulsed Doppler echocardiography in the left ventricular outflow tract to record simultaneously mitral valve inflow and aortic outflow (mitral-aorta), from which the time delay from atrial systole to ventricular systole could be inferred. AVB-I° was diagnosed when this fetal mechanical Doppler PR interval was found to be >150 ms (16).

DCM was defined as increased size of the left ventricle or multiple chambers in the absence of chamber wall hypertrophy with associated decreased contractility on echocardiogram (11, 12); endocardial fibroelastosis as the presence of abnormal areas of echogenicity on the endocardial surface of the cardiac chambers and/or valve leaflets on echocardiogram or endocardial fibrosis on biopsy or autopsy. Hydrops fetalis was defined as an abnormal accumulation of fluid in at least two fetal compartments (11, 12).

In each center, autoantibodies tests were performed in a referral laboratory certified for diagnosis.

Statistical Evaluation

Categorical variables were reported as proportion and/or percentage, while continuous variables as mean (±SD) values. Fisher's exact test or Chi-square test for categorical variables and Student's t-test or Wilcoxon-Mann-Whitney test for continuous variables were applied as appropriate. Multivariate analysis was not performed due to limited number of cases collected. $P <$

0.05 were considered significant and Odds Ratio (OR) with 95% Confidence Interval (95% CI) was indicated.

RESULTS

Patients

By May 2018, the registry included 89 cases of CHB from 85 patients who had 88 pregnancies. The 85 women were Caucasian (n = 79, 92.9%), African (n = 3, 3.5%), Asian (n = 2, 2.3%), and Afro-Caribbean (n = 1, 1.2%) (**Table 2**). An organ-specific autoimmune disease was diagnosed in 12 women: autoimmune thyroiditis (n = 8, 9.4%), celiac disease (n = 3, 3.5%), multiple sclerosis (n = 1, 1.2%).

Sixty patients reported previous pregnancies, without previous documented cases of CHB, except for one case of cutaneous NL. When their first child with CHB was diagnosed, 46 mothers (54.1%) fulfilled the classification criteria for CTDs: undifferentiated connective-tissue disease (UCTD) (n = 24, 28.2%), SS (n = 18, 21.2%), SLE (n = 4, 4.7%), whereas the others were considered as anti-SSA/Ro carriers. Few cases of acquired cardiovascular risk factors were collected: two patients were smokers, one suffered from hypertension and obesity, and one had diabetes mellitus.

Four cases of multiple pregnancies were collected: three were spontaneous dichorionic biamniotic twins, with one affected, and one unaffected fetus for each pair. The other multiple pregnancy was a triplet gestation after *in vitro* fertilization: two out the three fetuses were affected by CHB (one III and one II degree) and one unaffected. The triplet pregnancy has already been described (17).

TABLE 2 | Demographic information.

Maternal demography	N = 85 (%)
ETHNICITY	
Caucasian	79 (92.9)
African	3 (3.5)
Asian	2 (2.3)
Afro-Caribbean	1(1.2)
MATERNAL DIAGNOSIS AT CHB DETECTION	
Undifferentiated Connective Tissue Disease	24 (28.2)
Sjögren's Syndrome	18 (21.2)
Systemic Lupus Erythematosus	4 (4.7)
Carriers of anti-SSA/Ro	24 (28.2)
Carriers of anti-SSA/Ro + anti-SSB/La	15 (17.6)
ASSOCIATED ORGAN-SPECIFIC AUTOIMMUNE DISEASE	
Autoimmune thyroiditis	8 (9.4)
Celiac disease	3 (3.5)
Multiple sclerosis	1(1.2)
None/Unknown	73 (85.6)
AUTOANTIBODIES PROFILE	
Anti-SSA/Ro	85 (100)
Anti-SSB/La	50 (58.8)

CHB, congenital heart block.

Including the triplet pregnancy, three gestations that occurred after assisted reproductive technology procedures were collected.

All mothers were anti-SSA/Ro positive by inclusion criteria, and SSB/La antibodies were present in 58.8%. AntiRo52 status was available in 58.8% of the mothers, and all were positive.

The mean age at conception was 31.5 years (SD 5.3, range 22–42), 84 cases (94.4%) were diagnosed *in utero* at a median term of 21 gestational weeks (gw) (SD 4, range 17–38) and five (5.6%) were diagnosed in the neonatal period (15). CHB was initially incomplete in 24 fetuses (five with alternating II-III degree, two with alternating I-II degree, and 17 II degree). Considering the highest degree of CHB shown by the fetus/child, 71 (66 *in utero* and 5 neonatal) (79.8%) third-degree (complete) CHB, 18 (20.2%) second-degree CHB were included (**Table 2**).

Fetal/Neonatal Outcomes

Among the 89 cases, 73 (82%) children were born alive at a mean gestational week (gw) of 35.3 (SD 3.0, range 28–41), 7 elective terminations of pregnancy (TOP) were performed at a mean term of 22 gw, and nine intra-uterine fetal deaths occurred at a mean term of 26 gw (**Table 3**). All the cases of TOP were CHB grade III. **Table 4** reports the univariate statistical comparison of clinical and demographic features among survivors at birth and the deceased. By univariate analysis, factors associated with fetal death were pleural effusion (p = 0.005, OR > 100; CI 95% 2.88->100) and hydrops (p = 0.003, OR = 14.09; CI 95% 2.01–122).

The five cases diagnosed in the perinatal period or within the neonatal period (0–27 days after birth) occurred in the 1970–1980s: all these five newborns had III degree CHB; four of them received a pacemaker at a mean age of 7.2 years (range 2–18).

Treatment

Prior to CHB identification, only a limited number of patients were receiving treatments (**Table 5**), in all cases for maternal disease: nine were treated with low dose aspirin (LDA), eight with not-fluorinated steroids, seven with hydroxychloroquine (HCQ), and one with immunosuppressive therapy (**Table 5**).

TABLE 3 | Outcomes of 89 cases of CHB.

Pregnancy outcome	N = 89 (%)
Live birth	73 (82)
Intrauterine fetal death	9 (10.1)
Termination of pregnancy	7 (7.8)
CHB DETECTION	
In utero	84 (94.2)
CHB GRADE	
II degree	18 (20.2)
III degree	71 (79.8)
OVERALL MORTALITY	**23 (25.8)**
In utero	16 (18)
Neonatal	5 (5.6)
Childhood	2 (2.2)

TABLE 4 | Comparison of clinical and demographic features among children born alive and fetuses died *in utero*.

	Live birth $n = 68$ (%)	Deceased $n = 16$ (%)	*p*-value
***IN UTERO* DETECTED PATIENTS (84 CASES)**			
Maternal diagnosis of CTD	37 (54.4)	7 (43.7)	0.44
Non-Caucasian ethnicity	4 (5.4)	2 (12.5)	0.31
Maternal age at conception (SD)	31 (6.03)	32 (4.16)	0.76
Type of conception			
Spontaneous	64 (94.1)	16 (100.0)	0.73
Assisted reproduction techniques	4 (5.9)	0	
Timing of pregnancy			
Planned	21 (30.9)	6 (37.5)	0.767
Unplanned/unknown	47 (69.1)	10 (62.5)	
Gestational age at detection (gw) (SD)	22.8 (4.7)	20.7 (1.0)	0.27
Ventricular rate at nadir ≤50 bpm ($n = 73$)	21 (36.2)	6 (40)	0.78
Mean ventricular rate at nadir bpm (SD) ($n = 73$),	44.7 (27.9)	43.5 (30.8)	0.41
CHB grade ($n = 84$)			
II degree	16 (23.5)	2 (12.5)	0.3
III degree	52 (76.5)	14 (87.5)	
Impaired left ventricular function ($n = 71$)	5 (8.9)	3 (18.7)	0.35
Dilated cardiomyopathy ($n = 74$)	10 (12.6)	3 (27.3)	0.39
Hydrops ($n = 82$)	2 (3.0)	5 (31.2)	0.003*
Pleural effusion ($n = 81$)	0	3 (18.7)	0.005**
Pericardial effusion ($n = 81$)	8 (12.3)	5 (31.2)	0.12
Endocardial fibroelastosis ($n = 81$)	1 (1.5)	2 (13.3)	0.09
Intrauterine growth restriction ($n = 75$)	12 (19.3)	3 (23.1)	0.71
Oligohydramnios ($n = 84$)	5 (7.8%)	0	0.58

*CTD, connective tissue disease; gw, gestational week; bpm, beats per minute; *OR, 14.09; CI 95% 2.01–122, **OR > 100; CI 95% 2.88->100.*

TABLE 5 | Therapy before and after CHB detection.

	Live birth $n = 73$ (%)	Deceased $n = 16$ (%)	*p*-value
THERAPY BEFORE CHB DETECTION			
LDA	6 (8.2)	3 (16.6)	0.36
Non-fluorinated steroids	6 (8.2)	2 (12.5)	0.67
Hydroxychloroquine	7 (9.6)	0	0.33
DMARDs	0 (0)	1 (6.2)	0.19
MATERNAL THERAPY AFTER FETAL CHB DETECTION ($n = 84$)			
	Live birth $n = 68$ (%)	**Deceased $n = 16$ (%)**	***p*-value**
Any treatment	50 (73.5)	10 (62.5)	0.46
Fluorinated steroids	50 (73.5)	10 (62.5)	0.46
Intravenous Immunoglobulin	18 (26.4)	2 (12.5)	0.41
Plasma exchange	16 (23.5)	1 (6.2)	0.28
Other (beta-mimetics)	6 (8.9)	1 (6.2)	0.81
CHB VARIATION DURING/AFTER THERAPY ($n = 60$)			
	Live birth treated $n = 50$ (%)	**Deceased treated $n = 10$ (%)**	***p*-value**
Regression	5 (10)	0	0.74
Progression	3 (6)	1 (10)	
Unchanged	38 (76)	8 (80)	
Unknown	4 (8)	1 (10)	

LDA, low dose aspirin; DMARDS, immunosuppressive therapy.

After CHB detection, fluorinated steroids (FS) were administered in 60 (71.4%) pregnancies, with a mean total duration of treatment of 9.5 weeks (range 4–18 weeks). Twenty steroid-treated fetuses (33%) received intravenous immunoglobulin (IVIg) and 17 (28.3%) received cycles with plasma exchange as well. Sixteen newborns received IVIg at birth.

Effects of treatments in the 60 treated pregnancies were analyzed and in the majority of the cases no variation in the progression of CHB was observed (46 cases, 76.7%) (**Table 5**).

CHB was initially incomplete in 24 fetuses, all of them were treated at least with FS; five cases of regression from grade II CHB was observed. In detail: one change occurred from II degree to variable CHB (alternating between I and II degree), two from II to I degree and two regression from II degree to no CHB. Three out of the five fetuses were treated with a combined protocol composed by fluorinated steroids plus plasmapheresis plus IVIg, 1 received dexamethasone plus plasmapheresis, and one only dexamethasone.

Fourteen cases of newborns small for gestational age, five cases of intrauterine growth retardation, four cases of olygohydramnios, one case of maternal hypertension were recorded in the 60 mothers treated with FS; these complications may be related to the treatment with FS, particularly olygohydramnios and hypertension.

Postnatal Outcomes

Among the 73 live births, five newborns died within 10 days after birth (**Table 6**). These five children were born prematurely and in four cases death occurred even if a pacemaker was placed at birth.

Out of the remaining 68 children, two died later, one due to late onset DCM at the age of 21 months after a PM placed at birth, and 1 at the age of 6 years for a sudden death, probably due to a thrombotic event, however autopsy was not performed. Another child underwent cardiac transplantation at the age of 17 months for late onset DCM in 2003, and at present he is doing well.

Overall DCM was recorded in six cases at birth, while two cases of late onset DCM were observed (2.2%) (see **Table 1**). All the children with DCM were permanently paced, and two of them died (25%).

Overall a PM was placed in 51 of the 73 children born alive (69.8%): 19 (37.2%) at birth, 10 (19.6%) within the first month of life, 11 (21.5%) within the first year of life, and 11 later (21.5%).

TABLE 6 | Pregnancy outcome and postnatal follow-up in pregnancies ended with a live birth.

Pregnancy outcome	Live birth $n = 73$ (%)
Medium gestational week of delivery (SD) ($n = 70$)	35.3 (3.0)
Delivery ($n = 73$)	
Cesarean section	58 (82.3)
Vaginal	12 (17.1)
unknown	3 (6)
Preterm deliveries <37 weeks	53 (72.6)
Preterm deliveries <34 weeks	26 (35.6)
Sex ($n = 71$)	
Female	44 (62)
Male	27 (38)
Medium weight at birth (grams) (SD) ($n = 69$)	1776.5 (523.5)
Medium length (cm) (SD) ($n = 40$)	40.5 (5.8)
APGAR (1–10) ($n = 55$)	8.5 (1)
DCM at birth ($n = 72$)	5 (7.0)
POSTNATAL OUTCOME	
At birth/Neonatal PM implantation	29 (39.7)
Neonatal death	5 (6.8)
Infant/childhood PM implantation	22 (30.1)
Infant/childhood death	2 (3.1)
Overall PM pacing	51 (69.8)
Overall mortality	23 (25.8)

DCM, dilated cardiomyopathy; PM, pacemaker.

Within the first year of life, more than 50% of the surviving children were paced (40 children, 54.8%).

Recurrence

After the index pregnancy, 14 women had 17 subsequent pregnancies (reviewed in **Table 7**): three were complicated by a CHB therefore the recurrence rate in our cohort was 17.6%. Nine patients received treatments during 10 pregnancies (58.8%): hydroxychloroquine in 1, IVIg alone in 1, not-fluorinated steroids (for maternal indication) alone in 3, not-fluorinated steroids and IVIg in 3, IVIg and HCQ in 1, and IVIg with plasmapheresis and fluorinated steroids in 1. Non fluorinated steroids and HCQ were administered before pregnancy, fluorinated steroids were introduced at conception in two cases, and IVIG and plasmapheresis were started from week 12 (see **Table 7** for details).

Adverse events possibly related with a prolonged use of steroids (maternal hypertension, intra-uterine growth restriction, oligohydramnios) occurred in three. The recurrence rate was not statistically different in mothers who received steroids compared to those who did not (28.6 vs. 11.1%, respectively, $p = 0.55$), but the numbers are low. All the three recurrences of CHB occurred after an index pregnancy complicated with fetal or neonatal death due to a complete CHB.

Maternal Follow-Up

At the time of index pregnancy, 39 patients were considered as asymptomatic autoantibodies carriers. Two years after the latest pregnancy, 11 patients of them developed signs/symptoms that fulfilled the criteria for connective tissue disease: six cases of UCTD and five of SS. In six patients, a chronic treatment was required: oral steroids in four, HCQ in three, and methotrexate in one.

DISCUSSION

This paper describes the first data from the Italian Registry of neonatal cardiac lupus syndrome, including 89 retrospective cases of CHB associated with anti-SSA/Ro and/or anti-SSB/La antibodies. This registry was created in order to collect the cases diagnosed and treated in different Centers, some of them with a longstanding interest in this rare condition. Although some of the cases included in this registry have been already published (17–20), this remains the first effort to analyze all the data as a collaborative national study.

The results that were obtained are in many aspects in line with the published large retrospective studies (**Table 1**) (9–13). The number of cases of complete and incomplete CHB (79.8 vs. 20.2%) and the cumulative probability of pacemaker implantation, almost 70%, were very similar to already published data (1, 9–13) (see **Table 1**).

The risk of fetal mortality in the present cohort was 18% and the overall mortality was 25.8%, slightly higher in our cohort than reported in other publications (see **Table 1**). On statistical analysis, several risks factors that were associated or had a trend toward an increased risk for mortality were confirmed. The presence of hydrops and fetal serositis are well established risk factors for adverse outcome, confirmed in several previous papers (1, 11, 12). No other risk factors were identified in our cases, in particular fetal mortality was not associated with a maternal diagnosis of SLE or SS at the time of pregnancy or a specific ethnicity as previously reported (11).

Some confusion existed in the past on the definition of "congenital" heart block, with some cases detected after birth; for this reason a multidisciplinary group proposed to define congenital heart block as an atrioventricular block diagnosed *in utero*, at birth or within the neonatal period (15) and in the present report five cases were diagnosed after birth.

In our registry data on subsequent pregnancies after a case of CHB were also collected; recurrence rate of CHB was 17.6%, strikingly similar to what found (17.4%) (7) in the American Research Registry for Neonatal Lupus; in our registry all the three fetuses with recurrent CHB were born alive.

Till date, the management of CHB remains very controversial and there are no generalized recommendations on how to treat CHB or if a prophylactic treatment is required during pregnancy. Various treatment approaches have been reported, including steroids, plasmapheresis, IVIg, several immunosuppressive agents, and hydroxychloroquine (21). Fluorinated steroids (FS) could cross the placenta because they are only partially inactivated by 11ß-hydroxysteroid dehydrogenase complex expressed in syncytial trophoblast cells and have satisfactory bioavailability to the fetus (22), and are the drugs with the largest clinical experience. Side effects of high dose

TABLE 7 | Subsequent pregnancies after an index pregnancy complicated with CHB: treatment and pregnancy outcomes.

	Index pregnancy outcome	Maternal diagnosis	Year of pregnancy	Fetal ECHO	Treatment	Pregnancy outcome	Pregnancy complications
Pt 1	CHB III degree, born alive	SS	2005	yes	Prednisolone 28 mg/w IVIg 400mg/kg every 3 w between 12 and 24th gw	Born alive, without CHB	no
Pt 2	CHB III degree, neonatal detection, infant death	SS	1978	yes	no	Neonatal CHB III degree	no
Pt 3	CHB III degree, born alive	Carrier anti-SSA/Ro	2014	yes	no	Born alive, without CHB	no
Pt 4	CHB III degree, infant death	UCTD	2003	yes	no	Born alive, without CHB	no
			2006	yes	no	Born alive, without CHB	no
Pt 5	CHB II degree, born alive	SS	2007	yes	IVIg 400 mg/kg every 3 w between 12 and 24th gw HCQ 200 mg/daily	Born alive, without CHB	no
Pt 6	CHB III degree, TOP	UCTD	2006	yes	Prednisone 35 mg/w; IVIg 400 mg/kg every 3 w between 12 and 24th gw	Born alive, without CHB	Polyhydramnios
			2008	yes	Prednisone 25 mg/w; IVIg 400 mg/kg every 3 w between 12 amd 24h gw	Born alive, without CHB	Maternal hypertension
Pt 7	CHB III degree, TOP	SS	2002	yes	Prednisone 35 mg/w;	Born alive, without CHB	no
			2009	yes	no	Born alive, without CHB	no
Pt 8	CHB III degree, intra-uterine fetal death	Carrier SSA/Ro +SSB/La	2012	yes	Betametasone 28 mg/w, IVIg 1 g/kg every 2 w for 13w, Plasmapheresis for 14 w	CHB II degree	Olygo-anydramnios
Pt 9	CHB III degree, born alive	UCTD	1999	yes	Betametasone 10 mg/w	Born alive, without CHB	IUGR, maternal hypertension
Pt 10	CHB III degree, intra-uterine fetal death	Carrier SSA/Ro +SSB/La	2001	yes	Dexametasone 28 mg/w	CHB III degree	PM at birth
Pt 11	CHB III degree, TOP	UCTD	2007	yes	IVIg400 mg/kg every 3 w between 12 and 24th gw	Born alive, without CHB	
Pt 12	CHB III degree, born alive	Carrier SSA/Ro +SSB/La	2015	yes	no	Born alive, without CHB	
Pt 13	CHB III degree, intra-uterine fetal death	UCTD	2014	yes	HCQ	Born alive, without CHB	Oligohydramnios

We did not include in the table one case that ended with an early termination of pregnancy required by parents at 11 gw. ECHO, echocardiography; HCQ, hydroxychloroquine; TOP, termination of pregnancy; PM, pacemaker; UCTD, undifferentiated connective tissue disease; SS, Sjögren Syndrome; IUGR, intra-uterine growth restriction; IVIg, intravenous immunoglobulin; HCQ, hydroxychloroquine.

FS during pregnancy may be important: increased blood pressure, osteopenia, osteonecrosis, susceptibility to infections, gestational diabetes, premature rupture of the membranes and olygohydramnios. In the present study 60 women were treated with FS: olygohydramnios occurred in 6.6% of cases, intrauterine growth retardation in 8.3% and hypertension in 1.7%.

Retrospective data over a wide time span ranging from the 1970s through 2017 were collected in the present study, therefore the treatment strategies were very heterogeneous. Steroids resulted as the most used drugs, reaching the highest rate compared with other registries (see **Table 1**) and this result confirms that there is no consensus regarding treatment with steroids. Moreover, in many occasions, it depends on the historical approach followed in the single center (23): some centers treated no patients, irrespective of the fetal status, whereas in others hospitals FS were used almost in all cases. The most consistent data on the possible efficacy in CHB were published by Jaeggi et al. (24) in 2004. The authors reported a higher one-year survival rate and less complications or features associated with NL in 21 treated complete CHB compared with 11 patients who did not receive FS. This study, however, displays some limitations. Firstly, the authors compared fetuses from two different eras: the historical cohort from 1990 to 1996 did not receive steroids, whereas all fetuses between 1997 and 2003 were treated. A second important limitation was the higher rate of risk factors for a poor prognosis present in the untreated cohort. Subsequent works did not confirm these findings (10–12, 25). In fact, we also did not find any significant differences on fetal mortality between the groups treated and not with FS, which is consistent with the large international series.

In particular Izmirly et al. (25) compared 71 fetuses with isolated CHB who received FS within 1 week of detection with 85 who received no treatment and evaluated the development of EFE, dilated CMP, hydrops, mortality, and PM implantation. These authors observed that FS did not significantly prevent development of disease beyond the atrio-ventricular node [adjusted Hazard Risk (HR) = 0.90; $p = 0.77$], nor reduce mortality ($HR = 1.63$; $p = 0.47$), or forestall/prevent PM implantation ($HR = 0.87$; $p = 0.53$), so they concluded that no evidence supports fluorinated steroids to prevent disease progression or death in isolated CHB.

Another possible indication for the use of FS is for the prevention of the evolution from incomplete to complete CHB. Whereas, complete CHB is considered irreversible, regression from incomplete block after treatment has been described (10, 11, 26–28). In our cohort an improvement was observed in five cases, all treated with FS and three treated with a combination therapy recently published (29). In brief, in that paper (29) the authors wanted to summarize the possible effects of each single procedure: they demonstrated that plasmapheresis could remove anti/SSA-Ro autoantibodies (30), FS could reduce local inflammation and IVIg could limit the effects of autoantibodies. They used this approach in 12 patients with second or third degree CHB. No variation occurred in the six cases with complete CHB, whereas an improvement occurred in 50% of second degree CHB. The authors reported no side effects in the fetuses or in the mothers, proposing this combination therapy as a therapeutic option in second degree CHB. Unfortunately, since such improvement has been observed also in the absence of any treatment (12) or only with FS, it is not possible to draw any definite conclusion. The recent paper by Cuneo et al. (28) underlines as timing may very relevant for a possible therapeutical windows.

Several hypotheses have been proposed showing the potential usefulness of IVIG to prevent cardiac tissue damage: firstly increasing the elimination of maternal autoantibodies through IVIG saturation, secondly decreasing placental transport of autoantibodies through FcγRn leading to the modulation of inhibitory signaling on macrophages, with consequent reduction of the inflammatory response and fibrosis. This explain the patients treated during pregnancies and the 16 newborns treated immediately after birth (31–33).

There are no specific guidelines for the prevention of recurrence of CHB in subsequent pregnancies and this explains the extreme heterogeneity of treatment that was observed in this cohort, ranging from only clinical and echocardiography monitoring to combined therapies during pregnancy. Non-fluorinated steroids do not cross the placenta and would not be useful at all. Intravenous immunoglobulin has been proposed in the prevention of recurrence in small case series and in two prospective studies that were performed in Europe and in United States (34, 35) with a similar protocol (400 mg/kg every 3 weeks from 12 to 24 gw). Four of our cases were included in the European trial. Both the studies were terminated early because of an unchanged prevalence of recurrence and it was concluded that IVIg at the proposed dose was ineffective at reducing the recurrence rate of cardiac NL.

In the last years, the use of HCQ was shown to be a possible approach to the secondary prevention of the recurrence of CHB. Retrospective analysis from an international cohort (36) reported a higher recurrence rate in pregnancies not treated with HCQ compared with those treated with HCQ. In our study only a limited number of pregnancies were exposed to HCQ not allowing any possible further analysis. However, since the use of HCQ is compatible with pregnancy (37) and is generally a well-tolerated drug, it may be proposed in patients with known antibody positivity.

Our study has several limitations. Data were collected retrospectively and in some pregnancies not all of the data were available, which limits the power of our statistical analysis. It is well established that the distinction between II and III degree AV block *in utero* may be difficult, problematic and time consuming and, when revised centrally, some diagnoses of II degree might be reclassified as III degree and viceversa (13). For this paper it was not possible to reassess the diagnosis centrally therefore some complete CHB could be misdiagnoses as incomplete (13). CHB cases whose mothers were anti-SSA/Ro negative were not included (17). This first report of the registry is mainly driven by rheumatological centers, and some geographical Italian regions are not represented; only the centers whose ethical committees approved the study enrolled cases for this initial analysis. This peculiarity might also explain why in our registry the majority of the mothers already had a diagnosis of CTD at the time of the index pregnancy, an evidence that differs from other experiences. The syndrome of course requires a multidisciplinary approach, not only for the clinical management of each case but also for the systematic collection of the data and their analysis. Pediatric cardiologists and gynecologists play a fundamental role in the management of this condition, and it is planned to involve them in further collections and analyses of data.

In conclusion, this is the first preliminary report of the data from the Italian Registry of neonatal cardiac lupus syndrome, that was established in 2016. Italian centers showed an heterogenous pattern of management of CHB fetuses, with some centers treating all cases with FS and some centers treating no cases. The establishment of this registry might help to share the data, to make more homogenous the management of this rare condition and to stimulate further multidisciplinary studies.

AUTHOR CONTRIBUTIONS

AB, AT, MF, and LA: designed the study. MF, SC, VC, and LA: created the registry on RedCap platform. MF, TB, AB, SB, FC, RC, SD, ED, EE, FF, MGe, MGo, AH, AL, LM, AMi, PM, AM, MMo, MMu, MeP, MaP, RP, VR, AR, CT, MT, LT, and SZ: evaluated the patients. MF, TB, ABo, SB, FC, ED, EE, MGe, AH, AMi, MeP, MaP, VR, CT, BB, and MT: recruited the patients. MF, LA, AB, and AT: wrote the manuscript. All the co-authors reviewed the manuscript.

FUNDING

MF received a Grant from the Italian Society for Rheumatology (SIR) entitled Progetti di ricerca nell'ambito delle malattie reumatiche a carattere cronico infiammatorio, ad esclusione della valutazione clinica degli effetti dei farmaci as a support for the creation of this project.

ACKNOWLEDGMENTS

We wish to thank Dr. Ornella Milanesi, Cardiologia Pediatrica, Dipartimento di Salute della Donna e del Bambino, Università di Padova, Italy, and Dr. Gabriele Vignati, UO Cardiologia Pediatrica, Dipartimento Materno Infantile, ASST Ospedale Niguarda, Milano, Italy for their precious assistance. We are grateful to the children and their families for generous participation in the study.

REFERENCES

1. Brito-Zeron P, Izmirly PM, Ramos-CasalsM, Buyon JP, Khamastha M. The clinical spectrum of autoimmune congenital heart block. *Nat Rev Rheumatol.* (2015) 11:301–12. doi: 10.1038/nrrheum.2015.29
2. Buyon JP, Clancy RM. Maternal autoantibodies and congenital heart block: mediators, markers, and therapeutic approach. *Semin Arthritis Rheum.* (2003) 33:140–54. doi: 10.1016/j.semarthrit.2003.09.002
3. Ho YS, Esscher E, Anderson RH, Michaëlsson M. Anatomy of congenital complete heart block and relation to maternal anti-Ro antibodies. *Am J Cardiol.* (1986) 58:291–4. doi: 10.1016/0002-9149(86) 90064-0
4. Reichlin M, Brucato A, Frank MB, Maddison PJ, McCubbin VR, Wolfson-Reichlin M, et al. Concentration of autoantibodies to native 60-kd Ro/SS-A and denatured 52-kd Ro/SS-A in eluates from the heart of a child who died with congenital complete heart block. *Arthritis Rheum.* (1994) 37:1698–703. doi: 10.1002/art.1780371120
5. Brucato A, Frassi M, Franceschini F, Cimaz R, Faden D, Pisoni MP, et al. Risk of congenital complete heart block in newborns of mothers with anti-Ro/SSA antibodies detected by counterimmunoelectrophoresis: a prospective study of 100 women. *Arthritis Rheum.* (2001) 44:1832–5. doi: 10.1002/1529-0131(200108)44:8<1832::AID-ART320>3.0.CO;2-C
6. Costedoat-Chalumeau N, Amoura Z, Lupoglazoff JM, Huong DL, Denjoy I, Vauthier D, et al. Outcome of pregnancies in patients with anti-SSA/Ro antibodies: a study of 165 pregnancies, with special focus on electrocardiographic variations in the children and comparison with a control group. *Arthritis Rheum.* (2004) 50:3187–94. doi: 10.1002/art.20554
7. Llanos C, Izmirly PM, Katholi M, Katholi M, Clancy RM, Friedman DM, et al. Recurrence rates of cardiac manifestations associated with neonatal lupus and maternal/fetal risk factors. *Arthritis Rheum.* (2009) 60:3091–7. doi: 10.1002/art.24768
8. Julkunen H, Eronen M. The rate of recurrence of isolated congenital heart block: a population based study. *Arthritis Rheum.* (2001) 44:487–8. doi: 10. 1002/1529-0131(200102)44:2<487::AID-ANR70>3.0.CO;2-D
9. Lopes LM, Tavares GM, Damiano AP, Lopes MA, Aiello VD, Schultz R, et al. Perinatal outcome of fetal atrioventricular block: one-hundred-sixteen cases from a single institution. *Circulation.* (2008) 118:1268–75. doi: 10.1161/CIRCULATIONAHA.107.735118
10. Eliasson H, Sonesson SE, Sharland G, Granath F, Simpson JM, Carvalho JS, et al Isolated atrioventricular block in the fetus: a retrospective, multinational, multicenter study of 175 patients. *Circulation.* (2011) 124:1919–26. doi: 10.1161/CIRCULATIONAHA.111.041970
11. Izmirly PM, Saxena A, Kim MY, Wang D, Sahl SK, Llanos C, et al. Maternal and fetal factors associated with mortality and morbidity in a multi-racial/ethnic registry of anti-SSA/Ro-associated cardiac neonatal lupus. *Circulation.* (2011) 124:1927–35. doi: 10.1161/CIRCULATIONAHA.111.033894
12. Levesque K, Morel N, Maltret A, Baron G, Masseau A, Orquevaux P, et al. Description of 214 cases of autoimmune congenital heart block: results of the French neonatal lupus syndrome. *Autoimmun Rev.* (2015) 14:1154–60. doi: 10.1016/j.autrev.2015.08.005
13. Van den Berg NW, Slieker MG, van Beynum IM, Bilardo CM, de Bruijn D, Clur SA, et al. Fluorinated steroids do not improve outcome of isolated atrioventricular block. *Int J Cardiol.* (2016) 225:167–71. doi: 10.1016/j.ijcard.2016.09.119
14. Brucato A, Tincani A, Fredi M, Breda S, Ramoni V, Morel N, et al. Should we treat congenital heart block with fluorinated corticosteroids? *Autoimmun Rev.* (2017) 16:1115–8. doi: 10.1016/j.autrev.2017.09.005
15. Brucato A, Jonzon A, Friedman D, Allan LD, Vignati G, Gasparini M, et al. Proposal for a new definition of congenital complete atrioventricular block. *Lupus.* (2003) 12:427–35. doi: 10.1191/0961203303lu408oa
16. Friedman DM, Kim MY, Copel JA, Davis C, Phoon CK, Glickstein JS, et al. Utility of cardiac monitoring in fetuses at risk for congenital heart block: the PR Interval and Dexamethasone Evaluation (PRIDE) prospective study. *Circulation.* (2008) 117:485–93. doi: 10.1161/CIRCULATIONAHA.107.707661
17. Fesslova V, Mannarino S, Salice P, Boschetto C, Trespidi L, Acaia B, et al. Neonatal lupus: fetal myocarditis progressing to atrioventricular block in triplets. *Lupus.* (2003) 12:775–8. doi: 10.1191/0961203303lu441cr
18. Fesslova V, Vignati G, Brucato A, De Sanctis M, Butera G, Pisoni MP, et al. The impact of treatment of the fetus by maternal therapy on the fetal and postnatal outcomes for fetuses diagnosed with isolated complete atrioventricular block. *Cardiol Young.* (2009) 19:282–90. doi: 10.1017/S10479511090 04053
19. Brucato A, Grava C, Bortolati M, Ikeda K, Milanesi O, Cimaz R, et al. Congenital heart block not associated with anti-Ro/La antibodies: comparison with anti-Ro/La-positive cases. *J Rheumatol.* (2009) 36:1744–8. doi: 10.3899/jrheum.080737
20. Hoxha A, Ruffatti A, Ambrosi A, Ottosson V, Hedlund M, Ottosson L, et al. Identification of discrete epitopes of Ro52p200 and association with fetal cardiac conduction system manifestations in a rodent model. *Clin Exp Immunol.* (2016) 186:284–91. doi: 10.1111/cei.12854
21. Brucato A, Cimaz R, Caporali R, Ramoni V, Buyon J. Pregnancy outcomes in patients with autoimmune diseases and anti-Ro/SSA antibodies. *Clin Rev Allergy Immunol.* (2011) 40:27–41. doi: 10.1007/s12016-009-8190-6
22. Quinkler M, Oelkers W, Diederich S. Clinical implications of glucocorticoid metabolism by 11 Beta-hydroxysteroid dehydrogenases in target tissues. *Eur J Endocrinol.* (2001) 144:87–97. doi: 10.1530/eje.0.1440087

23. Buyon JP, Clancy RM, Friedman DM. Cardiac manifestations of neonatal lupus erythematosus: guidelines to management, integrating clues from the bench and bedside. *Nat Clin Pract Rheumatol.* (2009) 5:139–48. doi: 10.1038/ncprheum1018
24. Jaeggi ET, Fouron JC, Silverman ED, Ryan G, Smallhorn J, Hornberger LK. Transplacental fetal treatment improves the outcome of prenatally diagnosed complete atrioventricular block without structural heart disease. *Circulation.* (2004) 110:1542–8. doi: 10.1161/01.CIR.0000142046.58632.3A
25. Izmirly PM, Saxena A, Sahl SK, Shah U, Friedman DM, Kim MY, et al. Assessment of fluorinated steroids to avert progression and mortality in anti-SSA/Ro-associated cardiac injury limited to the fetal conduction system. *Ann Rheum Dis.* (2016) 75:1161–5. doi: 10.1136/annrheumdis-2015-208311
26. Saleeb S, Copel J, Friedman D, Buyon JP. Comparison of treatment with fluorinated glucocorticoids to the natural history of autoantibodyassociated congenital heart block: retrospective review of the Research Registry for Neonatal Lupus. *Arthritis Rheum.* (1999) 42:2335–45.
27. Theander E, Brucato A, Gudmundsson S, Salomonsson S, Wahren-Herlenius M, Manthorpe R. Primary Sjogren's syndrome: treatment of fetal incomplete atrioventricular block with dexamethasone. *J Rheumatol.* (2001) 28:373–6.
28. Cuneo BF, Sonesson SE, Levasseur S, Moon-Grady AJ, Krishnan A, Donofrio MT. Home monitoring for fetal heart rhythm during anti-ro pregnancies. *J Am Coll Cardiol.* (2018) 72:1940–51. doi: 10.1016/j.jacc.2018.07.076
29. Ruffatti A, Cerutti A, Favaro M, Del Ross T, Calligaro A, Hoxha A, et al. Plasmapheresis, intravenous immunoglobulins and bethametasone - a combined protocol to treat autoimmune congenital heart block: a prospective cohort study. *Clin Exp Rheumatol.* (2016) 34:706–13.
30. Tonello M, Ruffatti A, Marson P, Tison T, Marozio L, Hoxha A, et al. Plasma exchange effectively removes 52- and 60-kDa anti-Ro/SSA and anti-La/SSB antibodies in pregnant women with congenital heart block. *Transfusion.* (2015) 55:1782–6. doi: 10.1111/trf.13046
31. Hansen RJ, Balthasar JP. Effects of intravenous immunoglobulin on platelet count and antiplatelet antibody disposition in a rat model of autoimmune thrombocytopenia. *Blood.* (2002) 100:2087–93.
32. Hansen RJ, Balthasar JP. Intravenous immunoglobulin mediates an increase in anti-platelet antibody clearance via the FcRn receptor. *Thromb Haemost.* (2002) 88:898–9. doi: 10.1055/s-0037-1613331
33. Samuelsson A, Towers TL, Ravetch JV. Anti-inflammatory activity of IVIG mediated through the inhibitory Fc receptor. *Science.* (2001) 291:484–6. doi: 10.1126/science.291.5503.484
34. Friedman DM, Llanos C, Izmirly PM, Brock B, Byron J, Copel J, et al. Evaluation of fetuses in a study of intravenous immunoglobulin as preventive therapy for congenital heart block: results of a multicenter, prospective, open-label clinical trial. *Arthritis Rheum.* (2010) 62:1138–46. doi: 10.1002/art.27308
35. Pisoni CN, Brucato A, Ruffatti A, Espinosa G, Cervera R, Belmonte-Serrano M, et al. Failure of intravenous immunoglobulin to prevent congenital heart block: findings of a multicenter, prospective, observational study. *Arthritis Rheum.* (2010) 62:1147–52. doi: 10.1002/art.27350
36. Izmirly PM, Costedoat-Chalumeau N, Pisoni CN, Espinosa G, Cervera R, Belmonte-Serrano M, et al. Maternal use of hydroxychloroquine is associated with a reduced risk of recurrent anti-SSA/Ro-antibody-associated cardiac manifestations of neonatal lupus. *Circulation.* (2012) 126:76–82. doi: 10.1161/CIRCULATIONAHA.111.089268
37. Götestam Skorpen C, Hoeltzenbein M, Tincani A, Fischer-Betz R, Elefant E, Chambers C, et al. The EULAR points to consider for use of antirheumatic drugs before pregnancy, and during pregnancy and lactation. *Ann Rheum Dis.* (2016) 75:795–810. doi: 10.1136/annrheumdis-2015-208840

5

Targeting Inflammation to Prevent Cardiovascular Disease in Chronic Rheumatic Diseases: Myth or Reality?

*Elena Bartoloni, Alessia Alunno, Valentina Valentini, Filippo Luccioli, Eleonora Valentini, Giuliana Maria Concetta La Paglia, Maria Comasia Leone, Giacomo Cafaro, Elisa Marcucci and Roberto Gerli**

Rheumatology Unit, Department of Perugia, University of Perugia, Perugia, Italy

Correspondence:
Roberto Gerli
roberto.gerli@unipg.it

Evidence for increased risk of cardiovascular morbidity and mortality in chronic inflammatory rheumatic diseases has accumulated during the last years. Traditional cardiovascular risk factors contribute in part to the excess of cardiovascular risk in these patients and several mechanisms, including precocious acceleration of subclinical atherosclerotic damage, inflammation, and immune system deregulation factors, have been demonstrated to strictly interplay in the induction and progression of atherosclerosis. In this setting, chronic inflammation is a cornerstone of rheumatic disease pathogenesis and exerts also a pivotal role in all stages of atherosclerotic damage. The strict link between inflammation and atherosclerosis suggests that cardiovascular risk may be reduced by rheumatic disease activity control. There are data to suggest that biologic therapies, in particular TNFα antagonists, may improve surrogate markers of cardiovascular disease and reduce CV adverse outcome. Thus, abrogation of inflammation is considered an important outcome for achieving not only control of rheumatic disease, but also reduction of cardiovascular risk. However, the actual effect of anti-rheumatic therapies on atherosclerosis progression and CV outcome in these patients is rather uncertain due to great literature inconsistency. In this paper, we will summarize some of the main mechanisms linking the inflammatory pathogenic background underlying rheumatic diseases and the vascular damage observed in these patients, with a particular emphasis on the pathways targeted by currently available therapies. Moreover, we will analyze current evidence on the potential atheroprotective effects of these treatments on cardiovascular outcome pointing out still unresolved questions.

Keywords: rheumatic disease, inflammation, cardiovascular disease, atherosclerosis, biologic therapies, rheumatoid arthritis, psoriatic arthritis, ankylosing spondylitis

INTRODUCTION

The long-term prognosis of chronic inflammatory rheumatic diseases (RDs), such as rheumatoid arthritis (RA), psoriatic arthritis (PsA), and ankylosing spondylitis (AS), is significantly influenced by increased risk of cardiovascular (CV) morbidity and mortality. In a large population-based, observational study, CV events resulted the third most frequent comorbidity in RA patients after depression and asthma (1). However, the evidence that screening and management of CV comorbidities in these patients is far from optimal deserves attention considering that high prevalence of atherosclerosis seems to occur yet in the earliest stages of the disease and also in young subjects free from CV risk factors, as demonstrated in particular in RA patients (2).

Chronic RDs and atherosclerotic endothelial damage share a similar inflammatory pathogenic background and multiple mechanisms contribute to subclinical atherosclerosis in these patients (3). It is demonstrated that disease-related inflammatory and immune mechanisms have a pivotal role in the pathogenesis of atherosclerosis and CV risk and that the contribution of traditional CV risk factors is at least as important as disease-specific factors (4). Indeed, prevalence of classic CV risk factors is higher in these patients in comparison to general population (5–8). In particular, hypertension, and diabetes mellitus represent two major factors to monitor in RD patients, both being associated with other CV comorbidities, disease activity and increased risk of CV events (5–9).

As inflammation is a cornerstone of the pathogenesis of systemic RDs and considering its pivotal role in driving all stages of atherosclerosis, it is compelling to hypothesize that controlling the pathways that induce synovial and systemic inflammation may provide benefit on CV risk in these patients (10). Although inconsistency in results between studies mainly due to different study design and different outcome measures, there are data suggesting that biologic therapies, in particular tumor necrosis factor-α inhibitors (TNFα-i), improve surrogate markers of subclinical atherosclerosis. Moreover, better control of RA activity has recently been associated with fewer CV events (11, 12). In a recent prospective study, failure in achieving disease activity control increased from 4- to 8-fold the risk to develop subclinical atherosclerosis and CV events at 1 year of follow-up (13). Although it is quite difficult to provide an actual long-term estimation of CV risk due to the lack of validated scores, tight, and sustained control of RD activity is necessary to effectively prevent CV disease development. Treat-to-target and abrogation of inflammation are now considered two main outcomes for achieving RD control. In addition, effective pharmacological treatment could favor physical activity, with consequent decrease of risk of obesity, diabetes, hypertension, and at least, CV disease. It is to note, however, that introduction of biologic agents is less frequent in RA patients with multiple concomitant comorbidities, although with active disease, and that some medications commonly used in these patients, such as corticosteroids (CS) and non-steroidal anti-inflammatory drugs, are known to enhance CV risk (14). In particular, some drugs may exert a dual effect. Indeed, if short-term CS treatment may lead to initial beneficial effect due to rapid suppression of inflammatory burden, it is well-known that long-term side effects of CS therapy may have a net adverse association with CV disease risk (15). Of consequence, the real effect of non-biologic and biologic therapy on CV risk and outcome in these patients is still uncertain.

In this perspective, a literature search was performed to identify articles investigating medium- and long-term effect of non-biologic and biologic therapies on subclinical atherosclerosis measures and CV outcome in patients with RA, PsA, and AS. Articles were identified in PubMed by using Mesh terms and keywords. Search was restricted to English language.

INFLAMMATION: A LINK BETWEEN ATHEROSCLEROSIS AND RHEUMATIC DISEASES

The definite demonstration that atherosclerosis is a dynamic process greatly driven by inflammatory factors has highlighted interesting pathogenic links between atherosclerotic arterial wall damage and inflammatory mechanisms underlying the pathogenesis of systemic RDs (16) (**Figure 1**). Systemic inflammation contributes to all stages of atherosclerosis starting from activation of endothelial layer and recruitment of inflammatory cells within arterial layer to monocyte differentiation and foam cell formation, with subsequent plaque development. Moreover, these molecules promote apoptosis of arterial smooth muscle cells, matrix degradation, and fibrosis with subsequent destabilization and rupture of atherosclerotic plaques. Immune dysregulation, through the involvement of T lymphocytes, contributes to amplification of inflammatory response driving atherosclerotic damage. T helper (Th)1 cells, in particular, secrete several cytokines, such as interferon (IFN)γ, interleukin (IL)-2, IL-12, IL-18, and TNFα, which contribute to vascular endothelial damage and plaque progression (17). Interestingly, these cytokines, in particular TNFα, IL-6, and IL-18, have been associated with endothelial dysfunction, carotid atherosclerosis, CV morbidity, and risk of CV events and mortality in patients with systemic RDs (18). Among inflammatory biomarkers, C-reactive protein (CRP), IL-6, IL-1, and TNFα have been extensively studied and employed as predictive tools of CV risk and future CV events (16, 17, 19). Strong evidence supports the direct role of these molecules in contributing to atherogenesis by favoring endothelial dysfunction, vascular oxidative stress, foam cell formation, and atherosclerotic plaque destabilization (16, 17, 19). In addition, pro-inflammatory cytokines may induce atherosclerosis causing an alteration of lipid profile. In particular, TNFα and IL 6 have been shown to induce a pro-atherogenic profile and insulin resistance in patients with RDs (18).

Given the importance of pro-inflammatory cytokines in atherosclerosis and CV disease risk, effective modulation of inflammatory response in systemic RDs is expected to reduce risk and incidence of CV events and multiple pathways have been identified as potential therapeutic targets for the prevention and treatment of CV disease. In this setting, canakinumab, an inhibitor of IL-1β, was associated with significant reduction of recurrent CV events in patients with previous myocardial

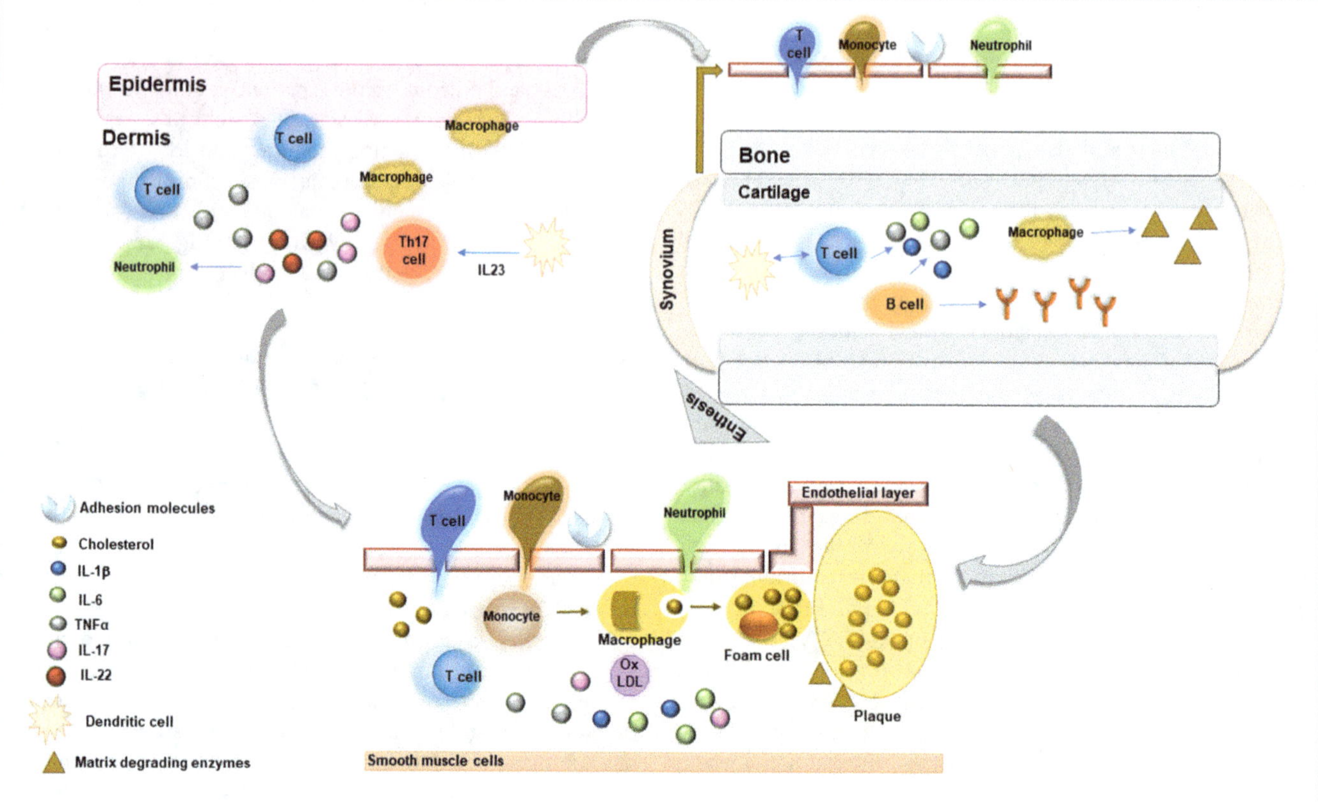

FIGURE 1 | Common inflammatory mechanisms driving the pathogenesis of chronic rheumatic diseases and athrosclerosis.

infarction and persistently elevated CRP levels (20). Three doses of canakinumab were tested and only the 150 mg dose reduced the relative risk of composite CV endpoint by 15%, mainly driven by a 24% reduction of relative risk of myocardial infarction. No significant reduction in CV death was observed and canakinumab was associated with an increased risk of fatal infection and sepsis. Surely, given the modest absolute clinical benefit, routine use of canakinumab in patients with previous myocardial infarction is not justified until more data are available.

On the other hand, in systemic RDs, randomized controlled trials (RCT)s of disease-modifying anti-rheumatic drugs (DMARDs), and biologic anti-cytokine therapies have not been powered to detect the impact of these agents on the modification of subclinical atherosclerosis and CV disease risk. Of consequence, data on the effect of these therapies on CV outcome in patients with RDs have been mainly driven by observational and pharmaco-epidemiological studies which suggest that close control of inflammation and disease activity in RDs may favorably affect some CV disease risk factors, reducing the rate of progression of subclinical atherosclerosis and the incidence of CV events (12) (**Table 1**).

DO ANTI-RHEUMATIC THERAPIES LOWER THE RISK OF ACCELERATED ATHEROSCLEROSIS?

Endothelial dysfunction, a potentially reversible step in atherosclerosis development, and structural vascular wall damage, assessed either as intima-media thickness (IMT) and carotid plaque, are considered important predictors of subsequent CV events in the general population as well as in patients with RA (21, 22). Multiple mechanisms, including systemic inflammatory burden, have been implicated in the pathophysiology of micro and macro-vascular endothelial dysfunction in patients with RDs and different methods are employed to detect precocious atherosclerosis in these patients (23). Thus, therapies reducing inflammation and disease activity are expected to improve vascular function and, possibly, arterial wall organic damage. In this setting, however, no definite conclusions can be driven on the effect of anti-rheumatic therapies on vascular endothelial function in inflammatory RDs. Multiple variables, including differences in study design, population enrolled, disease duration, instrumental technique employed in the assessment of subclinical atherosclerosis, length of follow-up, class of biologic drug used and concomitant therapies, hamper data interpretation and explain the high variability of study results. However, analysis of data derived by meta-analysis and systematic reviews, observational studies, and few RCTs allows to highlight some observations.

Conventional DMARDs

- Hydroxychloroquine (HCQ) has been associated with lower risk of diabetes mellitus (24), a better lipid profile characterized by reduced low-density lipoprotein and tryglyceride levels (25) and antithrombotic effect on platelet aggregation. Moreover, *in vitro* studies demonstrated a potential vasoprotective

TABLE 1 | Effect of non-biologic and biologic drugs on CV risk in RD patients.

Drug	Lipid profile	Metabolic syndrome	PWV	AIx	ED	IMT	Plaque	CV events
RHEUMATOID ARTHRITIS								
HCQ	Improve							↓
MTX	Improve	↓						↓
TNFα-i	Worsen/neutral		↓		↓	↓		↓
TCZ	Worsen		↓	↓	↓	↔	↔	↔
ABT	Neutral		↔	↔		↔	↔	↓
RTX	Neutral		↔	↔		↓		↔
PSORIATIC ARTHRITIS								
TNFα-i	Worsen/neutral							
UST								↔
SEC								↔
ANKYLOSING SPONDYLITIS								
TNFα-i	Worsen/neutral			↔		↔		
SEC								↔

HCQ, hydroxychloroquine; MTX, methotrexate; TNFα-I, tumor necrosis factorα inhibitors; TCZ, tocilizumab; ABT, abatacept; RTX, rituximab; UST, ustekinumab; SEC, secuckinumab; PWV, pulse wave velocity; AIx, augmentation index; ED, endothelial dysfunction; IMT, intima-media thickness; CV, cardiovascular.
↓, significantly decreased; ↔, no significant effect.

effect by reduction of vascular endothelial adhesion molecule expression (26). Despite this beneficial evidence on lipid and glucose homeostasis, no studies explored the effects of HCQ on surrogate markers of atherosclerosis. Interestingly, a recent meta-analysis demonstrated that patients with RA and systemic connective diseases assuming HCQ are characterized by a significant reduction of CV events in comparison to non-HCQ users (27).

- Methotrexate (MTX) has several favorable effects on markers of CV damage. In particular, MTX therapy has been associated with improvement in reverse cholesterol transport (28), reduction of foam cell formation (29), down-regulation of adhesion molecule expression on endothelial surface (30), and reduced risk of metabolic syndrome (31). Moreover, response to MTX therapy is associated with reduction of circulating cytokines, including TNFα, IL-6, and IL-1, which exert atherogenic activity. Effects of MTX on measures of subclinical atherosclerosis has been explored in few studies showing a favorable response in atherosclerosis progression (32–34). In a recent observational study, 6-month MTX monotherapy was associated with a more pronounced favorable effect on endothelial function in comparison to TNFα-i ± MTX in a cohort of RD patients (35). The effect was independent of disease activity improvement. However, the small number of patients enrolled and the method used to detect atherosclerosis progression (change in Reactive Hyperemic Index) suggest caution in data interpretation.

TNFα Inhibitors

- Short and medium-term studies demonstrated that TNFα-i are effective in improving arterial stiffness, evaluated as reduction of pulse wave velocity (PWV), and endothelial dysfunction, expressed as improvement in flow-mediated vasodilation (FMD), in RA patients, thus suggesting a link between chronic inflammation and endothelial dysfunction and arterial stiffness (11, 36, 37).
- TNFα-i therapy is associated with prevention or reversion of IMT progression in RD patients responding to treatment in studies with up to 5-year follow-up (36). The effect on IMT seems more relevant in RA patients with early disease (38).
- A beneficial effect on measures of microvascular endothelial dysfunction has been depicted in a small cohort of AS patients following 1 month of etanercept therapy, thus suggesting that suppression of inflammation is associated with rapid reversal of microvascular dysfunction in these patients (39). On the other hand, no effect of TNFα-i treatment has been detected on arterial stiffness and augmentation index (AIx) in wider cohorts of AS patients, suggesting that different disease-specific mechanims may contribute to endothelial impairment (40).
- AIx, a composite measure of arterial stiffness and speed of reflected wave from peripheral vascular resistances, usually does not change following TNFα-i therapy (36, 37). Intriguingly, this may suggest that arterial stiffness, a surrogate measure of macrovacular function, is more sensitive to inflammatory burden in RDs in comparison to other vascular functional parameters.
- Different TNFα-i may exert different effects on subclinical atherosclerosis. In this setting, adalimumab and etanercept have been associated with significant reduction of arterial stiffness in RA patients, while no change in the same measure was detected following infliximab administration (40). However, the limited number of studies does not allow to demonstrate a clear class-specific effect of TNFα-i on endothelial function in these patients (11).

Other Non-TNFα-i Therapies

Very few data are available on the effect of other non-TNFα-i targeted therapies on subclinical vascular endothelial damage.

Inhibition of IL-6, a potent inflammatory cytokine inducing hepatic acute phase reactant production, has been associated with improvement of endothelial function, expressed as FMD, arterial stiffness and AIx, in open-label RCTs (40, 41). Interestingly, no changes in carotid IMT were reported (42), suggesting that rapid suppression of inflammation exerts more pronounced effect on endothelial function and that longer follow-up may be needed to detect significant changes of structural arterial wall damage. Conversely, B-cell blockade with rituximab was associated with improvement of carotid IMT in a pilot study without exerting significant effect on arterial stiffness and AIx in open label studies (43–45). Despite studies on atherosclerosis-prone mice demonstrated a favorable effect of abatacept in atherogenesis reduction, treatment with abatacept in humans was not associated with an improvement of surrogate measures of subclinical atherosclerosis, including aortic stiffness, AIx, carotid IMT, and plaques (40, 46).

DO ANTI-RHEUMATIC THERAPIES LOWER THE RISK OF CARDIOVASCULAR EVENTS?

Conventional DMARDs

- Although no RCT explored the independent effect of MTX on major CV outcomes, robust evidence supports that patients treated with MTX are characterized by a significant lower risk of all CV events, myocardial infarction and stroke in comparison to RD patients not receiving MTX (12, 47, 48). The effect was more evident in responders to therapy and the pooled relative reduction resulted 28% for all CV events and 19% for myocardial infarction (12). Moreover, the evidence was stronger for overall reduction of CV morbidity and mortality and weaker for stroke risk reduction (12).
- As observed with MTX, no randomized studies evaluated the risk of CV diseases in RD patients treated with non-MTX non-biologic therapies. Observational data suggest that long exposure to leflunomide and sulfasalazine may be associated with a reduced risk of all CV events and myocardial infarction (38, 46).

TNFα Inhibitors

- Meta-analysis of cohort studies demonstrated that use of TNFα-i in RA patients is associated with a 30% relative reduction in all CV events and a 41% reduction of myocardial infarction in comparison to other non-biologic therapies (12). Subsequent systematic literature review of different studies confirmed the safety of biologic therapies in RDs patients with respect to CV outcome (40). However, the high variability in study design, CV outcome definition, populations enrolled and disease activity hamper data interpretation and makes it difficult to compare results among studies (40).
- As observed for MTX, the favorable effect on CV outcome may depend on clinical response since a lower incidence of myocardial infarction has been observed in responders to therapy (49).
- A recent prospective study with a longer follow-up (median 5 years) demonstrated that TNFα-i therapy in RA patients is associated with a significant reduction of 39% in the risk of myocardial infarction in comparison to DMARD therapy (50). This is the first demonstration that duration of TNFα-i exposure may be associated with reduction of CV risk in these patients and suggests that stable suppression of inflammation and disease activity control are mandatory targets in the prevention of CV disease risk.
- A prospective analysis of the same cohort depicted that, compared to DMARDs, ever-exposure to TNFα-i therapy is not associated to a significant effect on the risk of first ischemic stroke over a median period of 5 years. Although not statistically significant, there was a trend toward a reduction in mortality at 30 days and at 1 year following the event among patients treated with TNFα-i at stroke occurrence compared to the other group (51). This may suggest different and still unexplored pathogenic mechanims underlying ischemic cerebrovascular events in RA patients.

Other Non-TNFα-i Therapies

- Unfavorable lipid profile has been observed following TCZ therapy. However, pooled analysis of clinical trials and post-marketing safety data suggest that the CV disease risk in TCZ users is comparable to the risk associated with other biologic therapies (52–54). Indeed, a clear inverse relationship, known as the "lipid paradox," has been demonstrated between lipid levels and CV risk in RA patients with an increased risk of CV disease also in patients with low total cholesterol and low-density lipoprotein (LDL) levels in the setting of active inflammation (55). Despite the global increase in LDL, total cholesterol, and triglyceride levels following the reduction of inflammatory burden, a favorable anti-inflammatory change of high-density lipoprotein composition and function has been demonstrated following tocilizumab administration, thus suggesting its positive net effect on CV risk (56).
- Abatacept may be associated with lower risk of myocardial infarction in comparison with TNFα-i. A retrospective study enrolling RA patients initiating biologic therapies, patients treated with abatacept were characterized by a lower risk of myocardial infarction in comparison to patients on TNFα-i therapy (57). Interestingly, these data have been recently confirmed in a large population-based cohort of RA patients demonstrating that abatacept was associated with a significant 29% reduced risk of a CV composite endopoint (myocardial infarction, stroke/transient ischemic attack, and coronary revascularization) when compared with TNFα-i therapy, in particular in patients with diabetes mellitus (58).
- Data on CV outcome in patients treated with rituximab are scarce. Observational studies did not observe significant differences in CV event rates in patients treated with rituximab in comparison to TNFα-i therapy or abatacept (40, 46).
- The period passed from the introduction of anti IL-12/23 targeted therapies is too short to draw hypothesis on their effect on CV outcome (40, 59).

OPEN QUESTIONS AND FUTURE DIRECTIONS

Despite broad evidence suggests that non-biologic and biologic therapies may be associated with a reduced risk of CV events and more favorable CV outcome in RD patients, several points should be considered in data interpretation, suggesting caution in their feasibility.

- The high variability in study designs and inclusion/exclusion criteria, in disease characteristics (grade of activity, seropositivity, duration, concomitant CV risk factors, concomitant therapies as non-steroidal anti-inflammatory drugs), in CV event definition, and in cohort enrolled represent a major limit to consider.
- The median follow-up of almost all studies was too short to effectively detect a significant reduction of long-term CV events. Similarly, the variable follow-up across studies makes it difficult to verify the durability of therapy effect on subclinical atherosclerosis measure improvement.
- The application in many studies of surrogate markers of atherosclerosis to estimate CV disease risk due to the low number of CV events, which limited statistical significance detection, remains an important limit in the interpretation of study results.
- Further studies are needed to investigate if the reduction of CV risk is a direct effect of these targeted therapies on atherosclerotic process or an indirect manifestation of the general reduction of systemic inflammation and disease activity.
- Research should focus on evaluation of drug-specific class effects on CV disease risk in order to enable better and personalized use of targeted therapies according to patient CV risk phenotype and disease characteristics.
- Further studies are needed to more deeply elucidate the contribution of inflammation to the pathophysiology of atherosclerosis in RDs and to identify specific non-invasive biomarkers to be employed as tool to identify patients with higher CV risk and guide therapy selection.
- The effect of targeted therapies on CV risk as well as pathogenic mechanisms leading to atherosclerotic damage in patients with SA and PsA should be further investigated.
- Larger, prospective studies with longer follow-up and RCTs with hard CV end-points are urgently needed to better characterize the CV outcome in these patients.
- Specific CV disease screening by validated CV risk score in RD patients should be implemented in order to quantify the CV long-term outcome and guide the better primary and secondary CV preventive therapeutic strategy.
- Despite advances in the treatment of these chronic RDs and better control of disease activity, CV-related mortality remains elevated in these patients. Under-recognition and suboptimally treatment of CV risk factors in association with the unavailability of validated treatment recommendations represent major causes for the lack of proper CV risk management in usual clinical care.

AUTHOR CONTRIBUTIONS

EB wrote the whole manuscript. RG revised and approved the final manuscript draft. All Authors revised and approved the manuscript.

REFERENCES

1. Dougados M, Soubrier M, Antunez A, Balint P, Balsa A, Buch MH, et al. Prevalence of comorbidities in rheumatoid arthritis and evaluation of their monitoring: results of an international, cross-sectional study (COMORA). *Ann Rheum Dis.* (2014) 73:62–8. doi: 10.1136/annrheumdis-2013-204223
2. Bartoloni E, Alunno A, Bistoni O, Gerli R. How early is the atherosclerotic risk in rheumatoid arthritis? *Autoimmun Rev.* (2010) 9:701–7. doi: 10.1016/j.autrev.2010.06.001
3. Bartoloni E, Shoenfeld Y, Gerli R. Inflammatory and autoimmune mechanisms in the induction of atherosclerotic damage in systemic rheumatic diseases: two faces of the same coin. *Arthritis Care Res.* (2011) 63:178–83. doi: 10.1002/acr.20322
4. Crowson CS, Rollefstad S, Ikdahl E, Kitas G, van Riel PL, Gabriel S, et al. Impact of risk factors associated with cardiovascular outcomes in patients with rheumatoid arthritis. *Ann Rheum Dis.* (2018) 77:48–54. doi: 10.1136/annrheumdis-2017-211735
5. Bartoloni E, Alunno A, Valentini V, Luccioli F, Valentini E, La Paglia G, et al. Role of inflammatory diseases in hypertension. *High Blood Press Cardiovasc Prev.* (2017) 24:353–61. doi: 10.1007/s40292-017-0214-3
6. Bartoloni E, Alunno A, Valentini V, Valentini E, La Paglia GCM, Leone MC, et al. The prevalence and relevance of traditional cardiovascular risk factors in primary Sjögren's syndrome. *Clin Exp Rheumatol.* (2018) 36(Suppl. 112):113–120.
7. Bartoloni E, Alunno A, Gerli R. Hypertension as a cardiovascular risk factor in autoimmune rheumatic diseases. *Nat Rev Cardiol.* (2018) 15:33–44. doi: 10.1038/nrcardio.2017.118
8. Ruscitti P, Ursini F, Cipriani P, Ciccia F, Liakouli V, Carubbi F, et al. Prevalence of type 2 diabetes and impaired fasting glucose in patients affected by rheumatoid arthritis: results from a cross-sectional study. *Medicine* (2017) 96:e7896. doi: 10.1097/MD.0000000000007896
9. Crepaldi G, Scirè CA, Carrara G, Sakellariou G, Caporali R, Hmamouchi I, et al. Cardiovascular comorbidities relate more than others with disease activity in rheumatoid arthritis. *PLoS ONE* (2016) 11:e0146991. doi: 10.1371/journal.pone.0146991
10. Geovanini GR, Libby P. Atherosclerosis and inflammation: overview and updates. *Clin Sci.* (2018) 132:1243–52. doi: 10.1042/CS20180306
11. Ursini F, Leporini C, Bene F, D'Angelo S, Mauro D, Russo E, et al. Anti-TNF-alpha agents and endothelial function in rheumatoid arthritis: a systematic review and meta-analysis. *Sci Rep.* (2017) 7:5346. doi: 10.1038/s41598-017-05759-2
12. Roubille C, Richer V, Starnino T, McCourt C, McFarlane A, Fleming P, et al. The effects of tumour necrosis factor inhibitors, methotrexate, non-steroidal anti-inflammatory drugs and corticosteroids on cardiovascular events in rheumatoid arthritis, psoriasis and psoriatic arthritis: a systematic review and meta-analysis. *Ann Rheum Dis.* (2015) 74:480–9. doi: 10.1136/annrheumdis-2014-206624
13. Ruscitti P, Cipriani P, Masedu F, Romano S, Berardicurti O, Liakouli V, et al. Increased cardiovascular events and subclinical atherosclerosis in rheumatoid arthritis patients: 1 Year prospective single centre study. *PLoS ONE* (2017) 12:e0170108. doi: 10.1371/journal.pone.0170108
14. Radner H, Yoshida K, Hmamouchi I, Dougados M, Smolen JS, Solomon DH. Treatment patterns of multimorbid patients with rheumatoid arthritis: results from an international cross-sectional study. *J Rheumatol.* (2015) 42:1099–104. doi: 10.3899/jrheum.141534

15. Bartoloni E, Alunno A, Santoboni G, Gerli R. Beneficial cardiovascular effects of low-dose glucocorticoid therapy in inflammatory rheumatic diseases. *J Rheumatol.* (2012) 39:1758–60. doi: 10.3899/jrheum.120192
16. Raggi P, Genest J, Giles JT, Rayner KJ, Dwivedi G, Beanlands RS, et al. Role of inflammation in the pathogenesis of atherosclerosis and therapeutic interventions. *Atherosclerosis* (2018) 276:98–108. doi: 10.1016/j.atherosclerosis.2018.07.014
17. Moriya J. Critical roles of inflammation in atherosclerosis. *J Cardiol.* (2018) 73:22–7. doi: 10.1016/j.jjcc.2018.05.010
18. Arida A, Protogerou AD, Kitas GD, Sfikakis PP. Systemic inflammatory response and atherosclerosis: the paradigm of chronic inflammatory rheumatic diseases. *Int J Mol Sci.* (2018) 19:1890. doi: 10.3390/ijms19071890
19. Avan A, Tavakoly Sany SB, Ghayour-Mobarhan M, Rahimi HR, Tajfard M, Ferns G. Serum C-reactive protein in the prediction of cardiovascular diseases: overview of the latest clinical studies and public health practice. *J Cell Physiol.* (2018) 233:8508–25. doi: 10.1002/jcp.26791
20. Ridker PM, Everett BM, Thuren T, MacFadyen JG, Chang WH, Ballantyne C, et al. Antiinflammatory therapy with canakinumab for atherosclerotic disease. *N Engl J Med.* (2017) 377:1119–31. doi: 10.1056/NEJMoa1707914
21. Gutterman DD, Chabowski DS, Kadlec AO, Durand MJ, Freed JK, Ait-Aissa K, et al. The human microcirculation: regulation of flow and beyond. *Circ. Res.* (2016) 118:157–72. doi: 10.1161/CIRCRESAHA.115.305364
22. Evans MR, Escalante A, Battafarano DF, Freeman GL, O'Leary DH, del Rincón I. Carotid atherosclerosis predicts incident acute coronary syndromes in rheumatoid arthritis. *Arthritis Rheum.* (2011) 63:1211–20. doi: 10.1002/art.30265
23. Bordy R, Totoson P, Prati C, Marie C, Wendling D, Demougeot C. Microvascular endothelial dysfunction in rheumatoid arthritis. *Nat Rev Rheumatol.* (2018) 14:404–20. doi: 10.1038/s41584-018-0022-8
24. Solomon DH, Massarotti E, Garg R, Liu J, Canning C, Schneeweiss S. Association between disease-modifying antirheumatic drugs and diabetes risk in patients with rheumatoid arthritis and psoriasis. *JAMA* (2011) 305:2525–31. doi: 10.1001/jama.2011.878
25. Morris SJ, Wasko MC, Antohe JL, Sartorius JA, Kirchner HL, Dancea S, et al. Hydroxychloroquine use associated with improvement in lipid profiles in rheumatoid arthritis patients. *Arthritis Care Res.* (2011) 63:530–4. doi: 10.1002/acr.20393
26. Le NT, Takei Y, Izawa-Ishizawa Y, Heo KS, Lee H, Smrcka AV, et al. Identification of activators of ERK5 transcriptional activity by high-throughput screening and the role of endothelial ERK5 in vasoprotective effects induced by statins and antimalarial agents. *J Immunol.* (2014) 193:3803–15. doi: 10.4049/jimmunol.1400571
27. Mathieu S, Pereira B, Tournadre A, Soubrier M. Cardiovascular effects of hydroxychloroquine: a systematic review and meta-analysis. *Ann Rheum Dis.* (2018) 77:e65. doi: 10.1136/annrheumdis-2017-212668
28. Reiss AB, Carsons SE, Anwar K, Rao S, Edelman SD, Zhang H, et al. Atheroprotective effects of methotrexate on reverse cholesterol transport proteins and foam cell transformation in human THP-1 monocyte/macrophages. *Arthritis Rheum.* (2008) 58:3675–83. doi: 10.1002/art.24040
29. Ronda N, Greco D, Adorni MP, Zimetti F, Favari E, Hjeltnes G, et al. Newly identified antiatherosclerotic activity of methotrexate and adalimumab: complementary effects on lipoprotein function and macrophage cholesterol metabolism. *Arthritis Rheumatol.* (2015) 67:1155–64. doi: 10.1002/art.39039
30. Hjeltnes G, Hollan I, Forre O, Wiik A, Lyberg T, Mikkelsen K, et al. Serum levels of lipoprotein(a) and E-selectin are reduced in rheumatoid arthritis patients treated with methotrexate or methotrexate in combination with TNF-alpha-inhibitor. *Clin Exp Rheumatol.* (2013) 31:415–21.
31. Kerekes G, Nurmohamed MT, Gonzalez-Gay MA, Seres I, Paragh G, Kardos Z, et al. Rheumatoid arthritis andmetabolic syndrome. *Nat Rev Rheumatol.* (2014) 10:691–6. doi: 10.1038/nrrheum.2014.121
32. Vandhuick T, Allanore Y, Borderie D, Louvel JP, Fardellone P, Dieude P, et al. Early phase clinical and biological markers associated with subclinical atherosclerosis measured at 7 years of evolution in an early inflammatory arthritis cohort. *Clin Exp Rheumatol.* (2016) 34:58–67.
33. Kim HJ, Kim MJ, Lee CK, Hong YH. Effects of methotrexate on carotid intima-media thickness in patients with rheumatoid arthritis. *J Korean Med Sci.* (2015) 30:1589–96. doi: 10.3346/jkms.2015.30.11.1589
34. Guin A, Chatterjee Adhikari M, Chakraborty S, Sinhamahapatra P, Ghosh A. Effects of disease modifying anti-rheumatic drugs on subclinical atherosclerosis and endothelial dysfunction which has been detected in early rheumatoid arthritis: 1-year follow-up study. *Semin Arthritis Rheum.* (2013) 43:48–54. doi: 10.1016/j.semarthrit.2012.12.027
35. Deyab G, Hokstad I, Whist JE, Smastuen MC, Agewall S, Lyberg T, et al. Methotrexate and anti-tumor necrosis factor treatment improves endothelial function in patients with inflammatory arthritis. *Arthritis Res Ther.* (2017) 19:232. doi: 10.1186/s13075-017-1439-1
36. Tam LS, Kitas GD, González-Gay MA. Can suppression of inflammation by anti-TNF prevent progression of subclinical atherosclerosis in inflammatory arthritis? *Rheumatology* (2014) 53:1108–19. doi: 10.1093/rheumatology/ket454
37. Dulai R, Perry M, Twycross-Lewis R, Morrissey D, Atzeni F, Greenwald S. The effect of tumor necrosis factor-α antagonists on arterial stiffness in rheumatoid arthritis: a literature review. *Semin Arthritis Rheum.* (2012) 42:1–8. doi: 10.1016/j.semarthrit.2012.02.002
38. Zekanecz Z, Kerekes G, Végh E, Kardos Z, Baráth Z, Tamási L, et al. Autoimmune atherosclerosis in 3D: how it develops, how to diagnose and what to do. Autoimmun Rev. (2016) 15:756–69. doi: 10.1016/j.autrev.2016.03.014
39. van Eijk IC, Peters MJ, Serné EH, van der Horst-Bruinsma IE, Dijkmans BA, Smulders YM, et al. Microvascular function is impaired in ankylosing spondylitis and improves after tumour necrosis factor alpha blockade. *Ann Rheum Dis.* (2009) 68:362–6. doi: 10.1136/ard.2007.086777
40. Nurmohamed M, Choy E, Lula S, Kola B, DeMasi R, Accossato P. The impact of biologics and tofacitinib on cardiovascular risk factors and outcomes in patients with rheumatic disease: a systematic literature review. *Drug Saf.* (2018) 41:473–88. doi: 10.1007/s40264-017-0628-9
41. Protogerou AD, Zampeli E, Fragiadaki K, Stamatelopoulos K, Papamichael C, Sfikakis PP. A pilot study of endothelial dysfunction and aortic stiffness after interleukin-6 receptor inhibition in rheumatoid arthritis. *Atherosclerosis* (2011) 219:734–6. doi: 10.1016/j.atherosclerosis.2011.09.015
42. Kume K, Amano K, Yamada S, Hatta K, Ohta H, Kuwaba N. Tocilizumab monotherapy reduces arterial stiffness as effectivelyvas etanercept or adalimumab monotherapy in rheumatoid arthritis: an open-label randomized controlled trial. *J Rheumatol.* (2011) 38:2169–71. doi: 10.3899/jrheum.110340
43. Kerekes G, Soltesz P, Der H, Veres K, Szabo Z, Vegvari A, et al. Effects of rituximab treatment on endothelial dysfunction, carotid atherosclerosis, and lipid profile in rheumatoid arthritis. *Clin Rheumatol.* (2009) 28:705–10. doi: 10.1007/s10067-009-1095-1
44. Provan SA, Berg IJ, Hammer HB, Mathiessen A, Kvien TK, Semb AG. The impact of newer biological disease modifying anti-rheumatic drugs on cardiovascular risk factors: a 12-month longitudinal study in rheumatoid arthritis patients treated with rituximab, abatacept and tociliziumab. *PLoS ONE* (2015) 10:e0130709. doi: 10.1371/journal.pone.0130709
45. Mathieu S, Pereira B, Dubost JJ, Lusson JR, Soubrier M. No significant change in arterial stiffness in RA after 6 months and 1 year of rituximab treatment. *Rheumatology* (2012) 51:1107–11. doi: 10.1093/rheumatology/kes006
46. Giles J. Rheumatoid arthritis pharmacotherapies: do they have anti-atherosclerotic activity? *Curr Rheumatol Rep.* (2016) 18:27. doi: 10.1007/s11926-016-0578-8
47. Micha R, Imamura F, Wyler von Ballmoos M, Solomon DH, Hernàn M, Ridker P, et al. Systematic review and meta-analysis of methotrexate use and risk of cardiovascular disease. *Am J Cardiol.* (2011) 108:1362–70. doi: 10.1016/j.amjcard.2011.06.054
48. De Vecchis R, Baldi C, Palmisani L. Protective effects of methotrexate against ischemic cardiovascular disorders in patients treated for rheumatoid arthritis or psoriasis: novel therapeutic insights coming from a meta-analysis of the literature data. *Anatol J Cardiol.* (2016) 16:2–9. doi: 10.5152/akd.2015.6136
49. Dixon WG, Watson KD, Lunt M, Hyrich KL, British Society for Rheumatology Biologics Register Control Centre Consortium, Silman AJ, et al. Reduction in the incidence ofmyocardial infarction in patients with rheumatoid arthritis who respond to anti-tumor necrosis factor alpha therapy: results from the British Society for Rheumatology Biologics Register. *Arthritis Rheum.* (2007) 56:2905–12. doi: 10.1002/art.22809
50. Low AS, Symmons DP, Lunt M, Mercer LK, Gale CP, Watson KD, et al. Relationship between exposure to tumour necrosis factor inhibitor

therapy and incidence and severity of myocardial infarction in patients with rheumatoid arthritis. *Ann Rheum Dis.* (2017) 76:654–660. doi: 10.1136/annrheumdis-2016-209784
51. Low AS, Lunt M, Mercer LK, Watson KD, Dixon WG, Symmons DP, et al. Association between ischemic stroke and tumor necrosis factor inhibitor therapy in patients with rheumatoid arthritis. *Arthritis Rheumatol.* (2016) 68:1337–45. doi: 10.1002/art.39582
52. Xie F, Yun H, Levitan EB, Muntner P, Curtis JR. Tocilizumab and the risk of cardiovascular disease: a direct comparison among biologic disease-modifying antirheumatic drugs for rheumatoid arthritis patients. *Arthritis Care Res.* (2018). doi: 10.1002/acr.23737. [Epub ahead of print].
53. Kim SC, Solomon DH, Rogers JR, Gale S, Klearman M, Sarsour K, et al. No difference in cardiovascular risk of tocilizumab versus abatacept for rheumatoid arthritis: a multi-database cohort study. *Semin Arthritis Rheum.* (2018). doi: 10.1016/j.semarthrit.2018.03.012. [Epub ahead of print].
54. Generali E, Carrara G, Selmi C, Verstappen S, Zambon A, Bortoluzzi A, et al. Comparison of the risks of hospitalisation for cardiovascular events in patients with rheumatoid arthritis treated with tocilizumab and etanercept. *Clin Exp Rheumatol.* (2018) 36:310–13.
55. Myasoedova E. Lipids and lipid changes with synthetic and biologic disease-modifying antirheumatic drug therapy in rheumatoid arthritis: implications for cardiovascular risk. *Curr Opin Rheumatol.* (2017) 29:277–84. doi: 10.1097/BOR.0000000000000378
56. McInnes IB, Thompson L, Giles JT, Bathon JM, Salmon JE, Beaulieu AD, et al. Effect of interleukin-6 receptor blockade on surrogates of vascular risk in rheumatoid arthritis: MEASURE, a randomised, placebo-controlled study. *Ann Rheum Dis.* (2015) 74:694–702. doi: 10.1136/annrheumdis-2013-204345
57. Zhang J, Xie F, Yun H, Chen L, Muntner P, Levitan EB, et al. Comparative effects of biologics on cardiovascular risk among older patients with rheumatoid arthritis. *Ann Rheum Dis.* (2016) 75:1813–8. doi: 10.1136/annrheumdis-2015-207870
58. Kang EH, Jin Y, Brill G, Lewey J, Patorno E, Desai RJ, et al. Comparative cardiovascular risk of Abatacept and Tumor Necrosis Factor Inhibitors in patients with rheumatoid arthritis with and without diabetes mellitus: A multidatabase cohort study. *J Am Heart Assoc.* (2018) 7:e007393. doi: 10.1161/JAHA.117.007393
59. Welsh P, Grassia G, Botha S, Sattar N, Maffia P. Targeting inflammation to reduce cardiovascular disease risk: a realistic clinical prospect? *Br J Pharmacol.* (2017) 174:3898–913. doi: 10.1111/bph.13818

6

Non-Cytotoxic Cardiac Innate Lymphoid Cells are a Resident and Quiescent Type 2-Commited Population

*William Bracamonte-Baran[1], Guobao Chen[1], Xuezhou Hou[2], Monica V. Talor[1], Hee Sun Choi[1], Giovanni Davogustto[3], Heinrich Taegtmeyer[3], Jungeun Sung[4], David Joel Hackam[5], David Nauen[1] and Daniela Čiháková[1,2]**

[1] Department of Pathology, School of Medicine, Johns Hopkins University, Baltimore, MD, United States, [2] W. Harry Feinstone Department of Molecular Microbiology and Immunology, Bloomberg School of Public Health, Johns Hopkins University, Baltimore, MD, United States, [3] Division of Cardiology, Department of Internal Medicine, University of Texas Medical School at Houston, Houston, TX, United States, [4] School of Medicine, Institute of Genetic Medicine, Johns Hopkins University, Baltimore, MD, United States, [5] Division of General Pediatric Surgery, Johns Hopkins University and Bloomberg Children's Center, Johns Hopkins Hospital, Baltimore, MD, United States

***Correspondence:**
Daniela Čiháková
cihakova@jhmi.edu
Orcid.org/0000-0002-8713-2860

Innate lymphoid cells (ILC) are a subset of leukocytes with lymphoid properties that lack antigen specific receptors. They can be stimulated by and exert their effect via specific cytokine axes, whereas Natural Killers (NK) cells are the only known cytotoxic member of this family. ILCs are considered key in linking the innate and adaptive response in physiologic and pathologic environments. In this study, we investigated the properties of non-cytotoxic cardiac ILCs in physiologic, inflammatory, and ischemic conditions. We found that in healthy humans and mice, non-cytotoxic cardiac ILCs are predominantly a type 2-committed population with progenitor-like features, such as an absence of type-specific immunophenotype, intermediate GATA3 expression, and capacity to transiently express Pro-myelocytic Leukemia Zinc Finger protein (PLZF) upon activation. During myocarditis and ischemia, in both human and mice, cardiac ILCs differentiated into conventional ILC2s. We found that cardiac ILCs lack IL-25 receptor and cannot become inflammatory ILC2s. We found a strong correlation between IL-33 production in the heart and the ability of cardiac ILCs to become conventional ILC2s. The main producer of IL-33 was a subset of CD29+Sca-1+ cardiac fibroblasts. ILC2 expansion and fibroblast-derived IL-33 production were significantly increased in the heart in mouse models of infarction and myocarditis. Despite its progenitor-like status in healthy hearts, cardiac ILCs were unable to become ILC1 or ILC3 *in vivo* and *in vitro*. Using adoptive transfer and parabiosis, we demonstrated that the heart, unlike other organs such as lung, cannot be infiltrated by circulating ILCs in adulthood even during cardiac inflammation or ischemia. Thus, the ILC2s present during inflammatory conditions are derived from the heart-resident and quiescent steady-state population. Non-cytotoxic cardiac ILCs are a resident population of ILC2-commited cells, with undifferentiated progenitor-like features in steady-state conditions and an ability to expand and develop pro-inflammatory type 2 features during inflammation or ischemia.

Keywords: innate lymphoid cells, IL-33, heart, myocarditis, myocardial infarction, fibroblasts

INTRODUCTION

Innate lymphoid cells (ILCs), formerly named nuocytes (1), are a subset of leukocytes with lymphoid properties in terms of their responsiveness and cytokine production, but lack antigen specific receptors (2–4). ILCs are considered to play a key role in the cross-talk between the innate and adaptive immune responses, thus providing a functional link between them (5).

Three classic subsets of ILCs have been described, named ILCs type 1 (ILC1s), type 2 (ILC2s), and type 3 (ILC3s), based on their functional profiles (3). ILCs plasticity and capacity of trans-differentiation have been widely reported (6–8). Non-cytotoxic ILC1s mirror and complement Th1 response, as those cells are stimulated by IL-12, and express IFNγ and TNFα upon activation (9, 10). ILC1s development depends on the transcription nuclear factor Tbet (11). The main role of ILC1's is assisting in the anti-viral response in a non-cytotoxic manner, thus supporting the Th1 response (12–14). Natural Killer (NK) cells are considered the only known cytotoxic subtype of ILCs, belong to the type 1 subset, and display significant functional and phenotypic differences as compared with non-cytotoxic ILCs (12).

ILC2s are classic mediators of the Th2 response and have been associated with typical Th2 processes, like anti-helmintic and allergic responses in the gastrointestinal and respiratory tracts (15–19). In addition, ILC2s were shown to be involved in tissue remodeling in the lung and liver and also play a role in regulation of the lipid metabolism in adipose tissues (20–24). The main products of ILC2s are IL-5 and IL-13, which contribute to eosinophils and other granulocytes maturation in the bone marrow and their chemotaxis. ILC2s characteristic nuclear transcription factor is GATA3 (17, 25–28). The main stimulator of classic ILC2s is IL-33, a cytokine known to be produced as an alarmin by a wide range of cells, such as endothelial cells during cellular stress and noxious conditions (29–32). In lung tissues, a subset of inflammatory ILC2s (i-ILC2s) was described that specifically responds to IL-25 stimulation but not IL-33 and has a combination of ILC2 and ILC3-like properties (33–35).

ILC3s contribute to the Th17 response by producing IL-17A and GM-CSF in response to IL-23 and IL-1β stimulation (36, 37). ILC3s differentiation is dependent on the nuclear factor Rorγt (38). This ILC subset is involved in anti-bacteria responses but is also linked to autoimmune diseases such as psoriasis, inflammatory bowel disease, and ankylosing spondylitis (39–41).

ILCs originate in the bone marrow from common lymphoid progenitors that give rise to common helper innate lymphoid progenitors (CHILP), which progress to ILCs progenitors (ILCPs) (25, 42, 43). ILCPs finally differentiate into classic ILC1s, ILC2s, or ILC3s, depending on the specific cytokine milieu in the target organ (25). Moreover, several stages of differentiation were described between ILCPs and classically differentiated ILCs. A first example are ILC2 progenitors, which have been found predominantly in the bone marrow, but also described in murine liver tissues (44). ILC2 progenitors have been described to have a Lineage^{neg}Sca-1^{+}Id2^{+}GATA3^{+} phenotype, with upregulation of ILC type 2-associated genes as *Klrg1, Il2rα, Ccr9* (27, 44–46). The second example are peripheral human multipotent ILCPs, which lack type-specific phenotype but express CD117 (cKit) (47). Peripheral ILCPs are a circulating population that has been described as being able to infiltrate organs such as liver, lung, and cord blood, and its final fate is determined by tissue-specific microenvironments, being able to differentiate into ILC1s, ILC2s, and ILC3s (47). The development of ILCs depends on the expression of the IL-2 receptor common γ-chain (γc), whereas recombinant activating gene (RAG) is not required (48). GATA3, although considered characteristic of fully differentiated classic ILC2s, is also required for the development of ILCPs (49). In addition, a nuclear factor—the Pro-myelocytic Leukemia Zinc Finger Protein (PLZF)—is needed for the development of ILCPs and its differentiation into specific ILC types. PLZF is known to be transiently expressed during ILCP activation and differentiation (42, 49). Although it was reported that PLZF gene expression (*Zbtb16*) is transversally decreased in ILC2 progenitors as compared to earlier progenitors (44), its complex expression dynamics over time during ILC development has not been completely elucidated.

Little is known about non-cytotoxic cardiac ILCs. Their identity, origin, phenotype, and functionality has not been studied so far. We have previously described the role NK cells in myocarditis (50, 51). Thus, in this study we seek to comprehensively characterize non-cytotoxic cardiac ILCs, their function and behavior during heart inflammatory diseases.

Compared with other organs in which ILCs have been described, the heart has unique histological, cellular, and functional properties. Volumetrically, the heart is mainly a muscular organ, lacking a classic epithelium, but rather having an extensive endothelial layer in the endocardium and a serosal epithelium, which constitute the pericardium (52). Multiple type of mesenchymal and bone marrow derived cells reside in the heart, generating a complex microenvironment (53). The lineage and origins of cardiac cells are complex and not entirely understood (52). We and others have shown that cardiac fibroblasts are active contributors to cardiac inflammation by producing GM-CSF, CCL2, or CCL11 (54–58). Interestingly, IL-33 is produced by cardiac endothelial cells during pressure overload (30).

In this study, we evaluated non-cytotoxic cardiac ILCs in healthy human and mouse hearts and in ischemic cardiomyopathy and myocarditis. We found that cardiac ILCs

Abbreviations: CCR-, C-C chemokine receptor; CHILP, common helper-like innate lymphoid progenitor; cKit, proto-oncogene tyrosine-protein kinase Kit (synonym of CD117 and mast/stem cell growth factor receptor); CD, cluster of differentiation; CRTH2, chemoattractant Receptor-homologous molecule expressed on T-Helper type 2 cells (synonymous of DP2, Prostaglandin D_2 receptor 2); EAM, experimental autoimmune myocarditis; GATA3, G-A-T-A sequence-recognizing transcription factor 3; Id2, DNA-binding protein inhibitor 2; i-ILC, inflammatory innate lymphoid cell; ILC, innate lymphoid cell; ILCP, innate lymphoid cell progenitor; KLRG1, killer cell lectin-like receptor subfamily G member 1; LVAD, left ventricle assist device; MFI, geometric mean fluorescence intensity; MI, myocardial infarction; NK, natural killer; PBMC, peripheral blood mononuclear cell; PLZF, pro-myelocytic leukemia zinc finger protein; Rorγt, retinoic acid receptor alpha-related orphan receptor gamma; Tbet, T-box transcription factor TBX21; tSNE, t-distributed stochastic neighbor embedding; γc, IL-2 receptor common gamma chain.

are an ILC2-commited population. Under normal conditions, the cardiac ILC population was mainly undifferentiated with an incomplete ILC2 phenotype, while lacking ILC1 and ILC3 markers. During ischemia and myocarditis cardiac ILCs differentiated into ILC2s but not ILC1s and ILC3s. The number of ILC2s in the heart was associated with an increase of IL-33 production by cardiac fibroblasts. Furthermore, we found that non-cytotoxic cardiac ILCs are strictly cardiac resident cells during adulthood and circulating ILCs and ILCPs are unable to seed heart tissues.

RESULTS

Innate Lymphoid Cells Type 2 Are Predominant in Heart of Patients With Ischemic Cardiomyopathy or Myocarditis

We used multiparameter flow cytometry to comprehensively characterize non-cytotoxic cardiac ILCs in human endomyocardial biopsy samples. Biopsies were taken from ischemic cardiomyopathy ($n = 5$) and myocarditis ($n = 5$) patients with heart failure during left ventricular assist device (LVAD) implantation. Both groups displayed similar clinical, hemodynamic, and echocardiographic features. The only significant difference between the groups was a lower mean age of the myocarditis patients (**Table 1**). Controls were rapid autopsy specimens from deceased patients without any cardiac pathology ($n = 4$). To exclude all lymphocytes, myeloid cells, other classic leukocytes subsets including CD11b^{+} NK cells, and other potential CD45^{dim} cells, we used a Lineage channel containing CD3, TCRαβ, CD20, CD11c, CD11b, CD123, BDCA2, CD14, FcεR1α, CD31, and CD34 in the flow cytometry gating strategy. Among CD45^{+}Lineage^{neg} cells, non-cytotoxic ILCs were characterized as CD127 (IL-7R)$^{+}$ (**Figure 1A** and **Supplementary Figure 1**). CD11b^{+} NK cells, a cytotoxic ILC1 subset, were excluded from this analysis with the Lineage cocktail, whereas CD11b^{neg} NK cells were excluded from the non-cytotoxic ILC analysis by gating on CD127^{+}CD56^{neg}NKp44^{neg} cells (59) (**Figure 1** and **Supplementary Figure 1**). Non-cytotoxic ILC immunophenotypes were determined as ILC1 Tbet^{+}, ILC2 CRTH2^{+}, ILC3 Rorγt^{+}IL23R^{+}, or CD56^{+} (**Figure 1A** and **Supplementary Figure 1**) (59). The undifferentiated ILC population was CD127^{+}CD45^{+}Lineage^{neg} but also negative for all other cell type-specific markers such as CD56, NKp44, CRTH2, Rorγt, and IL23R (**Figure 1A** and **Supplementary Figure 1**). A significant proportion of non-cytotoxic ILCs was undifferentiated in normal controls, as well as in ischemic cardiomyopathy and myocarditis. The undifferentiated ILC population was predominant in normal controls, representing around 75% of the ILCs (**Figures 1B,C**). In ischemic cardiomyopathy and myocarditis, the undifferentiated ILC population decreased to about 25%, and ILC2 became the dominant population, representing around 65% of total ILCs (**Figures 1B,C**). That shift of undifferentiated ILCs to ILC2s was accompanied by minimal changes in non-cytotoxic ILC1 and ILC3 subpopulations (**Figures 1B,C**). In order to comprehensively characterize the entire ILC population

TABLE 1 | Clinical and hemodynamic characteristics of patients.

Variable	Ischemic cardiomyopathy	Myocarditis	Intergroup *P*
Number of patients	5	5	-
% of males	100%	100%	-
Age (years)	62.40 ± 2 .73	35.00 ± 8.32	0.01
Height (cm)	173.60 ± 2.22	180.60 ± 3.04	0.10
Weight (Kg)	81.68 ± 5.41	96.42 ± 5.66	0.09
EF (%)	21.00 ± 2.44	16.00 ± 1.00	0.09
LVIDd (cm)	7.20 ± 0.21	7.25 ± 0.30	0.89
LVPWd (cm)	1.06 ± 0.02	0.87 ± 0.08	0.05
IVSd (cm)	0.94 ± 0.09	0.90 ± 0.08	0.76
BNP (pg/mL)	971.60 ± 531.10	1285.00 ± 536.70	0.71
Troponin level	5/5 <0.15 pg/m	2/2 available <0.15 pg/mL	-
Patients going to OHT	5/5	4/5 (1 patient to Jarvik)	-
Days on LVAD	339.80 ± 50.70	688.00 ± 208.10	0.14

EF, Ejection fraction; LVIDd, Left ventricular internal diameter end diastole; LVPWd, Left ventricular posterior wall end diastole; IVSdL, Interventricular septum end diastole; BNP, Brain natriuretic peptide; OHT, Orthotopic heart transplant; LVAD, Left ventricular assist device.

and clearly dissect NK cells from the non-cytotoxic ILCs, we performed similar flow cytometry analyses in autopsy myocardial specimens, but placing CD11b in a separated channel out of the Lineage cocktail (**Supplementary Figure 2**). We confirmed that cardiac NK cells are mutually exclusive of non-cytotoxic ILCs, displaying a CD11b^{+}CD56^{+}NKp44^{neg}CD127^{neg} profile. Conversely, non-cytotoxic ILCs were strictly CD127^{+}. Following this alternative strategy, we found identical pattern of non-cytotoxic cardiac ILCs in the human heart. There were no ILC1 and ILC3 while 20% of cardiac ILC2s population were CRTH2^{+} ILC2s. The non-cytotoxic cardiac ILCs were mainly undifferentiated ILCs (~80%) (**Supplementary Figure 2**).

To better understand and validate the ILC2 and undifferentiated ILCs phenotype observed in the heart based on CRTH2 expression, we performed immunophenotyping of healthy human PBMCs ($n = 3$), (**Supplementary Figure 3**). We found a population of activated NKp44^{+}CD127^{neg}CD56^{+}Tbet^{+} population distinct from non-cytotoxic circulating ILCs, which were mainly comprised of ILC2s (~60%) which homogenously expressed CRTH2. No undifferentiated ILC population was found in clear contrast to its dominant presence in the heart (**Supplementary Figure 3**).

Since cardiac ILCs are an extremely infrequent population, we performed analyzes of the immunophenotype clustering pattern of the non-cytotoxic cardiac ILC subpopulations using t-distributed Stochastic Neighbor Embedding (tSNE), a machine learning algorithm of dimensional reduction, in order to validate the conventional gating analyses. The clustering pattern in tSNE plots is considered a strong supportive evidence of the feasibility of those small subsets (60, 61). tSNE analyses were performed on concatenates of all the samples for each group, and a robust nucleated clustering of undifferentiated ILCs and ILC2s was observed (See Methods for technical details). ILC2 pattern in

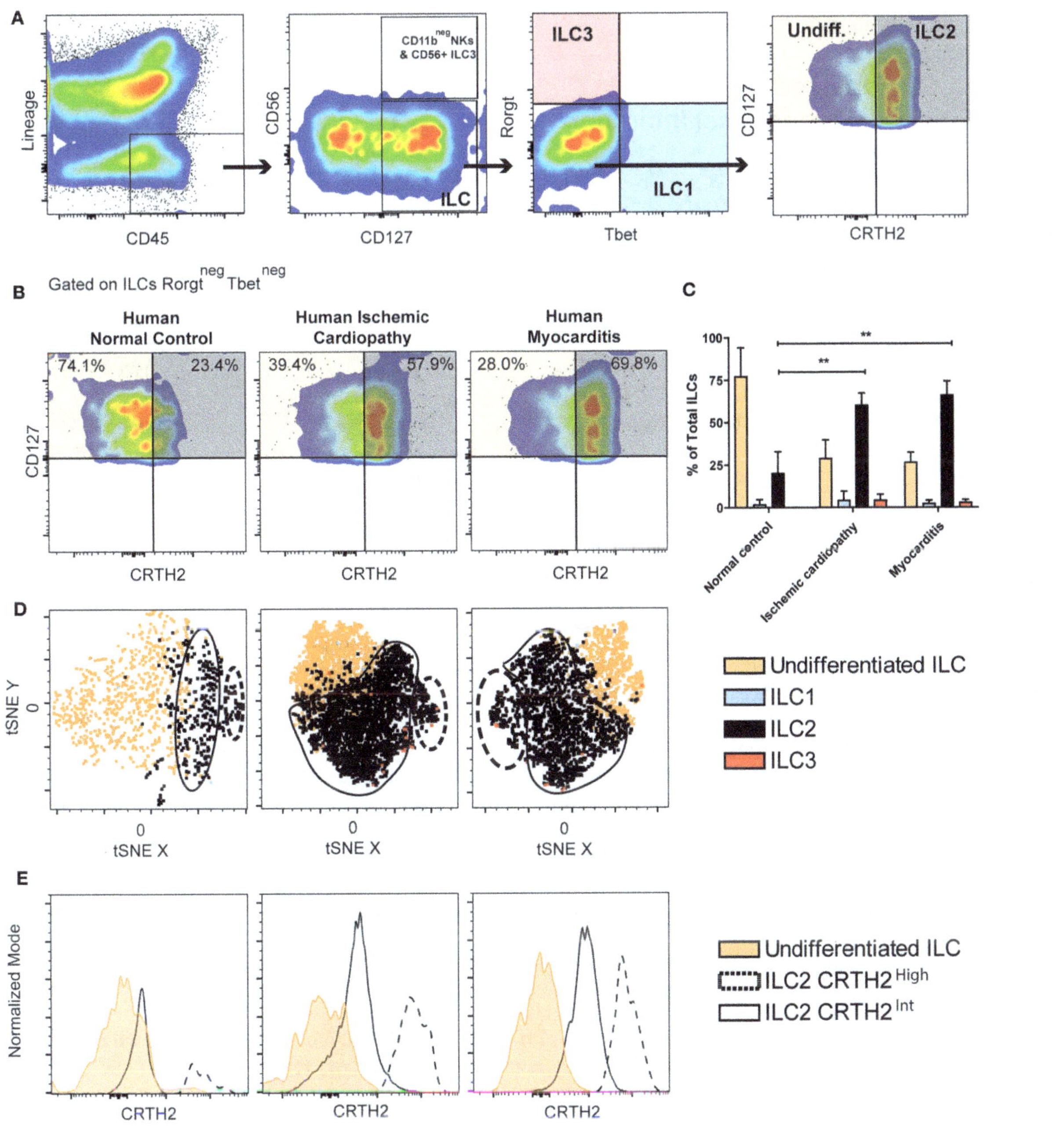

FIGURE 1 | Majority of human ILCs are undifferentiated in healthy hearts, whereas ILC2s predominate in ischemic cardiomyopathy and myocarditis. **(A)** Human cardiac ILCs gating strategy, ILCs were defined as $CD45^{+}Lineage^{neg}CD127^{+}$, NK cells as $CD56^{+}NKp44^{+}$, non-cytotoxic ILC1s (blue) as $Tbet^{+}$, ILC2s (gray) as $CRTH2^{+}GATA3^{int-high}$, ILC3s (transparent red) as $Ror\gamma t^{+}IL\text{-}23R^{+}$.Undifferentiated ILCs (transparent orange) were defined as ILCs negative for all type-specific markers. **(D)** Representative flow cytometry plots showing median examples of the profile of undifferentiated ILCs and ILC2s gated in $Ror\gamma t^{neg}$ $Tbet^{neg}$ ILCs. **(C)** Frequency of ILC subsets in healthy human hearts, ischemic cardiomyopathy and myocarditis. **(D)** tSNE clustering analyses of ILCs immunophenotypes. **(E)** Comparison of CRTH2 expression in two distinctive ILC2s population in normal hearts, ischemic cardiomyopathy and myocarditis. Data show $n = 5$ for ischemic cardiomyopathy, $n = 5$ for myocarditis and $n = 4$ for controls. tSNE plots are concatenates of all the samples for group. Bar graphs shows Mean and SD. Statistics were calculated using Dunnett's test. $^{**}P < 0.01$.

both ischemic cardiomyopathy and myocarditis showed two distinctive and significantly populated clusters (**Figure 1D**). The difference between those two clusters was the magnitude of CRTH2 expression (**Figure 1E**). We found an increase in the proportion of cells belonging to the cluster with a higher expression of CRTH2 in both diseases (**Figures 1D,E**). Thus, we observed increased proportion of the ILC2 population in the heart of patients with chronic ischemic cardiomyopathy and myocarditis, in contrast to a predominantly undifferentiated ILC profile in healthy human hearts.

Cardiac ILC2 Population Increases in Murine Models of Myocardial Infarction and Myocarditis

Next, we examined murine cardiac ILCs in two models of cardiac diseases, myocardial infarction (MI) and experimental autoimmune myocarditis (EAM), using the flow cytometry approach. Severity of EAM at day 21 was assessed with standard histology (H&E, **Supplementary Figure 4A**). The gating strategy followed the same rationale as human experiments, while using the standardized markers for mouse ILCs. Mouse ILCs were defined as $CD45^{+}Lineage^{neg}CD90^{+}$, where the Lineage was CD3, TCRβ, CD5, CD19, CD11b, CD11c, GR1, FcεR1α, CD31, and TER119, to exclude other $CD45^{+}$ populations, erythroid and endothelial cells. The $CD11b^{+}$ NK population was excluded by the presence of CD11b in the Lineage cocktail. Downstream in the gating strategy, $CD11b^{neg}$ NK cells were identified by NKp46 positivity and further Rorγt evaluation. Within the non-cytotoxic ILCs ($CD45^{+}Lineage^{neg}CD90^{+}NKp46^{neg}$) the classic subpopulations were characterized as $Tbet^{+}$ ILC1s, $ST2^{+}KLRG1^{+}GATA3^{int-high}$ ILC2s, $Ror\gamma t^{+}$ ILC3s and $Tbet^{neg}Ror\gamma t^{neg}ST2^{low}KLRG1^{neg-int}$ undifferentiated ILCs population (**Figure 2A**). We did not find differences in the composition of the cardiac ILCs compartment between naïve, mock immunized and sham surgery controls (**Supplementary Figure 4B**). Within the $CD90^{+}NKp46^{+}$ population we did not found Rorγt, which excluded the existence of $NKp46^{+}$ ILC3s (**Supplementary Figure 4C**). The ILC population did not express Rorγt or IL25R nor hyper-high levels of KLRG1 (**Figure 2A** and **Supplementary Figure 4D**). Thus, we ruled out an inflammatory ILC (i-ILC2) and ILC3 identity (**Figures 2A,B** and **Supplementary Figure 4D**). Unlike peripheral ILCPs (47), the cardiac ILC population was CD117 (cKit) negative (**Supplementary Figure 4D**). Around 75% of cardiac ILCs were undifferentiated in naïve controls, resembling the findings in human endomyocardial biopsy samples (**Figures 1B, 2B**). We found a significant increase of ILC2 to about 45% of total cardiac ILC population in MI, paralleled by a decrease in the undifferentiated ILC population (**Figures 2B–C**). The proportion of ILC1s and ILC3s was negligible. In EAM, although the flow cytometry plot showed a qualitatively more robust ILC2 differentiation with stronger ST2 expression, the increase in the proportion of this population was not statistically significant relative to controls (**Figures 2B–C**). Nevertheless, the absolute ILC count in the heart demonstrated a significant increase in both, undifferentiated and ILC2s in EAM as compared to controls (**Supplementary Figures 4C,D**). In fact, the increase in the absolute number of cardiac ILC2 in MI was comparable to that in EAM (**Supplementary Figure 4E**). In EAM, the undifferentiated population also expanded significantly (**Supplementary Figure 4F**). ILC2s had a higher GATA3 expression as compared with undifferentiated ILCs in all conditions, although undifferentiated ILCs intermediately express GATA3 (**Figure 2D**). GATA3 mean fluorescent intensity (MFI) expression in EAM and MI was normalized to the mean GATA3 MFI of naïve controls. The normalized GATA3 expression by ILC2s in naïve hearts was 1.5 higher than the mean of undifferentiated ILCs (**Figure 2E**). In MI and EAM hearts, we observed a 2.5-fold upregulation of GATA3 in the expanded ILC2 population, compared to undifferentiated ILCs (**Figure 2E**). To confirm the reliability of such a small population, we validated the conventional gating strategy with tSNE analyses of concatenated samples for each experimental group, following the same approach used with human samples. We also found a robust clustering of the undifferentiated and ILC2 population, thus supporting the homogeneity of each subset and ruling out significant noise interference (**Figure 2F**).

In order to precisely discriminate NK cells from non-cytotoxic ILCs, we analyzed non-cytotoxic ILCs and NK cells in the hearts of WT Balb/c mice, placing CD11b and CD3 out of the Lineage cocktail (**Supplementary Figure 5A**). We found that the vast majority of NK cells were $CD11b^{+}CD90^{neg}CD122^{+}$. Importantly, the $CD11b^{neg}CD90^{+}NKp46^{+}$ population was strictly an NK population and not an ILC3 subset, as it displayed a downstream $CD122^{+}Ror\gamma t^{neg}$ status, thus confirming again the absence of ILC3 in murine heart tissues (**Supplementary Figure 5A**). With this alternative gating strategy, we found an identical pattern amongst non-cytotoxic ILCs as in the previous experiments, with predominance of undifferentiated ILCs over ILC2s (**Supplementary Figure 5B**).

Despite we observed a significantly more robust expansion of ILC2s percentagewise during myocarditis in humans as compared with murine EAM, the predominance of undifferentiated ILCs and the overall composition of this compartment in naïve mouse hearts resembled the human controls. Also, a similar expansion of differentiated ILC2s was observed in murine and human ischemic heart diseases. Thus, our findings suggest that heart ILCs are a quiescent and phenotypically undifferentiated population which develop ILC type 2 features during inflammatory processes such as ischemia and autoimmunity.

A Subset of Cardiac Fibroblasts Express IL-33 During MI and EAM

IL-33 is the main stimulus for ILC2 differentiation and expansion (33, 62). We found that in both humans and mice, ILC2 expanded during cardiac ischemia and myocarditis despite the differences in the initial insult. We used a knock-in IL-33 reporter mouse strain ($il33^{citrine/+}$) to determine the source of IL-33 during MI and EAM. A small proportion of cardiac resident cells constitutively express IL-33 in naïve state (**Figure 3A**). The number of IL-33-producing cardiac cells significantly expanded during MI and EAM, about 6-fold and 10-fold, respectively (**Figure 3A**). In all conditions, the predominant IL-33^{+} cells were $CD45^{neg}CD31^{neg}CD29^{+}$ cardiac fibroblasts (**Figure 3A**). Within the cardiac fibroblasts, the IL-33 production was restricted to the Sca-1^{+} subset (**Figure 3B**). The proportion of IL-33^{+} cells among fibroblasts showed a 20-fold increase in MI and EAM compared to controls (**Figure 3C**). tSNE analysis demonstrates a well-defined cluster of Sca-1^{+} cardiac fibroblasts, representing

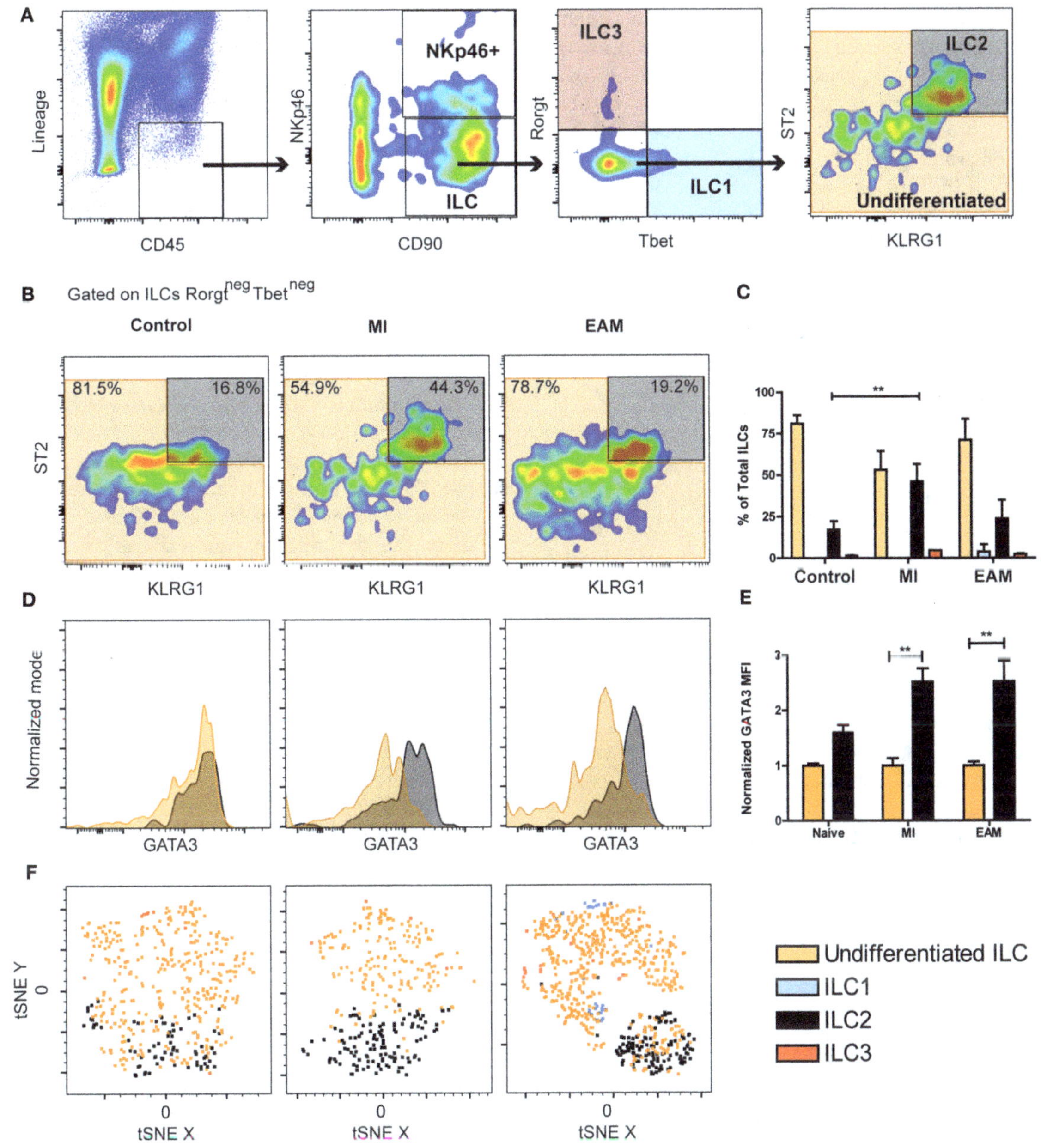

FIGURE 2 | Undifferentiated ILCs are predominant in naïve mice hearts, while the ILC2 compartment expands during MI and EAM. **(A)** Mouse cardiac ILCs gating strategy, defining ILCs as $CD45^{+}Lineage^{neg}CD90^{+}$, $CD11b^{neg}$ NK cells and $NKp46^{+}$ ILC3s as $CD90^{+}NKp46^{+}$, non-cytotoxic ILC1s (blue) as $Tbet^{+}$, ILC2s (gray) as $ST2^{+}KLRG1^{+}GATA3^{int-high}$, ILC3s (transparent red) as $Roryt^{+}$. Undifferentiated ILCs (transparent orange) as ILCs negative for all ILC type-specific markers. **(B)** Representative flow cytometry plots show median examples of the profile of undifferentiated ILCs and ILC2s in naïve, MI and EAM hearts gated on $Roryt^{neg}$ $Tbet^{neg}$ ILCs. Frequency of ILC types in naïve, MI, EAM hearts. **(D)** Representative flow cytometry histograms show GATA3 expression on ILC2s (black) and undifferentiated ILCs (orange). **(E)** Normalized GATA3 MFI in naïve, MI, and EAM hearts. **(F)** tSNE analysis shows ILC2 clustering (black) within the undifferentiated population (orange). Plots, including tSNE analyses, show concatenates of all mice in each group of 1 of 3 independent experiments (n = 4–5 group / experiment). Bar graphs shows Mean and SD. Statistics for **(C,E)** calculated by Dunnett's test. $^{**}P < 0.01$.

about 50% of total $CD29^{+}$ fibroblasts (**Supplementary Figure 6**). The sub-population of IL-33^{+} fibroblasts was entirely restricted to the cluster of Sca-1^{+} fibroblasts (**Supplementary Figure 6**). We used microscopy flow cytometry (ImageStream) to verify the reliability of the signal of the IL-33 reporter molecule (citrine) and visually corroborate the conventional flow cytometry results. We confirmed the predominance of Sca-1^{+} fibroblasts as the source of IL-33. The IL-33/citrine signal showed the expected homogeneous intracellular pattern, thus ruling out auto-fluorescence phenomena. Even within the IL-33^{+} cells, the citrine intensity was dimmer in controls as compared with MI and EAM (**Figures 3D–F**). The absolute number of ILC2s in the heart showed a linear correlation with the proportion of IL-33 producing cells amongst total cellularity in all conditions (**Figure 3G**), whereas the ILC2s' absolute count had an exponential correlation with the proportion of IL-33$^+$ cells within the fibroblasts (**Figure 3H**). These results strongly suggest that, regardless of the type of noxa (autoimmune or ischemic), IL-33 is produced by a subset of cardiac fibroblasts during tissue damage, leading to a differentiation of quiescent cardiac ILCs and expansion of the ILC2 compartment.

Naïve Cardiac ILCs Are a Type-2 Committed Population With Restricted Plasticity

To evaluate the functional capacity and plasticity of the predominantly undifferentiated non-cytotoxic ILC population in a naïve mouse heart, we performed *in vitro* differentiation experiments. We FACS sorted CD45$^+$Lineage^{neg}CD90$^+$NKp46^{neg} ILCs from naïve mice hearts. Then, ILCs were stimulated with different cytokines for 6 days to induce type-specific differentiation. To induce ILC1 differentiation, we used recombinant cytokines IL-2+IL-7+IL-12, to generate ILC2s we used IL-2+IL-7+IL-33 and for ILC3 induction, IL-2+IL-7+IL-23. As controls we included plain media and IL-2+IL-7 only. ILCs in media only were undifferentiated with mild expression of Ki67 and no expression of the PLZF (**Figure 4A**). Unspecific stimulation with IL-2+IL-7 induced a moderate activation of cardiac ILCs, characterized by co-expression of Ki67 and PLZF (**Figure 4A**), but no significant Rorγt, Tbet, or ST2 and KLRG1 expression (**Figures 4B,C**). The proportion of ILC2s under stimulation with IL-2+IL-7 was slightly higher than plain media (**Figure 4C**). ILCs stimulated with type 1, 2, and 3 differentiating conditions were activated (**Figure 4A**), reaching statistical significance in every case in respect to the media control (**Figure 4D**). Nevertheless, the proportion of activated PLZF$^+$Ki67$^+$ cells was significantly higher with the IL-33 stimulation as compared to controls as well as IL-12 and IL-23 conditions (**Figure 4D**). Unexpectedly, IL-12 and IL-23 were unable to induce ILC1 and ILC3 differentiation, respectively (**Figure 4B**). No differences were observed between controls, stimulation with IL-23 and IL-1β (**Supplementary Figures 7A–E**). IL-33, in conjunction to IL-2+IL-7, induced a robust ILC2 differentiation (**Figures 4A,C,E**). Finally, as a functional readout, the main ILC1, 2, and 3 cytokines were analyzed in the supernatants by ELISA. Congruent with the immunophenotype, neither IFNγ, TNFα nor IL-17A increased in any of the conditions and remain at basal levels (**Figure 4F** and **Supplementary Figure 7F**). IL-33 induced a marked and significant production of IL-5 and IL-13 (**Figure 4F**).

The monotonic PLZF/Ki67 co-expression (~85%) achieved only in IL-33 conditions suggests that the entire non-cytotoxic cardiac ILC population, including the undifferentiated ones, have a type 2-biased functionality evidenced by responsiveness to IL33. To rule out the possibility of exclusive expansion of already differentiated ILC2 during this experiments, we FACS sorted CD45$^+$Lineage^{neg}CD90$^+$NKp46^{neg}ST2$^+$ cardiac ILCs and culture them with IL-2+IL-7+IL-33 for 6 days. That small subset failed to significantly proliferate and differentiate (**Supplementary Figure 7G**), thus strongly suggesting that undifferentiated ILC population, or at least a subset of them, can differentiate to a full ILC2 status, but not to ILC1 or ILC3 phenotype.

These results confirm that naïve non-cytotoxic cardiac ILC population is committed with an ILC2 fate and functionality, despite its undifferentiated status in steady-state conditions.

Naïve Cardiac ILCs Transiently Express PLZF Upon Activation and ILC2 Differentiation

PLZF has been described as a nuclear factor transiently expressed by subsets of ILC progenitors during activation, including the subset of ILC2-commited progenitors (42). As naïve cardiac ILCs were predominantly undifferentiated but ILC2-commited, we decided to perform timeline *in vitro* experiments to study the dynamics of their activation and steady-state properties. We determined the kinetics of Ki67 and PLZF expression to address the naïve cardiac ILCs' proliferation capacity and progenitor features (**Figure 5A**). Also, we analyzed the progression of the ILC2-associated transcription factor GATA3 (**Figure 5B**) and the evolution of ILC2 phenotype (**Figure 5C**) over time under the influence of IL-33. Naïve cardiac ILCs CD45$^+$Lineage^{neg}CD90$^+$NKp46^{neg} were FACS sorted and cultured *in vitro* with IL-2+IL-7+IL-33, and its phenotypic and functional changes assessed on days 1, 3, 5, and 7. The activation dynamics showed a low baseline ILCs activation at day 1. Ki67$^+$PLZF$^+$ co-expression progressively increased, reaching significance at day 3 and peaking at day 5 (**Figures 5A,D**), when a monotonic co-expression was achieved. PLZF and Ki67 levels abruptly decayed after day 5, returning to baseline levels by day 7, demonstrating a pattern of transient PLZF expression after cytokine-induced activation (**Figures 5A,D**). GATA3, however, showed different kinetics than PLZF, as it progressively increased, reaching a plateau at day 5 and persisting significantly elevated at day 7 (**Figures 5B,E**). The ILC2 phenotype developed progressively in terms of KLRG1 and ST2 co-expression, following a quasi-linear dynamic after day 3 (**Figures 5C,F**). Finally, the production of IL-5 and IL-13 increased in parallel following an exponential pattern (**Figure 5G**). Therefore, we found that cardiac ILCs, in addition to having an undifferentiated phenotype and negligible cytokine production in resting conditions, display a progenitor-like activation pattern, implying transient expression of PLZF. This behavior suggests an incomplete, yet biased, differentiation in normal conditions, compatible with a committed progenitor status.

Cardiac ILCs Are a Strictly Resident Population

To differentiate resident vs. infiltrating status of cardiac non-cytotoxic ILCs, we performed adoptive transfer experiments. Bone marrow ILC progenitors, Lineage^{neg}CD45$^+$Id2$^+$Sca-1$^+$

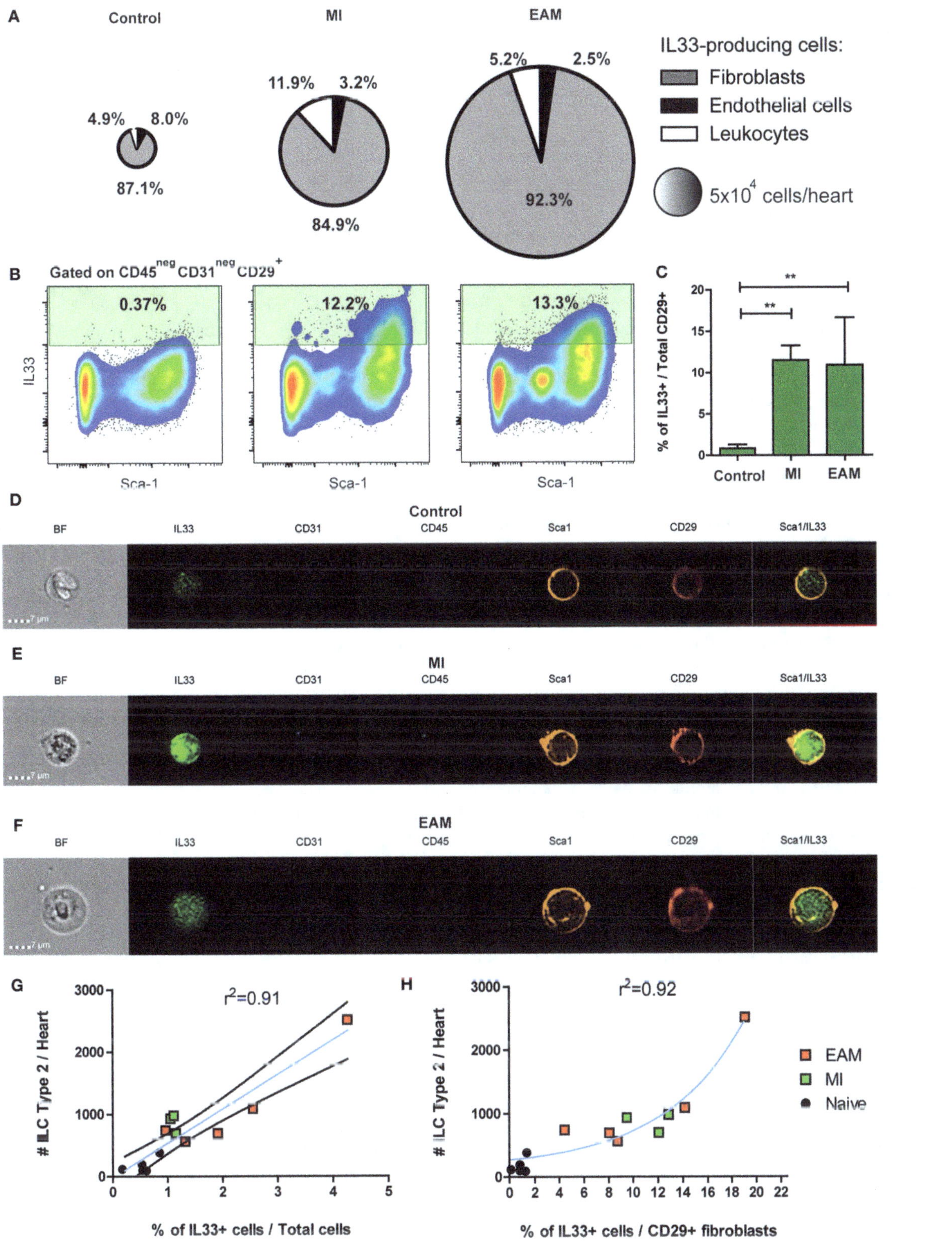

FIGURE 3 | IL-33 is expressed by cardiac fibroblasts during MI and EAM. **(A)** Pie charts represent the percentage and total number of the heart IL-33-producing population and its composition in naïve, MI, and EAM hearts. Charts are based on concatenates of all mice in a group. **(B)** Representative flow plots of IL-33 expression by $CD45^{neg}CD31^{neg}CD29^{+}$ fibroblasts are shown for all conditions. Median examples are shown. **(C)** Frequency of IL-33 producing cardiac fibroblasts

(Continued)

FIGURE 3 | in naïve, MI and EAM hearts. **(D–F)** Representative examples of Microscopy flow cytometry (ImageStream) single cells images, showing the pattern of IL-33, Sca-1, and CD29 expression in cardiac fibroblasts. Representative examples of 500–1,500 events per sample are shown. **(G)** Linear regression of absolute number of ILC2s and percentage of IL-33$^+$ cells in naïve, MI, and EAM hearts analyzed together. Blue line shows linear function and black lines the 95% confidence interval. **(H)** Regression plot shows an exponential correlation between absolute number of ILC2s and percentage of IL-33$^+$ cells amongst fibroblasts, represented by the blue line. Data of 1 of 2 independent experiments, $n = 5$ for controls and EAM, $n = 3$ for MI. Bar graphs shows Mean and SD. Correlations estimated using Pearson r. Statistic difference of means were calculated with Dunnett's test. $^{**}P < 0.01$.

cells were FACS sorted from semi-allogeneic $H2^{b/d}$ $Id2^{GFP}$ reporter mice and transferred into $RAG2^{-/-}$ $\gamma c^{-/-}$ $H2^{d}$ mice, allowing to track the transferred ILCs based on $H2\text{-}K^{b}$ expression (**Figure 6A**). After 28 days of the transference, no heart-infiltrating ILCs were detected, but we found a small but well-defined infiltrating ILC population in lung tissues (**Figures 6B,C**). To further investigate the origin of cardiac ILCs, we performed parabiosis experiments. In this experimental setting, CD45.1 mice underwent EAM induction (on days 0 and 7), and were surgically paired to CD45.2 naïve mice on day 2. Pairs with a mock immunized CD45.1 mouse and naïve CD45.1 were used as controls (**Figure 6D**). In naïve parabionts, the chimeric cells were CD45.1, whereas in mock and EAM parabionts, the chimeric cells were tracked based on CD45.2 expression (**Figure 6E**). We checked establishment of leukocyte chimerism in peripheral blood at day 14 in every case, finding a successful engraftment of 30–40% (not shown). On day 21, all groups had leukocyte chimerism in their hearts, about 20% in naïve parabionts and 35–40% in mock and EAM parabionts (**Figures 6F,G**). Nevertheless, the chimerism in the cardiac ILC compartment was disproportionately low as compared with the total leukocyte engraftment. In all conditions, the chimeric ILCs represented about 5% of the heart ILC population (**Figures 6F,G**). Leukocyte mixed chimerism also occurred in lungs, with 50% engraftment in naïve parabionts and about 20% in mock and EAM parabionts. In naïve parabionts, the specific pulmonary ILC engraftment was also disproportionally low as compared with the leukocyte chimerism, representing about 8% of the ILC population compared to 50% of leukocyte population. Conversely, in mock and EAM mice, both known to have systemic inflammation due to use of CFA as adjuvant (63), the ILC engraftment in the lungs was proportional and not statistically different as compared to the whole leukocyte chimerism, representing both 20–30% of the ILC and leukocyte compartments, respectively (**Figures 6H,I**). Lung engraftment demonstrated the intrinsic infiltrative capacity of circulating ILCs. These adoptive transfer and parabiosis results suggest that heart is a unique niche with resident ILCs that are not replenished from blood ILCs even during cardiac inflammation during myocarditis or after ischemia.

DISCUSSION

ILCs are a subset of leukocytes which play a key role in multiple immune processes, providing a link between the innate and the adaptive responses (2). Originally, ILCs were considered patrollers of mucosa- and epithelium-associated tissues, such as the respiratory tract, gut, and skin (15). Further investigation has revealed their presence and physiologic importance in organs, such as the liver and adipose tissue, having an impact even in modulating metabolic processes (20, 21, 23). In this paper, we investigated characteristics of heart ILCs.

We found that in normal human heart and naïve mouse tissues, cardiac ILCs lack a well-defined immunophenotype, and we denoted them as undifferentiated. Those ILCs did not express ILC1 nor ILC3 markers. In normal human hearts, the majority of cardiac ILCs were undifferentiated as they did not express the ILC2-specific marker CRTH2 (64). In naïve mice, the predominant undifferentiated cardiac ILCs expressed intermediate levels of GATA3 and variable levels of KLRG1. They did not express ST2 as conventional ILC2s do. Undifferentiated ILCs neither expressed high levels of KLRG1, IL25R (IL-17RB), nor Rorγt as is characteristic for inflammatory ILC2s (i-ILC2s) (34). The predominance of ILCs without a fully mature phenotype in normal hearts is different from the typical complete ILC differentiation described in organs such as the skin, lung, and gut (65). Our findings support the concept that normal ILCs status depends on an organ-specific milieu leading to a tissue-specific ILC training, a phenomenon previously described as "ILC-poiesis" (47).

Inflammation associated with ischemic cardiomyopathy is considered to be modulated by a monocyte/macrophage response and a cytotoxic, Th1, Th17, and Treg responses (54, 55, 66–70). Autoimmune myocarditis predominantly exhibits Th1 and Th17 responses during the inflammatory phase, with Th17 activity being required for the progression to dilated cardiomyopathy (DCM) in chronic stages (58, 71, 72).

We found a robust increase of classic ILC2s, which replaced a majority of the undifferentiated ILC population in a group of patients with both ischemic- and myocarditis- end-stage heart failure. Remarkably, almost no ILC1s and ILC3s were detected, despite the differences in the etiology of both diseases and the fact that both Th17 and Th1 responses are essential for their pathogenesis. We found significant similarities in the non-cytotoxic ILC compartment between human and murine hearts in steady-state and ischemic conditions. Regarding myocarditis, the expansion of ILC2s was significantly more robust in human cardiomyopathy than in murine EAM, which might be an evidence for inter-species differences. This finding could be also influenced, by the chronicity of the analyzed human myocarditis as compared with the EAM model.

ILCs are influenced by the complex interaction of microbiota, external environment, stromal, parenchymal, and immune cells (9, 73, 74). Our experimental data strongly suggest that cardiac ILCs are biased toward an ILC2 fate, regardless of the differences in the pathologic T cell milieu and despite the undifferentiated ILC status in steady-state physiologic conditions. Furthermore, IL-33 reporter mice showed a massive

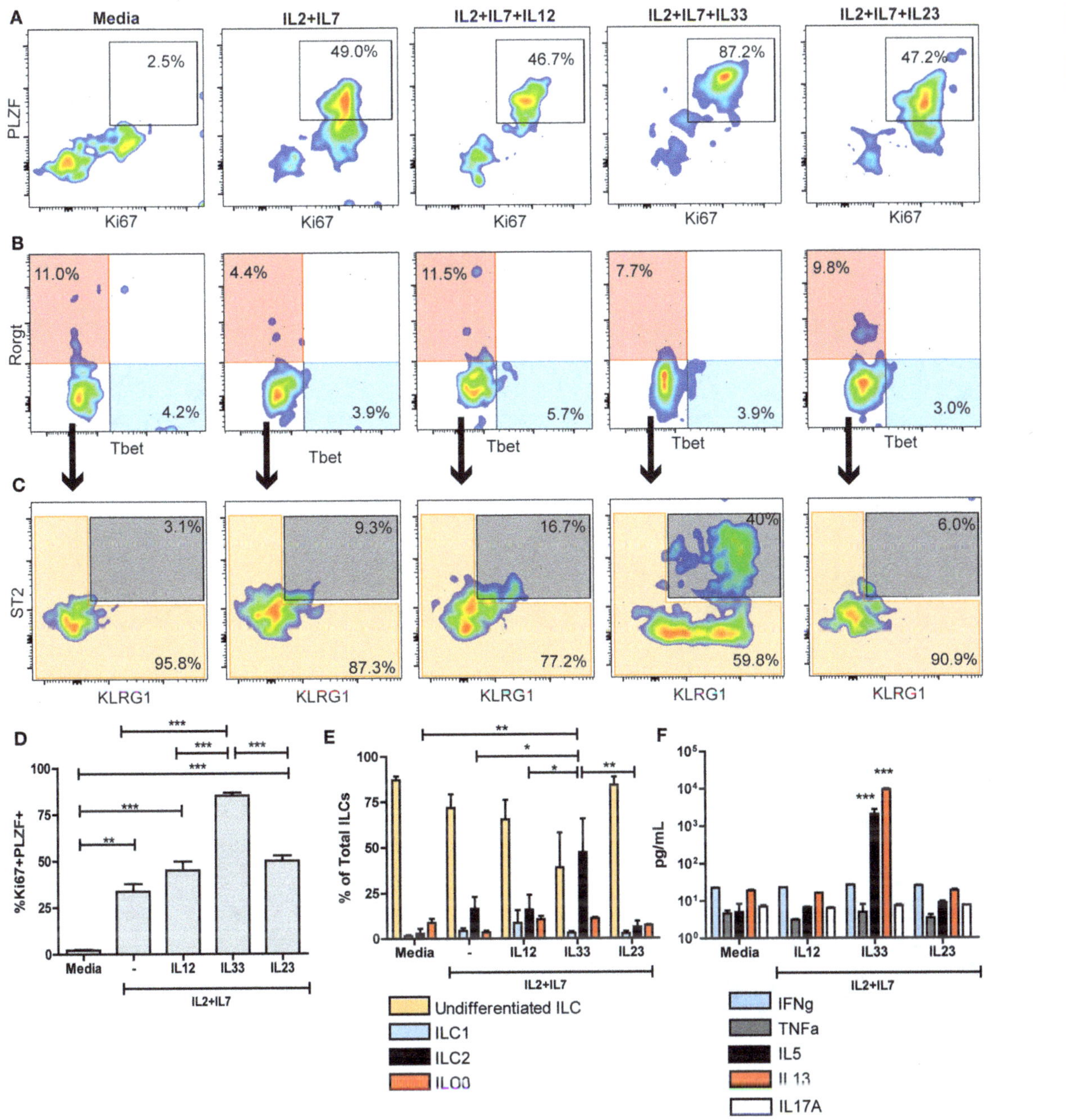

FIGURE 4 | Naïve cardiac ILCs are an ILC type-2 committed population. **(A)** PLZF/Ki67 activation pattern of ILCs under different *in vitro* conditions: Media, IL-2+IL-7, IL-2+IL-7+IL-12 (to induce ILC1s), IL-2+IL-7+IL-33 (to induce ILC2s) and IL-2+IL-7+IL-23 (to induce ILC3s). **(B)** Flow cytometry plots show ILC1 (blue) and ILC3 (transparent red) differentiation under different conditions, based on Rorγt and Tbet expression. **(C)** Plots show undifferentiated ILCs (transparent orange) and ILC2s (gray) compartments after *in vitro* stimulation, based on KLRG1 and ST2 expression. **(D)** Comparison of PLZF^{+}Ki67^{+} activated population in different conditions. **(E)** Comparison of different ILC subpopulations after *in vitro* stimulation. **(F)** Comparison of cytokine profile determined by ELISA under different stimulating conditions. In F, ***indicates significance of both bars with respect to all other conditions. Flow cytometry plots show median representative examples. Graphics show results of 1 of 4 independent experiments, each one made in triplicates for each condition. Bar graphs shows Mean and SD. Statistics calculated with one-way ANOVA and Bonferroni *post-test*. *P < 0.05; **P < 0.01; ***P < 0.001.

increase in IL-33 production by Sca-1^{+} cardiac fibroblasts during ischemia and myocarditis, which was correlated with an expansion of the ILC2 compartment. These findings complement our previous reports about the immunologic importance of Sca-1^{+} cardiac fibroblasts and its role in inflammatory heart diseases, such as the influence of Sca-1^{+} cardiac fibroblasts in the development of heart failure via secretion of GM-CSF (55).

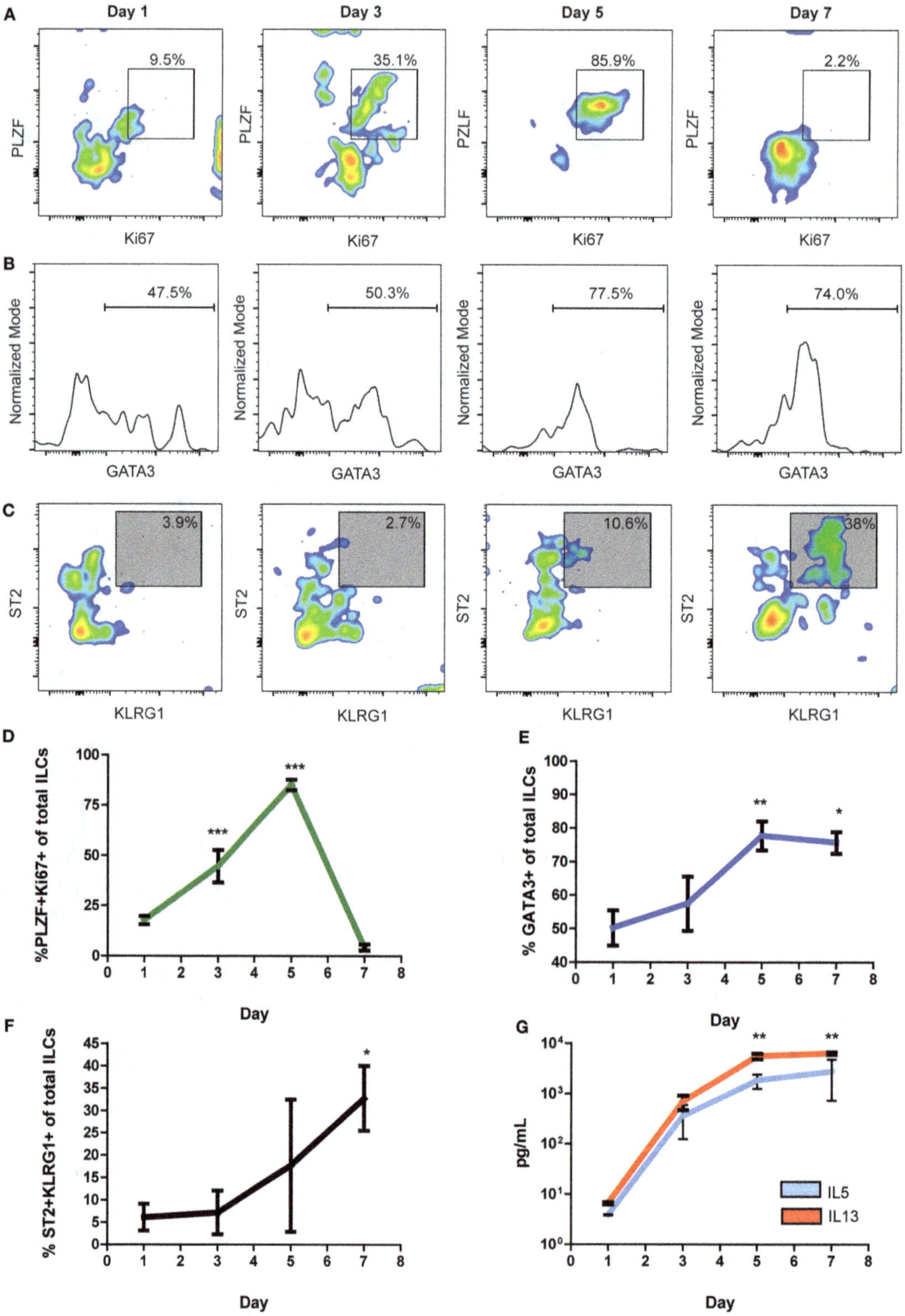

FIGURE 5 | Undifferentiated naïve cardiac ILCs transiently express PLZF upon activation. **(A)** Timeline of PLZF$^+$Ki67$^+$ activation pattern under *in vitro* ILC2-differentiating conditions, IL-2+IL-7+IL-33. **(B)** Progression of GATA3 expression, showing the gate of GATA3$^+$ ILCs. **(C)** Time course of ILC2 phenotype development, based on KLRG1 and ST2 co-expression. **(D)** Graph representing the evolution of the PLZF$^+$Ki67$^+$ co-expression. **(E)** Timeline of GATA3

(Continued)

FIGURE 5 | expression during *in vitro* IL-33 stimulation. **(F)** Time curve showing the progression of ILC2 phenotype development. **(G)** Curve showing the evolution of IL-5 (blue) and IL-13 (red) production under IL-2+IL-7+IL-33 stimulation, as measured by ELISA of supernatants. Graphics show results of 1 of 2 independent experiments, each one made in triplicates for each condition. Asterisks represent the statistical significance of each time-point with respect to day 1-baseline values. Dots and whiskers show Mean and SD. Statistics calculated with one-way ANOVA and Bonferroni *post-test*. $^{*}P < 0.05$; $^{**}P < 0.01$; $^{***}P < 0.001$.

We propose that, regardless of the triggers and initial noxa, cardiac fibroblasts produce IL-33 as an alarmin, inducing the final differentiation of the ILC2-biased population. Thus, in the heart, the ILC2 development is not restricted to Th2-predominant inflammatory processes. This ILC cardiac-specific feature might lead to diversification and deviation of the immune response, and contribute with an innate component in acute and chronic inflammatory heart diseases.

In addition, we found the existence of a baseline low levels of IL-33 production in heart tissues in normal physiologic conditions. We hypothesize that this is one of the components of the heart micro-environment that generates the ILC2-bias of the quiescent undifferentiated cardiac ILCs. Similar phenomenon seems to occur in the lung, but in this case the exposure to external environment leads to complete ILC2 differentiation (74).

In vitro experiments demonstrated that activation of undifferentiated cardiac ILCs was characterized by a transient co-expression of Ki67 and PLZF, as described for ILC progenitors (42, 43). Nevertheless, cardiac ILCs did not express CD117 (cKit) nor have multipotent capacity, unlike the peripheral ILCPs present in cord blood, lung, and liver (47). Despite the fact that cardiac ILCs expressed PLZF under the influence of only IL-2 and IL-7, the presence of IL-33 in the milieu was strictly required for final ILC2 development. As a consequence, the phenotype and functionality of cardiac ILCs are not compatible with previously described peripheral ILCPs. Conversely, cardiac ILCs are a non-multipotent population that retain restricted progenitor-like features, such as the capacity to express PLZF and lack of completely differentiated phenotype in normal conditions.

The residence and infiltration properties of ILCs are still a matter of debate. The preferential role of tissue resident ILCs in early stages of the inflammatory responses is widely accepted (15). Nevertheless, their migratory and infiltrative capacities have also been described (47, 65). We showed here, using adoptive transfer experiments of bone marrow derived-ILC progenitors, that ILCs have an intrinsic infiltrative capacity in adult lymphoid-deficient mice RAG2$^{-/-}$ $\gamma c^{-/-}$, as was evident in lung tissues. Conversely, bone-marrow-derived ILC progenitors were unable to seed the heart. Similarly, we demonstrated that circulating chimeric ILCs were able to populate lungs in naïve, mock and EAM parabionts, but were unable to seed heart tissues. These findings suggest that heart is a restricted niche for ILCs, and the limited traffic is a heart-specific phenomenon rather than an intrinsic feature of migratory ILCs.

Overall, our study shows that the heart is a unique niche in terms of the ILC compartment. Cardiac ILCs seem to be strictly resident population in adulthood. It remains to be elucidated in which stage of fetal development or early life the heart is populated by ILCs, a complicated conundrum due to the complexity of the embryologic development of the heart (52). Cardiac ILC resident population is constituted by quiescent ILC2-committed undifferentiated cells, which remain in resting status in physiologic conditions. Importantly, heart inflammation of multiple etiologies and Th skewness, such as ischemia and autoimmunity, activates a fibroblast-IL-33-ILC axis, which induces activation and differentiation of ILC2s.

IL-33 production in heart has been shown in other pathologic conditions, such as pressure overload (30). Soluble ST2, thought to be a homeostatic neutralizing molecule, has been described as a biomarker of heart failure of any etiology (75, 76). These facts prompt us to propose the existence of a heart stroma/parenchima-IL-33-resident ILC axis that deserves to be explored as a biomarker and potential therapeutic target for multiple inflammatory heart diseases. Our data show that important features, such as the balance between tissue resident and infiltrating ILCs, their status in physiologic conditions, and their final fate do not depend only on intrinsic ILC's cellular capacities, but also on organ-specific properties and microenvironments. In this regard, our findings are aligned with recent theoretical proposals about the dynamic changes of the innate lymphoid compartment over time and in tight association with organ-specific and microenvironmental features (77), which might have implications in physiologic homeostasis and pathologic processes.

MATERIALS AND METHODS

Human Samples

Heart Samples

Endomyocardial biopsies from the apex of the left ventricle were obtained from patients with end stage heart failure (American Heart Association, AHA, stage D) due to chronic ischemic cardiomyopathy or secondary to progression of myocarditis-related cardiomyopathy undergoing implantation of LVAD devices at the Texas Heart Institute. Informed consent was obtained from human subjects and the study protocol was approved by the Committee for the Protection of Human Subjects (University of Texas Health Science Center at Houston. IRB #HSC-MS-05-0074) as previously described (78). Samples were properly preserved in cryovials embedded in liquid nitrogen (−190°C) and then kept at −80°C in the tissue bank at the Texas Heart Institute, Houston, TX. Aliquots of the samples were shipped frozen and processed for flow cytometry in Dr. Ciháková lab, at Johns Hopkins University, Department of Pathology, Baltimore, MD. Reported diagnoses correspond to clinical charts, based on standard histology (H&E), clinical presentation, hemodynamic parameters, and routine clinical biochemical and serology parameters. Patient's information of all samples was processed with random non-linked code relabeling in a database at the time of preservation. Furthermore, for

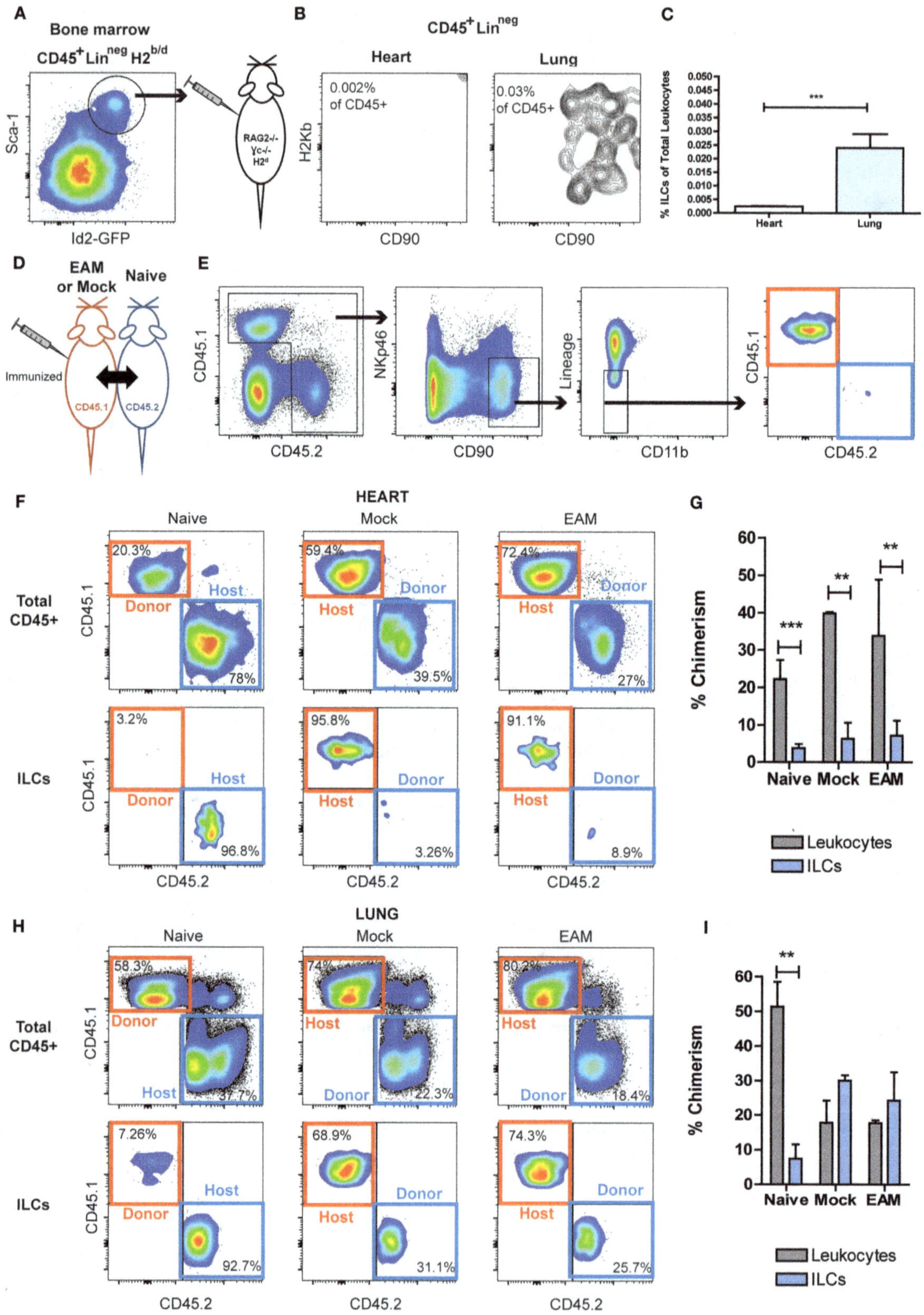

FIGURE 6 | Circulating ILCs cannot infiltrate heart tissues. **(A)** FACS sorting strategy of bone marrow ILC progenitors, CD45$^+$Lineage^{neg}Id2$^+$Sca1$^+$, transferred into RAG2$^{-/-}\gamma c^{-/-}$. **(B)** Flow cytometry plots of infiltrating H2K^b ILCs in heart and lung. **(C)** Bar graphs comparing the detectable infiltrating ILC population in heart and lung. **(D)** Scheme of parabiosis experiment. **(E)** Gating strategy used to analyze ILC population at the peak of EAM, using a naïve parabiont as

(Continued)

FIGURE 6 | representative example. In naïve pairs the infiltrating ILCs were CD45.1 (red boxes), and in Mock and EAM pairs the infiltrating ILCs were CD45.2 (blue boxes). **(F)** Flow cytometry plots showing the source of leukocytes and ILCs in heart. **(G)** Bar graphs comparing the proportion of infiltrating ILCs and leukocytes in heart. **(H)** Flow cytometry plots showing the source of leukocytes and ILCs in lung. **(I)** Bar graphs comparing the proportion of infiltrating ILCs and leukocytes in lung tissues. Naïve $n = 8$, EAM $n = 3$, Mock $n = 2$. Bar graphs shows Mean and SD. Statistics were calculated with Student t **(C)** and one-way ANOVA and Bonferroni *post-test* **(G–I)**. $^{**}P < 0.01$, $^{***}P < 0.001$.

each sample, a separate random non-linked code was assigned for the analyses process. Autopsy samples were obtained upon request, with a time of ischemia of 16–24 h from the Department of Pathology, Johns Hopkins Hospital, aliquot and frozen in cryovials at −80°C.

Blood Samples

Approximately eight milliliters of blood was drawn under aseptic conditions from consenting healthy volunteers from the basilic vein in the cubital fossae, and collected in CPT™ cell tubes (BD Vacutainer, Ref# 362753). Then, tubes were spin at room temperature (~21°C) at 1,800 g for 30 min without deceleration. Then the layer of PBMCs was gently removed, transferred into conical tubes and washed in PBS. After adjusting cell concentration, the PBMCs were processed in fresh for immunostaining.

Mice

All purchased mice were obtained at 6–10 weeks old, and all mice used for experiments were 8–10 weeks old for EAM, mock and naïve conditions and 9–11 weeks old for MI and sham surgery. We purchased the following strains from Jackson labs: WT Balb/cJ mice (JAX000651), CD45.1 WT Balb/cJ mice (JAX006584), RAG2$^{-/-}\gamma c^{-/-}$ mice on Balb/c background (JAX014593), Id2 reporter mouse on C57BL/6 background (B6.129S(Cg)-Id2tm2.1Blh/ZhuJ, JAX016224). Those C57BL/6 Id2 reporters were crossed with CD45.1 Balb/c (JAX006584) to obtain semi-allogeneic H2$^{b/d}$ CD45.1^{+} Id2$^{GFP/+}$ reporter mice in F1. Genotyping of Id2 alleles was done by PCR following vendor instructions (primers: common forward CAAGAAGGTGACCAAGATGGA; common TCTGGGCAGTGGCGTACTT; forward mutant GATCACTCTCGGCATGGACG), and H2 haplotyping and CD45.1 cogenic expression by FACS. *il-33*$^{citrine/citrine}$ mice on Balb/c background (*Il33*^{tm1Anjm}) (79) were obtained from Dr. Andrew McKenzie, MRC Center Cambridge). To obtain IL-33 citrine reporter animals (*heterozygous il-33*$^{citrine/+}$), we crossed Balb/c *il-33*$^{citrine/citrine}$ mice with WT Balb/cJ mice; whereas functionally IL-33 KO mice were obtained by following a homozygous x homozygous crossing scheme (*il-33*$^{citrine/citrine}$ × *il-33*$^{citrine/citrine}$). For terminal experiments, mice were euthanized by cervical dislocation after achievement of deep anesthesia status with a single intra-peritoneal dose of Avertin (Tribromoethanol 2.5% w/v; dose of 0.02 mL/gram of body weight).

EAM Induction

To induce EAM, we injected mice with 125 μg of α-myosin heavy chain peptide (MyHCα614-629, Ac-SLKLMATLFSTYASAD) emulsified in CFA supplemented with 4 mg/mL heat-killed *Mycobacterium tuberculosis* strain H37Ra on days 0 and 7. On day 0, mice also received a dose of 500 ng pertussis toxins intraperitoneally (57, 71, 80).

EAM Histology Assessments

Myocarditis severity was evaluated by histology on day 21. Heart tissues were fixed in SafeFix solution, paraffin embedded and then cut in 5 μm serial sections. Sections were stained with H&E and ventricular inflammation was evaluated with light microscopy, and scores from two independent evaluators (DC and WBB) were averaged using the following criteria: grade 0, no inflammation; grade 1, <10% of the heart section is involved; grade 2, 10–25%; grade 3, 25–50%; grade 4, 50–75%; grade 5, >75% (57).

Myocardial Infarction

To induce MI, we performed permanent ligation of the left anterior descending coronary artery or to a sham operation without ligation. Briefly, mice were anesthetized with 3.5% isoflurane, endotracheal intubation performed and then mechanical ventilation started and kept throughout the operation via small animal ventilator (Harvard Apparatus, model 845). Pre-operational analgesics (0.05 mg/kg Buprenorphine) and paralytics (1 mg/kg Succinylcholine) were administrated prior to operation. A thoracotomy was performed on the 3rd or 4th intercostal space. A 8-0-polyethylene suture was advanced sub-epicardially and perpendicular to the left anterior descending coronary artery. For permanent occlusion, a ligation was done around the artery. The immediate impact was verified by myocardial bleaching and decreased contractility below the occlusion. The chest and skin were closed with a 6-0 nylon suture. Those procedures were performed by the same surgeon, who was also blinded to the experimental design (GC). Mice that died during recovery from anesthesia were excluded from the analysis. Sham-operated animals underwent a similar procedure but without coronary artery ligation (55).

Flow Cytometry (FACS), Imaging Flow Cytometry (ImageStream), and FACS Sorting

Human myocardial biopsy samples weight ranged between 80 and 300 mg. Mouse heart and lungs were perfused *in situ* with PBS using a peristaltic pump (Rainin PR-1), via left and right ventricles for 5–6 min or until the organs looked bleached and pale. In murine experiments approximately half of mice hearts (sagittal cut) were used for FACS, having a weight between 70 and 90 mg; whereas the remaining cardiac tissues were used for histology. Heart and lung FACS specimens were cut in fragments of ~2 mm^3. Fragments were placed in GentleMACS C Tubes (Miltenyi Biotec) in 5 mL of enzymatic digestion buffer: Hank's Balanced Salt Solution [HBSS] supplemented with 600 U/mL

Collagenase II and 60 U/mL DNase I (Worthington). Afterwards, samples were digested for 30 min at 37°C in an ellipsoid shaker, and then further mechanically dissociated with GentleMACS (Miltenyi Biotec). Cell suspension was filtered through a 40 μm cell strainer. Finally, cells were washed and re-suspended in PBS, cell count estimated with hemocymeter counting and then concentration adjusted to 10^6-10^7 cells/150–200 μL of PBS. Viability of cells was determined using a Live/Dead staining of nitrogenated products (Thermofisher). Prior to immunostaining, samples were treated for 5 min with unconjugated Fc Receptor Binding Inhibitor (αCD16/32 for mice, Biolegend; and pan-Fc blocker for human samples, eBioscience). Surface immunostaining was performed using standard protocols, concentrations and times of incubation suggested by vendors of the fluorochrome-labeled antibodies (eBiosciences, BD Biosciences and BioLegend). For intracellular cytokine staining, cells were fixed and then permeabilized with appropriated nuclear staining reagents from eBiosciences. Experimental FACS data were acquired with an LSR II (BD Biosciences) or ImageStream MK-II (Millipore). Gates were stablished based on proper Fluorescent Minus One (FMO) Controls for markers with incomplete separation (**Supplementary Figure 8**). For FACS sorting the processing steps were identical. Heart ILCs $CD45^+CD31^{neg}Lineage^{neg}CD90^+$ were sorted using a FACSAria II Cell Sorter (BD Biosciences) and collected in HBSS + 10% FBS. Data were analyzed with FlowJo v10.4 (Tree Star), tSNE algorithm embedded in FlowJo v10.4 (Tree Star) and for Imaging Flow cytometry we used Ideas v6.0 (Millipore). tSNE analyses were performed on concatenates of all samples belonging to determinate experimental group, using 1,000 iterations with the following parameters: Perplexity 20, Theta 0.5, and Learning rate of 200.

Fluorescent Antibodies

Anti-human Abs: GATA3 (PE-Cy7), Tbet (PerCP-Cy5.5), CD56 (PE-Texas Red), IL23R (PE), CD3, TCRαβ, TCRγδ, CD19, CD20, CD1a, CD11b, CD11c, CD123, BDCA2, CD14, FcεR1a (FITC), CD127 (BV711), NKp44 (BV605), CRTH2 (BV421), CD117 (APC-Cy7), CD4 (AF700), Rorγt (APC), CD45 (BUV395).

Anti-mouse Abs: PLZF (PE-Cy7), GATA3 (PerCP-Cy5.5), CD45 (PE-Texas Red), CD3, CD8, CD5, TCRβ, CD19, CD11b, CD11c, GR1, TER119, CD31, FcεRIα (FITC), Ki67 (BV605), ST2 (BV421), KLRG1 (APC-Cy7), CD4 (AF700), CD90 (BUV395), CD11b (APC), NKp46 (BV711), IL25R (PE).

In vitro Culture

For *in vitro* experiments, hearts from 10 naïve Balb/cJ WT mice were processed and pooled. After sorting cardiac ILCs, cells were washed and resuspended in standard lymphoid cell-appropriated media: RPMI + L-glutamate + non-essential aminoacids + sodium piruvate + penicillin/streptomycin. Cells were placed in round bottom 96-well plates in a concentration of ≈600–800 cells/well/200 μL. Recombinant IL-2, IL-7, IL-33, IL-12, IL-23, IL-1β (Biolegend) were added at a concentration of 20 ng/mL. At the end of the pre-established time of culture, cells were spin down (300 g × 8 min), harvested, washed and stained for FACS as described above. Supernatants were collected for ELISA analysis (IL-5, IL-13, IL-17A, TNFα, IFNγ, R&D Systems).

Adoptive Transfer of ILCs

Bone marrow cells were obtained by flushing mechanically the content of the femurs of Id2 reporter mice. Both femurs were harvested for each mouse, and 10 mice pooled for each transfer experiment. In brief, both femoral epiphysis were surgically removed after euthanasia of a donor mice. Then, using a 22G needle and a syringe loaded with 4 mL of PBS, the bone marrow was flushed into a 15 mL conical tube. After washing and standard treatment with ACK buffer, the single cell suspension was handled as described for FACS staining. Then, using FACSAria II, the $CD45^+Lineage^{negative}Sca\text{-}1^+Id2^+$ ILCPs were FACS sorted as described above. Finally, cells were resuspended at a concentration of 10^4 ILCPs ($CD45^+Lin^{negative}Sca\text{-}1^+Id2^+$) per 200 μL of RPMI and injected intravenously in mice retro-orbitally.

Parabiosis Surgery

Mice were anesthetized with inhaled isoflurane, 4.0–5.0%. Maintenance anesthesia was kept during surgery with intramuscular injections of ketamine (80 mg/kg) and xylazine (16 mg/kg). For complementary analgesia buprenorphine (0.1 mg/kg) was intraperitoneally injected concurrent to initial analgesia, and 12 h postoperatively. Longitudinal incisions in the skin and subcutaneous tissues were made through the skin starting from the elbow joint and extended down to the knee joint. In order to promote skin anastomosis, a continuous 5-0 absorbable Vicryl suture was also used through the muscular layer to connect the pairs. Non-absorbable 4-0 discontinuous sutures were made to attach corresponding subcutaneous tissues between parabionts. Surgical stapler was used to connect the skins of the pairs. Baytril (Enrofloxacin) was used upon the completion of the procedure as antibiotic prophylaxis. All parabiosis surgeries were done by one surgeon (JS). Animals were provided with moistened chow and gel food diet supplement every other day until sacrifice on days 19–20 after the parabiosis. Mice were daily evaluated for signs of pain and discomfort. In the set of experiments reported in this study, no additional analgesia doses were required. The establishment of mixed chimerism was evaluated on day 14 after the surgery in peripheral blood by FACS using CD45.1 and CD45.2 immunostaining of PBMCs.

Statistical Analyses

Comparison between groups was estimated as follows: (a) two independent groups using Student t, (b) three or more independent experimental groups using one-way ANOVA plus Bonferroni's *post-test*, (c) two experimental groups in respect to a single control group using Dunnetts's test. Significance of numerical correlations was calculated with Pearson r of best-fitting mathematical functions. Shapiro-Wilk test was used to verify Gaussian distribution prior to further statistical analysis. We used non-parametric U-Mann Whitney for comparison of histological scores between 2 groups. In every case $\alpha = 0.05$ and $\beta = 0.20$

(Potency = 80%) were used as thresholds to estimate significance. All calculations were made using GraphPad Prism v6.0.

AUTHOR CONTRIBUTIONS

WB-B conceptualization, designed experiments, performed the experiments, analyzed data, wrote the manuscript, funding acquisition. GC, XH, MT, HC, and GD performed some experiments, gathered clinical data. HT conceptualization, obtained human cardiac biopsy samples. JS and DH helped to designed and perform parabiosis experiments. DN conceptualization, gathered clinical data. DČ conceptualization, designed experiments, analyzed data, wrote the manuscript, main funding acquisition. All authors approved the manuscript.

ACKNOWLEDGMENTS

This work was supported by National Institutes of Health/National Heart, Lung, and Blood Institute grants R01HL118183, R01HL136586, R01HL113008 to DČ and 5R01-HL-61483 to HT; American Heart Association AWRP Winter 2017 Grant-in-Aid (17GRNT33700274) to DČ; American Heart Association Postdoctoral Fellowship (16POST31330012) to WB-B; American Autoimmune Related Disease Association Young Investigator Award 2016 to WB-B; American Heart Association AWRP Winter 2017 Grant-in-Aid (17GRNT33700274) and Johns Hopkins Catalyst Award to DČ. Matthew Poyner MVP Memorial Myocarditis Research Fund to Nisha Gilotra and DČ; Johns Hopkins Autoimmune Disease Research Center O'Leary-Wilson Fellowship and Johns Hopkins Bloomberg School of Public Health Richard J and Margaret Conn Himelfarb Student Support fund, and Katherine E. Welsh Fellowship to XH; Myocarditis Foundation Postdoctoral Fellowship (90072351) to GC, and American Heart Association 2016 Predoctoral Fellowship to HC. We acknowledge the invaluable contribution of Dr. Andrew McKenzie for providing the *il-33$^{citrine/citrine}$* mice (*Il33^{tm1Anjm}*), Xiaoling Zhang, JHU Ross Flow Cytometry Core, for support on cell sorting experiments and Julie Schaub for mouse colony management. We also thank David Hughes, Megan Wood and Martin Cihák for manuscript edits, as well as Taejoon Won, Nicola Diny, William J. Burlingham, and Paulina Chalan for insightful analyses, critiques and discussions.

SUPPLEMENTARY MATERIAL

Supplementary Figure 1 | Flow cytometry gating strategy for human ILCs. Basic gating strategy of human cardiac ILCs. FSC and SSC parameters allowed an initial morphologic gate and exclusion of doublets. Live/Dead Aqua dye was used to exclude dead cells and cells with incompetent membrane. ILCs were defined CD45$^+$Lineage^{neg}CD127$^+$. The Tbet^{neg}Rorγ^{neg} population was also negative for NKp44 and IL-23R.

Supplementary Figure 2 | Comprehensive analysis of cardiac ILCs, including NK cells and non-cytotoxic ILC population. **(A)** Gating strategy in which CD11b was excluded of the Lineage cocktail. NK cells were CD45$^+$CD11b$^+$CD56$^+$ CD127^{neg} and predominantly NKp44^{neg}. Non-cytotoxic ILCs were defined as Lineage^{neg}CD11b^{neg}CD56^{neg}CD127$^+$. **(B)** Bar graphs showing the proportion of CD45$^+$Lineage^{neg} cells represented by NK cells and the non-cytotoxic ILC subsets.

Supplementary Figure 3 | Analysis of circulating ILCs in peripheral blood. Basic gating strategy used to analyze non-cytotoxic ILCs and NK cells in PBMCs. CD11b was removed from the Lineage cocktail. Activated NK cells were defined as NKp44$^+$CD56$^+$Tbet$^+$, whereas non-cytotoxic ILCs were CD127$^+$NKp44^{neg}. ILC3s (red) were IL23R+Tbetint, ILC1 (blue) were Tbet+ and ILC2s (orange) were defined based on CRTH2 expression (FMO control is shown in dashed histogram).

Supplementary Figure 4 | Expansion of absolute number of ILC2s during MI and EAM. **(A)** Representative H&E ventricular histology images of EAM and mock immunized mice, and histology scores. **(B)** Bar graphs showing the similarity of ILC compartment composition in naïve, mock immunized and sham surgery controls. **(C)** Flow cytometry analysis of Rorγt and FcεR1a in NKp46$^+$CD90$^+$ ILCs. **(D)** Flow cytometry plots showing cKit and IL25R expression in total heart's ILCs population. **(E)** Absolute number of murine cardiac ILC2s in control, MI and EAM hearts. **(F)** Absolute number of undifferentiated ILC in control, MI, EAM hearts. Flow plots show concatenates of representative examples of 1 of 3 independent experiments, where $n = 5$ for naïve controls and EAM, $n = 4$ for MI in this experiment, and $n = 2$–3 mock and sham. Bar graphs shows Mean and SD. Statistics were calculated using Dunnett's test. $^*P < 0.05$. $^{**}P < 0.01$.

Supplementary Figure 5 | Comprehensive analysis of murine ILC compartment including NK cells and non-cytotoxic ILCs. **(A)** Basic gating strategy followed to analyze murine cardiac ILCs and NK cells. CD11b and CD3 were placed in independent channels out of the Lineage cocktail. Classic NK cells were CD11b$^+$CD90^{neg}NKp46$^+$CD122$^+$. CD11b^{neg} NK cells were CD90$^+$NKp46$^+$CD122$^+$. Non-cytotoxic were defined ILC1s (blue) as Tbet$^+$, ILC2s (gray) as ST2$^+$KLRG1$^+$, ILC3s (transparent red) as Rorγt$^+$. Undifferentiated ILCs (transparent orange) as ILCs negative for all ILC type-specific markers. **(B)** Bar graphs showing the proportion of total leukocytes (CD45$^+$ cells) represented by the NK and non-cytotoxic ILC subsets.

Supplementary Figure 6 | tSNE analysis of cardiac fibroblast population shows restriction of IL-33$^+$ cells to Sca-1$^+$ cardiac fibroblast cluster. tSNE plots of cardiac fibroblasts and IL-33 production in naïve hearts, MI and EAM. It shows Sca-1^{neg} cells in gray, Sca-1$^+$ in orange, and IL-33$^+$ events in green. Majority of IL-33$^+$ events (green) overlap with Sca-1$^+$ cluster (orange).

Supplementary Figure 7 | *In vitro* responses to IL-23 are comparable to IL-1β and *in vitro* culture of ST2+ non-cytotoxic ILCs. **(A–C)** Flow plots showing phenotypic differentiation *in vitro* of naïve heart ILCs under control IL-2+IL-7+IL-1β differentiation condition. **(D,E)** Bar graphs comparing cardiac ILCs differentiation under control, IL-23- and IL-1β-inducing type 3 conditions. **(F)** ELISA results showing the cytokine production profile of cardiac ILCs under control, IL-23- and IL-1β-inducing type 3 conditions. **(G)** Flow cytometry plots gated on live cells, showing the cellularity retrieved after a 6-day culture of ST2+ non-cytotoxic ILCs in IL-2+IL-7+IL-33 conditions. Flow cytometry plots show median representative examples. Graphics show results of 1 of 2–4 independent experiments, each one made in triplicates for each condition. Bar graphs shows Mean and SD. Statistics calculated with one-way ANOVA and Bonferroni *post-test*.

Supplementary Figure 8 | Fluorescence Minus One (FMO) controls. Representative examples of histogram overlay of FMO controls (gray) with stained cardiac ILCs (open red histogram) used to set flow cytometry gates in human **(A)** and mouse **(B)** experiments.

REFERENCES

1. Neill DR, Wong SH, Bellosi A, Flynn RJ, Daly M, Langford TK, et al. Nuocytes represent a new innate effector leukocyte that mediates type-2 immunity. *Nature.* (2010) 464:1367–70. doi: 10.1038/nature08900
2. Artis D, Spits H. The biology of innate lymphoid cells. *Nature.* (2015) 517:293–301. doi: 10.1038/nature14189
3. Eberl G, Colonna M, Di Santo JP, McKenzie AN. Innate lymphoid cells. Innate lymphoid cells: a new paradigm in immunology. *Science.* (2015) 348:aaa6566. doi: 10.1126/science.aaa6566
4. Hwang YY, McKenzie AN. Innate lymphoid cells in immunity and disease. *Adv Exp Med Biol.* (2013) 785:9–26. doi: 10.1007/978-1-4614-6217-0_2
5. Symowski C, Voehringer D. Interactions between innate lymphoid cells and cells of the innate and adaptive immune system. *Front Immunol.* (2017) 8:1422. doi: 10.3389/fimmu.2017.01422
6. Bal SM, Bernink JH, Nagasawa M, Groot J, Shikhagaie MM, Golebski K, et al. IL-1β, IL-4 and IL-12 control the fate of group 2 innate lymphoid cells in human airway inflammation in the lungs. *Nat Immunol.* (2016) 17:636–45. doi: 10.1038/ni.3444
7. Bernink JH, Krabbendam L, Germar K, de Jong E, Gronke K, Kofoed-Nielsen M, et al. Interleukin-12 and–23 control plasticity of CD127(+) group 1 and Group 3 innate lymphoid cells in the intestinal lamina propria. *Immunity.* (2015) 43:146–60. doi: 10.1016/j.immuni.2015.06.019
8. Silver JS, Kearley J, Copenhaver AM, Sanden C, Mori M, Yu L, et al. Inflammatory triggers associated with exacerbations of COPD orchestrate plasticity of group 2 innate lymphoid cells in the lungs. *Nat Immunol.* (2016) 17:626–35. doi: 10.1038/ni.3443
9. Cortez VS, Robinette ML, Colonna M. Innate lymphoid cells: new insights into function and development. *Curr Opin Immunol.* (2015) 32:71–7. doi: 10.1016/j.coi.2015.01.004
10. Fuchs A, Vermi W, Lee JS, Lonardi S, Gilfillan S, Newberry RD, et al. Intraepithelial type 1 innate lymphoid cells are a unique subset of IL-12- and IL-15-responsive IFN-γ-producing cells. *Immunity.* (2013) 38:769–81. doi: 10.1016/j.immuni.2013.02.010
11. Zhang J, Marotel M, Fauteux-Daniel S, Mathieu AL, Viel S, Marcais A, et al. T-bet and Eomes govern differentiation and function of mouse and human NK cells and ILC1. *Eur J Immunol.* (2018) 48:738–50. doi: 10.1002/eji.201747299
12. Seillet C, Belz GT, Huntington ND. Development, homeostasis, and heterogeneity of NK cells and ILC1. *Curr Top Microbiol Immunol.* (2016) 395:37–61. doi: 10.1007/82_2015_474
13. Spits H, Bernink JH, Lanier L. NK cells and type 1 innate lymphoid cells: partners in host defense. *Nat Immunol.* (2016) 17:758–64. doi: 10.1038/ni.3482
14. Weizman OE, Adams NM, Schuster IS, Krishna C, Pritykin Y, Lau C, et al. ILC1 confer early host protection at initial sites of viral infection. *Cell.* (2017) 171:e712. doi: 10.1016/j.cell.2017.09.052
15. Gasteiger G, Fan X, Dikiy S, Lee SY, Rudensky AY. Tissue residency of innate lymphoid cells in lymphoid and nonlymphoid organs. *Science.* (2015) 350:981–5. doi: 10.1126/science.aac9593
16. Gold MJ, Antignano F, Halim TY, Hirota JA, Blanchet MR, Zaph C, et al. Group 2 innate lymphoid cells facilitate sensitization to local, but not systemic, TH2-inducing allergen exposures. *J Allergy Clin Immunol.* (2014) 133:1142–8. doi: 10.1016/j.jaci.2014.02.033
17. Jia Y, Fang X, Zhu X, Bai C, Zhu L, Jin M, et al. IL-13(+) type 2 innate lymphoid cells correlate with asthma control status and treatment response. *Am J Respir Cell Mol Biol.* (2016) 55:675–83. doi: 10.1165/rcmb.2016-0099OC
18. KleinJan A, Klein Wolterink RG, Levani Y, de Bruijn MJ, Hoogsteden HC, van Nimwegen M, et al. Enforced expression of Gata3 in T cells and group 2 innate lymphoid cells increases susceptibility to allergic airway inflammation in mice. *J Immunol.* (2014) 192:1385–94. doi: 10.4049/jimmunol.1301888
19. Nausch N, Mutapi F. Group 2 ILCs: a way of enhancing immune protection against human helminths? *Parasite Immunol.* (2018) 40:e12450. doi: 10.1111/pim.12450
20. Bordon Y. Immunometabolism. ILC2s skew the fat. *Nat Rev Immunol.* (2015) 15:67. doi: 10.1038/nri3805
21. Brestoff JR, Kim BS, Saenz SA, Stine RR, Monticelli LA, Sonnenberg GF, et al. Group 2 innate lymphoid cells promote beiging of white adipose tissue and limit obesity. *Nature.* (2015) 519:242–6. doi: 10.1038/nature14115
22. Chalubinski M, Luczak E, Wojdan K, Gorzelak-Pabis P, Broncel M. Innate lymphoid cells type 2 - emerging immune regulators of obesity and atherosclerosis. *Immunol Lett.* (2016) 179:43–6. doi: 10.1016/j.imlet.2016.09.007
23. McHedlidze T, Waldner M, Zopf S, Walker J, Rankin AL, Schuchmann M, et al. Interleukin-33-dependent innate lymphoid cells mediate hepatic fibrosis. *Immunity.* (2013) 39:357–71. doi: 10.1016/j.immuni.2013.07.018
24. Monticelli LA, Sonnenberg GF, Abt MC, Alenghat T, Ziegler CG, Doering TA, et al. Innate lymphoid cells promote lung-tissue homeostasis after infection with influenza virus. *Nat Immunol.* (2011) 12:1045–54. doi: 10.1038/ni.2131
25. Diefenbach A, Colonna M, Koyasu S. Development, differentiation, and diversity of innate lymphoid cells. *Immunity.* (2014) 41:354–65. doi: 10.1016/j.immuni.2014.09.005
26. Guo L, Huang Y, Chen X, Hu-Li J, Urban JFJr, Paul WE. Innate immunological function of TH2 cells *in vivo*. *Nat Immunol.* (2015) 16:1051–9. doi: 10.1038/ni.3244
27. Hoyler T, Klose CS, Souabni A, Turqueti-Neves A, Pfeifer D, Rawlins EL, et al. The transcription factor GATA-3 controls cell fate and maintenance of type 2 innate lymphoid cells. *Immunity.* (2012) 37:634–48. doi: 10.1016/j.immuni.2012.06.020
28. Van Gool F, Molofsky AB, Morar MM, Rosenzwajg M, Liang HE, Klatzmann D, et al. Interleukin-5-producing group 2 innate lymphoid cells control eosinophilia induced by interleukin-2 therapy. *Blood.* (2014) 124:3572–6. doi: 10.1182/blood-2014-07-587493
29. Cayrol C, Girard JP. IL-33: an alarmin cytokine with crucial roles in innate immunity, inflammation and allergy. *Curr Opin Immunol.* (2014) 31:31–7. doi: 10.1016/j.coi.2014.09.004
30. Chen WY, Hong J, Gannon J, Kakkar R, Lee RT. Myocardial pressure overload induces systemic inflammation through endothelial cell IL-33. *Proc Natl Acad Sci USA.* (2015) 112:7249–54. doi: 10.1073/pnas.1424236112
31. Liew FY, Girard JP, Turnquist HR. Interleukin-33 in health and disease. *Nat Rev Immunol.* (2016) 16:676–89. doi: 10.1038/nri.2016.95
32. Xu J, Guardado J, Hoffman R, Xu H, Namas R, Vodovotz Y, et al. IL33-mediated ILC2 activation and neutrophil IL5 production in the lung response after severe trauma: a reverse translation study from a human cohort to a mouse trauma model. *PLoS Med.* (2017) 14:e1002365. doi: 10.1371/journal.pmed.1002365
33. Camelo A, Rosignoli G, Ohne Y, Stewart RA, Overed-Sayer C, Sleeman MA, et al. IL-33, IL-25, and TSLP induce a distinct phenotypic and activation profile in human type 2 innate lymphoid cells. *Blood Adv.* (2017) 1:577–89. doi: 10.1182/bloodadvances.2016002352
34. Huang Y, Guo L, Qiu J, Chen X, Hu-Li J, Siebenlist U, et al. IL-25-responsive, lineage-negative KLRG1(hi) cells are multipotential 'inflammatory' type 2 innate lymphoid cells. *Nat Immunol.* (2015) 16:161–9. doi: 10.1038/ni.3078
35. Huang Y, Paul WE. Inflammatory group 2 innate lymphoid cells. *Int Immunol.* (2016) 28:23–8. doi: 10.1093/intimm/dxv044
36. Melo-Gonzalez F, Hepworth MR. Functional and phenotypic heterogeneity of group 3 innate lymphoid cells. *Immunology.* (2017) 150:265–75. doi: 10.1111/imm.12697
37. Pearson C, Thornton EE, McKenzie B, Schaupp AL, Huskens N, Griseri T, et al. ILC3 GM-CSF production and mobilisation orchestrate acute intestinal inflammation. *Elife.* (2016) 5:e10066. doi: 10.7554/eLife.10066
38. Sawa S, Cherrier M, Lochner M, Satoh-Takayama N, Fehling HJ, Langa F, et al. Lineage relationship analysis of ROR-gammat+ innate lymphoid cells. *Science.* (2010) 330:665–9. doi: 10.1126/science.1194597
39. Lo BC, Gold MJ, Hughes MR, Antignano F, Valdez Y, Zaph C, et al. The orphan nuclear receptor ROR α and group 3 innate lymphoid cells drive fibrosis in a mouse model of Crohn's disease. *Sci Immunol.* (2016) 1:eaaf8864. doi: 10.1126/sciimmunol.aaf8864
40. Teunissen MB, Munneke JM, Bernink JH, Spuls PI, Res PC, Te Velde A, et al. Composition of innate lymphoid cell subsets in the human skin: enrichment of NCR(+) ILC3 in lesional skin and blood of psoriasis patients. *J Invest Dermatol.* (2014) 134:2351–60. doi: 10.1038/jid.2014.146
41. Villanova F, Flutter B, Tosi I, Grys K, Sreeneebus H, Perera GK, et al. Characterization of innate lymphoid cells in human skin and blood demonstrates increase of NKp44+ ILC3 in psoriasis. *J Invest Dermatol.* (2014) 134:984–91. doi: 10.1038/jid.2013.477

42. Constantinides MG, McDonald BD, Verhoef PA, Bendelac A. A committed precursor to innate lymphoid cells. *Nature.* (2014) 508:397–401. doi: 10.1038/nature13047
43. Harly C, Cam M, Kaye J, Bhandoola A. Development and differentiation of early innate lymphoid progenitors. *J Exp Med.* (2018) 215:249–62. doi: 10.1084/jem.20170832
44. Seillet C, Mielke LA, Amann-Zalcenstein DB, Su S, Gao J, Almeida FF, et al. Deciphering the innate lymphoid cell transcriptional program. *Cell Rep.* (2016) 17:436–47. doi: 10.1016/j.celrep.2016.09.025
45. Halim TY, Steer CA, Matha L, Gold MJ, Martinez-Gonzalez I, McNagny KM, et al. Group 2 innate lymphoid cells are critical for the initiation of adaptive T helper 2 cell-mediated allergic lung inflammation. *Immunity.* (2014) 40:425–35. doi: 10.1016/j.immuni.2014.01.011
46. Walker JA, McKenzie AN. Development and function of group 2 innate lymphoid cells. *Curr Opin Immunol.* (2013) 25:148–55. doi: 10.1016/j.coi.2013.02.010
47. Lim AI, Li Y, Lopez-Lastra S, Stadhouders R, Paul F, Casrouge A, et al. Systemic human ILC precursors provide a substrate for tissue ILC differentiation. *Cell.* (2017) 168:e1010. doi: 10.1016/j.cell.2017.02.021
48. Walker JA, Barlow JL, McKenzie AN. Innate lymphoid cells–how did we miss them? *Nat Rev Immunol.* (2013) 13:75–87. doi: 10.1038/nri3349
49. Fang D, Zhu J. Dynamic balance between master transcription factors determines the fates and functions of CD4 T cell and innate lymphoid cell subsets. *J Exp Med.* (2017) 214:1861–76. doi: 10.1084/jem.20170494
50. Ong S, Ligons DL, Barin JG, Wu L, Talor MV, Diny N, et al. Natural killer cells limit cardiac inflammation and fibrosis by halting eosinophil infiltration. *Am J Pathol.* (2015) 185:847–61. doi: 10.1016/j.ajpath.2014.11.023
51. Ong S, Rose NR, Cihakova D. Natural killer cells in inflammatory heart disease. *Clin Immunol.* (2017) 175:26–33. doi: 10.1016/j.clim.2016.11.010
52. Meilhac SM, Lescroart F, Blanpain C, Buckingham ME. Cardiac cell lineages that form the heart. *Cold Spring Harb Perspect Med.* (2014) 4:a013888. doi: 10.1101/cshperspect.a013888
53. Bani D, Nistri S. New insights into the morphogenic role of stromal cells and their relevance for regenerative medicine. lessons from the heart. *J Cell Mol Med.* (2014) 18:363–70. doi: 10.1111/jcmm.12247
54. Anzai A, Choi JL, He S, Fenn AM, Nairz M, Rattik S, et al. The infarcted myocardium solicits GM-CSF for the detrimental oversupply of inflammatory leukocytes. *J Exp Med.* (2017) 214:3293–310. doi: 10.1084/jem.20170689
55. Chen G, Bracamonte-Baran W, Diny NL, Hou X, Talor MV, Fu K, et al. Sca-1(+) cardiac fibroblasts promote development of heart failure. *Eur J Immunol.* (2018) 48:1522–38. doi: 10.1002/eji.201847583
56. Diny NL, Hou X, Barin JG, Chen G, Talor MV, Schaub J, et al. Macrophages and cardiac fibroblasts are the main producers of eotaxins and regulate eosinophil trafficking to the heart. *Eur J Immunol.* (2016) 46:2749–60. doi: 10.1002/eji.201646557
57. Wu L, Diny NL, Ong S, Barin JG, Hou X, Rose NR, et al. Pathogenic IL-23 signaling is required to initiate GM-CSF-driven autoimmune myocarditis in mice. *Eur J Immunol.* (2015) 46:582–92. doi: 10.1002/eji.201545924
58. Wu L, Ong S, Talor MV, Barin JG, Baldeviano GC, Kass DA, et al. Cardiac fibroblasts mediate IL-17A-driven inflammatory dilated cardiomyopathy. *J Exp Med.* (2014) 211:1449–64. doi: 10.1084/jem.20132126
59. Spits H, Artis D, Colonna M, Diefenbach A, Di Santo JP, Eberl G, et al. Innate lymphoid cells–a proposal for uniform nomenclature. *Nat Rev Immunol.* (2013) 13:145–9. doi: 10.1038/nri3365
60. Chester C, Maecker HT. Algorithmic tools for mining high-dimensional cytometry data. *J Immunol.* (2015) 195:773–9. doi: 10.4049/jimmunol.1500633
61. Mair F, Hartmann FJ, Mrdjen D, Tosevski V, Krieg C, Becher B. The end of gating? An introduction to automated analysis of high dimensional cytometry data. *Eur J Immunol.* (2016) 46:34–43. doi: 10.1002/eji.201545774
62. Stier MT, Zhang J, Goleniewska K, Cephus JY, Rusznak M, Wu L, et al. IL-33 promotes the egress of group 2 innate lymphoid cells from the bone marrow. *J Exp Med.* (2018) 215:263–81. doi: 10.1084/jem.20170449
63. Fontes JA, Barin JG, Talor MV, Stickel N, Schaub J, Rose NR, et al. Complete Freund's adjuvant induces experimental autoimmune myocarditis by enhancing IL-6 production during initiation of the immune response. *Immun Inflamm Dis.* (2017) 5:163–76. doi: 10.1002/iid3.155
64. Hazenberg MD, Spits H. Human innate lymphoid cells. *Blood.* (2014) 124:700–9. doi: 10.1182/blood-2013-11-427781
65. Kim CH, Hashimoto-Hill S, Kim M. Migration and tissue tropism of innate lymphoid cells. *Trends Immunol.* (2016) 37:68–79. doi: 10.1016/j.it.2015.11.003
66. Dutta P, Nahrendorf M. Monocytes in myocardial infarction. *Arterioscler Thromb Vascul Biol.* (2015) 35:1066–70. doi: 10.1161/ATVBAHA.114.304652
67. Fang L, Moore XL, Dart AM, Wang LM. Systemic inflammatory response following acute myocardial infarction. *J Geriatr Cardiol.* (2015) 12:305–12. doi: 10.11909/j.issn.1671-5411.2015.03.020
68. Heidt T, Courties G, Dutta P, Sager HB, Sebas M, Iwamoto Y, et al. Differential contribution of monocytes to heart macrophages in steady-state and after myocardial infarction. *Circul Res.* (2014) 115:284–95. doi: 10.1161/CIRCRESAHA.115.303567
69. Liu J, Wang H, Li J. Inflammation and inflammatory cells in myocardial infarction and reperfusion injury: a double-edged sword. *Clin Med Insights Cardiol.* (2016) 10:79–84. doi: 10.4137/CMC.S33164
70. Van der Borght K, Scott CL, Nindl V, Bouche A, Martens L, Sichien D, et al. Myocardial infarction primes autoreactive T cells through activation of dendritic cells. *Cell Rep.* (2017) 18:3005–17. doi: 10.1016/j.celrep.2017.02.079
71. Baldeviano GC, Barin JG, Talor MV, Srinivasan S, Bedja D, Zheng D, et al. Interleukin-17A is dispensable for myocarditis but essential for the progression to dilated cardiomyopathy. *Circul Res.* (2010) 106:1646–55. doi: 10.1161/CIRCRESAHA.109.213157
72. Bracamonte-Baran W, Cihakova D. Cardiac autoimmunity: myocarditis. *Adv Exp Med Biol.* (2017) 1003:187–221. doi: 10.1007/978-3-319-57613-8_10
73. Minton K. Innate lymphoid cells: ILC diversity maintained by microbiota. *Nat Rev Immunol.* (2016) 16:593. doi: 10.1038/nri.2016.101
74. Saluzzo S, Gorki ADB, Rana MJ, Martins R, Scanlon S, Starkl K, et al. First-breath-induced type 2 pathways shape the lung immune environment. *Cell Rep.* (2017) 18:1893–905. doi: 10.1016/j.celrep.2017.01.071
75. Kohli P, Bonaca MP, Kakkar R, Kudinova AY, Scirica BM, Sabatine MS, et al. Role of ST2 in non-ST-elevation acute coronary syndrome in the MERLIN-TIMI 36 trial. *Clin Chem.* (2012) 58:257–66. doi: 10.1373/clinchem.2011.173369
76. Sabatine MS, Morrow DA, Higgins LJ, MacGillivray C, Guo W, Bode C, et al. Complementary roles for biomarkers of biomechanical strain ST2 and N-terminal prohormone B-type natriuretic peptide in patients with ST-elevation myocardial infarction. *Circulation.* (2008) 117:1936–44. doi: 10.1161/CIRCULATIONAHA.107.728022
77. Kotas ME, Locksley RM. Why innate lymphoid cells? *Immunity.* (2018) 48:1081–90. doi: 10.1016/j.immuni.2018.06.002
78. Razeghi P, Young ME, Alcorn JL, Moravec CS, Frazier OH, Taegtmeyer H. Metabolic gene expression in fetal and failing human heart. *Circulation.* (2001) 104:2923–31. doi: 10.1161/hc4901.100526
79. Wong SH, Walker JA, Jolin HE, Drynan LF, Hams E, Camelo A, et al. Transcription factor RORα is critical for nuocyte development. *Nat Immunol.* (2012) 13:229–36. doi: 10.1038/ni.2208
80. Cihakova D, Sharma RB, Fairweather D, Afanasyeva M, Rose NR. Animal models for autoimmune myocarditis and autoimmune thyroiditis. *Methods Molecul Med.* (2004) 102:175–93. doi: 10.1385/1-59259-805-6:175

7

Autoimmune Calcium Channelopathies and Cardiac Electrical Abnormalities

Yongxia Sarah Qu[1,2*], *Pietro Enea Lazzerini*[3], *Pier Leopoldo Capecchi*[3], *Franco Laghi-Pasini*[3], *Nabil El Sherif*[2] *and Mohamed Boutjdir*[2,4]

[1] *Department of Cardiology, New York Presbyterian Brooklyn Methodist Hospital, Brooklyn, NY, United States,* [2] *VA New York Harbor Healthcare System and State University of New York Downstate Medical Center, Brooklyn, NY, United States,* [3] *Department of Medical Sciences, Surgery and Neurosciences, University of Siena, Siena, Italy,* [4] *NYU School of Medicine, New York, NY, United States*

Correspondence:
Yongxia Sarah Qu
ysq9001@nyp.org

Patients with autoimmune diseases are at increased risk for developing cardiovascular diseases, and abnormal electrocardiographic findings are common. Voltage-gated calcium channels play a major role in the cardiovascular system and regulate cardiac excitability and contractility. Particularly, by virtue of their localization and expression in the heart, calcium channels modulate pace making at the sinus node, conduction at the atrioventricular node and cardiac repolarization in the working myocardium. Consequently, emerging evidence suggests that calcium channels are targets to autoantibodies in autoimmune diseases. Autoimmune-associated cardiac calcium channelopathies have been recognized in both sinus node dysfunction atrioventricular block in patients positive for anti-Ro/La antibodies, and ventricular arrhythmias in patients with dilated cardiomyopathy. In this review, we discuss mechanisms of autoimmune-associated calcium channelopathies and their relationship with the development of cardiac electrical abnormalities.

Keywords: calcium channel, autoantibodies, autoimmune, channelopathy, cardiac electrical abnormalities

INTRODUCTION

Voltage gated calcium channels (VGCCs) are macromolecular complexes which include the main pore forming α_1-subunits, the accessory β, $\alpha_2\delta$, and γ-subunits (1–4). In the heart, VGCCs mediate calcium (Ca) influx in response to membrane depolarization and modulate excitability, contraction, hormonal secretion and gene transcription (1–6). There are many pathologies, both genetic and acquired, involving VGCCs. Mutations in VGCCs cause dysfunctions of Ca channels, resulting in abnormal excitation of the cardiomyocyte, and cardiac arrhythmias (2, 6–8), which contribute substantially to morbidity and mortality. Among the different pathophysiological mechanisms of arrhythmogenesis, a new area of interest has recently emerged and is related to autoimmune-associated Ca channel dysfunction (autoimmune Ca channelopathies) in cardiac arrhythmias (9–12). This review summarizes the recent findings on the roles of cardiac Ca channels in autoantibodies-associated cardiac arrhythmias.

VOLTAGE-GATED CALCIUM CHANNELS IN THE HEART

L-type and T-type Ca channels are the two major classes of VGCCs in the heart. The L-type Ca channel is a high voltage-activated, long-lasting, and the T-type channel is characterized by a low voltage-activated, transient-type channel (2, 3, 5, 6, 13, 14). There are 10 isoforms of mammalian genes encoding the α_1 subunit. (5, 15–18). *CACNA1S, CACNA1C, CACNA1D,* and *CACNA1F* encode α_{1S}, α_{1C}, α_{1D}, and α_{1F} subunits (L-type Ca channels) respectively. *CACNA1A, CACNA1B,* and *CACNA1E* encode α_{1A}, α_{1B}, and α_{1E} subunits (P/Q-, N-, and R-types), respectively, (19–21). The T-type Ca channels α_{1G}, α_{1H}, and α_{1I} subunits are encoded by *CACNA1G, CACNA1H,* and *CACNA1I,* respectively, (22–24). Among these channels, the L-type Ca channels α_{1C} and α_{1D} isoforms and the T-type Ca channels α_{1G} and α_{1H} isoforms are the major VGCCs expressed in the heart (25–27). The features and tissue distribution of the L-type and T-type Ca channels are summarized in **Table 1**.

L-type Ca Channels in the Heart

α_{1C} L-type Ca Channel

Cardiac α_{1C} L-type VGCC is a protein complex comprised of α_{1C}, β_2, and α_2/δ subunits. The α_1 subunit is the pore-forming subunit, which determines the major features of the channel, such as ion selectivity, activation-inactivation and the sensitivity to Ca channel blockers (3, 6, 15, 16). The β_2 and α_2/δ accessory subunits play important roles in the regulation of the biophysical properties of Ca channels (36). The α_{1C} VGCC is universally expressed in the heart and plays a critical role in excitation–contraction coupling, impulse generation in sinus node (SAN) and its conduction in the atrioventricular node (AVN). The Ca ions entering the cardiomyocytes through α_{1C} VGCCs also shape the plateau phase of the ventricular action potential and induce the release of Ca from the sarcoplasmic reticulum (calcium induced-calcium release) which initiates the myocardial contraction (1, 6, 36).

α_{1D} L-type Ca Channel

In contrast to the ubiquitously expressed α_{1C} VGCCs in the heart, α_{1D} VGCCs are restricted to the supraventricular tissue of the adult heart, with the highest expression in the atria, SAN, and AVN, but they are not expressed in the normal adult ventricles (5, 28, 37–42). In the fetal heart, however, α_{1D} VGCCs are expressed throughout the heart including the ventricles, atria, SAN, and AVN (39). While α_{1C} VGCCs activate at more positive (−40 and −30 mV) potentials, α_{1D} VGCCs activate between −60 and −40 mV at a range of diastolic depolarization of the SAN (28, 42). This unique feature allows α_{1D} VGCCs to play an important role in the automaticity of SAN pacemaker cells (29, 43, 44). The unexpected SAN dysfunction reported in mice lacking α_{1D} VGCCs was the first evidence of their importance in heart automaticity (28, 42, 44). Deletion of the α_{1D} VGCC gene impairs pace making in the SAN and atrioventricular conduction in the AVN but has no effect on myocardial contractility (42, 44).

T-type Ca Channels in the Heart

There are 3 isoforms of T-type VGCC: α_{1G} (23, 45), α_{1H} (24), and α_{1I} (45, 46). Among them, α_{1G} and α_{1H} are the major isoforms in the myocardium and their expression is developmentally regulated (17, 30, 31). While α_{1H} T-type VGCC constitutes the predominant isoform in embryonic heart tissue (32); α_{1G} T-type VGCC expression increases during the perinatal period and reaches its maximal level in adulthood. In adult SAN, α_{1G} expression is higher than α_{1H} T-type VGCC (26, 27, 33). In contrast to α_{1D} L-type VGCC, which requires accessary subunits for normal gating, α_{1G} or α_{1H} subunits expression alone exhibit native T-type Ca channel properties (17, 47, 48). In addition, T-type VGCCs open at significantly more negative membrane potentials that overlap the pacemaker potentials of SAN cells (30, 49). The threshold for activation is −70 to −60 mV, and the channel is fully activated at −30 to −10 mV (17, 31, 49). T-type VGCCs are expressed in the SAN (34), the AVN (50), and the Purkinje fibers (51, 52), supporting their roles in the generation of the diastolic depolarization, the automaticity of SAN and the impulse conduction of the heart (30, 31, 53, 54). Indeed, homozygous transgenic mice lacking α_{1G} VGCC exhibit first-degree atrioventricular block (AVB) and bradycardia (25). Collectively, both L-type, and T-type Ca channels by virtue of their tissue-specific localization can modulate automaticity, conduction and repolarization, and as such, agents and compounds like autoantibodies (discussed below) which interact and target these channels are expected to affect the electrical activity of the heart.

AUTOANTIBODIES-ASSOCIATED CARDIAC CALCIUM CHANNELOPATHIES

Autoimmune disorders and cardiovascular disorders are associated with significant morbidity and mortality and are a major health problem both in the USA and worldwide. While the field of "cardio-immunology" is being formally established, recent and emerging advances in this area indicate that autoantibodies play an important role in the development of cardiac arrhythmias.

Autoantibodies Against Ca Channel and Ventricular Arrhythmias: Anti-α_{1C} Subunit Antibody

Autoimmunity is one of the main mechanisms involved in the pathogenesis of dilated cardiomyopathy (DCM) (55–57). Sudden death caused by ventricular arrhythmias is one of the leading causes of death in patients with DCM (58–60). Results from previous studies indicated that the VGCC plays an important role in the pathogenesis of DCM (11, 61, 62). The function of VGCCs in DCM is affected either by autoantibodies directed against the regulatory pathway/accessary subunits or autoantibodies targeting the pore forming α_1 subunit itself. Several autoantibodies indirectly affecting the L-type VGCCs have been identified in patients with DCM (63–65). The presence of antibody against the β-adrenoceptor

TABLE 1 | Features of Ca channels in the heart.

Channel	Gene	Activation	Distribution	Developmental change	Function
α_{1C} VGCC	Cav1.2	−40 mV	Ubiquitous	Increase with developmental stage	• Action potential in SAN and AVN, • Inotropy, contraction of atria and ventricles
α_{1D} VGCC	Cav1.3	−60 mV	SAN, AVN, Atria in adult heart; Ubiquitous in immature heart	Decrease with developmental stage	• Pace making, • AVN conduction • Atrial excitability
α_{1G} VGCC	Cav3.1	−70 mV	Supraventricular tissue, 30-fold more in SAN than in atria	Increase during development, maximal at adult stage	• Pacing making • AVN conduction
α_{1H} VGCC	Cav3.2	−70 mV	Supraventricular tissue	Predominant in embryonic stage	

references (6, 14, 15, 17, 18, 28–35).

was first reported in a patient with Chagas' disease by Sterin-Borda et al. (66). Ten years later, Wallukat and Wollenberger demonstrated the presence of an agonist-like anti-β1 adrenoceptor in DCM patients (67). Subsequent studies showed that these autoantibodies in DCM target the second extra-cellular loop of the β1-adrenoreptor (68), resulting in a positive chronotropic effect. Autoantibodies against β1-adrenoceptors were closely related to ventricular arrhythmias in patients with DCM (69). Anti-β1-adrenoceptor antibodies induced in an animal model caused action potential duration prolongation, with higher propensity for induction of early repolarization, promoting the development of ventricular arrhythmias which increased the risk of sudden death (69–71). Notably, Christ et al. (72) demonstrated that anti-β1 adrenoceptor antibodies increased L-Type Ca current, I_{Ca-L} in adult rat ventricular cells in concordance with the prolongation of the action potential duration. Autoantibodies against adenine nucleotide translocators, which cross-react with VGCCs, increases the Ca inflow which causes myocyte damage by Ca overload in DCM (73–75).

The evidence of the presence of agonist-like autoantibodies directly against the L-type VGCC α_{1C} subunits in DCM was demonstrated by Liao et al. (76) and Xiao et al. (11) subsequently demonstrated that autoantibodies against α_{1C} Ca channel are arrhythmogenic and lead to sudden cardiac death in patients with DCM. In a prospective study, the authors compared ventricular arrhythmias and sudden death in 80 patients with DCM and age- and gender-matched controls for 32 months. Autoantibodies against L-type α_{1C} subunits (anti-α_{1C}) were detected by ELISA in 39 patients with DCM (48.8%) and 5 controls (6.3%). Higher incidence of ventricular arrhythmias and sudden cardiac death was observed in anti-α_{1C} antibody-positive patients as compared to the antibody-negative patients. The presence of anti-α_{1C} antibodies was identified as the strongest independent predictor for sudden death in DCM (11). The arrhythmogenic effect of anti-α_{1C} antibodies was reproduced in a rat model (11). Perfusion of affinity purified anti-α_{1C} antibodies lead to ventricular arrhythmias by action potential duration prolongation and triggered activity (11). This effect was blocked by pre-incubating the anti-α_{1C} antibodies with its specific peptide and Ca channel blockers, indicating the specificity of the arrhythmogenic effect of the anti-α_{1C} antibodies (11). To further investigate the underlying mechanism of the anti-α_{1C} antibodies, Xiao et al. using immunofluorescent approach demonstrated that anti-α_{1C} antibodies were able specifically to bind to the Ca channel on the myocyte, enhancing the channel's activities (hence the agonist-like effect). In a prospective study, Yu et al. (62) recruited 2096 patients with congestive heart failure, of which 841 dilated cardiomyopathy patients (DMC) 1,255 ischemic cardiomyopathy (ICM) patients, and 834 controls. By the end of a median follow up of 52 months, 102 cases of DCM had sudden cardiac death. Interestingly, the rate of anti-Ca channel antibody in DCM was significantly higher in DCM patients compared to controls. After adjusting for risk factor including age, left ventricular ejection fraction (LVEF), hypertension, diabetes, New York Heart Association (NYHA) functional classification, QTc, and medications, Cox regression analysis revealed that the presence of anti-Ca channel antibodies still remains an independent risk factor for sudden cardiac death in DCM patients. In conclusion, there are novel agonist-like anti-α_{1C} Ca channel antibodies in patients with DCM, which prolong action potential duration and QT interval, induce early after depolarizations, and ventricular tachycardia, eventually leading to sudden cardiac death. These antibodies could serve as novel clinical markers and as positive predictor of sudden death in DCM (**Figure 1**) (61, 62).

Autoimmune-Associated Brady-Arrhythmias and Conduction Abnormalities: Cardiac L-type Ca Channels and Anti-ro Antibodies

While presence of the anti-α_{1C} Ca channel antibody is identified as a strong predictor for ventricular arrhythmias and sudden cardiac death in DCM (11), its role has not been well-established in other autoimmune-associated cardiac electrical abnormalities. The best studied disease caused by autoantibody related L-type Ca channel dysfunction is autoimmune-associated congenital heart block (CHB) characterized by AVB, and sinus bradycardia (10, 35, 77–80). CHB is a conduction abnormality that affects structurally normal hearts of fetuses and/or newborn to mothers with autoantibodies against the intracellular ribonucleoproteins SSA-Ro and SSB-La (10, 79, 80). The hallmark of CHB is

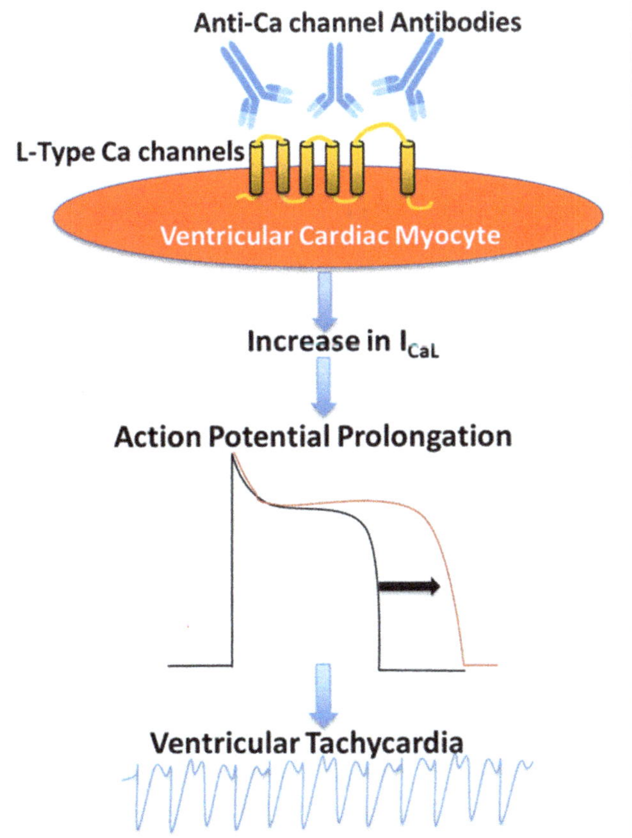

FIGURE 1 | Proposed mechanism of the pathogenic role of anti-Ca channels autoantibodies in Dilated Cardiomyopathy. Anti-Ca channels autoantibodies target L-type Ca channels in the ventricular myocyte resulting in an increase in L-type Ca current (I_{CaL}) which in turn leads to action potential prolongation and ventricular arrhythmias.

various degrees of AVB, with complete AVB being the most common, for which more than 60% of affected children require lifelong pacemakers (81), and carries mortality rate up to 30% (81, 82). Because anti-Ro antibodies are the most prevalent autoantibodies in CHB (83–85), anti-La antibodies are not discussed in this review. There are 2 subtypes of anti-Ro autoantibodies: anti-52 and anti-60 kD SSA/Ro (collectively termed anti-Ro antibodies in this review). Anti-Ro antibodies result from an autoimmune response to the SSA-Ro antigen, which is an intracellular ribonucleoprotein that is not accessible to the circulating anti-Ro antibodies in the normal cardiac myocyte, likely because of their large size. Anti-Ro antibodies are more prevalent in certain autoimmune diseases including Sjögren's syndrome, systemic lupus erythematosus, scleroderma, rheumatoid arthritis, systemic sclerosis, and myositis (86, 87). Intriguingly, these anti-Ro antibodies are also present in the general healthy population (87–89). The incidence of CHB is about 1:11,000 (81, 90); however, this incidence dramatically increases to about 5% in anti-Ro positive mothers and up to 18% in subsequent pregnancies thereby affecting the decision to have a second child (79, 81). The causal relationship of anti-Ro antibodies to the development of CHB was reproduced in both active and passive mice models of CHB (81, 91–93). Various degree of AVB developed in pups born to female mice immunized with recombinant 52 SSA/Ro protein (active immunization) (81, 93, 94). Transfer of anti-Ro antibodies from mothers with CHB children (anti-Ro antibody positive IgG) directly into timely pregnant mice also resulted in first degree AVB and, surprisingly, sinus bradycardia in about 70% of the pups (passive immunization) (91). Similarly, clinical data (95, 96) also confirmed similar sinus bradycardia in newborns of mothers with anti-Ro antibody positive IgG, indicating that the spectrum of CHB extends beyond AVN to also affect SAN.

Anti-Ro Antibody Positive IgG Inhibits Both α_{1C} and α_{1D} Ca Currents

As mentioned above, the hallmark of CHB is AVB. The conduction of the impulse through the AVN depends critically on α_{1C} Ca current, I_{Ca-L}, which activates at more positive (−40 and −30 mV) potentials (97). It is logical to speculate that anti-Ro antibody positive IgG might target α_{1C} Ca channel to disturb the electrical conduction at AVN as seen in CHB. Anti-Ro antibody positive IgG and affinity purified anti-52 Ro antibodies from mothers with CHB children, but not anti-Ro antibody negative IgG from healthy mothers, inhibited I_{Ca-L} in isolated SAN, AVN cells, Purkinje fibers and in ventricular cells by 50–59% (77, 78, 98–100). In addition, anti-Ro antibody positive IgG had no effect on K currents (the transient outward current, I_{to} and the inward rectifier, I_{K1}), or the Na current (I_{Na}), indicating its specificity toward Ca channels (98). To exclude the possibility of potential contamination from other ion currents, α_{1C} Ca channels expressed in Xenopus oocytes were similarly inhibited about 50% by anti-Ro antibody positive IgG (92, 99, 100).

While inhibition of α_{1C} I_{Ca-L} could account for the AVB seen in CHB, the contribution of α_{1C} I_{Ca-L} to diastolic depolarization of the SA node is generally considered to be minor. SAN pacemaker depolarization occurs between −60 and −40 mV; however α_{1C} I_{Ca-L} activates at more positive (−40 and −30 mV) potentials (101). Knockout of the α_{1D} Ca channel, which activates at −60 and −40 mV in mice, results in significant sinus bradycardia and AVB (28, 42, 102), a phenotype reminiscent to that seen in CHB. Mangoni et al. (44) showed I_{Ca-L} in SAN cells was decreased by 75% in α_{1D} Ca channel knockout mice compared with wild-type mice, which indicates that the contribution of the α_{1D} Ca channel to total I_{Ca-L} is significant in the mouse SA node cell. Furthermore, our previous studies demonstrated that both α_{1D} Ca channel transcripts and proteins are expressed in human fetal heart and in adult rabbit SAN (39, 40). Collectively, these data suggest that α_{1D}, along with α_{1C}, contribute to form I_{Ca-L}, playing a critical role in pace making activity in SAN and are a potential target by anti-Ro antibodies. Because there are no biophysical methods or specific blockers to separate α_{1D} from α_{1C} I_{CaL} in native cells, the specific effect of anti-Ro antibodies on α_{1D} I_{Ca-L} has been challenging. Initial studies were carried out in expression systems to allow individual expression of α_{1D} I_{Ca-L} to characterize the effect of anti-Ro antibody positive IgG. Anti-Ro antibody positive IgG from mothers with CHB children inhibited α_{1D} I_{Ca-L} by about 43% in tsA201 cells and about 33% in Xenopus oocytes (40, 77,

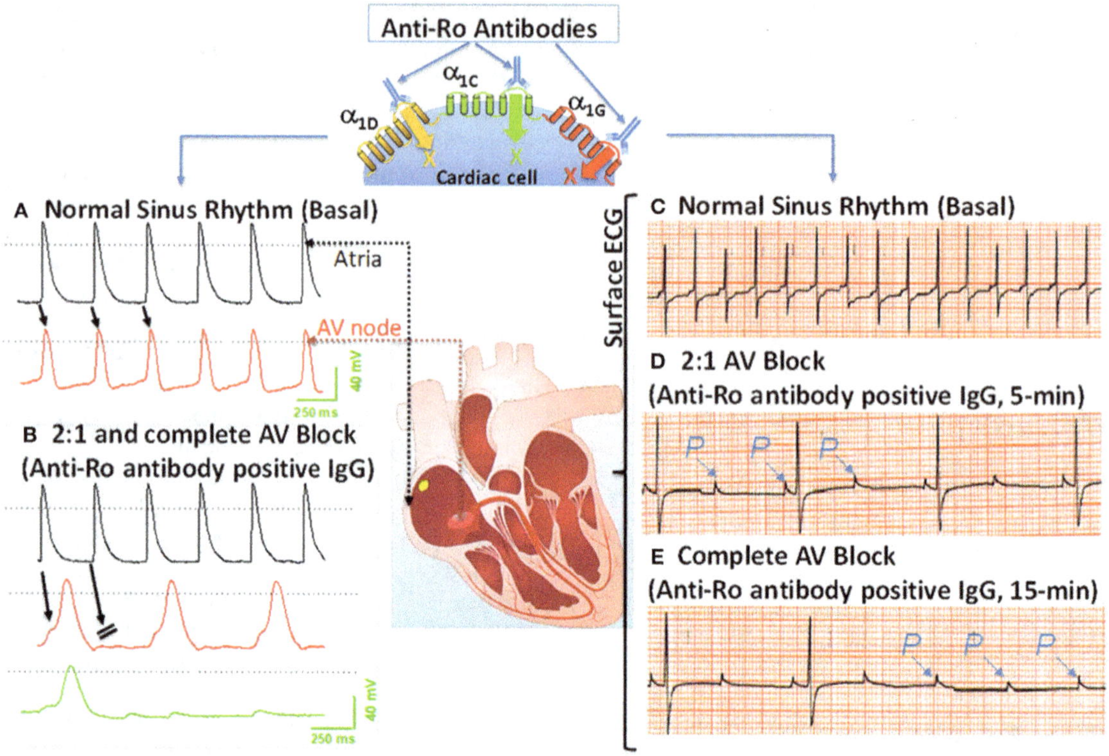

FIGURE 2 | Effects of anti-Ro antibodies from mothers of children with congenital heart block on an isolated multicellular AV nodal preparation (left) and Langendorff perfused whole heart (Right). **(A)** Simultaneous control action potentials from the crista terminalis (black tracing) and the AV node area (red tracing). **(B)** Superfusion of the preparation with positive IgG (800 μg/mL) for 10 min resulted in 2:1 AV block (indicated by the arrows) which progressed to near complete inhibition of the AV node action potential by 15 min **(B)**, (green tracing). **(C)** ECG was recorded by the conventional ECG machine in lead I, except for the use of silver wires at the recording end of the leads. One lead was inserted in the atrium, the second in the left ventricle near the apex, and the third in Tyrode's solution (ground). "P" indicates, the P wave and on the ECG. Regular sinus rhythm (horizontal scale, 50 mm/s and vertical scale: 5 mm/mV) at 300 beats/min in Tyrode's solution. **(D)** After 5 min of perfusion with positive IgG (800 μg/mL), there was bradycardia associated with a 2:1 second degree AV block that degenerated into complete AV block by 15 min of IgG perfusion **(E)**. The sectioned heart in the middle panel illustrates the location of the microelectrode recordings.

78, 92, 99, 100). To overcome this limitation of using expression systems, our group has tested the effect of anti-Ro antibodies on α_{1D} I_{Ca-L} in native neonatal cardiomyocytes, in which the α_{1C} gene was effectively silenced by lentivirus. Adding anti-Ro antibody positive IgG resulted in 35% reduction of α_{1D} I_{Ca-L} in naïve cardiomyocytes (103), similar to the results seen using expression systems.

Because anti-Ro antibodies inhibit both α_{1C} and α_{1D} I_{Ca-L}, it is anticipated that anti-Ro antibodies will cause both sinus bradycardia and AVB. Further experimental evidence using isolated multicellular AVN preparations (**Figures 2A,B**) and Langendorff-perfused whole hearts (**Figures 2C–E**) demonstrated that anti-Ro antibody positive IgG resulted in bradycardia associated with 2:1 AVB then complete third degree AVB as recorded by surface EG. In contrast, perfusion of the AVN preparation or whole heart with control anti-Ro antibody negative IgG had no effect on ECG parameters (78). The sinus bradycardia and AVB were also demonstrated in Langendorff-perfused human hearts by our group (77) and by others (104, 105). Similar findings were obtained using the optical mapping technique, which allows simultaneous recording of voltage action potentials at multiple areas of the heart including the AVN area. Perfusion of hearts with anti-Ro antibody positive IgG revealed the sites of conduction abnormalities at the sinoatrial junction and AVN, thereby confirming the site of action for these autoantibodies (106).

In summary, α_{1D} and α_{1C} Ca channels both contribute to total I_{Ca-L} in the heart, with α_{1D} Ca channels playing a more critical role in the SAN and α_{1C} Ca channels in the AVN. Anti-Ro antibodies inhibit I_{Ca-L} emanating from both α_{1D} and α_{1C}, resulting in AVB and sinus bradycardia seen in CHB. This causal relationship was confirmed by reproducing active and passive mice CHB models by induction of anti-Ro antibodies (active immunization) or passive transfer of the anti-Ro positive maternal IgG into pregnant mice (passive immunization). Altogether, anti-Ro autoantibodies' inhibition of Ca channels are causally related to the development of CHB, but the low incidence of CHB children born to anti-Ro antibodies positive mothers suggest that additional factor(s) may be necessary to contribute to the full spectrum of CHB.

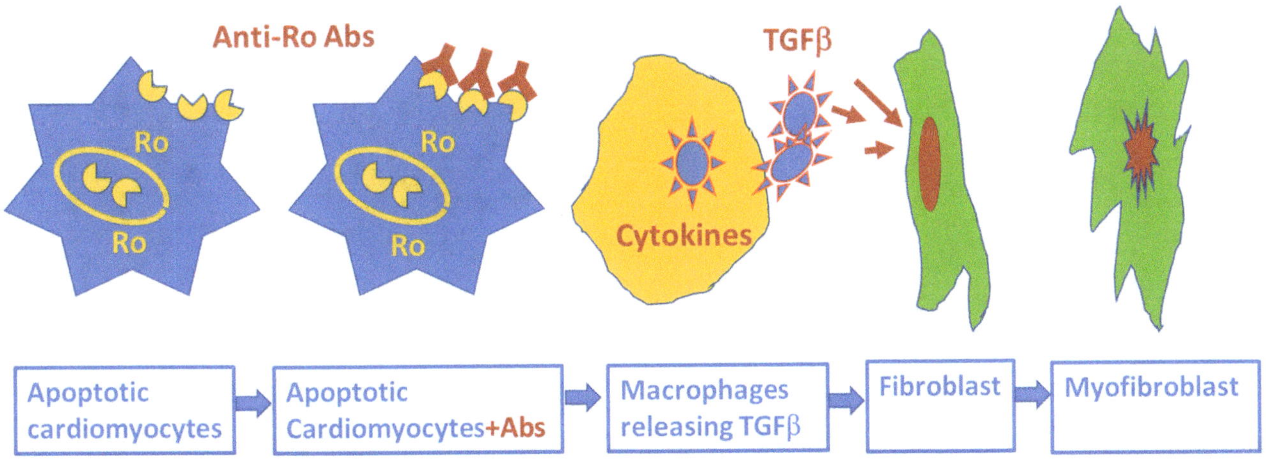

FIGURE 3 | Schematic representation of alternative mechanism of linking anti-Ro antibodies to the development of atrioventricular block: fetal cardiomyocytes undergoing "physiological" apoptosis cause the surface translocation of the intracellular located Ro antigens. Circulating maternal anti-Ro antibodies which can cross the placenta, subsequently bind to the translocated Ro antigens at the cell surface; provoke the secretion of proinflammatory cytokines such as TGFβ from macrophages. Excessive TGFβ secretion activates fibroblasts leading to scars promoting myofibroblasts in the Atrioventricular node, resulting in atrioventricular block.

Anti-ro Antibody Positive IgG Inhibits Ca Currents by Binding Directly to the Pore Forming Subunit of the Ca Channels

As pointed out earlier, anti-Ro antibody positive IgG cannot cross the sarcolemma of a normal fetal cardiac myocyte, and hence one can suspect that its effects are not directly mediated through its antigen, SSA/Ro, but rather via sarcolemma targets such as Ca channels. Evidence for direct interaction between anti-Ro antibodies and Ca channels is provided by the direct binding of anti-Ro antibodies on the pore forming α_1 subunit of VGCC, resulting in inhibition of I_{CaL}. Indeed, using immunostaining and Western blots, it was demonstrated that anti-Ro antibody positive IgG binds directly to the Ca channels' α_1 subunit (99, 107). In a subsequent study, purified GST fusion proteins corresponding to the extracellular loop S5–S6 of each of the four domains that form the pore of the α_{1D} subunit were expressed and their reactivity to anti-Ro antibody positive IgG was tested. Fourteen percent of anti-Ro antibody positive IgG reacted specifically with the extracellular loop S5-S6 of the first domains of the α_{1D} subunit, as demonstrated by both ELISA and Western blots (108). L-type Ca channels' inhibition by anti-Ro antibodies is one of the mechanisms for the electrocardiographic abnormalities seen in CHB. The resulting formulation of the "Ca channel hypothesis" was based on the above experimental findings and was driven by the fact that AVN electrogenesis depends on the L-type Ca channels. Inhibition of this channel will ultimately lead to AVB, as seen in CHB. The "Ca channel hypothesis" states that circulating maternal antibodies directly cross react with L-type Ca channel pore forming protein α_1-subunit, inhibiting the currents and leading to the development of AVB (97).

T-type Ca Channel and Autoimmune-Associated Congenital Heart Block

T-type α_{1G} VGCCs subtype participates with α_{1H} in regulating electrical conduction through the AVN (18, 27, 31, 34). α_{1G} VGCC is highly expressed in the AVN in human hearts (27, 31, 32). Homozygous α_{1G} knockout mice exhibit first-degree AVB and bradycardia, a phenotype seen in CHB (25). These findings suggest α_{1G} VGCC as an additional potential cross-reactive target with anti-Ro antibody positive IgG in the development of CHB. Hu et al. demonstrated that anti-Ro antibody positive IgG decreased both I_{CaL} and T-type Ca current (I_{Ca-T}) without affecting the delayed rectifier K current, I_K, and the funny current, I_f, in rabbit SAN cells (98). The average inhibition of I_{Ca-T} by anti-Ro antibody positive IgG was 31.4% at −40 mV and 44.1% at −20 mV in rabbit SAN cells (98). In addition, although anti-Ro antibody positive IgG inhibited the α_{1H} I_{CaT} expressed in the Xenopus oocyte (100), α_{1H} Ca channel knockout mice have no ECG changes (109), likely secondary to the low level of α_{1H} expression in the human neonatal AVN cells (107). These findings support the conclusion that the α_{1G} Ca channel is the target for anti-Ro antibody positive IgG. Strindberg et al. demonstrated α_{1G} mRNA and proteins in human fetal hearts and that α_{1G} I_{Ca-T} rather than α_{1H} I_{Ca-T} is the dominant current in the AVN in newborns (107). Experimental data using immunoprecipitation, Western blot and immunofluorescent staining have demonstrated accessibility of anti-Ro antibody positive IgG to the α_{1G} epitope on the surfaces on the cardiomyocytes in the human fetal heart (107). Reactivity to α_{1G} T-type VGCC was significantly higher in CHB maternal sera compared to controls. Binding epitope of anti-Ro antibody positive IgG was mapped to the extracellular S5–S6 portion of repeat I of α_{1G} subunit (aa305–319; designated as p305). Using the patch-clamp technique, the authors also demonstrated that anti-Ro antibody positive IgG inhibited I_{Ca-T} in isolated mice SAN cells (107). Taken together, these results indicate that anti-Ro antibody positive IgG readily target an extracellular epitope of α_{1G} T-type VGCC and inhibit the current in human fetal cardiomyocytes, thus contributing to the development of AVB as seen in CHB.

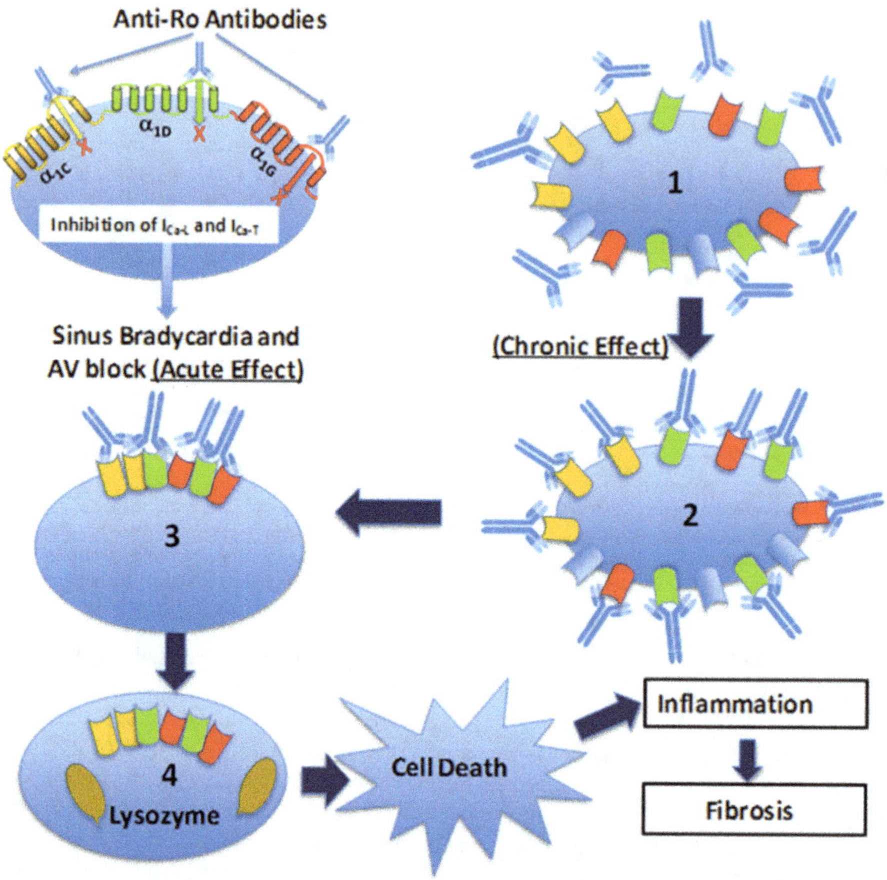

FIGURE 4 | Schematic illustration of the Ca channel hypothesis. Maternal anti-Ro antibodies cross react and bind to α_{1C} (yellow), α_{1D} (green), and α_{1G} (red) Ca channels in the fetal human heart, inhibit all three Ca currents leading to sinus bradycardia and atrioventricular (AV) block (acute effect). Furthermore, fetal heart Ca channels are exposed *chronically* (chronic effect) (1) to maternal anti-Ro antibodies during pregnancy. Binding of anti-Ro antibodies to Ca channels (2), can cause cross-linking of the adjacent ion channels by the two Fab arms of IgG (3) to increase the internalization of the channel/antibody complex and thereby decrease of the channel density on the cell membrane. Internalized Ca channels are lysed by lysosomes (4). If the number of Ca channels on cell surface decreased to a critical level, then cell death will occur. Cell death, *per se*, could trigger inflammation subsequent to leukocytic influx resulting in damage of the surrounding healthy myocytes such as in sinoatrial node and AV node which can cause permanent sinus bradycardia and AV block.

Anti-52kD Ro antibodies are present in 80% of mothers of children with CHB; however, the risk of having CHB children is low, with only 1–2% in single anti-Ro antibody positive pregnancies (84). Markham et al. investigated if reactivity with p305 (anti-Ro/p305) can be used clinically to more accurately predict CHB in anti-Ro antibody positive patients (110). Using anti-Ro antibody positive IgG and with multiple control groups, reactivity was determined and compared for binding to anti-Ro/p305. In mothers carrying anti-Ro antibodies, positive anti-Ro/p305 antibodies were detected in 3/59 (5%) CHB pregnancies, 4/30 (13%) unaffected pregnancies with a CHB-sibling, and 0/42 (0%) of unaffected pregnancies with no CHB-sibling. Similarly, using umbilical blood from 61 CHB and 41 healthy with CHB-sibling, in which reactivity would unambiguously substantiate exposure to maternal antibody, no association of anti-Ro/p305 with CHB was detected. These data indicate that anti-Ro/p305 reactivity in pregnant anti-Ro antibody-positive patients is not a robust maternal marker for assessing increased risk of CHB (110).

As described above, it is well-recognized that maternal anti-Ro antibody is associated with the development of the congenial AVB, at least in part resulting from an inhibitory cross-reaction with L- and T-type Ca channels. More recent, studies demonstrated that 10–60% of anti-Ro-positive subjects are at increased risk of developing QTc prolongation as a result of anti-Ro antibodies' interference with K channels, (111–115) resulting in complex ventricular arrhythmia, (116, 117) including Torsade's de Pointes (TdP) (118, 119). Lazzerini et al. (119) recently evaluated 25 consecutive patients who experienced TdP, where anti-Ro antibody was present in 15 out of 25 patients. Purified anti-Ro positive IgG from TdP patients cross-reacted with the Human Ether-a-go-go-related Gene (hERG) K channel and significantly inhibited the resulting current, IKr. This observation indicates that anti-Ro antibodies may represent a novel, clinically silent risk factors for TdP. To date, studies on the association of anti-Ro antibodies and atrial fibrillation are scarce. In our previous study (120), we were able to induce atrial fibrillation in the α_{1D} knockout mice but not in the wild-type mice. One can speculate that the unique atrial specific distribution of α_{1D} Ca channel, together with the documented inhibitory effect of the anti-Ro antibodies on the α_{1D} Ca channels, may suggest that anti-Ro positive patients might be at increased risk of having atrial fibrillation, warranting further investigations.

CONCLUSIONS AND FUTURE DIRECTIONS

Cardiac Ca channels, including both L- and T-type Ca channels, play critical roles in the impulse generation in the SAN, the conduction through the AVN and the development of arrhythmias. Autoantibodies targeting Ca channels have been identified in 2 major pathologies, DCM and CHB. In addition, several autoantibodies are directly related to sudden death in patients with DCM, including anti-N/K-ATPase, anti-M2 muscarinic acetylcholine receptors, and anti-β1 receptor antibodies, indirectly affecting the L-type VGCCs. Early risk stratification to effectively prevent adverse outcomes in DCM has been challenging. Recent studies confirmed the presence of autoantibodies directly against Ca channel α_{1C} subunit in DCM, which was identified as a strong predictor for ventricular arrhythmias and sudden cardiac death, indicating that anti-α_{1C} Ca channel antibodies might be a valuable biomarker to predict sudden death in DCM.

The association of anti-Ro autoantibodies with CHB is generally accepted, but the predictive value of these autoantibodies is still low despite overwhelming experimental data demonstrating causality between anti-Ro antibodies and electrocardiographic abnormalities seen in CHB (**Figure 2**). This indicates that anti-Ro antibodies are necessary, but not sufficient, for inducing the clinical electrocardiographic phenotype. To date, two hypotheses have been proposed to explain the molecular mechanism(s) by which maternal anti-Ro antibodies lead to the development of CHB in the fetal hearts (79, 121). The "apoptosis hypothesis" (**Figure 3**) suggests that intracellular antigens translocate to the surface of cardiomyocytes undergoing apoptosis during physiological remodeling, thereby exposing the antigens to the circulating maternal anti-Ro antibodies. Binding of anti-Ro antibodies to the cell surface antigens promotes pro-inflammatory and pro-fibrotic responses (122, 123), causing the fibrosis of the AVN, which eventually leads to the development of the irreversible AVB (124, 125). The "Ca channel hypothesis" explained in this review is based on molecular mimicry, whereby anti-Ro antibodies directly cross-react and subsequently inhibit the cardiac Ca channels' activity, thereby causing sinus bradycardia and AVB (77, 78, 108) (**Figure 4**). This occurs by anti-Ro autoantibodies binding to Ca channels and the resulting inhibition of I_{CaL} (Acute effect, **Figure 4**). The subsequent cross-linkage and downregulation of Ca channels and lysis by lysosomes followed by intracellular Ca dysregulation leads to cell death/apoptosis, inflammation, and fibrosis of the AVN (**Figure 4**). The ultimate proof of direct autoantibodies' involvement in CHB is provided by the identification of the site of action on the different subunits of cardiac Ca channels (126–128), including α_{1C} and α_{1D} subunits of L-type VGCCs and α_{1G} subunit of T-type VGCCs (**Figure 4**). Although autoantibodies are utilized as diagnostic or prognostic markers in other pathologies, unfortunately, to date, there is no specific maternal marker for assessing the increased risk of having CHB children during an anti-Ro positive pregnancy. It is possible that, instead of having a single CHB-inducing antibody specificity, future studies may focus on several different specificities that may act synergistically to induce AVB in fetal hearts.

Peptide-based therapeutic approaches are one of the growing classes of novel therapeutic agents. The development of short non-immunogenic peptides and their use as decoy targets for pathogenic autoantibodies is expected to minimize and/or prevent autoantibody association with ion channels and their functions. This therapeutic path awaits further development and progress.

AUTHOR CONTRIBUTIONS

All authors listed have made a substantial, direct and intellectual contribution to the work, and approved it for publication.

REFERENCES

1. Rougier JS, Abriel H. Cardiac voltage-gated calcium channel macromolecular complexes. *Biochim Biophys Acta.* (2016) 1863:1806–12.doi: 10.1016/j.bbamcr.2015.12.014
2. Betzenhauser MJ, Pitt GS, Antzelevitch C. Calcium channel mutations in cardiac arrhythmia syndromes. *Curr Mol Pharmacol.* (2015) 8:133–42. doi: 10.2174/1874467208666150518114857
3. Dolphin AC. Calcium channel diversity: multiple roles of calcium channel subunits. *Curr Opin Neurobiol.* (2009) 19:237–44. doi: 10.1016/j.conb.2009.06.006
4. Catterall WA. Signaling complexes of voltage-gated sodium and calcium channels. *Neurosci Lett.* (2010) 486:107–16. doi: 10.1016/j.neulet.2010.08.085
5. Mesirca P, Torrente AG, Mangoni ME. Functional role of voltage gated Ca(2+) channels in heart automaticity. *Front Physiol.* (2015) 6:19. doi: 10.3389/fphys.2015.00019
6. Zamponi GW, Striessnig J, Koschak A, Dolphin AC. The physiology, pathology, and pharmacology of voltage-gated calcium channels and their future therapeutic potential. *Pharmacol Rev.* (2015) 67:821–70. doi: 10.1124/pr.114.009654
7. Zhang Q, Chen J, Qin Y, Wang J, Zhou L. Mutations in voltage-gated L-type calcium channel: implications in cardiac arrhythmia. *Channels.* (2018) 12:201–18. doi: 10.1080/19336950.2018.1499368
8. Venetucci L, Denegri M, Napolitano C, Priori SG. Inherited calcium channelopathies in the pathophysiology of arrhythmias. *Nat Rev Cardiol.* (2012) 9:561–75. doi: 10.1038/nrcardio.2012.93
9. Lee HC, Huang KT, Wang XL, Shen WK. Autoantibodies and cardiac arrhythmias. *Heart Rhythm.* (2011) 8:1788–95. doi: 10.1016/j.hrthm.2011.06.032
10. Lazzerini PE, Capecchi PL, Laghi-Pasini F, Boutjdir M. Autoimmune cardiac channelopathies: the heart of the matter. *Nat Rev Cardiol.* (2017) 14:566. doi: 10.1038/nrcardio.2017.111
11. Xiao H, Wang M, Du Y, Yuan J, Cheng X, Chen Z, et al. Arrhythmogenic autoantibodies against calcium channel lead to sudden death in idiopathic dilated cardiomyopathy. *Eur J Heart Fail.* (2011) 13:264–70. doi: 10.1093/eurjhf/hfq198

12. Durante A, Bronzato S. The increased cardiovascular risk in patients affected by autoimmune diseases: review of the various manifestations. *J Clin Med Res.* (2015) 7:379–84. doi: 10.14740/jocmr2122w
13. Nilius B, Hess P, Lansman JB, Tsien RW. A novel type of cardiac calcium channel in ventricular cells. *Nature.* (1985) 316:443–6. doi: 10.1038/316443a0
14. Bean BP. Two kinds of calcium channels in canine atrial cells. differences in kinetics, selectivity, and pharmacology. *J Gen Physiol.* (1985) 86:1–30. doi: 10.1085/jgp.86.1.1
15. Catterall WA. Voltage-gated calcium channels. *Cold Spring Harb Perspect Biol.* (2011) 3:a003947. doi: 10.1101/cshperspect.a003947
16. Dolphin AC. Voltage-gated calcium channels and their auxiliary subunits: physiology and pathophysiology and pharmacology. *J Physiol.* (2016) 594:5369–90. doi: 10.1113/JP272262
17. Perez-Reyes E. Molecular physiology of low-voltage-activated t-type calcium channels. *Physiol Rev.* (2003) 83:117–61. doi: 10.1152/physrev.00018.2002
18. Cribbs L. T-type calcium channel expression and function in the diseased heart. *Channels.* (2010) 4:447–52. doi: 10.4161/chan.4.6.12870
19. Nowycky MC, Fox AP, Tsien RW. Three types of neuronal calcium channel with different calcium agonist sensitivity. *Nature.* (1985) 316:440–3. doi: 10.1038/316440a0
20. Mintz IM, Adams ME, Bean BP. P-type calcium channels in rat central and peripheral neurons. *Neuron.* (1992) 9:85–95. doi: 10.1016/0896-6273(92)90223-Z
21. Namkung Y, Smith SM, Lee SB, Skrypnyk NV, Kim HL, Chin H, et al. Targeted disruption of the Ca2+ channel beta3 subunit reduces N- and L-type Ca2+ channel activity and alters the voltage-dependent activation of P/Q-type Ca2+ channels in neurons. *Proc. Natl. Acad. Sci. U.S.A.* (1998) 95:12010–5. doi: 10.1073/pnas.95.20.12010
22. Lambert RC, McKenna F, Maulet Y, Talley EM, Bayliss DA, Cribbs LL, et al. Low-voltage-activated Ca2+ currents are generated by members of the CavT subunit family (alpha1G/H) in rat primary sensory neurons. *J Neurosci.* (1998) 18:8605–13. doi: 10.1523/JNEUROSCI.18-21-08605.1998
23. Perez-Reyes E, Cribbs LL, Daud A, Lacerda AE, Barclay J, Williamson MP, et al. Molecular characterization of a neuronal low-voltage-activated T-type calcium channel. *Nature.* (1998) 391:896–900. doi: 10.1038/36110
24. Cribbs LL, Lee JH, Yang J, Satin J, Zhang Y, Daud A, et al. Cloning and characterization of alpha1H from human heart, a member of the T-type Ca2+ channel gene family. *Circ Res.* (1998) 83:103–9. doi: 10.1161/01.RES.83.1.103
25. Mangoni ME, Traboulsie A, Leoni AL, Couette B, Marger L, Le Quang K, et al. Bradycardia and slowing of the atrioventricular conduction in mice lacking CaV3.1/alpha1G T-type calcium channels. *Circ Res.* (2006) 98:1422–30. doi: 10.1161/01.RES.0000225862.14314.49
26. Mizuta E, Shirai M, Arakawa K, Hidaka K, Miake J, Ninomiya H, et al. Different distribution of Cav3.2 and Cav3.1 transcripts encoding T-type Ca(2+) channels in the embryonic heart of mice. *Biomed Res.* (2010) 31:301–5. doi: 10.2220/biomedres.31.301
27. Monteil A, Chemin J, Bourinet E, Mennessier G, Lory P, Nargeot J. Molecular and functional properties of the human alpha(1G) subunit that forms T-type calcium channels. *J Biol Chem.* (2000) 275:6090–100. doi: 10.1074/jbc.275.9.6090
28. Koschak A, Reimer D, Huber I, Grabner M, Glossmann H, Engel J, et al. alpha 1D (Cav1.3) subunits can form l-type Ca2+ channels activating at negative voltages. *J Biol Chem.* (2001) 276:22100–6. doi: 10.1074/jbc.M101469200
29. Baig SM, Koschak A, Lieb A, Gebhart M, Dafinger C, Nurnberg G, et al. Loss of Ca(v)1.3 (CACNA1D) function in a human channelopathy with bradycardia and congenital deafness. *Nat Neurosci.* (2011) 14:77–84. doi: 10.1038/nn.2694
30. Ono K, Iijima T. Pathophysiological significance of T-type Ca2+ channels: properties and functional roles of T-type Ca2+ channels in cardiac pacemaking. *J Pharmacol Sci.* (2005) 99:197–204. doi: 10.1254/jphs.FMJ05002X2
31. Vassort G, Talavera K, Alvarez JL. Role of T-type Ca2+ channels in the heart. *Cell Calcium.* (2006) 40:205–20. doi: 10.1016/j.ceca.2006.04.025
32. Ferron L, Capuano V, Deroubaix E, Coulombe A, Renaud JF. Functional and molecular characterization of a T-type Ca(2+) channel during fetal and postnatal rat heart development. *J Mol Cell Cardiol.* (2002) 34:533–46. doi: 10.1006/jmcc.2002.1535
33. Bohn G, Moosmang S, Conrad H, Ludwig A, Hofmann F, Klugbauer N. Expression of T- and L-type calcium channel mRNA in murine sinoatrial node. *FEBS Lett.* (2000) 481:73–6. doi: 10.1016/S0014-5793(00)01979-7
34. Hagiwara N, Irisawa H, Kameyama M. Contribution of two types of calcium currents to the pacemaker potentials of rabbit sino-atrial node cells. *J Physiol.* (1988) 395:233–53. doi: 10.1113/jphysiol.1988.sp016916
35. Benitah JP, Gomez AM, Fauconnier J, Kerfant BG, Perrier E, Vassort G, et al. Voltage-gated Ca2+ currents in the human pathophysiologic heart: a review. *Basic Res Cardiol.* (2002) 97 (Suppl. 1):I11–8. doi: 10.1007/s0039502 00023
36. Striessnig J, Pinggera A, Kaur G, Bock G, Tuluc P. L-type Ca(2+) channels in heart and brain. *Wiley Interdiscip Rev Membr Transp Signal.* (2014) 3:15–38. doi: 10.1002/wmts.102
37. Pinggera A, Lieb A, Benedetti B, Lampert M, Monteleone S, Liedl KR, et al. CACNA1D *de novo* mutations in autism spectrum disorders activate Cav1.3 L-type calcium channels. *Biol Psychiatry.* (2015) 77:816–22. doi: 10.1016/j.biopsych.2014.11.020
38. Srivastava U, Aromolaran AS, Fabris F, Lazaro D, Kassotis J, Qu Y, et al. Novel function of alpha1D L-type calcium channel in the atria. *Biochem Biophys Res Commun.* (2017) 482:771–6. doi: 10.1016/j.bbrc.2016.11.109
39. Qu Y, Karnabi E, Ramadan O, Yue Y, Chahine M, Boutjdir M. Perinatal and postnatal expression of Cav1.3 alpha1D Ca(2)(+) channel in the rat heart. *Pediatr Res.* (2011) 69:479–84. doi: 10.1203/PDR.0b013e318217a0df
40. Qu Y, Baroudi G, Yue Y, Boutjdir M. Novel molecular mechanism involving alpha1D (Cav1.3) L-type calcium channel in autoimmune-associated sinus bradycardia. *Circulation.* (2005) 111:3034–41. doi: 10.1161/CIRCULATIONAHA.104.517326
41. Marionneau C, Couette B, Liu J, Li H, Mangoni ME, Nargeot J, et al. Specific pattern of ionic channel gene expression associated with pacemaker activity in the mouse heart. *J Physiol.* (2005) 562:223–34. doi: 10.1113/jphysiol.2004.074047
42. Platzer J, Engel J, Schrott-Fischer A, Stephan K, Bova S, Chen H, et al. Congenital deafness and sinoatrial node dysfunction in mice lacking class D L-type Ca2+ channels. *Cell.* (2000) 102:89–97. doi: 10.1016/S0092-8674(00)00013-1
43. Striessnig J, Koschak A. Exploring the function and pharmacotherapeutic potential of voltage-gated Ca2+ channels with gene knockout models. *Channels.* (2008) 2:233–51. doi: 10.4161/chan.2.4.5847
44. Mangoni ME, Couette B, Bourinet E, Platzer J, Reimer D, Striessnig J, et al. Functional role of L-type Cav1.3 Ca2+ channels in cardiac pacemaker activity. *Proc. Natl. Acad. Sci. U.S.A.* (2003) 100:5543–8. doi: 10.1073/pnas.0935295100
45. Lee JH, Daud AN, Cribbs LL, Lacerda AE, Pereverzev A, Klockner U, et al. Cloning and expression of a novel member of the low voltage-activated T-type calcium channel family. *J Neurosci.* (1999) 19:1912–21. doi: 10.1523/JNEUROSCI.19-06-01912.1999
46. Catterall WA, Perez-Reyes E, Snutch TP, Striessnig J. International Union of Pharmacology. XLVIII. Nomenclature and structure-function relationships of voltage-gated calcium channels. *Pharmacol Rev.* (2005) 57:411–25. doi: 10.1124/pr.57.4.5
47. Dolphin AC, Wyatt CN, Richards J, Beattie RE, Craig P, Lee JH, et al. The effect of alpha2-delta and other accessory subunits on expression and properties of the calcium channel alpha1G. *J Physiol.* (1999) 519:35–45. doi: 10.1111/j.1469-7793.1999.0035o.x
48. Dubel SJ, Altier C, Chaumont S, Lory P, Bourinet E, Nargeot J. Plasma membrane expression of T-type calcium channel alpha(1) subunits is modulated by high voltage-activated auxiliary subunits. *J Biol Chem.* (2004) 279:29263–9. doi: 10.1074/jbc.M313450200
49. Chiang CS, Huang CH, Chieng H, Chang YT, Chang D, Chen JJ, et al. The Ca(v)3.2 T-type Ca(2+) channel is required for pressure overload-induced cardiac hypertrophy in mice. *Circ Res.* (2009) 104:522–30. doi: 10.1161/CIRCRESAHA.108.184051
50. Liu DQ, Zhou SS, Zhao DH, Sheng BH. Effects of furyl-dihydropyridine on action potential ventricular myocardium of rabbit *in vivo* and isolated guinea pig left atrium *in vitro*. *Zhongguo Yao Li Xue Bao.* (1993) 14:164–7.

51. Hirano Y, Fozzard HA, January CT. Characteristics of L- and T-type Ca2+ currents in canine cardiac Purkinje cells. *Am J Physiol.* (1989) 256:H1478–92. doi: 10.1152/ajpheart.1989.256.5.H1478
52. Tseng GN, Boyden PA. Multiple types of Ca2+ currents in single canine Purkinje cells. *Circ Res.* (1989) 65:1735–50. doi: 10.1161/01.RES.65.6.1735
53. Nilius B. Possible functional significance of a novel type of cardiac Ca channel. *Biomed Biochim Acta.* (1986) 45:K37–45.
54. Nilius B, Talavera K, Verkhratsky A. T-type calcium channels: the never ending story. *Cell Calcium.* (2006) 40:81–8. doi: 10.1016/j.ceca.2006.04.011
55. Liao YH, Fu M. Autoimmunity in the pathogenesis of cardiomyopathy. *J Autoimmun.* (2001) 16:1–2. doi: 10.1006/jaut.2000.0466
56. MacLellan WR, Lusis AJ. Dilated cardiomyopathy: learning to live with yourself. *Nat Med.* (2003) 9:1455–6. doi: 10.1038/nm1203-1455
57. Jahns R, Boivin V, Schwarzbach V, Ertl G, Lohse MJ. Pathological autoantibodies in cardiomyopathy. *Autoimmunity.* (2008) 41:454–61. doi: 10.1080/08916930802031603
58. Felker GM, Thompson RE, Hare JM, Hruban RH, Clemetson DE, Howard DL, et al. Underlying causes and long-term survival in patients with initially unexplained cardiomyopathy. *N Engl J Med.* (2000) 342:1077–84. doi: 10.1056/NEJM200004133421502
59. Braunwald E. Expanding indications for beta-blockers in heart failure. *N Engl J Med.* (2001) 344:1711–2. doi: 10.1056/NEJM200105313442210
60. Klein GJ, Krahn AD, Skanes AC, Yee R, Gula LJ. Primary prophylaxis of sudden death in hypertrophic cardiomyopathy, arrhythmogenic right ventricular cardiomyopathy, and dilated cardiomyopathy. *J Cardiovas Electrophys.* (2005) 16 (Suppl. 1):S28–34. doi: 10.1111/j.1540-8167.2005.50116.x
61. Xiao H, Wang M, Du Y, Yuan J, Zhao G, Tu D, et al. Agonist-like autoantibodies against calcium channel in patients with dilated cardiomyopathy. *Heart Vessels.* (2012) 27:486–92. doi: 10.1007/s00380-011-0176-7
62. Yu H, Pei J, Liu X, Chen J, Li X, Zhang Y, et al. Calcium channel autoantibodies predicted sudden cardiac death and all-cause mortality in patients with ischemic and nonischemic chronic heart failure. *Dis Markers.* (2014) 2014:796075. doi: 10.1155/2014/796075
63. Deubner N, Berliner D, Schlipp A, Gelbrich G, Caforio AL, Felix SB, et al. Cardiac beta1-adrenoceptor autoantibodies in human heart disease: rationale and design of the Etiology, Titre-Course, and Survival (ETiCS) Study. *Eur J Heart Fail.* (2010) 12:753–62. doi: 10.1093/eurjhf/hfq072
64. Jahns R. Autoantibodies against cardiac troponin I: friend or foe? *Eur J Heart Fail.* (2010) 12:645–8. doi: 10.1093/eurjhf/hfq098
65. Heymans S, Hirsch E, Anker SD, Aukrust P, Balligand JL, Cohen-Tervaert JW, et al. Inflammation as a therapeutic target in heart failure? a scientific statement from the translational research committee of the heart failure association of the European Society of Cardiology. *Eur J Heart Fail.* (2009) 11:119–29. doi: 10.1093/eurjhf/hfn043
66. Sterin-Borda L, Cossio PM, Gimeno MF, Gimeno AL, Diez C, Laguens RP, et al. Effect of chagasic sera on the rat isolated atrial preparation: immunological, morphological and function aspects. *Cardiovasc Res.* (1976) 10:613–22. doi: 10.1093/cvr/10.6.613
67. Wallukat G, Wollenberger A. Effects of the serum gamma globulin fraction of patients with allergic asthma and dilated cardiomyopathy on chronotropic beta adrenoceptor function in cultured neonatal rat heart myocytes. *Biomed Biochim Acta.* (1987) 46:S634–9.
68. Magnusson Y, Marullo S, Hoyer S, Waagstein F, Andersson B, Vahlne A, et al. Mapping of a functional autoimmune epitope on the beta 1-adrenergic receptor in patients with idiopathic dilated cardiomyopathy. *J Clin Invest.* (1990) 86:1658–63. doi: 10.1172/JCI114888
69. Iwata M, Yoshikawa T, Baba A, Anzai T, Mitamura H, Ogawa S. Autoantibodies against the second extracellular loop of beta1-adrenergic receptors predict ventricular tachycardia and sudden death in patients with idiopathic dilated cardiomyopathy. *J Am Coll Cardiol.* (2001) 37:418–24. doi: 10.1016/S0735-1097(00)01109-8
70. Magnusson Y, Wallukat G, Waagstein F, Hjalmarson A, Hoebeke J. Autoimmunity in idiopathic dilated cardiomyopathy. characterization of antibodies against the beta 1-adrenoceptor with positive chronotropic effect. *Circulation.* (1994) 89:2760–7. doi: 10.1161/01.CIR.89.6.2760
71. Magnusson Y, Hjalmarson A, Hoebeke J. Beta 1-adrenoceptor autoimmunity in cardiomyopathy. *Int J Cardiol.* (1996) 54:137–41. doi: 10.1016/0167-5273(96)02590-9
72. Christ T, Wettwer E, Dobrev D, Adolph E, Knaut M, Wallukat Get al. Autoantibodies against the beta1 adrenoceptor from patients with dilated cardiomyopathy prolong action potential duration and enhance contractility in isolated cardiomyocytes. *J Mol Cell Cardiol.* (2001) 33:1515–25. doi: 10.1006/jmcc.2001.1414
73. Schulze K, Heineman FW, Schultheiss HP, Balaban RS. Impairment of myocardial calcium homeostasis by antibodies against the adenine nucleotide translocator. *Cell Calcium.* (1999) 25:361–70. doi: 10.1054/ceca.1999.0039
74. Liao YH. Functional analysis of autoantibodies against ADP/ATP carrier from dilated cardiomyopathy. *Int J Cardiol.* (1996) 54:165–9. doi: 10.1016/0167-5273(96)02594-6
75. Liao YH, Cheng LX, Dai SP, Tu YS. Autoantibodies against ADP/ATP carrier from patients with dilated cardiomyopathy increase activity of voltage-dependent Ca channels in isolated cardiac myocytes. *Blood Press Supple.* (1996) 3:41–4.
76. Liao YH, Yuan J. Progress in the research of targets for the molecular immunotherapy in dilated cardiomyopathy. *Zhonghua yi xue za zhi.* (2006) 86:1158–60. doi: 10.3760/j:issn:0376-2491.2006.17.003
77. Boutjdir M, Chen L, Zhang ZH, Tseng CE, DiDonato F, Rashbaum W, et al. Arrhythmogenicity of IgG and anti-52-kD SSA/Ro affinity-purified antibodies from mothers of children with congenital heart block. *Circ Res.* (1997) 80:354–62. doi: 10.1161/01.RES.80.3.354
78. Boutjdir M, Chen L, Zhang ZH, Tseng CE, El-Sherif N, Buyon JP. Serum and immunoglobulin G from the mother of a child with congenital heart block induce conduction abnormalities and inhibit L-type calcium channels in a rat heart model. *Pediatr Res.* (1998) 44:11–9. doi: 10.1203/00006450-199807000-00002
79. Boutjdir M. Molecular and ionic basis of congenital complete heart block. *Trends Cardiovasc Med.* (2000) 10:114–22. doi: 10.1016/S1050-1738(00)00059-1
80. Lazzerini PE, Capecchi PL, Guideri F, Acampa M, Selvi E, Bisogno S, et al. Autoantibody-mediated cardiac arrhythmias: mechanisms and clinical implications. *Basic Res Cardiol.* (2008) 103:1–11. doi: 10.1007/s00395-007-0686-8
81. Miranda-Carus ME, Boutjdir M, Tseng CE, DiDonato F, Chan EK, Buyon JP. Induction of antibodies reactive with SSA/Ro-SSB/La and development of congenital heart block in a murine model. *J Immunol.* (1998) 161:5886–92.
82. Brucato A, Franceschini F, Buyon JP. Neonatal lupus: long-term outcomes of mothers and children and recurrence rate. *Clin Exp Rheumatol.* (1997) 15:467–73.
83. Buyon JP, Winchester RJ, Slade SG, Arnett F, Copel J, Friedman D, et al. Identification of mothers at risk for congenital heart block and other neonatal lupus syndromes in their children. comparison of enzyme-linked immunosorbent assay and immunoblot for measurement of anti-SS-A/Ro and anti-SS-B/La antibodies. *Arthritis Rheum.* (1993) 36:1263–73. doi: 10.1002/art.1780360911
84. Brucato A, Frassi M, Franceschini F, Cimaz R, Faden D, Pisoni MP, et al. Risk of congenital complete heart block in newborns of mothers with anti-Ro/SSA antibodies detected by counterimmunoelectrophoresis: a prospective study of 100 women. *Arthritis Rheum.* (2001) 44:1832–5. doi: 10.1002/1529-0131(200108)44:8<1832::AID-ART320>3.0.CO;2-C
85. Gordon P, Khamashta MA, Rosenthal E, Simpson JM, Sharland G, Brucato A, et al. Anti-52 kDa Ro, anti-60 kDa Ro, and anti-La antibody profiles in neonatal lupus. *J Rheumatol.* (2004) 31:2480-7.
86. Franceschini F, Cavazzana I. Anti-Ro/SSA and La/SSB antibodies. *Autoimmunity.* (2005) 38:55–63. doi: 10.1080/08916930400022954
87. Satoh M, Chan EK, Ho LA, Rose KM, Parks CG, Cohn RD, et al. Prevalence and sociodemographic correlates of antinuclear antibodies in the United States. *Arthritis Rheum.* (2012) 64:2319–27. doi: 10.1002/art.34380
88. Hayashi N, Koshiba M, Nishimura K, Sugiyama D, Nakamura T, Morinobu S, et al. Prevalence of disease-specific antinuclear antibodies in general population: estimates from annual physical examinations of residents of

a small town over a 5-year period. *Mod Rheumatol.* (2008) 18:153–60. doi: 10.1007/s10165-008-0028-1
89. Guo YP, Wang CG, Liu X, Huang YQ, Guo DL, Jing XZ, et al. The prevalence of antinuclear antibodies in the general population of china: a cross-sectional study. *Curr Ther Res Clin Exp.* (2014) 76:116–9. doi: 10.1016/j.curtheres.2014.06.004
90. Siren MK, Julkunen H, Kaaja R. The increasing incidence of isolated congenital heart block in Finland. *J Rheumatol.* (1998) 25:1862–4.
91. Mazel JA, El-Sherif N, Buyon J, Boutjdir M. Electrocardiographic abnormalities in a murine model injected with IgG from mothers of children with congenital heart block. *Circulation.* (1999) 99:1914–8. doi: 10.1161/01.CIR.99.14.1914
92. Xiao GQ, Qu Y, Hu K, Boutjdir M. Down-regulation of L-type calcium channel in pups born to 52 kDa SSA/Ro immunized rabbits. *FASEB J.* (2001) 15:1539–45. doi: 10.1096/fj.01-0052com
93. Salomonsson S, Sonesson SE, Ottosson L, Muhallab S, Olsson T, Sunnerhagen M, et al. Ro/SSA autoantibodies directly bind cardiomyocytes, disturb calcium homeostasis, and mediate congenital heart block. *J Exp Med.* (2005) 201:11–7. doi: 10.1084/jem.20041859
94. Suzuki H, Silverman ED, Wu X, Borges C, Zhao S, Isacovics B, et al. Effect of maternal autoantibodies on fetal cardiac conduction: an experimental murine model. *Pediatr Res.* (2005) 57:557–62. doi: 10.1203/01.PDR.0000155947.82365.E4
95. Menon A, Silverman ED, Gow RM, Hamilton RM. Chronotropic competence of the sinus node in congenital complete heart block. *Am J Cardiol.* (1998) 82:1119–21. doi: 10.1016/S0002-9149(98)00569-4
96. Brucato A, Cimaz R, Catelli L, Meroni P. Anti-Ro-associated sinus bradycardia in newborns. *Circulation.* (2000) 102:E88–9. doi: 10.1161/01.CIR.102.11.e88
97. Mendez C, Zipes DP. Possible ionic mechanism of the action potentials of the atrioventricular node of rabbits. *Bol Estud Med Biol.* (1974) (Suppl 1):67–80.
98. Hu K, Qu Y, Yue Y, Boutjdir M. Functional basis of sinus bradycardia in congenital heart block. *Circ Res.* (2004) 94:e32–8. doi: 10.1161/01.RES.0000121566.01778.06
99. Qu Y, Xiao GQ, Chen L, Boutjdir M. Autoantibodies from mothers of children with congenital heart block downregulate cardiac L-type Ca channels. *J Mol Cell Cardiol.* (2001) 33:1153–63. doi: 10.1006/jmcc.2001.1379
100. Xiao GQ, Hu K, Boutjdir M. Direct inhibition of expressed cardiac l- and t-type calcium channels by IGG from mothers whose children have congenital heart block. *Circulation.* (2001) 103:1599–604. doi: 10.1161/01.CIR.103.11.1599
101. Takimoto K, Li D, Nerbonne JM, Levitan ES. Distribution, splicing and glucocorticoid-induced expression of cardiac alpha 1C and alpha 1D voltage-gated Ca2+ channel mRNAs. *J Mol Cell Cardiol.* (1997) 29:3035–42. doi: 10.1006/jmcc.1997.0532
102. Matthes J, Yildirim L, Wietzorrek G, Reimer D, Striessnig J, Herzig S. Disturbed atrio-ventricular conduction and normal contractile function in isolated hearts from Cav1.3-knockout mice. *Naunyn Schmiedebergs Arch Pharmacol.* (2004) 369:554–62. doi: 10.1007/s00210-004-0940-7
103. Karnabi E, Qu Y, Mancarella S, Yue Y, Wadgaonkar R, Boutjdir M. Silencing of Cav1.2 gene in neonatal cardiomyocytes by lentiviral delivered shRNA. *Biochem Biophys Res Commun.* (2009) 384:409–14. doi: 10.1016/j.bbrc.2009.04.150
104. Hamilton RM, Lee-Poy M, Kruger K, Silverman ED. Investigative methods of congenital complete heart block. *J Electrocardiol.* (1998) 30:69–74. doi: 10.1016/S0022-0736(98)80035-6
105. Garcia S, Nascimento JH, Bonfa E, Levy R, Oliveira SF, Tavares AV, et al. Cellular mechanism of the conduction abnormalities induced by serum from anti-Ro/SSA-positive patients in rabbit hearts. *J Clin Invest.* (1994) 93:718–24. doi: 10.1172/JCI117025
106. Restivo M, Kozhevnikov DO, Boutjdir M. Optical mapping of activation patterns in an animal model of congenital heart block. *Am J Physiol Heart Circ Physiol.* (2001) 280:H1889–95. doi: 10.1152/ajpheart.2001.280.4.H1889
107. Strandberg LS, Cui X, Rath A, Liu J, Silverman ED, Liu X, et al. Congenital heart block maternal sera autoantibodies target an extracellular epitope on the alpha1G T-type calcium channel in human fetal hearts. *PLoS ONE.* (2013) 8:e72668. doi: 10.1371/journal.pone.0072668
108. Karnabi E, Qu Y, Wadgaonkar R, Mancarella S, Yue Y, Chahine M, et al. Congenital heart block: identification of autoantibody binding site on the extracellular loop (domain I, S5-S6) of alpha(1D) L-type Ca channel. *J Autoimmun.* (2010) 34:80–6. doi: 10.1016/j.jaut.2009.06.005
109. Chen CC, Lamping KG, Nuno DW, Barresi R, Prouty SJ, Lavoie JL, et al. Abnormal coronary function in mice deficient in alpha1H T-type Ca2+ channels. *Science.* (2003) 302:1416–8. doi: 10.1126/science.1089268
110. Markham AJ, Rasmussen SE, Salmon JE, Martinez-Ortiz W, Cardozo TJ, Clancy RM, et al. Reactivity to the p305 epitope of the alpha1G T-type calcium channel and autoimmune-associated congenital heart block. *J Am Heart Assoc.* (2015) 4:e001836. doi: 10.1161/JAHA.115.001836
111. Cimaz R, Stramba-Badiale M, Brucato A, Catelli L, Panzeri P, Meroni PL. QT interval prolongation in asymptomatic anti-SSA/Ro-positive infants without congenital heart block. *Arthritis Rheum.* (2000) 43:1049–53. doi: 10.1002/1529-0131(200005)43:5<1049::AID-ANR13>3.0.CO;2-X
112. Cimaz R, Meroni PL, Brucato A, Fesstova V, Panzeri P, Goulene K, et al. Concomitant disappearance of electrocardiographic abnormalities and of acquired maternal autoantibodies during the first year of life in infants who had QT interval prolongation and anti-SSA/Ro positivity without congenital heart block at birth. *Arthritis Rheum.* (2003) 48:266–8. doi: 10.1002/art.10700
113. Bourre-Tessier J, Clarke AE, Huynh T, Bernatsky S, Joseph L, Belisle P, et al. Prolonged corrected QT interval in anti-Ro/SSA-positive adults with systemic lupus erythematosus. *Arthritis Care Res.* (2011) 63:1031–7. doi: 10.1002/acr.20470
114. Lazzerini PE, Capecchi PL, Acampa M, Morozzi G, Bellisai F, Bacarelli MR, et al. Anti-Ro/SSA-associated corrected QT interval prolongation in adults: the role of antibody level and specificity. *Arthritis Care Res.* (2011) 63:1463–70. doi: 10.1002/acr.20540
115. Tufan AN, Sag S, Oksuz MF, Ermurat S, Coskun BN, Gullulu M, et al. Prolonged Tpeak-Tend interval in anti-Ro52 antibody-positive connective tissue diseases. *Rheumatol Int.* (2017) 37:67–73. doi: 10.1007/s00296-016-3488-1
116. Lazzerini PE, Capecchi PL, Guideri F, Bellisai F, Selvi E, Acampa M, et al. Comparison of frequency of complex ventricular arrhythmias in patients with positive versus negative anti-Ro/SSA and connective tissue disease. *Am J Cardiol.* (2007) 100:1029–34. doi: 10.1016/j.amjcard.2007.04.048
117. Duke C, Stuart G, Simpson JM. Ventricular tachycardia secondary to prolongation of the QT interval in a fetus with autoimmune mediated congenital complete heart block. *Cardiol Young.* (2005) 15:319–21. doi: 10.1017/S1047951105000673
118. Nakamura K, Katayama Y, Kusano KF, Haraoka K, Tani Y, Nagase S, et al. Anti-KCNH2 antibody-induced long QT syndrome: novel acquired form of long QT syndrome. *J Am Coll Cardiol.* (2007) 50:1808–9. doi: 10.1016/j.jacc.2007.07.037
119. Lazzerini PE, Yue Y, Srivastava U, Fabris F, Capecchi PL, Bertolozzi I, et al. Arrhythmogenicity of anti-Ro/SSA antibodies in patients with torsades de pointes. *Circ Arrhythm Electrophysiol.* (2016) 9:e003419. doi: 10.1161/CIRCEP.115.003419
120. Mancarella S, Yue Y, Karnabi E, Qu Y, El-Sherif N, Boutjdir M. Impaired Ca2+ homeostasis is associated with atrial fibrillation in the alpha1D L-type Ca2+ channel KO mouse. *Am J Physiol Heart Circ Physiol.* (2008) 295:H2017–24. doi: 10.1152/ajpheart.00537.2008
121. Izmirly P, Saxena A, Buyon JP. Progress in the pathogenesis and treatment of cardiac manifestations of neonatal lupus. *Curr Opin Rheumatol.* (2017) 29:467–72. doi: 10.1097/BOR.0000000000000414
122. Clancy RM, Neufing PJ, Zheng P, O'Mahony M, Nimmerjahn F, Gordon TP, et al. Impaired clearance of apoptotic cardiocytes is linked to anti-SSA/Ro and -SSB/La antibodies in the pathogenesis of congenital heart block. *J Clin Invest.* (2006) 116:2413–22. doi: 10.1172/JCI27803
123. Brito-Zerón P, Izmirly PM, Ramos-Casals M, Buyon JP, Khamashta MA. The clinical spectrum of autoimmune congenital heart block. *Nat Rev Rheumatol.* (2015) 11:301–12. doi: 10.1038/nrrheum.2015.29
124. Litsey SE, Noonan JA, O'Connor WN, Cottrill CM, Mitchell B. Maternal connective tissue disease and congenital heart block. demonstration of immunoglobulin in cardiac tissue. *N Engl J Med.* (1985) 312:98–100. doi: 10.1056/NEJM198501103120206
125. Ho SY, Esscher E, Anderson RH, Michaelsson M. Anatomy of congenital complete heart block and relation to maternal anti-Ro antibodies. *Am J Cardiol.* (1986) 58:291–4. doi: 10.1016/0002-9149(86)90064-0

126. Tonello M, Ruffatti A, Favaro M, Tison T, Del Ross T, Calligaro A, et al. Maternal autoantibody profiles at risk for autoimmune congenital heart block: a prospective study in high-risk patients. *Lupus Sci Med.* (2016) 3:e000129. doi: 10.1136/lupus-2015-000129
127. Reed JH, Clancy RM, Lee KH, Saxena A, Izmirly PM, Buyon JP. Umbilical cord blood levels of maternal antibodies reactive with p200 and full-length Ro 52 in the assessment of risk for cardiac manifestations of neonatal lupus. *Arthritis Care Res.* (2012) 64:1373–81. doi: 10.1002/acr.21704
128. Izmirly PM, Saxena A. In search of an antibody specificity highly predictive of congenital heart block. *Lupus Sci Med.* (2016) 3:e000154. doi: 10.1136/lupus-2016-000154

8

DPP-4 Inhibitors as Potential Candidates for Antihypertensive Therapy: Improving Vascular Inflammation and Assisting the Action of Traditional Antihypertensive Drugs

Jianqiang Zhang[1], *Qiuyue Chen*[1], *Jixin Zhong*[2], *Chaohong Liu*[3], *Bing Zheng*[1,4*] and *Quan Gong*[1,4*]

[1] *Department of Immunology, School of Medicine, Yangtze University, Jingzhou, China,* [2] *Cardiovascular Research Institute, Case Western Reserve University, Cleveland, OH, United States,* [3] *Department of Microbiology, School of Basic Medicine, Tongji Medical College, Huazhong University of Science & Technology, Wuhan, China,* [4] *Clinical Molecular Immunology Center, School of Medicine, Yangtze University, Jingzhou, China*

***Correspondence:**
Bing Zheng
hxzheng@yangtzeu.edu.cn
Quan Gong
gongquan1998@163.com

Dipeptidyl peptidase-4 (DPP-4) is an important protease that is widely expressed on the surface of human cells and plays a key role in immune-regulation, inflammation, oxidative stress, cell adhesion, and apoptosis by targeting different substrates. DPP-4 inhibitors (DPP-4i) are commonly used as hypoglycemic agents. However, in addition to their hypoglycemic effect, DPP-4i have also shown potent activities in the cardiovascular system, particularly in the regulation of blood pressure (BP). Previous studies have shown that the regulatory actions of DPP-4i in controlling BP are complex and that the mechanisms involved include the functional activities of the nerves, kidneys, hormones, blood vessels, and insulin. Recent work has also shown that inflammation is closely associated with the elevation of BP, and that the inhibition of DPP-4 can reduce BP by regulating the function of the immune system, by reducing inflammatory reactions and by improving oxidative stress. In this review, we describe the potential anti-hypertensive effects of DPP-4i and discuss potential new anti-hypertensive therapies. Our analysis indicated that DPP-4i treatment has a mild anti-hypertensive effect as a monotherapy and causes a significant reduction in BP when used in combined treatments. However, the combination of DPP-4i with high-dose angiotensin converting enzyme inhibitors (ACEI) can lead to increased BP. We suggest that DPP-4i improves vascular endothelial function in hypertensive patients by suppressing inflammatory responses and by alleviating oxidative stress. In addition, DPP-4i can also regulate BP by activating the sympathetic nervous system, interfering with the renin angiotensin aldosterone system (RAAS), regulating Na/H_2O metabolism, and attenuating insulin resistance (IR).

Keywords: DPP-4, DPP-4i, GLP-1, inflammation, cardiovascular effects, hypertension

INTRODUCTION

Dipeptidyl peptidase-4 (DPP-4), which is also referred to as adenosine deaminase complexing protein 2 (ADCP2), cluster of differentiation 26 (CD26), or adenosine deaminase binding protein (ADBP), is an important protease that is widely expressed on the surface of human cells. As a member of the leukocyte surface antigen family, DPP-4 plays an important role in the immune system, and can regulate inflammation, oxidative stress, cell adhesion, and apoptosis. Due to their inhibitory effects on T cell activation and function, DPP-4 inhibitors (DPP-4i) have been successfully evaluated *in vivo* as immunosuppressive therapies using animal models of rheumatoid arthritis (RA), multiple sclerosis (MS), and transplantation. Otherwise, it cleaves N-terminal two amino acids with alanine or proline in the penultimate position by way of its enzyme activity. The substrates of DPP-4 can be divided into three groups: regulatory peptide; chemokines and cytokines, and neuropeptides (1). The most well-known substrates are glucagon-like peptide 1 (GLP-1), neuropeptide Y (NPY), stromal-cell-derived factor-1 (SDF-1), substance P, and B-type natriuretic peptide (BNP) (1). In addition to catalytic functions, DPP4 also interacts with different types of ligands, including adenosine deaminase (ADA), caveolin-1, fibronectin, and C-X-C chemokine receptor type 4 (CXCR4) (1).

Due to the efficacy of GLP-1 upon blood glucose regulation, DPP-4i has gradually become a new anti-diabetic drug for the treatment of type 2 diabetes mellitus (T2DM). In addition to its activity against hyperglycemia, DPP-4i has shown beneficial cardiovascular effects including cardioprotective action, endothelial protection, and an anti-hypertensive effect. Both the EXamination of cArdiovascular outcoMes with alogliptIN vs. standard of carE in patients with type two diabetes mellitus and acute coronary syndrome (EXAMINE) study, and the Saxagliptin Assessment of Vascular Outcomes Recorded in Patients With Diabetes Mellitus-Thrombolysis in Myocardial Infarction 53 trialin (SAVOR-TIMI 53), examined the effects of DPP-4 inhibition on cardiovascular outcomes. However, these studies found no significant improvements in a range of safety endpoints for cardiovascular diseases (2, 3). Although its efficacy upon cardiovascular terminal events are not completely satisfactory, DPP-4i has shown beneficial cardiovascular benefits in many research studies, including the alleviation of vascular inflammation, the protection of endothelial cells, and the reduction of blood pressure (BP). For example, Leung et al. reported that DPP-4i could improve left ventricle systolic and diastolic function in T2DM (4). It has also been reported that alogliptin treatment results in a significant improvement of glomerular filtration rate (GFR) and left ventricular ejection fraction (LVEF) in patients with T2DM by increasing left ventricular systolic function (5). In another study, Read et al. reported that sitagliptin could remarkably improve cardiac ejection fraction (6). In addition, Jax et al. demonstrated that linagliptin treatment significantly improved microvascular function, but had no effect upon macrovascular function (7). Ida et al. provided evidence that trelagliptin treatment resulted in a visible increase of serum adiponectin level, which could regulate the function of vascular endothelial cells (8). Additional evidence has also suggested that DPP-4i can regulate BP. In the present review, describe the roles and mechanisms of DPP-4i in the improvement of hypertension, and discuss new anti-hypertensive therapies for T2DM patients or non-diabetics.

THE ROLE OF DPP-4 INHIBITORS IN HYPERTENSION

The first DPP-4 inhibitor, sitagliptin, was approved as an anti-hyperglycemic agent for T2DM in the United States of America in 2006. Since then, a range of other drugs have been developed and used clinically, including sitagliptin, vidagliptin, saxagliptin, alogliptin, and linagliptin. Compared with classical oral-hypoglycemic drugs, biguanides, thiazolidinediones, sulfonylureas, and alpha glucosidase inhibitors, patients receiving DPP-4i treatment have a lower incidence of hypoglycemic events and gain less weight. In addition to its outstanding glucose-lowering effect, DPP-4i have also shown non-metabolic functional activities, including anti-inflammatory effect and cardiovascular protection, particularly with regards to BP regulation.

Recent clinical trials and experimental studies have suggested that DPP-4i, can regulating cardiovascular function via different pathways directly, in either a direct or indirect manner. Extensive clinical studies have confirmed that DPP-4i exerts protective effects on hypertension patients. For example, sitagliptin and vildagliptin treatment could lower systolic blood pressure (SBP) independently of a reduction in blood glucose (9, 10). Some other studies showed that both SBP and diastolic blood pressure (DBP) were reduced after treatment with vildagliptin (11, 12). Furthermore, the hypotensive effect was not only limited to patients with diabetes, but also included other patients. For example, Hussain et al. found that sitagliptin significantly reduced BP in non-diabetic patients (13). Many other groups have provided evidence to support and therefore confirm this phenomenon (14). Consistent with these clinical trials, several recent studies have reported that DPP-4i can alleviate hypertensive conditions in animal models (15–19). In contrast, several studies have reported that humans or animals treated with DPP-4i do not show changes in BP when compared with placebo (4, 20, 21). Furthermore, some studies have demonstrated that a combination of DPP-4 and high-dose angiotensin converting enzyme inhibitors (ACEI) can actually increase blood pressure (22, 23). It is therefore very valuable to clarify the mechanism of BP regulation in response to DPP-4i, particularly in combined drug treatments (**Table 1**).

DPP-4 INHIBITORS AND BP REGULATION: POTENTIAL MECHANISMS

Primary hypertension is a cardiovascular syndrome characterized by elevated BP, and represents the leading cause of cardiovascular disease and stroke and the primary cause of death and disease burden worldwide (24). Hypertension is caused by the interaction of genetic factors with environmental factors, although there is no unified understanding of the

TABLE 1 | The regulatory effects of DPP-4i on blood pressure in the clinical researches and animal experiments.

Drugs	Subjects	Number	Duration	Effects	Date	References
Saxagliptin	Humans	102	48 w	SBP ↓ and DBP ↓	2018	(12)
Sitagliptin	Humans	454	24w	SBP ↓ and DBP ↓	2017	(14)
Vildagliptin	Humans	2108	24 w	SBP ↓ and DBP ↓	2016	(11)
Sitagliptin	Humans	70	12 w	SBP ↓ and DBP ↓	2016	(13)
Sitagliptin/ Vildagliptin/ Saxagliptin	Humans	25	48w	No effect	2016	(4)
Sitagliptin/ vildagliptin	Humans	51	12 w	SBP ↓	2016	(10)
Vildagliptin	Rats	48	4 w	DBP ↓	2016	(19)
Vildagliptin	Rats	17	1 w	SBP ↓	2015	(17)
Sitagliptin with enalapril (10 mg/kg)	Rats	12	3 w	SBP ↑ and DBP ↑	2015	(23)
Linagliptin	Rats	59	16 w	No effect	2013	(21)
Linagliptin	Mice	60	12 w	No effect	2012	(20)
Linagliptin	Rats	48	1 w	Mean BP ↓	2012	(15)
Saxagliptin	Rats	52	8 w	SBP↓ and DBP↓	2012	(18)
Sitagliptin	Rats	16	2 w	SBP↓	2012	(16)
Sitagliptin with enalapril (10/5 mg)	Humans	24	3 w	5 mg: BP↑ 10 mg: BP↓	2010	(22)

mechanisms involved. At present, the generally accepted mechanisms underlying hypertension are said to involve nerves, kidneys, hormones, blood vessels, and insulin resistance. In addition to these traditional mechanisms, it is widely believed that mild inflammation can lead to BP elevation and its associated cardiovascular complications. Current treatments for hypertension include angiotensin II (AngII) type 1 receptor blockers (ARB), angiotensin converting enzyme inhibitors (ACEIs), calcium channel antagonists, beta receptor blockers, and diuretics. Although the use of antihypertensive drugs has significantly improved the quality of life of patients and reduced the incidence and mortality of hypertension complications, half of all patients are still not optimistic about BP control (25). Therefore, it is particularly important to identify new candidates for antihypertensive treatment. In view of the beneficial effects of DPP-4i on blood pressure regulation, we aimed to review the effects of DPP-4i upon hypertension in association with the immune system, blood vessels, the nervous system, hormones, kidneys, and insulin resistance. We also attempt try to provide an effective strategy for anti-hypertensive therapy.

Immunological Mechanisms of DPP-4i Upon Hypertension

Many chronic diseases are closely related to non-specific inflammatory processes, such as insulin resistance, metabolic syndrome, T2DM, and coronary heart disease, which are associated with increased infiltration and cell proliferation of immune cells and the elevated release of inflammatory mediators. Recent data suggests that innate and adaptive immune systems contribute to low-grade inflammation and play a role in the development and progression of hypertension (26).

It has been found that DPP-4/CD26 participates in non-specific inflammation by predominantly regulating the activation and chemotaxis of mononuclear/macrophages, NK cells, and T cells. Inflammatory mediators secreted from these immune cells, such as chemokines, cytokines, adhesion molecules, and reactive oxygen species (ROS), can disturb the functional activity of the vascular endothelium (27), for example, by increasing the proliferation of smooth muscle cells and participating in vascular remodeling (28). da Silva Júnior et al. suggested that DPP-4 is associated with endothelial inflammation and microvascular function, and that DPP-4 can significantly increase blood flow (29). T lymphocytes have a general role in contributing to inflammatory responses associated with hypertension (30). Early studies showed that T cells can secret and deliver AngII via the endogenous renin-angiotensin system (RAS), therefore leading to an increase in BP (31, 32). The application of DPP-4i reduces the production of cytokines controlling the proliferation of T lymphocytes (33). In view of this, we hypothesize that DPP-4 inhibitors could show potential hypotensive effects by inhibiting T cell activation and function, and reduce the secretion of inflammatory cytokines. In addition, DPP-4i also inhibits inflammation by suppressing the activation and chemotaxis of monocytes and macrophages (34–36).

It is well-known that naive T cells are stimulated by antigen presentation by antigen-presenting cells (APCs), and T cells can differentiate into different types of effector T-cells: Th1 cells, Th2 cells, Th17 cells, and Treg cells (37). Activated T cells secrete a variety of inflammatory mediators. For example, studies have shown that Th17 cells have very high expression levels of DPP-4 (38), and that interleukin 17 (IL-17) secreted by Th17 cells initiates the progression of

AngII-induced hypertension (30). Saxagliptin was previously shown to inhibit the AngII-induced activation of a range of cardiac proinflammatory/profibrotic signaling intermediates, including interleukin 18 (IL-18), interleukin 17A (IL-17A), nuclear transcription factor-κB (NF-κB), and TLR4 (39). Interleukin 6 (IL-6) and tumor necrosis factor alpha (TNF-α) have been positively correlated with blood pressure (40, 41), and the inhibition of DPP-4 has been shown to down-regulate the expression of IL-6 and TNF-α (36, 42, 43). In contrast, Tinsley et al. found that interleukin 10 (IL-10), released by Treg cells, has beneficial effects in terms of reducing inflammation, ameliorating endothelial function, and lowering BP in hypertensive pregnant rats (44). Furthermore, the DPP-4 inhibitor MK0626 has been shown to increase IL-10 levels (34).

Inflammation and oxidative stress result in a series of vascular stress reactions, causing vascular endothelial dysfunction, which then leads to hypertension (45–47). The administration of DPP-4i inhibits the immune response and relieves oxidative stress (48–50). Mega et al. also found that the administration of sitagliptinin rats with T2DM reduced the levels of lipid peroxidation (51). Alam et al. suggested that sitagliptin can prevent inflammation and fibrosis of the heart and kidney by improving oxidative stress (52). Koibuchi et al. reported that the beneficial effects of linagliptin in cardiovascular injury appeared to be attributed to the reduction of oxidative stress and the downregulation of angiotensin converting enzyme (ACE) (53). Moreover, many studies were performed to explore the deeper mechanism. For example, Jo et al. showed that DPP-4i can restrain the activity of the nod-like receptor protein 3 (NLRP3) inflammasome by alleviating nicotinamide adenine dinucleotide phosphate (NADPH) oxidase 2-associated oxidative stress (43). Hu et al. further showed that the treatment of vascular endothelial cells with sitagliptin could inhibit the TNF-induced expression of vascular cell adhesion mole 1 (VCAM-1) mRNA (54). Other research showed that advanced glycation end products (AGE), and receptor of advanced glycation end products (RAGE), induces the release of ROS and stimulates DPP-4 expression from ECs by interacting with the mannose 6-phosphate/insulin-like growth factor II receptor (M6P/IGF-IIR) (55). GLP-1 inhibit AGE/RAGE-induced ROS release and inflammatory reactions via the cAMP pathway by targeting glucagon-like peptide 1 receptor (GLP-1R) (56). Consistent with this, linagliptin significantly inhibited AGE-induced ROS generation by increasing the expression of GLP-1 (55). DPP-4 inhibition via gemigliptin prevents the abnormal vascular remodeling induced by oxidative stress via the activation of nuclear factor erythroid-derived 2 (NF-E2)-related factor 2 (57). Liraglutide also exerts anti-inflammatory effects through the GLP-1R/cyclic adenosine monophosphate (cAMP) pathway via cascading cAMP-dependent protein kinase/Liver kinase B1 (PKA/LKB1), thereby increasing nitric oxide production and suppressing NF-κB (58). The activation of NF-κB can also be suppressed by DPP-4 inhibitor (59).

Investigating the regulatory activity of DPP-4 upon the inflammatory mediators and oxidative stress associated with elevated BP may provide us with good expectations for the future use of DPP-4i in the treatment of hypertension, especially in patients with inflammation. However, until now, there is still a deficiency in our understanding of the immunological mechanisms associated with DPP-4i and BP regulation. Further research is urgently required in this regard.

Vascular Mechanisms Underlying the Effect of DPP-4i on Hypertension

Vascular smooth muscle can be affected by various physical and chemical factors, resulting in either relaxation or contraction, thus causing effect upon BP. The structure and function of large arteries and arterioles play an important role in the pathogenesis of hypertension. Endothelial cells (ECs) covering the inner surface of the vascular wall can generate, activate, and release various vasoactive substances and regulate cardiovascular function, including nitric oxide (NO), prostacyclin (PGI2), endothelin-1 (ET-1), and endothelium-derived contracting factors (EDCF). However, other, non-endothelium derived substances, can also affect vascular smooth muscle cells and endothelial cells in different pathways.

NO is a crucial physiological signaling molecule in a diverse array of organ systems, and has important anti-inflammation effects, thereby exerting effect upon cardiovascular function, including vasodilation and endothelium protection. NO is synthesized by three types of NO synthase (NOS): endothelial NOS (eNOS), neuronal NOS (nNOS), and inducible NOS (60). Recent studies have shown that DPP-4 inhibitors can increase NO levels in hypertensive models (61–63). Linagliptin, a DPP-4 inhibitor, has been reported to upregulate eNOS and restore endothelium-dependent vasodilation (64, 65). Besides the direct vasodilative effects of NO/NOS, the vasodilation caused by DPP-4i also appears to be related to GLP-1. A previous meta-analysis provided evidence that GLP-1 analogs could significantly reduce sitting SBP, suggesting that GLP-1 may be associated with BP and vascular function (66). Consistent with this, other researchers have shown that GLP-1 can induce vasodilation (67–69). The vasodilatory response of GLP-1 may occur via two different pathways: GLP-1R-dependent and independent pathways. Hattori et al. reported that the activator of GLP-1 receptor liraglutide increased eNOS phosphorylation and NO production in a protein kinase-dependent manner (58). The metabolite of active GLP 1(7 36), GLP-1(9-36), is also known to have a vasodilatory effect via the NO/cyclic guanosine monophosphate (cGMP)-dependent mechanism (68). It has also been reported that insulin which was induced by GLP-1 could affect the diastolic function of the blood vessels via the nitric oxide pathway (70). Moreover, another study reported that the vasodilatory effects of GLP-1 are independent of insulin action (71). Other vasodilatory substances, such as a-type natriuretic peptide (ANP), cGMP, and cAMP can be induced by the GLP-1R agonist exenatide (72). In addition, BNP, another substrate of DPP-4, also possesses vasodilatation activity (73). We hypothesize that DPP-4i could simultaneously enhance the concentration of activated BNP, thus promoting vasodilatation.

In contrast, another substrate of DPP-4i, neuropeptide Y1-36 (NPY1-36), has shown potent vasoconstrictive effects. NPY is a Y1-receptor agonist released from the sympathetic nerve terminals. NPY1-36 can be converted to its inactive form NPY3-36 by DPP-4 (74). Stimulation of a sympathetic nerve leads to the release of NPY which has stronger vasoconstriction properties than norepinephrine (75). NPY1-36 causes vasoconstriction via Y1 receptors, whereas NPY3-36 is a selective Y2-receptor agonist without effect on vascular tone (76, 77). DPP-4i prevents the inactivation of NPY1-36 and exerts contraction effects which are dependent upon catecholamine (78, 79). Simultaneously, NPY can inhibit the activity of vasodilator substances and enhance vasoconstrictor substances, resulting in a significant increase in vasoconstriction (80). Prieto et al. previously showed that NPY elevates Ca^{2+} influx by stimulating L-type calcium channels, leading to the secretion and potentiation of noradrenaline (81). Other studies have also shown that NPY is able to hydrolyze phosphoric inositol on cell membranes into an inositol trisphosphate (IP3) signal substance, which can promote the release of calcium ions and increase the concentration of extracellular calcium ions (82). In addition, some studies have reported that vasoconstriction is affected by the sodium potassium pump; inhibition of this pump can change the polarization of the cell membrane, thereby regulating Na^+/Ca^{2+} exchange (83).

These studies gave us some insight into how DPP-4i causes effects upon the vascular endothelium. Further studies should now be performed to identify the precise mechanisms involved with the action of DPP-4i. We believe that the different efficacies of DPP-4i in regulating the function of vascular endothelial cell are possibly associated with the immunity of the human body, the distribution of cytokines, and the administration of drugs. The vasoconstriction of NPY is highly Ca^{2+}-dependent, thus suggesting that the combination of DPP-4i and Ca^{2+} antagonists can improve the situation. And Y1 receptor antagonists could also prevent the prohypertensive effect of NPY and possibly augment the antihypertensive effects of DPP-4i.

Neural Mechanisms of the Action of DPP-4i on Hypertension

The sympathetic nervous system (SNS) plays an important role in regulating the heart and other visceral organs. The activity of the sympathetic nerve is responsible for the physiological needs of the body when it is in a state of tension, causing constricted blood vessels, increased heart rate, dilated pupils, and reduced secretion of the digestive glands. Vasoconstriction is caused by noradrenaline activated alpha-1 adrenergic receptor released from sympathetic ganglion neurons. In contrast, Beta-1 receptors are mainly distributed in the heart, and can increase myocardial contractility, self-regulation, and conduction function. As a result of vasoconstriction and heart excitement by SNS activation, there is a consequential rise in BP.

Substance P is an important neuropeptide and acts as both a vasodilator and sympathetic activator; it can also be degraded by DPP-4. Previous research has shown that substance P is highly expressed in the heart. The expression of tachykinin precursor 1 (TAC1), the gene encoding substance P, was up-regulated when the BP is raised, indicating an involvement of substance P in high BP conditions (84). DPP-4 is a potent lyase of substance P and DPP-4i prevents the degradation of substance P from an activated state to an inactivated state. Concurrent with DPP-4 and ACEI, the intra-arterial administration of substance P stimulated the SNS (85). Further evidence was provided by another clinical study which suggested that sitagliptin could reduce BP under low-dose enalapril treatment without effects on cardiac rhythm and hormonal level, but increased hypertensive response in combination with high-dose enalapril accompanied by increasing heart rate and norepinephrine concentration. This result suggests that the SNS was activated during maximal ACEI and sitagliptin treatment (22). Consistent with the findings in humans, the same result was also found in spontaneously hypertensive rats (SHR) (86). One reasonable explanation for this is that high-dose ACEI and DPP-4i significantly reduced the degradation of substance P, due to the combined inhibition of ACE and DPP-4. Therefore, when combined with high doses of ACEI and DPP-4i, substance P may lead to sympathetic activation rather than vasodilation.

In addition, it has also been shown that BP can be elevated by GLP-1 and the GLP-1 receptor. Recent studies have demonstrated that GLP-1 and GLP-1R agonists induced a sustained elevation of BP in rodents (45, 87). This elevation in BP may have occurred as a result of the increased sympathetic activity by GLP-1 receptor activation in the central nervous system (88). Yamamoto et al. reported that centrally and peripherally administered GLP-1R agonists increased BP and heart rate by enhancing sympathetic activity in a dose-dependent manner (89). Similarly, Trahair et al. reported that intravenous GLP-1 administration attenuated the hypotensive response in healthy older individuals (90). In contrast, another study indicated that GLP-1 does not contribute to sympathetic activation (91).

In conclusion, the BP lowering effect of DPP-4i may be reduced by stimulating sympathetic activity via reducing degradation of GLP-1 and substance P when combined with ACEI, especially in high-dose ACEI. We suggest that combined treatment with agents that block the SNS could diminish the hypertensive effect of DPP-4i and that this effect may be enhanced by agents with no effect on the SNS.

Hormonal Mechanisms Underlying the Effect of DPP-4i on Hypertension

The renin angiotensin aldosterone system (RAAS) plays a role in regulating BP. Renin is secreted from the juxtaglomerular cells in the renal afferent arteriole, converting the angiotensinogen released by the liver into angiotensin I (AngI). Angiotensin I is subsequently converted to angiotensin II (AngII) by the angiotensin-converting enzyme (ACE) found on the surface of vascular endothelial cells, predominantly those of the lungs. AngII is the major effector of RAAS, acting on AngII receptor type 1 (AT1), causing contraction of the smooth muscle of the arteriole and stimulating the adrenocortical spherical band to secrete aldosterone. AngII receptor type 2 (AT2) is generally considered to be an antagonist of the AT1 receptor, regulating the relaxation of the smooth muscle (92). Aldosterone induced by AngII promoting the reabsorption of sodium and water from the kidney, can increase water retention, and norepinephrine secretion via positive feedback from the sympathetic end of the anterior membrane, eventually leading to an increase in BP.

Recent studies have shown that DPP-4i can exert antihypertensive effects by interfering with the function of the RAAS system. For example, in a previous study, teneligliptin ameliorated hypertension and comorbid cardiac remodeling in SHR by attenuating circulating AngII (93). Treatment with liraglutide and linagliptin during AngII infusion down-regulated the AT1 receptor and up-regulated AT2 receptor expression, suggesting that DPP-4i may reduce BP via the AngII receptor-mediated pathway (94). In addition, sodium/hydrogen exchanger 1 (NHE-1), a membrane-bound enzyme, is thought to be partly mediated by AngII and involved in modulating intracellular acidity; its activation would lead to intracellular Na^+ retention, thus enhancing Na^+/Ca^{2+} exchange and H_2O reabsorption (95, 96). Moreover, Kawase et al. found that teneligliptin suppressed NHE-1 expression, an effect that was enhanced by AngII, showing that DPP-4i could reduce BP by inhibiting the AngII-NHE-1 pathway (93). However, GLP-1 may also participate in regulating the function of RAAS. For example, Chaudhuri et al. showed that exenatide administration could lead to the reduction of renin, angiotensin II, and angiotensinogen in the plasma concentrations (72).

In addition, ACE inactivates substance P via the carboxy terminus. Combined treatment with high-dose ACEI and sitagliptin significantly increased BP by elevating the expression of substance P, while low-dose ACEI had no such effect (22). We suggest that when using combined treatments of DPP-4i and anti-hypertensive drugs targeting RAAS, then high-dose ACEIs should be avoided. Moreover, the important effect of the AngII receptor upon BP control should not be underestimated. We should also remember that treatment with both DPP-4i and ARB may exert synergistic anti-hypertensive effects.

Renal Mechanisms Underlying the Action of DPP-4i on Hypertension

Various factors act upon the renal system and cause water-sodium retention, thus increasing cardiac output and peripheral vascular resistance. Water and salt metabolism can regulate blood-volume by affecting plasma crystal osmotic pressure. Increased osmotic pressure leads to elevated blood volume and higher BP. There are many active substances that can affect the excretion of water and sodium in the kidneys, including BNP, anti-diuretic hormone, and aldosterone.

DPP-4 is also expressed in the renal proximal tubular brush border, where it regulates $Na+/H_2O$ reabsorption (97). DPP-4i exerts diuretic and natriuretic effects by inhibiting the activity of DPP-4 (98); sitagliptin was recently shown to reduce BP by increasing sodium excretion and reducing H_2O reabsorption (15). The hypotensive effect of DPP-4i seems to contribute to the reducing activity of NHE3, a Na+/H+ exchanger isoform responsible for reabsorption of $NaHCO_3$ and NaCl (15, 99). Researches have shown that exogenous treatment with GLP-1 can induce diuretic and natriuretic effects mediated by downregulation of the activity of NHE3 (100–102). This phenomenon indicates that the diuretic and natriuretic effects of DPP-4i are mediated by preventing the degradation of GLP-1. GLP-1 could increase the urinary excretion of cAMP, suggesting that cAMP signaling pathways may participate in this process (101). Crajoinas et al. demonstrated that GLP-1 activates the cAMP/PKA signaling pathway by binding to its receptor GLP-1R and by then phosphorylating the PKA consensus site of NHE3 (101). However, Girardi et al. suggested that the effect of DPP-4i in reducing NHE3 activity results from the inhibition of a tyrosine kinase signaling pathway rather than by activation of PKA (103). The natriuretic effect of teneligliptin was partially associated with GLP-1R, and the natriuretic effect was inhibited by the GLP-1R antagonist, exendin9-39; diuresis, however, was not affected (98). Ronn et al. previously showed that these diuretic and natriuretic effects cannot be fully inhibited by the GLP-1 inhibitor exendin9-39 in SHR, which lack the expression of GLP-1 receptors (104). These findings indicated the involvement of some other unknown pathways.

BNP is a member of the natriuretic peptide family which plays an important physiological role in maintaining cardiovascular and renal homeostasis (105). It is well-known that BNP has potent diuretic and natriuretic effects. DPP-4 converts BNP1-32 into its inactive form BNP3-32 (106) and can attenuate the diuretic and natriuretic effects of BNP1-32 (107). This means that DPP-4i can enhance the diuretic and natriuretic effects of BNP1-32. Another member of the natriuretic peptide family, A type natriuretic peptide (ANP), which also has diuresis activity, was shown to be stimulated by exenatide, a GLP-1 receptor agonist (72, 108). It has also been reported that exenatide and liraglutide induced an increased concentration of ANP through the GLP-1 receptor-dependent pathway (108). In addition, insulin induced by GLP-1 may also promote ANP secretion (72).

Generally, the diuretic and natriuretic effects of DPP-4i are associated with the reduced degradation of GLP-1 and BNP. Similarly, another natriuretic peptide, ANP, is increased via a GLP-1 pathway. Anti-hypertensive drugs, diuretics, are especially effective for elderly and obese hypertensive patients when monotherapy is not satisfactory, and can significantly reduce cardiac load. Combined treatment with diuretics and DPP-4i may amplify the effects of diuretics upon the reduction of BP and decreasing cardiac load.

Insulin Resistant Mechanisms Underlying the Action of DPP-4i on Hypertension

Insulin resistance (IR) is considered as a pathological condition in which cells fail to respond normally to the hormone insulin (109). Recently, it is generally believed that IR is common in patients with hypertension and plays a key role in cardiovascular complications. A body of evidence has indicated that IR is closely related to the occurrence and development of hypertension (110). Insulin acts directly on the vascular tissue, including endothelial cells (111), and smooth muscle cells (112). In patients with T2DM, extended treatment with insulin can significantly improve endothelial-dependent vasodilation (113). Drugs that improve insulin sensitivity have also shown beneficial effects in the control of BP (114). Insulin improves arterial endothelial function in healthy individuals but not in metabolic syndrome patients with IR; this phenomenon demonstrates that IR may be responsible for increased cardiovascular disease risk (70).

The administration of DPP-4 promotes IR (115, 116), and insulin sensitivity has been shown to be improved when DPP-4 was down-regulated (111, 117). Furthermore, clinical research has shown that DPP-4i can improve β cell activity and increase insulin release (118), and that the long term administration of DPP-4i can improve insulin sensitivity (119, 120). For example, Smits et al. found that GLP-1-based therapies, including exenatide or sitagliptin, could significantly lower BP in the same manner as insulin therapy (121), thus suggesting that the hypotensive effects of insulin may be associated with GLP-1 (122). Chen et al. further suggested that saxagliptin could upregulate nesfatin-1 secretion and ameliorate insulin resistance (12), while other research has demonstrated that nesfatin-1 increases the secretion of GLP-1 (123). Ahren et al. suggested that GLP-1 may increase insulin release via a cAMP-dependent pathway (83). Other investigators have suggested that a NOS-related pathway may also contribute to improve insulin release. NOS inhibitors, for example, NG-monomethyl-L-arginine (L-NMMA), and asymmetrical dimethylarginine, can both improve insulin sensitivity (124, 125). With an improvement of IR, initiated by the stimulatory production of NO from the endothelium, insulin gradually exhibits its vasodilatory action (111, 117).

In summary, IR disturbs the function of the vascular endothelium and weakens the anti-hypertensive effect of insulin. DPP-4i could reduce BP by improve IR, particularly in patients with T2DM. And with the improvement of IR, the vascular inflammation can be improved, thereby reducing the cardiovascular complications.

CONCLUSIONS

As a differentiation antigen on the surface of T cells, DPP-4/CD26 plays an important role in regulating the activation and chemotaxis of mononuclear-macrophages, NK cells, and T cells. DPP-4 inhibitors can regulate anti-inflammatory and anti-hypertensive effects by regulating the functions of these immune cells, especially T cells. We found that DPP-4i exhibits strong inhibitory effects on inflammation and oxidative stress, and a few studies provide direct evidence that DPP-4iDPP-4i reduces BP by regulating immune reactions. Moreover, the inflammatory factors regulated by DPP-4i are also closely associated with hypertension. We speculate that DPP-4i could reduce BP by regulating T cell activation, thus alleviating vascular inflammation and improving oxidative stress. However, due to the lack of research data at present, and because the mechanism underlying the action of DPP-4iDPP-4i upon BP is complex, further studies are now needed to identify the precise mechanism involved.

The substrates of DPP-4 plays an important role in regulating blood pressure. GLP-1, substance P, and BNP, commonly show a vasodilation effect, while NPY has a significant hypertensive effect. Our literature review indicated that the effect of vasoconstriction is closely associated with elevated calcium concentration. Thus, the combination of calcium antagonists may be a potent solution to resist the effect of vasoconstriction in DPP-4i treatment. In addition, the regulation of Na/H_2O

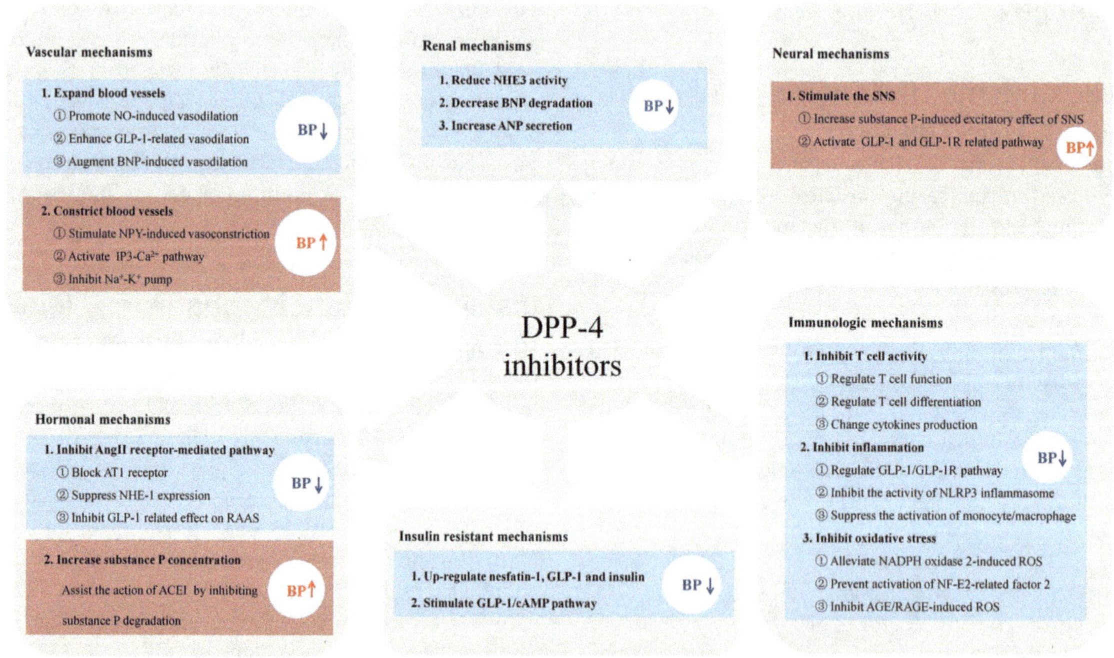

FIGURE 1 | The potential mechanisms of DPP-4i in regulating blood pressure. DPP-4i has shown unique advantages in regulating blood pressure in the six mechanisms, including the aspects of immune systems, blood vessel, nervous system, hormone, kidney, and insulin resistance.

metabolism, the reduction of circulating AngII levels, and improvements in insulin resistance, may all contribute to anti-hypertensive activities. In contrast, in some situations, particularly when combined with high-dose ACEI, DPP-4i may exhibit hypertensive effects by stimulating sympathetic activity and alleviating the degradation of GLP-1 and substance P. The hypertensive effects of DPP-4i may be diminished by agents that block the SNS and enhanced by hypotensive agents with no effect on the SNS (86). Furthermore, antihypertensive drugs that do not block the SNS may exhibit an increasing BP effect of DPP-4 inhibitors by lowering basal vascular tone (86).

In summary, the effects of DPP-4i on BP occur in a highly context-dependent manner, and the mechanisms of DPP4-i in regulating BP are summarized in **Figure 1**. DPP-4i has shown good anti-hypertensive potency and combined treatment has better effect than DPP-4i alone. However, combination with high-dose ACEI could increase blood pressure. DPP-4i has shown BP modulating effects in the aspect of five traditional etiological mechanisms of hypertension, indicating that DPP-4i has great potential as a combined therapy for the treatment of hypertension; this exploits the fact that a combination of drugs causes effects on different targets. For patients with diabetes and hypertension, the advantage of DPP-4i is that it regulates blood pressure and improves insulin resistance. In addition, DPP-4i can alleviate vascular inflammation in hypertension by regulating inflammatory responses and improving vascular endothelial function, thereby reducing the incidence of cardiovascular complications. When combining DPP-4i with ARB and diuretics, the improvement of cardiac load and ventricular remodeling can be augmented. Notably, the opposite effects of DPP-4i, that promote sympathetic activation and vasoconstriction, cannot be ignored when combined with anti-hypertensive drugs. High-dose ACEI with DPP-4i may diminish the effect of anti-hypertensive drugs due to increased sympathetic activation, while low-dose ACEI has no such effect. Anti-sympathetic drugs, such as β-blockers, may represent suitable candidates in combination with DPP-4 for the treatment of hypertension with which to prevent sympathetic activity. Vasoconstriction of NPY induced by DPP-4i can similarly elevate BP via a Ca^{2+}-dependent vasoconstrictive effect, thus suggesting that the combination of DPP-4i and Ca^{2+} antagonists can improve the situation.

Until now the specific etiological mechanism of hypertension has not yet been fully identified, and choosing the most appropriate and effective antihypertensive drugs is still a problem. Because it has multiple targets, DPP-4i would be a good choice with which to treat hypertension, especially in patients with chronic inflammatory diseases, such as coronary heart disease, diabetes mellitus, and hyperlipidemia. Because existing studies are still deficient, the specific mechanism of DPP-4i in regulating BP has not yet been completely clarified. Further investigations are now needed to illustrate the modulatory mechanisms and effects of DPP-4i on BP.

AUTHOR CONTRIBUTIONS

QG organized the article. JiaZ wrote the draft. QC drew the figure and table. BZ edited the language, figure and table. JixZ and CL revised the draft.

FUNDING

This work was supported by Natural Science Foundation of China (81670431) and Natural Science Foundation of Hubei Province (2015CFA080).

REFERENCES

1. Gong Q, Rajagopalan S, Zhong J. Dpp4 inhibition as a therapeutic strategy in cardiometabolic disease: Incretin-dependent and -independent function. *Int J Cardiol.* (2015) 197:170–9. doi: 10.1016/j.ijcard.2015.06.076
2. White WB, Wilson CA, Bakris GL, Bergenstal RM, Cannon CP, Cushman WC, et al. Angiotensin-converting enzyme inhibitor use and major cardiovascular outcomes in type 2 diabetes mellitus treated with the dipeptidyl peptidase 4 inhibitor alogliptin. *Hypertension.* (2016) 68:606–13. doi: 10.1161/HYPERTENSIONAHA.116.07797
3. Scirica BM, Bhatt DL, Braunwald E, Steg PG, Davidson J, Hirshberg B, et al. Saxagliptin and cardiovascular outcomes in patients with type 2 diabetes mellitus. *N Engl J Med.* (2013) 369:1317–26. doi: 10.1056/NEJMoa1307684
4. Leung M, Leung DY, Wong VW. Effects of dipeptidyl peptidase-4 inhibitors on cardiac and endothelial function in type 2 diabetes mellitus: a pilot study. *Diab Vasc Dis Res.* (2016) 13:236–43. doi: 10.1177/1479164116629352
5. Kato S, Fukui K, Kirigaya H, Gyotoku D, Iinuma N, Kusakawa Y, et al. Inhibition of DPP-4 by alogliptin improves coronary flow reserve and left ventricular systolic function evaluated by phase contrast cine magnetic resonance imaging in patients with type 2 diabetes and coronary artery disease. *Int J Cardiol.* (2016) 223:770–5. doi: 10.1016/j.ijcard.2016.08.306
6. Read PA, Khan FZ, Heck PM, Hoole SP, Dutka DP. DPP-4 inhibition by sitagliptin improves the myocardial response to dobutamine stress and mitigates stunning in a pilot study of patients with coronary artery disease. *Circ Cardiovasc Imaging.* (2010) 3:195–201. doi: 10.1161/CIRCIMAGING.109.899377
7. Jax T, Stirban A, Terjung A, Esmaeili H, Berk A, Thiemann S, et al. A randomised, active- and placebo-controlled, three-period crossover trial to investigate short-term effects of the dipeptidyl peptidase-4 inhibitor linagliptin on macro- and microvascular endothelial function in type 2 diabetes. *Cardiovasc Diabetol.* (2017) 16:13. doi: 10.1186/s12933-016-0493-3
8. Ida S, Murata K, Betou K, Kobayashi C, Ishihara Y, Imataka K, et al. Effect of trelagliptin on vascular endothelial functions and serum adiponectin level in patients with type 2 diabetes: a preliminary single-arm prospective pilot study. *Cardiovasc Diabetol.* (2016) 15:153. doi: 10.1186/s12933-016-0468-4
9. Ogawa S, Ishiki M, Nako K, Okamura M, Senda M, Mori T, et al. Sitagliptin, a dipeptidyl peptidase-4 inhibitor, decreases systolic blood pressure in Japanese hypertensive patients with type 2 diabetes. *Tohoku J Exp Med.* (2011) 223:133. doi: 10.1620/tjem.223.133
10. Duvnjak L, Blaslov K. Dipeptidyl peptidase-4 inhibitors improve arterial stiffness, blood pressure, lipid profile and inflammation parameters in patients with type 2 diabetes mellitus. *Diabetol Metab Syndr.* (2016) 8:26. doi: 10.1186/s13098-016-0144-6
11. Evans M, Schweizer A, Foley JE. Blood pressure and fasting lipid changes after 24 weeks' treatment with vildagliptin: a pooled analysis in >2,000 previously drug-naive patients with type 2 diabetes mellitus. *Vasc Health Risk Manag.* (2016) 12:337–40. doi: 10.2147/VHRM.S112148
12. Chen K, Zhuo T, Wang J, Mei Q. Saxagliptin upregulates nesfatin-1 secretion and ameliorates insulin resistance and metabolic profiles in type 2 diabetes mellitus. *Metab Syndr Relat Disord.* (2018) 16:336–41. doi: 10.1089/met.2018.0010

13. Hussain M, Atif MA, Ghafoor MB. Beneficial effects of sitagliptin and metformin in non-diabetic hypertensive and dyslipidemic patients. *Pak J Pharm Sci.* (2016) 29:2385–9.
14. Yuasa S, Sato K, Furuki T, Minamizawa K, Sakai H, Numata Y, et al. Primary care-based investigation of the effect of sitagliptin on blood pressure in hypertensive patients with type 2 diabetes. *J Clin Med Res.* (2017) 9:188–92. doi: 10.14740/jocmr2820w
15. Pacheco BP, Crajoinas RO, Couto GK, Davel AP, Lessa LM, Rossoni LV, et al. Dipeptidyl peptidase IV inhibition attenuates blood pressure rising in young spontaneously hypertensive rats. *J Hypertens.* (2011) 29:520–8. doi: 10.1097/HJH.0b013e328341939d
16. Liu L, Liu J, Wong WT, Tian XY, Lau CW, Wang YX, et al. Dipeptidyl peptidase 4 inhibitor sitagliptin protects endothelial function in hypertension through a glucagon-like peptide 1-dependent mechanism. *Hypertension.* (2012) 60:833–41. doi: 10.1161/HYPERTENSIONAHA.112.195115
17. Sufiun A, Rafiq K, Fujisawa Y, Rahman A, Mori H, Nakano D, et al. Effect of dipeptidyl peptidase-4 inhibition on circadian blood pressure during the development of salt-dependent hypertension in rats. *Hypertens Res.* (2015) 38:237–43. doi: 10.1038/hr.2014.173
18. Mason RP, Jacob RF, Kubant R, Ciszewski A, Corbalan JJ, Malinski T. Dipeptidyl peptidase-4 inhibition with saxagliptin enhanced nitric oxide release and reduced blood pressure and sICAM-1 levels in hypertensive rats. *J Cardiovasc Pharmacol.* (2012) 60:467–73. doi: 10.1097/FJC.0b013e31826be204
19. Sivasinprasasn S, Sa-Nguanmoo P, Pongkan W, Pratchayasakul W, Chattipakorn SC, Chattipakorn N. Estrogen and DPP4 inhibitor, but not metformin, exert cardioprotection via attenuating cardiac mitochondrial dysfunction in obese insulin-resistant and estrogen-deprived female rats. *Menopause.* (2016) 23:894–902. doi: 10.1097/GME.0000000000000640
20. Alter ML, Ott IM, von Websky K, Tsuprykov O, Sharkovska Y, Krause-Relle K, et al. DPP-4 inhibition on top of angiotensin receptor blockade offers a new therapeutic approach for diabetic nephropathy. *Kidney Blood Press Res.* (2012) 36:119–30. doi: 10.1159/000341487
21. Chaykovska L, Alter ML, von Websky K, Hohmann M, Tsuprykov O, Reichetzeder C, et al. Effects of telmisartan and linagliptin when used in combination on blood pressure and oxidative stress in rats with 2-kidney-1-clip hypertension. *J Hypertens.* (2013) 31:2290–8, discussion 2299. doi: 10.1097/HJH.0b013e3283649b4d
22. Marney A, Kunchakarra S, Byrne L, Brown NJ. Interactive hemodynamic effects of dipeptidyl peptidase-IV inhibition and angiotensin-converting enzyme inhibition in humans. *Hypertension.* (2010) 56:728–33. doi: 10.1161/HYPERTENSIONAHA.110.156554
23. Jackson EK, Mi Z, Tofovic SP, Gillespie DG. Effect of dipeptidyl peptidase 4 inhibition on arterial blood pressure is context dependent. *Hypertension.* (2015) 65:238–49. doi: 10.1161/HYPERTENSIONAHA.114.04631
24. Lim SS, Vos T, Flaxman AD, Danaei G, Shibuya K, Adair-Rohani H, et al. A comparative risk assessment of burden of disease and injury attributable to 67 risk factors and risk factor clusters in 21 regions, 1990–2010: a systematic analysis for the global burden of disease study 2010. *Lancet.* (2012) 380:2224–60. doi: 10.1016/S0140-6736(12)61766-8
25. Animut Y, Assefa AT, Lemma DG. Blood pressure control status and associated factors among adult hypertensive patients on outpatient follow-up at University of Gondar Referral Hospital, northwest Ethiopia: a retrospective follow-up study. *Integr Blood Press Contr.* (2018) 11:37–46. doi: 10.2147/IBPC.S150628
26. Schiffrin EL. The immune system: role in hypertension. *Can J Cardiol.* (2013) 29:543–8. doi: 10.1016/j.cjca.2012.06.009
27. Leibowitz A, Schiffrin EL. Immune mechanisms in hypertension. *Curr Hypertens Rep.* (2011) 13:465–72. doi: 10.1007/s11906-011-0224-9
28. Virdis A, Schiffrin EL. Vascular inflammation: a role in vascular disease in hypertension? *Curr Opin Nephrol Hypertens.* (2003) 12:181–7. doi: 10.1097/00041552-200303000-00009
29. da Silva Júnior WS, Souza M, Nogueira Neto JF, Bouskela E, Kraemer-Aguiar LG. Constitutive DPP4 activity, inflammation, and microvascular reactivity in subjects with excess body weight and without diabetes. *Microvasc Res.* (2018) 120:94–9. doi: 10.1016/j.mvr.2018.07.005
30. Madhur MS, Lob HE, McCann LA, Iwakura Y, Blinder Y, Guzik TJ, et al. Interleukin 17 promotes angiotensin II-induced hypertension and vascular dysfunction. *Hypertension.* (2010) 55:500–7. doi: 10.1161/HYPERTENSIONAHA.109.145094
31. Jurewicz M, McDermott DH, Sechler JM, Tinckam K, Takakura A, Carpenter CB, et al. Human T and natural killer cells possess a functional renin-angiotensin system: further mechanisms of angiotensin II-induced inflammation. *J Am Soc Nephrol.* (2007) 18:1093–102. doi: 10.1681/ASN.2006070707
32. Hoch NE, Guzik TJ, Chen W, Deans T, Maalouf SA, Gratze P, et al. Regulation of T-cell function by endogenously produced angiotensin II. *Am J Physiol Regul Integr Comp Physiol.* (2009) 296:R208–16. doi: 10.1152/ajpregu.90521.2008
33. Schon E, Demuth HU, Eichmann E, Horst HJ, Korner IJ, Kopp J, et al. Dipeptidyl peptidase IV in human T lymphocytes. Impaired induction of interleukin 2 and gamma interferon due to specific inhibition of dipeptidyl peptidase IV. *Scand J Immunol.* (1989) 29:127–32. doi: 10.1111/j.1365-3083.1989.tb01108.x
34. Nistala R, Habibi J, Lastra G, Manrique C, Aroor AR, Hayden MR, et al. Prevention of obesity-induced renal injury in male mice by DPP4 inhibition. *Endocrinology.* (2014) 155:2266–76. doi: 10.1210/en.2013-1920
35. Shah Z, Kampfrath T, Deiuliis JA, Zhong J, Pineda C, Ying Z, et al. Long-term dipeptidyl-peptidase 4 inhibition reduces atherosclerosis and inflammation via effects on monocyte recruitment and chemotaxis. *Circulation.* (2011) 124:2338–49. doi: 10.1161/CIRCULATIONAHA.111.041418
36. Salim HM, Fukuda D, Higashikuni Y, Tanaka K, Hirata Y, Yagi S, et al. Teneligliptin, a dipeptidyl peptidase-4 inhibitor, attenuated pro-inflammatory phenotype of perivascular adipose tissue and inhibited atherogenesis in normoglycemic apolipoprotein-E-deficient mice. *Vascul Pharmacol.* (2017) 96–8:19–25. doi: 10.1016/j.vph.2017.03.003
37. Miossec P, Korn T, Kuchroo VK. Interleukin-17 and type 17 helper T cells. *N Engl J Med.* (2009) 361:888–98. doi: 10.1056/NEJMra0707449
38. Bengsch B, Seigel B, Flecken T, Wolanski J, Blum HE, Thimme R. Human Th17 cells express high levels of enzymatically active dipeptidylpeptidase IV (CD26). *J Immunol.* (2012) 188:5438–47. doi: 10.4049/jimmunol.1103801
39. Brown SM, Smith CE, Meuth AI, Khan M, Aroor AR, Cleeton HM, et al. Dipeptidyl peptidase-4 inhibition with saxagliptin ameliorates angiotensin II-induced cardiac diastolic dysfunction in male mice. *Endocrinology.* (2017) 158:3592–604. doi: 10.1210/en.2017-00416
40. Jia XQ, Xu S, Tian MR, Ma YY. The relationship between inflammatory factor expression and blood pressure and urinary protein in the placenta of gestational hypertension rats. *Exp Ther Med.* (2018) 16:3793–8. doi: 10.3892/etm.2018.6668
41. Crosswhite P, Sun Z. Ribonucleic acid interference knockdown of interleukin 6 attenuates cold-induced hypertension. *Hypertension.* (2010) 55:1484–91. doi: 10.1161/HYPERTENSIONAHA.109.146902
42. Esposito G, Cappetta D, Russo R, Rivellino A, Ciuffreda LP, Roviezzo F, et al. Sitagliptin reduces inflammation, fibrosis and preserves diastolic function in a rat model of heart failure with preserved ejection fraction. *Br J Pharmacol.* (2017) 174:4070–86. doi: 10.1111/bph.13686
43. Jo CH, Kim S, Park JS, Kim GH. Anti-inflammatory action of sitagliptin and linagliptin in doxorubicin nephropathy. *Kidney Blood Press Res.* (2018) 43:987–99. doi: 10.1159/000490688
44. Tinsley JH, South S, Chiasson VL, Mitchell BM. Interleukin-10 reduces inflammation, endothelial dysfunction, and blood pressure in hypertensive pregnant rats. *Am J Physiol Regul Integr Comp Physiol.* (2010) 298:R713–9. doi: 10.1152/ajpregu.00712.2009
45. Ussher JR, Drucker DJ. Cardiovascular actions of incretin-based therapies. *Circ Res.* (2014) 114:1788–803. doi: 10.1161/CIRCRESAHA.114.301958
46. Chan CT, Sobey CG, Lieu M, Ferens D, Kett MM, Diep H, et al. Obligatory role for B cells in the development of angiotensin II-dependent hypertension. *Hypertension.* (2015) 66:1023–33. doi: 10.1161/HYPERTENSIONAHA.115.05779
47. Gorrell MD, Wickson J, McCaughan GW. Expression of the rat CD26 antigen (dipeptidyl peptidase IV) on subpopulations of rat lymphocytes. *Cell Immunol.* (1991) 134:205–15. doi: 10.1016/0008-8749(91)90343-A
48. Rizzo MR, Barbieri M, Marfella R, Paolisso G. Reduction of oxidative stress and inflammation by blunting daily acute glucose fluctuations in patients

with type 2 diabetes: role of dipeptidyl peptidase-IV inhibition. *Diabetes Care.* (2012) 35:2076–82. doi: 10.2337/dc12-0199

49. Ervinna N, Mita T, Yasunari E, Azuma K, Tanaka R, Fujimura S, et al. Anagliptin, a DPP-4 inhibitor, suppresses proliferation of vascular smooth muscles and monocyte inflammatory reaction and attenuates atherosclerosis in male apo E-deficient mice. *Endocrinology.* (2013) 154:1260–70. doi: 10.1210/en.2012-1855
50. Hwang HJ, Chung HS, Jung TW, Ryu JY, Hong HC, Seo JA, et al. The dipeptidyl peptidase-IV inhibitor inhibits the expression of vascular adhesion molecules and inflammatory cytokines in HUVECs via Akt- and AMPK-dependent mechanisms. *Mol Cell Endocrinol.* (2015) 405:25–34. doi: 10.1016/j.mce.2015.01.025
51. Mega C, Lemos ETD, Vala H, Fernandes R, Oliveira J, Mascarenhas-Melo F, et al. Diabetic nephropathy amelioration by a low-dose sitagliptin in an animal model of type 2 diabetes (zucker diabetic fatty rat). *Exp. Diabetes Res.* (2015) 2011:162092. doi: 10.1155/2011/162092
52. Alam MA, Chowdhury MRH, Jain P, Sagor MAT, Reza HM. DPP-4 inhibitor sitagliptin prevents inflammation and oxidative stress of heart and kidney in two kidney and one clip (2K1C) rats. *Diabetol Metab Syndr.* (2015) 7:107. doi: 10.1186/s13098-015-0095-3
53. Koibuchi N, Hasegawa Y, Katayama T, Toyama K, Uekawa K, Sueta D, et al. DPP-4 inhibitor linagliptin ameliorates cardiovascular injury in salt-sensitive hypertensive rats independently of blood glucose and blood pressure. *Cardiovasc Diabetol.* (2014) 13:157. doi: 10.1186/s12933-014-0157-0
54. Hu Y, Liu H, Simpson RW, Dear AE. GLP-1-dependent and independent effects and molecular mechanisms of a dipeptidyl peptidase 4 inhibitor in vascular endothelial cells. *Mol Biol Rep.* (2013) 40:2273–9. doi: 10.1007/s11033-012-2290-8
55. Ishibashi Y, Matsui T, Maeda S, Higashimoto Y, Yamagishi S. Advanced glycation end products evoke endothelial cell damage by stimulating soluble dipeptidyl peptidase-4 production and its interaction with mannose 6-phosphate/insulin-like growth factor II receptor. *Cardiovasc Diabetol.* (2013) 12:125. doi: 10.1186/1475-2840-12-125
56. Ishibashi Y, Nishino Y, Matsui T, Takeuchi M, Yamagishi S. Glucagon-like peptide-1 suppresses advanced glycation end product-induced monocyte chemoattractant protein-1 expression in mesangial cells by reducing advanced glycation end product receptor level. *Metabolism.* (2011) 60:1271–7. doi: 10.1016/j.metabol.2011.01.010
57. Choi SH, Park S, Oh CJ, Leem J, Park KG, Lee IK. Dipeptidyl peptidase-4 inhibition by gemigliptin prevents abnormal vascular remodeling via NF-E2-related factor 2 activation. *Vascul Pharmacol.* (2015) 73:11–9. doi: 10.1016/j.vph.2015.07.005
58. Hattori Y, Jojima T, Tomizawa A, Satoh H, Hattori S, Kasai K, et al. A glucagon-like peptide-1 (GLP-1) analogue, liraglutide, upregulates nitric oxide production and exerts anti-inflammatory action in endothelial cells. *Diabetologia.* (2010) 53:2256–63. doi: 10.1007/s00125-010-1831-8
59. Shinjo T, Nakatsu Y, Iwashita M, Sano T, Sakoda H, Ishihara H, et al. DPP-IV inhibitor anagliptin exerts anti-inflammatory effects on macrophages, adipocytes, and mouse livers by suppressing NF-kappaB activation. *Am J Physiol Endocrinol Metab.* (2015) 309:E214–23. doi: 10.1152/ajpendo.00553.2014
60. Forstermann U, Sessa WC. Nitric oxide synthases: regulation and function. *Eur Heart J.* (2012) 33:829–37, 837a-837d. doi: 10.1093/eurheartj/ehr304
61. Mason RP, Jacob RF, Kubant R, Walter MF, Bellamine A, Jacoby A, et al. Effect of enhanced glycemic control with saxagliptin on endothelial nitric oxide release and CD40 levels in obese rats. *J Atheroscler Thromb.* (2011) 18:774–83. doi: 10.5551/jat.7666
62. Ishii M, Shibata R, Kondo K, Kambara T, Shimizu Y, Tanigawa T, et al. Vildagliptin stimulates endothelial cell network formation and ischemia-induced revascularization via an endothelial nitric-oxide synthase-dependent mechanism. *J Biol Chem.* (2014) 289:27235–45. doi: 10.1074/jbc.M114.557835
63. Shih CM, Chen YH, Lin YW, Tsao NW, Wu SC, Kao YT, et al. MK-0626, a dipeptidyl peptidase-4 inhibitor, improves neovascularization by increasing both the number of circulating endothelial progenitor cells and endothelial nitric oxide synthetase expression. *Curr Med Chem.* (2014) 21:2012–22. doi: 10.2174/09298673113206660273
64. Aroor AR, Sowers JR, Bender SB, Nistala R, Garro M, Mugerfeld I, et al. Dipeptidylpeptidase inhibition is associated with improvement in blood pressure and diastolic function in insulin-resistant male Zucker obese rats. *Endocrinology.* (2013) 154:2501–13. doi: 10.1210/en.2013-1096
65. Aroor AR, Sowers JR, Jia G, Demarco VG. Pleiotropic effects of the dipeptidylpeptidase-4 inhibitors on the cardiovascular system. *Am J Physiol Heart Circ Physiol.* (2014) 307:H477–92. doi: 10.1152/ajpheart.00209.2014
66. Katout M, Zhu H, Rutsky J, Shah P, Brook RD, Zhong J, et al. Effect of GLP-1 mimetics on blood pressure and relationship to weight loss and glycemia lowering: results of a systematic meta-analysis and meta-regression. *Am J Hypertens.* (2014) 27:130–9. doi: 10.1093/ajh/hpt196
67. Nystrom T, Gonon AT, Sjoholm A, Pernow J. Glucagon-like peptide-1 relaxes rat conduit arteries via an endothelium-independent mechanism. *Regul Pept.* (2005) 125:173–7. doi: 10.1016/j.regpep.2004.08.024
68. Ban K, Noyan-Ashraf MH, Hoefer J, Bolz SS, Drucker DJ, Husain M. Cardioprotective and vasodilatory actions of glucagon-like peptide 1 receptor are mediated through both glucagon-like peptide 1 receptor-dependent and -independent pathways. *Circulation.* (2008) 117:2340–50. doi: 10.1161/CIRCULATIONAHA.107.739938
69. Basu A, Charkoudian N, Schrage W, Rizza RA, Basu R, Joyner MJ. Beneficial effects of GLP-1 on endothelial function in humans: dampening by glyburide but not by glimepiride. *Am J Physiol Endocrinol Metab.* (2007) 293:E1289–95. doi: 10.1152/ajpendo.00373.2007
70. Jahn LA, Hartline L, Rao N, Logan B, Kim JJ, Aylor K, et al. Insulin enhances endothelial function throughout the arterial tree in healthy but not metabolic syndrome subjects. *J Clin Endocrinol Metab.* (2016) 101:1198–206. doi: 10.1210/jc.2015-3293
71. Sjoberg KA, Holst JJ, Rattigan S, Richter EA, Kiens B. GLP-1 increases microvascular recruitment but not glucose uptake in human and rat skeletal muscle. *Am J Physiol Endocrinol Metab.* (2014) 306:E355–62. doi: 10.1152/ajpendo.00283.2013
72. Chaudhuri A, Ghanim H, Makdissi A, Green K, Abuaysheh S, Batra M, et al. Exenatide induces an increase in vasodilatory and a decrease in vasoconstrictive mediators. *Diabetes Obes Metab.* (2017) 19:729–33. doi: 10.1111/dom.12835
73. Komarek M, Bernheim A, Schindler R, Steden R, Kiowski W, Brunner-La Rocca HP. Vascular effects of natriuretic peptides in healthy men. *J Cardiovasc Pharmacol Ther.* (2004) 9:263–70. doi: 10.1177/107424840400900406
74. Pablo Huidobro-Toro J, Veronica Donoso M. Sympathetic co-transmission: the coordinated action of ATP and noradrenaline and their modulation by neuropeptide Y in human vascular neuroeffector junctions. *Eur J Pharmacol.* (2004) 500:27–35. doi: 10.1016/j.ejphar.2004.07.008
75. Onuoha GN, Nicholls DP, Alpar EK, Ritchie A, Shaw C, Buchanan K. Regulatory peptides in the heart and major vessels of man and mammals. *Neuropeptides.* (1999) 33:165–72. doi: 10.1054/npep.1999.0017
76. Jackson EK, Mi Z. Sitagliptin augments sympathetic enhancement of the renovascular effects of angiotensin II in genetic hypertension. *Hypertension.* (2008) 51:1637–42. doi: 10.1161/HYPERTENSIONAHA.108.112532
77. Dubinion JH, Mi Z, Zhu C, Gao L, Jackson EK. Pancreatic polypeptide-fold peptide receptors and angiotensin II-induced renal vasoconstriction. *Hypertension.* (2006) 47:545–51. doi: 10.1161/01.HYP.0000197033.54756.83
78. Andriantsitohaina R, Bian K, Stoclet JC, Bukoski RD. Neuropeptide Y increases force development through a mechanism that involves calcium entry in resistance arteries. *J Vasc Res.* (1993) 30:309–14. doi: 10.1159/000159011
79. Chen H, Fetscher C, Schafers RF, Wambach G, Philipp T, Michel MC. Effects of noradrenaline and neuropeptide Y on rat mesenteric microvessel contraction. *Naunyn Schmiedebergs Arch Pharmacol.* (1996) 353:314–23. doi: 10.1007/BF00168634
80. Bischoff A, Gerbracht A, Michel MC. Gender and hypertension interact to regulate neuropeptide Y receptor responsiveness. *Naunyn Schmiedebergs Arch Pharmacol.* (2000) 361:173–80. doi: 10.1007/s002109900175
81. Prieto D, Buus CL, Mulvany MJ, Nilsson H. Neuropeptide Y regulates intracellular calcium through different signalling pathways linked to a Y(1)-receptor in rat mesenteric small arteries. *Br J Pharmacol.* (2000) 129:1689–99. doi: 10.1038/sj.bjp.0703256

82. Spinazzi R, Andreis PG, Nussdorfer GG. Neuropeptide-Y and Y-receptors in the autocrine-paracrine regulation of adrenal gland under physiological and pathophysiological conditions (Review). *Int J Mol Med.* (2005) 15:3–13. doi: 10.3892/ijmm.15.1.3
83. Ahren B, Landin-Olsson M, Jansson PA, Svensson M, Holmes D, Schweizer A. Inhibition of dipeptidyl peptidase-4 reduces glycemia, sustains insulin levels, and reduces glucagon levels in type 2 diabetes. *J Clin Endocrinol Metab.* (2004) 89:2078–84. doi: 10.1210/jc.2003-031907
84. Dehlin HM, Manteufel EJ, Monroe AL, Reimer MH, Levick SP. Substance P acting via the neurokinin-1 receptor regulates adverse myocardial remodeling in a rat model of hypertension. *Int J Cardiol.* (2013) 168:4643–51. doi: 10.1016/j.ijcard.2013.07.190
85. Devin JK, Pretorius M, Nian H, Yu C, Billings FTt, Brown NJ. Substance P increases sympathetic activity during combined angiotensin-converting enzyme and dipeptidyl peptidase-4 inhibition. *Hypertension.* (2014) 63:951–7. doi: 10.1161/HYPERTENSIONAHA.113.02767
86. Jackson EK, Dubinion JH, Mi Z. Effects of dipeptidyl peptidase iv inhibition on arterial blood pressure. *Clin Exp Pharmacol Physiol.* (2008) 35:29–34. doi: 10.1111/j.1440-1681.2007.04737.x
87. Ussher JR, Drucker DJ. Cardiovascular biology of the incretin system. *Endocr Rev.* (2012) 33:187–215. doi: 10.1210/er.2011-1052
88. Griffioen KJ, Ruiqian W, Eitan O, Xin W, Mary Rachael LB, Yazhou L, et al. GLP-1 receptor stimulation depresses heart rate variability and inhibits neurotransmission to cardiac vagal neurons. *Cardiovasc Res.* (2011) 89:72–8. doi: 10.1093/cvr/cvq271
89. Yamamoto H. Glucagon-like peptide-1 receptor stimulation increases blood pressure and heart rate and activates autonomic regulatory neurons. *J Clin Invest.* (2002) 110:43–52. doi: 10.1172/JCI15595
90. Trahair LG, Horowitz M, Stevens JE, Feinle-Bisset C, Standfield S, Piscitelli D, et al. Effects of exogenous glucagon-like peptide-1 on blood pressure, heart rate, gastric emptying, mesenteric blood flow and glycaemic responses to oral glucose in older individuals with normal glucose tolerance or type 2 diabetes. *Diabetologia.* (2015) 58:1769–78. doi: 10.1007/s00125-015-3638-0
91. Devin JK, Pretorius M, Nian H, Yu C, Billings FTt, Brown NJ. Dipeptidyl-peptidase 4 inhibition and the vascular effects of glucagon-like peptide-1 and brain natriuretic peptide in the human forearm. *J Am Heart Assoc.* (2014) 3:e001075. doi: 10.1161/JAHA.114.001075
92. Stegbauer J, Coffman TM. New insights into angiotensin receptor actions: from blood pressure to aging. *Curr Opin Nephrol Hypertens.* (2011) 20:84–8. doi: 10.1097/MNH.0b013e3283414d40
93. Kawase H, Bando YK, Nishimura K, Aoyama M, Monji A, Murohara T. A dipeptidyl peptidase-4 inhibitor ameliorates hypertensive cardiac remodeling via angiotensin-II/sodium-proton pump exchanger-1 axis. *J Mol Cell Cardiol.* (2016) 98:37–47. doi: 10.1016/j.yjmcc.2016.06.066
94. Zhang LH, Pang XF, Bai F, Wang NP, Shah AI, McKallip RJ, et al. Preservation of glucagon-like peptide-1 level attenuates angiotensin II-induced tissue fibrosis by altering AT1/AT 2 receptor expression and angiotensin-converting enzyme 2 activity in rat heart. *Cardiovasc Drugs Ther.* (2015) 29:243–55. doi: 10.1007/s10557-015-6592-7
95. Reid AC, Mackins CJ, Seyedi N, Levi R, Silver RB. Coupling of angiotensin II AT1 receptors to neuronal NHE activity and carrier-mediated norepinephrine release in myocardial ischemia. *Am J Physiol Heart Circ Physiol.* (2004) 286:H1448–54. doi: 10.1152/ajpheart.01062.2003
96. Costa-Pessoa JM, Figueiredo CF, Thieme K, Oliveira-Souza M. The regulation of NHE(1) and NHE(3) activity by angiotensin II is mediated by the activation of the angiotensin II type I receptor/phospholipase C/calcium/calmodulin pathway in distal nephron cells. *Eur J Pharmacol.* (2013) 721:322–31. doi: 10.1016/j.ejphar.2013.08.043
97. von Websky K, Reichetzeder C, Hocher B. Physiology and pathophysiology of incretins in the kidney. *Curr Opin Nephrol Hypertens.* (2014) 23:54–60. doi: 10.1097/01.mnh.0000437542.77175.a0
98. Moroi M, Kubota T. Diuretic and natriuretic effects of dipeptidyl peptidase-4 inhibitor teneligliptin: the contribution of glucagon-like peptide-1. *J Cardiovasc Pharmacol.* (2015) 66:159–64. doi: 10.1097/FJC.0000000000000258
99. Girardi AC, Fukuda LE, Rossoni LV, Malnic G, Reboucas NA. Dipeptidyl peptidase IV inhibition downregulates Na+ - H+ exchanger NHE3 in rat renal proximal tubule. *Am J Physiol Renal Physiol.* (2008) 294:F414–22. doi: 10.1152/ajprenal.00174.2007
100. Rieg T, Gerasimova M, Murray F, Masuda T, Tang T, Rose M, et al. Natriuretic effect by exendin-4, but not the DPP-4 inhibitor alogliptin, is mediated via the GLP-1 receptor and preserved in obese type 2 diabetic mice. *Am J Physiol Renal Physiol.* (2012) 303:F963–71. doi: 10.1152/ajprenal.00259.2012
101. Crajoinas RO, Oricchio FT, Pessoa TD, Pacheco BP, Lessa LM, Malnic G, et al. Mechanisms mediating the diuretic and natriuretic actions of the incretin hormone glucagon-like peptide-1. *Am J Physiol Renal Physiol.* (2011) 301:F355–63. doi: 10.1152/ajprenal.00729.2010
102. Schlatter P, Beglinger C, Drewe J, Gutmann H. Glucagon-like peptide 1 receptor expression in primary porcine proximal tubular cells. *Regul Pept.* (2007) 141:120–8. doi: 10.1016/j.regpep.2006.12.016
103. Girardi AC, Knauf F, Demuth HU, Aronson PS. Role of dipeptidyl peptidase IV in regulating activity of Na+/H+ exchanger isoform NHE3 in proximal tubule cells. *Am J Physiol Cell Physiol.* (2004) 287:C1238–45. doi: 10.1152/ajpcell.00186.2004
104. Ronn J, Jensen EP, Wewer Albrechtsen NJ, Holst JJ, Sorensen CM. Glucagon-like peptide-1 acutely affects renal blood flow and urinary flow rate in spontaneously hypertensive rats despite significantly reduced renal expression of GLP-1 receptors. *Physiol Rep.* (2017) 5:e13503. doi: 10.14814/phy2.13503
105. Rubattu S, Sciarretta S, Valenti V, Stanzione R, Volpe M. Natriuretic peptides: an update on bioactivity, potential therapeutic use, and implication in cardiovascular diseases. *Am J Hypertens.* (2008) 21:733–41. doi: 10.1038/ajh.2008.174
106. Brandt I, Lambeir AM, Ketelslegers JM, Vanderheyden M, Scharpe S, De Meester I. Dipeptidyl-peptidase IV converts intact B-type natriuretic peptide into its des-SerPro form. *Clin Chem.* (2006) 52:82–7. doi: 10.1373/clinchem.2005.057638
107. Boerrigter G, Costello-Boerrigter LC, Harty GJ, Lapp H, Burnett JC, Jr. Des-serine-proline brain natriuretic peptide 3-32 in cardiorenal regulation. *Am J Physiol Regul Integr Comp Physiol.* (2007) 292:R897–901. doi: 10.1152/ajpregu.00569.2006
108. Kim M, Platt MJ, Shibasaki T, Quaggin SE, Backx PH, Seino S, et al. GLP-1 receptor activation and Epac2 link atrial natriuretic peptide secretion to control of blood pressure. *Nat Med.* (2013) 19:567–75. doi: 10.1038/nm.3128
109. Wang G. Raison d'etre of insulin resistance: the adjustable threshold hypothesis. *J R Soc Interface.* (2014) 11:20140892. doi: 10.1098/rsif.2014.0892
110. de Almeida AR, Monte-Alegre S, Zanini MB, Souza AL, Etchebehere M, Gontijo JA. Association between prehypertension, metabolic and inflammatory markers, decreased adiponectin and enhanced insulinemia in obese subjects. *Nutr Metab.* (2014) 11:25. doi: 10.1186/1743-7075-11-25
111. Zeng G, Quon MJ. Insulin-stimulated production of nitric oxide is inhibited by wortmannin. Direct measurement in vascular endothelial cells. *J Clin Invest.* (1996) 98:894–8. doi: 10.1172/JCI118871
112. Johansson GS, Arnqvist HJ. Insulin and IGF-I action on insulin receptors, IGF-I receptors, and hybrid insulin/IGF-I receptors in vascular smooth muscle cells. *Am J Physiol Endocrinol Metab.* (2006) 291:E1124–30. doi: 10.1152/ajpendo.00565.2005
113. Westerbacka J, Bergholm R, Tiikkainen M, Yki-Jarvinen H. Glargine and regular human insulin similarly acutely enhance endothelium-dependent vasodilatation in normal subjects. *Arterioscler Thromb Vasc Biol.* (2004) 24:320–4. doi: 10.1161/01.ATV.0000110444.59568.56
114. Ogihara T, Rakugi H, Ikegami H, Mikami H, Masuo K. Enhancement of insulin sensitivity by troglitazone lowers blood pressure in diabetic hypertensives. *Am J Hypertens.* (1995) 8:316–20. doi: 10.1016/0895-7061(95)96214-5
115. Baumeier C, Schluter L, Saussenthaler S, Laeger T, Rodiger M, Alaze SA, et al. Elevated hepatic DPP4 activity promotes insulin resistance and non-alcoholic fatty liver disease. *Mol Metab.* (2017) 6:1254–63. doi: 10.1016/j.molmet.2017.07.016
116. Horton ES, Silberman C, Davis KL, Berria R. Weight loss, glycemic control, and changes in cardiovascular biomarkers in patients with type 2 diabetes receiving incretin therapies or insulin in a large cohort database. *Diabetes Care.* (2010) 33:1759–65. doi: 10.2337/dc09-2062
117. Steinberg HO, Brechtel G, Johnson A, Fineberg N, Baron AD. Insulin-mediated skeletal muscle vasodilation is nitric oxide dependent. a novel

action of insulin to increase nitric oxide release. *J Clin Invest.* (1994) 94:1172–9. doi: 10.1172/JCI117433

118. Fehmann HC, Hering BJ, Wolf MJ, Brandhorst H, Brandhorst D, Bretzel RG, et al. The effects of glucagon-like peptide-I (GLP-I) on hormone secretion from isolated human pancreatic islets. *Pancreas.* (1995) 11:196–200. doi: 10.1097/00006676-199508000-00014
119. Kern M, Kloting N, Niessen HG, Thomas L, Stiller D, Mark M, et al. Linagliptin improves insulin sensitivity and hepatic steatosis in diet-induced obesity. *PLoS ONE.* (2012) 7:e38744. doi: 10.1371/journal.pone.0038744
120. Kim MK, Chae YN, Ahn GJ, Shin CY, Choi SH, Yang EK, et al. Prevention and treatment effect of evogliptin on hepatic steatosis in high-fat-fed animal models. *Arch Pharm Res.* (2017) 40:268–81. doi: 10.1007/s12272-016-0864-z
121. Smits MM, Tonneijck L, Muskiet MH, Hoekstra T, Kramer MH, Diamant M, et al. The effects of GLP-1 based therapies on postprandial haemodynamics: two randomised, placebo-controlled trials in overweight type 2 diabetes patients. *Diabetes Res Clin Pract.* (2017) 124:1–10. doi: 10.1016/j.diabres.2016.12.011
122. Rohrborn D, Bruckner J, Sell H, Eckel J. Reduced DPP4 activity improves insulin signaling in primary human adipocytes. *Biochem Biophys Res Commun.* (2016) 471:348–54. doi: 10.1016/j.bbrc.2016.02.019
123. Ayada C, Turgut G, Turgut S, Guclu Z. The effect of chronic peripheral nesfatin-1 application on blood pressure in normal and chronic restraint stressed rats: related with circulating level of blood pressure regulators. *Gen Physiol Biophys.* (2015) 34:81–8. doi: 10.4149/gpb2014032
124. Fujimoto M, Shimizu N, Kunii K, Martyn JA, Ueki K, Kaneki M. A role for iNOS in fasting hyperglycemia and impaired insulin signaling in the liver of obese diabetic mice. *Diabetes.* (2005) 54:1340–8. doi: 10.2337/diabetes.54.5.1340
125. Sydow K, Mondon CE, Schrader J, Konishi H, Cooke JP. Dimethylarginine dimethylaminohydrolase overexpression enhances insulin sensitivity. *Arterioscler Thromb Vasc Biol.* (2008) 28:692–7. doi: 10.1161/ATVBAHA.108.162073

9

Increased Expression of miR-146a in Valvular Tissue from Patients with Aortic Valve Stenosis

Jana Petrkova [1,2], Jana Borucka [1,3], Martin Kalab [4], Petra Klevcova [1], Jaroslav Michalek [5], Milos Taborsky [2] and Martin Petrek [1,3,6*]*

[1] Department of Pathological Physiology, Faculty of Medicine Dentistry, Palacky University, Olomouc, Czechia, [2] Internal Medicine I - Cardiology, Palacky University and University Hospital, Olomouc, Czechia, [3] Faculty of Medicine and Dentistry, Institute of Molecular and Translational Medicine, Palacky University, Olomouc, Czechia, [4] Department of Cardiac Surgery, Palacky University and University Hospital, Olomouc, Czechia, [5] Department of Clinical and Molecular Pathology, Faculty of Medicine and Dentistry, Palacky University, Olomouc, Czechia, [6] Laboratory of Cardiogenomics, University Hospital Olomouc, Olomouc, Czechia

***Correspondence:**
Jana Petrkova
jana.petrkova@fnol.cz
Martin Petrek
martin.petrek@fnol.cz

miR-146a has been implicated in the regulation of the immune response as well as in inflammatory process of atherosclerosis. In the present study, we have investigated the expression of miR-146a and its targets, TLR4 a IRAK1, in aortic valve stenosis. A total of 58 patients with aortic stenosis (non- and atherosclerotic; tissue obtained during standard aortic valve replacement) were enrolled. The relative expression of mir-146a was higher in valvular tissue from patients with atherosclerosis compared to those without atherosclerosis ($p = 0.01$). Number of the IRAK1 and TLR4 transcripts did not differ between the investigated groups. There was a trend toward elevation of miR-146a expression in context of inflammatory infiltrate observed in the valvular tissue from patients with atherosclerosis ($p = 0.06$). In conclusion, in line with the acknowledged role of miR-146a in atherosclerotic inflammation, our data suggest it may be extended to the specific location of aortic valves in aortic stenosis.

Keywords: aortic stenosis, microRNA, IRAK1, TLR4, epigenetics

INTRODUCTION

Aortic valve stenosis represents the major cardiac valve disease which is characterized by inflammation, atherosclerosis, and calcification (1, 2). In addition to proatherogenic risk factors, mechanical forces, metabolic alteration, and environmental effects [rev. e.g., by Pasipoularides (3) and Cho et al. (4)], genetic and namely epigenetic mechanism have been recently nominated to play a role in aortic stenosis pathogenesis (5). In general, as reviewed by Menon and Lincoln (6) or Kishore and Petrek (7), epigenetic mechanisms exert their regulatory effects via processes of methylation, histone modification, and also activities of small non-coding RNAs—miRNAs.

Reflecting miRNAs effects as master regulators of gene expression in physiological and pathophysiological processes encompassing also cardiovascular system [reviewed e.g., by Kishore et al. (8)], it is relevant to address possible involvement of miRNAs as epigenetic factors involved in pathogenesis of aortic stenosis, including its atherosclerotic component. In this context, miR-146a could be a plausible candidate: apart from its proinflammatory/atherogenic properties (9, 10), miR-146a has been shown to be an important element in controlling signaling pathways including NF-kB, TRAF6, and IRAK1 (11, 12). These genes encode two key adapter molecules downstream of cytokine and Toll-like receptors (TLR) that have been involved in development of atherosclerosis (13), and recently also implicated in pathogenesis of aortic valve disease (14).

To investigate a plausible role of this candidate miRNA in aortic valve stenosis, we, therefore, investigated the expression of miR-146a in valvular tissues obtained from patients undergoing standard aortic valve replacement. We also determined the expression of Toll-like receptor (TLR)-4 and the interleukin-1 receptor associated kinase 1 (IRAK1) mRNA as plausible targets of miR-146a. Analyzing the obtained data, we wished to reveal if there was any relationship between miR-146a, their targets and pathological processes in valvular tissues.

MATERIALS AND METHODS

Patients

Fifty-eight patients (for their characteristics see **Table 1**) with aortic valve stenosis have been enrolled, valvular tissue was obtained during standard aortic valve replacement (AVR); patients were enrolled on a consecutive basis, in time order of their AVR procedure. Presence of atherosclerosis was detected by angiography of coronary arteries prior the surgery; atherosclerosis was defined as more than 30% limitation of perfusion; 26 patients belonged to this category and 32 patients had non-altered perfusion. The patients who showed presence of inflammation, patients with systemic diseases and/or malignancies were excluded from the study. All patients have consented in writing to the participation in this study according to the Declaration of Helsinki and the Ethics committee of University Hospital and Faculty of Medicine, Palacky University Olomouc approved the study protocol.

TABLE 1 | Characteristics of study groups.

Parameter	Non-atherosclerotic	Atherosclerotic
Number (no.) of patients	32	26
Age (years)	68.6 (7.6)	71.0 (8.1)
Sex (Males/Females)	18/14	20/6
Cholesterol (mmol/L)	4.78 (1.20)	4.51 (1.03)
Triglycerides (mmol/L)	1.56 (1.15)	1.46 (0.71)
HDL (mmol/L)	1.33 (0.42)	1.33 (0.29)
LDL (mmol/L)	2.74 (1.15)	2.53 (0.88)
Height (cm)	168 (9.5)	166.7 (10.4)
Weight (kg)	83.1 (12.8)	84.7 (15.6)
BMI	29.4 (5.0)	30.5 (5.8)
Smoking (absolute no./from all patients) (%)	5/32 (15.6)	5/26 (19.2)
Inflammation, absolute no./from all assessed specimen (%)	19/29 (65.5)	13/23 (56.5)
Fibrosis, absolute no./from all assessed specimen (%)	16/31 (51.6)	11/26 (42.3)

Patients with aortic stenosis were divided based on assessment of coronary perfusion into two groups: those with non-altered perfusion (non-atherosclerotic) and with decreased perfusion (atherosclerotic), for details see section materials and methods.
If not specified otherwise, the values represent the mean and standard deviation (in brackets).
Terms "Inflammation" and "Fibrosis" refers to valvular tissue.

miRNA/mRNA Determination

The valvular tissue obtained during surgery was placed into RNA later solution to prevent RNA degradation. Subsequently, total RNA was extracted from aortic valvular tissues by *mir*Vana™ miRNA Isolation Kit; whole (complete, homogenized) tissue specimen were used for the extraction procedure For the miRNA detection, RNA was reverse transcribed using TaqMan MicroRNA Reverse Transcription kit and TaqMan MicroRNA Assays using a specific reverse primer and real time PCR was performed with primer-probe with specific primers for miR-146a (all so far mentioned reagents/kits/primers were from Life Technologies, Thermo Fisher Scientific, Waltham, MA, USA) and LightCycler 480 Probes Master (Roche Life Sciences, Indianapolis, IN, USA). Expression levels of miR-146a were normalized to RNU6B (Life Technologies, as above). Real time PCR was performed in Rotor Gene detection system (Corbett Research, Mortlake, NSW, Australia). Program was set up for holding at for 10 min, followed by 40 cycles consisting of for 15 s and for 60 s. TLR-4 and IRAK1 mRNA expression was determined by the same methodology, the probes used for the assessment of this gene were (TLR4 left primer: CTCTCCTGCGTGAGACCAG, TLR4 right primer: CAGCTCCATGCATTGATAAGTAA; IRAK1 left primer: tgcctggtgtacggcttc, IRAK1 right primer: ctgaggccaggagagaggt) obtained from Roche Applied Science (Penzberg, Germany). Expression levels of TLR4 and IRAK1 were normalized to GAPDH (left primer: agccacatcgctcagacac, right primer: gcccaatacgaccaaatcc).

Histopathological Examination

Tissue sections were evaluated by a histopathologist to assess presence of inflammatory infiltrate and fibrosis (absolute and relative values are shown in **Table 1**, bottom lines); the extent of infiltrate, if present, was semi-quantitated (grading + to + + ++). Standard procedure utilizing hematoxylin-eosin staining in formalin-fixed paraffin-embedded (FFPE) samples was utilized.

Statistical Analysis

The non-parametric Mann–Whitney *U*-test was performed to assess the relative expression of miR-146a, TLR4, and IRAK-1 transcripts and to test for differences between patient subgroups. Pearson's correlation coefficient was used to examine the relationship between miR-146a and TLR4 and miR-146a and IRAK1 expressions. $P < 0.05$ was considered statistically significant.

RESULTS

miR-146a was detected in 58 of 58 samples (100%). When the study subjects were separated based on angiography perfusion data into two subgroups, miR-146a was elevated in the aortic valve tissues from 26 patients with decreased coronary perfusion as a marker of atherosclerosis compared to 32 patients with non-altered perfusion, $p = 0.01$ (**Figure 1A**).

TLR-4 transcripts were detected in 47 of 58 samples (81%). TLR-4 mRNA expression did not differ between the atherosclerotic and non-atherosclerotic subjects ($p > 0.05$),

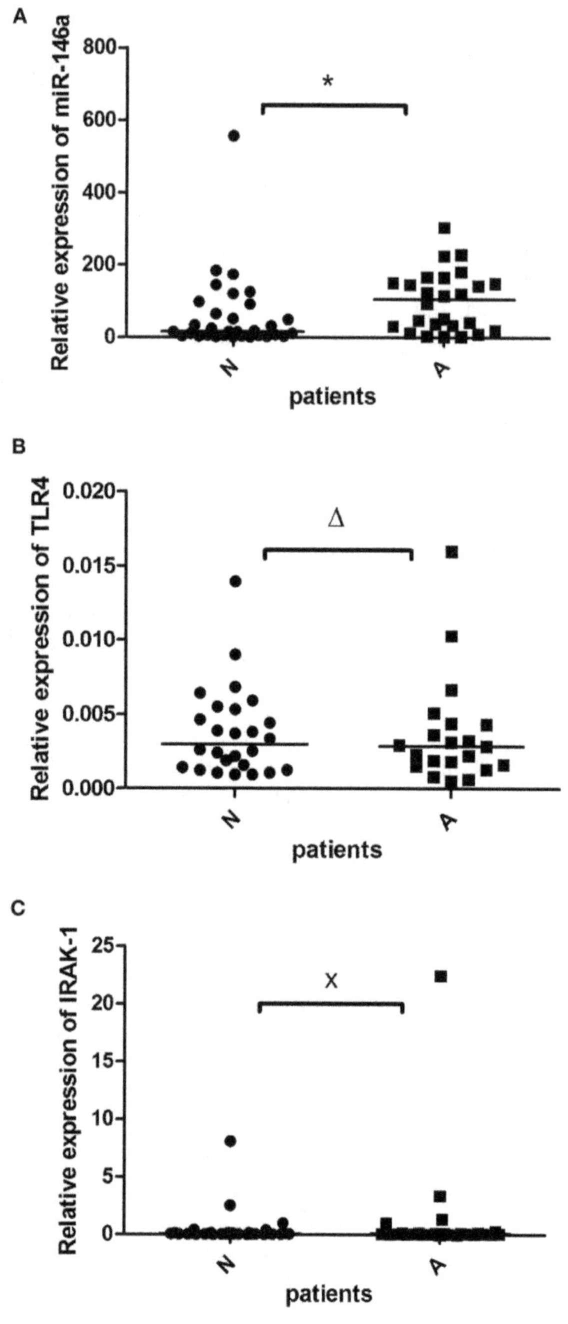

FIGURE 1 | The relative expression of miR-146a **(A)**, TLR4 m-RNA **(B)**, and IRAK1 m-RNA **(C)** in the valvular tissue obtained from patients with aortic stenosis with signs of atherosclerosis (A; $n = 26^{\neq}$) and without atherosclerosis (N; $n = 32^{\neq}$). The miR-146a expression was normalized to the RNU6B expression, expression of TLR-4 and IRAK1 was normalized to GADPH. The lines represent median values and the following symbols denote *P*-values: * = 0.01; Δ = 0.64; x = 0.57. ≠Note: for TLR4 **(B)** $N = 26$ and $A = 21$ patients.

Figure 1B. There was a trend to negative correlation ($r = -0.2$) between the miR-146a and TLR-4 mRNA expression ($p = 0.1$).

IRAK1 mRNA was detected in all 58 investigated samples (100%). There was no difference between IRAK1 mRNA relative

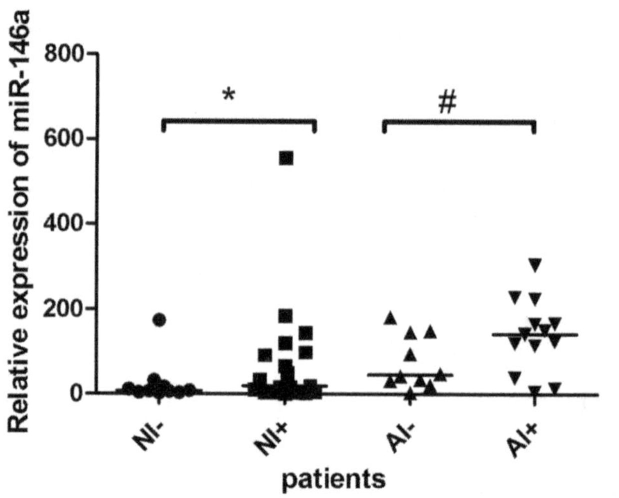

FIGURE 2 | The relative expression of miR-146a in the valvular tissue obtained from patients with aortic stenosis. Description of abbreviations designating patient subgroups: non-atherosclerotic patients with (NI+, $n = 19$) or without inflammatory cell infiltrate (NI-, $n = 10$); atherosclerotic patients with (AI+, $n = 13$) or without inflammatory cell infiltrate (AI-, $n = 10$). The lines represent median values and the symbols denote *P*-values: * = 0.10, # = 0.06.

expression in atherosclerotic and non-atherosclerotic subjects ($p > 0.05$), **Figure 1C**. There was no relationship between the miR-146a and IRAK1 mRNA expressions.

When study subjects were further sub-grouped according to absence/presence of inflammatory cellular infiltrate, a trend toward miR-146a elevation was observed in patients with infiltrated valvular tissue (**Figure 2**), this observation was more pronounced in atherosclerotic patients ($p = 0.06$) than in patients without atherosclerosis ($p = 0.1$). **Figure 3** shows representative examples of valvular histopathology.

DISCUSSION

This study investigated the expression of miR-146a and of its targets, TLR4 and IRAK1, in valvular tissue obtained from the patients with aortic valve stenosis. Upregulation of miR-146a expression in valvular tissue was observed in the subgroup of patients with decreased coronary perfusion as a marker of atherosclerosis. miR-146a expression tended to be elevated in those atherosclerotic patients whose valvular tissue contained inflammatory cell infiltrate. These findings extend the previous and recent reports (9, 10, 15, 16) about the role of miR-146a in atherosclerosis in general to the specific location in aortic valve stenosis. Overall, though obtained in a smaller scale study limited to patients, our data may implicate this non-coding miRNA, and in wider sense epigenetic factors, as eligible research targets in further investigations of pathogenesis of aortic valve disease.

miR-146a has been implicated in several key physiological processes including innate immune and inflammatory responses. It has been previously shown that upregulation of miR-146 family (miR-146a/b) regulated downstream toll-like receptor 4 (TLR4) signaling, IL-1 receptor associated kinase 1 (IRAK1), and

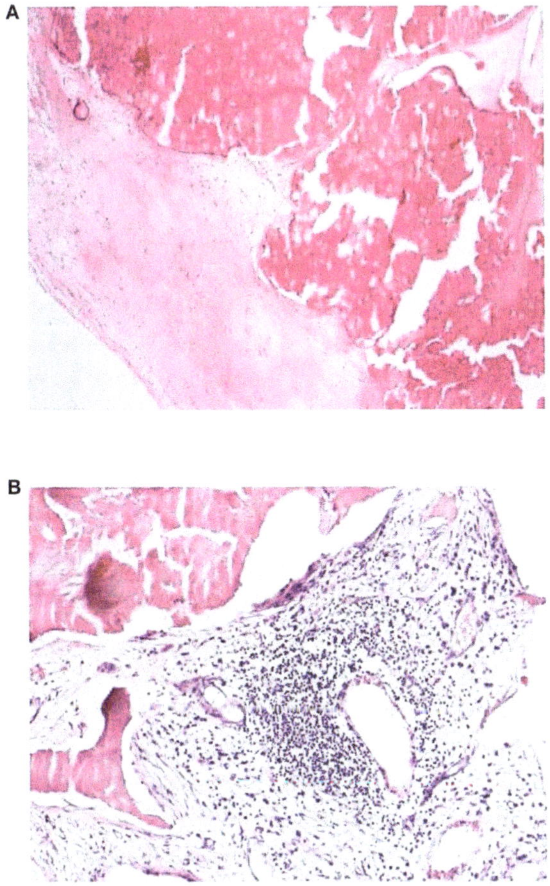

FIGURE 3 | (A, B) Aortic valve tissue histopathology HE, 40x **(A)**, 100x **(B)**; **A**: dystrophic calcification of valve, absence of inflammatory infiltration, **B**: presence of mononuclear (lymphoplasmacytic) inflammatory infiltration in connective tissue of aortic valve.

TNF-receptor associated factor-6 (TRAF6) through a negative-feedback regulation loop (11, 17). In this context, we analyzed expression of target genes miR-146a, specifically of the *TLR4* and *IRAK1* genes. There was, however, no difference between expression of the TLR4 and also of the IRAK transcripts between the groups of atherosclerotic and non atherosclerotic patients, only an insignificant inverse relationship between miR-146a and TLR4 mRNA expression could be described. While this observation is in contrast with some reports, e.g., of a correlation between miR-146a and TLR4, IRAK1 in patients with coronary artery disease (18), others have observed reduced expression of IRAK1 by upregulation of miR-146a, e.g., in psoriasis (19) and in senescent cells (20). It is, therefore, conceivable that expression and mutual relationship of miR-146a and its targets may reflect a specific localization of inflammatory processes. This suggestion implied from our primary analyses of miR-146a expression and TLR4 and IRAK transcripts should be, therefore, verified by further experiments, preferably with expanded collection of aortic valve samples, eventually of different stages, and also on protein level.

It should be also mentioned that the expression of both miR-146a and its targets is, on an individual basis, affected by variations in their gene sequences. Functional single nucleotide polymorphisms (SNPs) have been reported in *TLR4, IRAK1* genes (21, 22) and importantly they are also located in pre-miR146a—those were responsible not only for the establishment of diversity among individuals but also for changes in their expression and/or development of different disease phenotypes, including coronary heart disease (23–25).

Despite limitations of the present study (analysis of a single miRNA in a cohort comprising only patients with aortic valve stenosis, not subjects without this pathology), to our knowledge we present the first report plausibly implicating miR-146a in aortic valve stenosis. A spectrum of miRNAs, but not including miR-146a, has been recently found to be deregulated in patients with aortic stenosis [reviewed by Menon and Lincoln (6)]; miR-146a has also not been noted in microarray expression study combined with bioinformatics analyses (26), nor in a recent report by Duan et al. (27). In this context, it is desirable to conduct studies of miRNA-146a expression in extended cohorts including specimen from patients without valvular disease. These studies should address in greater detail presence and plausible role of miRNA-146a targets, preferably including *in situ* hybridization and/or immunohistochemistry experiments, also for characterizing the cellular infiltrate. If our data are validated and extended, there may be yet another plausible candidate for further studies of miRNAs involvement in aortal valve stenosis, which could also be explored on the level of exosomes and extracellular vesicles as recently proposed by Blaser and Aikawa (28).

ETHICS STATEMENT

All patients have consented in writing to the participation in this study in accordance with the Declaration of Helsinki and the Ethics committee of University Hospital and Faculty of Medicine, Palacky University Olomouc approved the study protocol.

AUTHOR CONTRIBUTIONS

The idea to investigate miRNA expression in aortic valves was initiated by JP, who set up the clinical design and also provided the patients with the help of MK and MT. JP also realized the logistics within the laboratory and pathology department. JB performed the RT-PCR expression analyses and, together with JP and MP, drafted the manuscript. PK determined TLR4. JM performed histopathological examination. The final version of the paper was prepared by JP and MP. MP is the author responsible for the integrity of the data. All authors approved the final version of the manuscript.

FUNDING

This work was supported in parts from projects IGA UP: LF_2018_015, LO1304 and RVO: 00098892.

REFERENCES

1. Mohler ER. Are atherosclerotic processes involved in aortic-valve calcification? *Lancet.* (2000) 356:524–5. doi: 10.1016/S0140-6736(00)02572-1
2. Thaden JJ, Nkomo VT, Enriquez-Sarano M. The global burden of aortic stenosis. *Prog Cardiovasc Dis.* (2014) 56:565–71. doi: 10.1016/j.pcad.2014.02.006
3. Pasipoularides A. Calcific aortic valve disease: part 1—molecular pathogenetic aspects, hemodynamics, and adaptive feedbacks. *J Cardiovasc Transl Res.* (2016) 9:102–18. doi: 10.1007/s12265-016-9679-z
4. Cho KI, Sakuma I, Sohn IS, Jo S-H, Koh KK. Inflammatory and metabolic mechanisms underlying the calcific aortic valve disease. *Atherosclerosis.* (2018) 277:60–5. doi: 10.1016/j.atherosclerosis.2018.08.029
5. Gošev I, Zeljko M, Durić Ž, Nikolić I, Gošev M, Ivčević S, et al. Epigenome alterations in aortic valve stenosis and its related left ventricular hypertrophy. *Clin Epigenet.* (2017) 9:106. doi: 10.1186/s13148-017-0406-7
6. Menon V, Lincoln J. The genetic regulation of aortic valve development and calcific disease. *Front Cardiovasc Med.* (2018) 5:162. doi: 10.3389/fcvm.2018.00162
7. Kishore A, Petrek M. Next-generation sequencing based HLA typing: deciphering immunogenetic aspects of sarcoidosis. *Front Genet.* (2018) 9:503. doi: 10.3389/fgene.2018.00503
8. Kishore A, Borucka J, Petrkova J, Petrek M. Novel insights into miRNA in lung and heart inflammatory diseases. *Mediators Inflamm.* (2014) 2014:1–27. doi: 10.1155/2014/259131
9. Cheng HS, Besla R, Li A, Chen Z, Shikatani EA, Nazari-Jahantigh M, et al. Paradoxical Suppression of atherosclerosis in the absence of microRNA-146a. *Circ Res.* (2017) 121:354–67. doi: 10.1161/CIRCRESAHA.116.310529
10. Nguyen M-A, Karunakaran D, Geoffrion M, Cheng HS, Tandoc K, Perisic Matic L, et al. Extracellular vesicles secreted by atherogenic macrophages transfer MicroRNA to inhibit cell migration. *Arterioscler Thromb Vasc Biol.* (2018) 38:49–63. doi: 10.1161/ATVBAHA.117.309795
11. Taganov KD, Boldin MP, Chang K-J, Baltimore D. NF-kappaB-dependent induction of microRNA miR-146, an inhibitor targeted to signaling proteins of innate immune responses. *Proc Natl Acad Sci USA.* (2006) 103:12481–6. doi: 10.1073/pnas.0605298103
12. Li S, Yue Y, Xu W, Xiong S. MicroRNA-146a represses Mycobacteria-induced inflammatory response and facilitates bacterial replication via targeting IRAK-1 and TRAF-6. *PLoS ONE.* (2013) 8:e81438. doi: 10.1371/journal.pone.0081438
13. Edfeldt K, Swedenborg J, Hansson GK, Yan ZQ. Expression of toll-like receptors in human atherosclerotic lesions: a possible pathway for plaque activation. *Circulation.* (2002) 105:1158–61. doi: 10.1161/circ.105.10.1158
14. García-Rodríquez C, Parra-Izquierdo I, Castaños-Mollor I, López J, San Román JA, Sánchez Crespo M. Toll-like receptors, inflammation, and calcific aortic valve disease. *Front Physiol.* (2018) 9:201. doi: 10.3389/fphys.2018.00201
15. Li J, Wan Y, Guo Q, Zou L, Zhang J, Fang Y, et al. Altered microRNA expression profile with miR-146a upregulation in CD4+ T cells from patients with rheumatoid arthritis. *Arthritis Res Ther.* (2010) 12:R81. doi: 10.1186/ar3006
16. Raitoharju E, Lyytikäinen L-P, Levula M, Oksala N, Mennander A, Tarkka M, et al. MiR-21, miR-210, miR-34a, and miR-146a/b are up-regulated in human atherosclerotic plaques in the tampere vascular study. *Atherosclerosis.* (2011) 219:211–7. doi: 10.1016/j.atherosclerosis.2011.07.020
17. Nazari-Jahantigh M, Wei Y, Schober A. The role of microRNAs in arterial remodelling. *Thromb Haemost.* (2012) 107:611–8. doi: 10.1160/TH11-12-0826
18. Takahashi Y, Satoh M, Minami Y, Tabuchi T, Itoh T, Nakamura M. Expression of miR-146a/b is associated with the Toll-like receptor 4 signal in coronary artery disease: effect of renin–angiotensin system blockade and statins on miRNA-146a/b and Toll-like receptor 4 levels. *Clin Sci.* (2010) 119:395–405. doi: 10.1042/CS20100003
19. Xia P, Fang X, Zhang Z-H, Huang Q, Yan K-X, Kang K-F, et al. Dysregulation of miRNA146a versus IRAK1 induces IL-17 persistence in the psoriatic skin lesions. *Immunol. Lett.* (2012) 148:151–62. doi: 10.1016/j.imlet.2012.09.004
20. Bhaumik D, Scott GK, Schokrpur S, Patil CK, Orjalo AV, Rodier F, et al. MicroRNAs miR-146a/b negatively modulate the senescence-associated inflammatory mediators IL-6 and IL-8. *Aging.* (2009) 1:402–11. doi: 10.18632/aging.100042
21. Noreen M, Shah MAA, Mall SM, Choudhary S, Hussain T, Ahmed I, et al. TLR4 polymorphisms and disease susceptibility. *Inflamm Res.* (2012) 61:177–88. doi: 10.1007/s00011-011-0427-1
22. Zhu J, Mohan C. Toll-like receptor signaling pathways—therapeutic opportunities. *Mediators Inflamm.* (2010) 2010:781235. doi: 10.1155/2010/781235
23. Gong J, Tong Y, Zhang H-M, Wang K, Hu T, Shan G, et al. Genome-wide identification of SNPs in microRNA genes and the SNP effects on microRNA target binding and biogenesis. *Hum Mutat.* (2012) 33:254–63. doi: 10.1002/humu.21641
24. Xiong X-D, Cho M, Cai X-P, Cheng J, Jing X, Cen J-M, et al. A common variant in pre-miR-146 is associated with coronary artery disease risk and its mature miRNA expression. *Mutat Res.* (2014) 761:15–20. doi: 10.1016/j.mrfmmm.2014.01.001
25. He Y, Yang J, Kong D, Lin J, Xu C, Ren H, et al. Association of miR-146a rs2910164 polymorphism with cardio-cerebrovascular diseases: a systematic review and meta-analysis. *Gene.* (2015) 565:171–9. doi: 10.1016/j.gene.2015.04.020
26. Wang H, Shi J, Li B, Zhou Q, Kong X, Bei Y. MicroRNA expression signature in human calcific aortic valve disease. *Biomed Res Int.* (2017) 2017:4820275. doi: 10.1155/2017/4820275
27. Duan C, Cao Z, Tang F, Jian Z, Liang C, Liu H, et al. miRNA-mRNA crosstalk in myocardial ischemia induced by calcified aortic valve stenosis. *Aging.* (2019) 11:448–66. doi: 10.18632/aging.101751
28. Blaser MC, Aikawa E. Roles and regulation of extracellular vesicles in cardiovascular ineral metabolism. *Front Cardiovasc Med.* (2018) 5:187. doi: 10.3389/fcvm.2018.00187

10

Connexin 43 Hemichannel Activity Promoted by Pro-Inflammatory Cytokines and High Glucose Alters Endothelial Cell Function

*Juan C. Sáez[1,2], Susana Contreras-Duarte[1,3], Gonzalo I. Gómez[4], Valeria C. Labra[4], Cristian A. Santibañez[4], Rosario Gajardo-Gómez[4], Beatriz C. Avendaño[4], Esteban F. Díaz[4], Trinidad D. Montero[4], Victoria Velarde[1] and Juan A. Orellana[4]**

[1] Departamento de Fisiología, Pontificia Universidad Católica de Chile, Santiago de Chile, Chile, [2] Instituto de Neurociencias, Centro Interdisciplinario de Neurociencias de Valparaíso, Universidad de Valparaíso, Valparaíso, Chile, [3] Departamento de Ginecología y Obstetricia, Escuela de Medicina, Facultad de Medicina, Pontificia Universidad Católica de Chile, Santiago, Chile, [4] Departamento de Neurología, Escuela de Medicina and Centro Interdisciplinario de Neurociencias, Facultad de Medicina, Pontificia Universidad Católica de Chile, Santiago, Chile

***Correspondence:**
Juan A. Orellana
jaorella@uc.cl

The present work was done to elucidate whether hemichannels of a cell line derived from endothelial cells are affected by pro-inflammatory conditions (high glucose and IL-1β/TNF-α) known to lead to vascular dysfunction. We used EAhy 926 cells treated with high glucose and IL-1β/TNF-α. The hemichannel activity was evaluated with the dye uptake method and was abrogated with selective inhibitors or knocking down of hemichannel protein subunits with siRNA. Western blot analysis, cell surface biotinylation, and confocal microscopy were used to evaluate total and plasma membrane amounts of specific proteins and their cellular distribution, respectively. Changes in intracellular Ca^{2+} and nitric oxide (NO) signals were estimated by measuring FURA-2 and DAF-FM probes, respectively. High glucose concentration was found to elevate dye uptake, a response that was enhanced by IL-1β/TNF-α. High glucose plus IL-1β/TNF-α-induced dye uptake was abrogated by connexin 43 (Cx43) but not pannexin1 knockdown. Furthermore, Cx43 hemichannel activity was associated with enhanced ATP release and activation of p38 MAPK, inducible NO synthase, COX_2, PGE_2 receptor EP_1, and $P2X_7/P2Y_1$ receptors. Inhibition of the above pathways prevented completely the increase in Cx43 hemichannel activity of cells treated high glucose and IL-1β/TNF-α. Both synthetic and endogenous cannabinoids (CBs) also prevented the increment in Cx43 hemichannel opening, as well as the subsequent generation and release of ATP and NO induced by pro-inflammatory conditions. The counteracting action of CBs also was extended to other endothelial alterations evoked by IL-1β/TNF-α and high glucose, including increased ATP-dependent Ca^{2+} dynamics and insulin-induced NO production. Finally, inhibition of Cx43 hemichannels also prevented the ATP release from endothelial cells treated with IL-1β/TNF-α and high glucose. Therefore, we propose that reduction of hemichannel activity could represent a strategy against the activation of deleterious pathways that lead to endothelial dysfunction and possibly cell damage evoked by high glucose and pro-inflammatory conditions during cardiovascular diseases.

Keywords: connexins, endothelium, inflammation, cytokines, gap junctions

INTRODUCTION

The endothelial cell lining of vessels walls plays central roles in regulating vascular homeostasis, such as the maintenance of vessel integrity, supply of oxygen and nutrients to underlying tissues and promotion of a well-balanced redox and immune environment (1). Under physiological conditions, endothelial cells maintain a proper interface barrier between blood and tissue; surveilling and combating possible perturbations of invading pathogens or endogenous threats in response to tissue damage (2). The endothelium rapidly reacts to acute damage by modulating blood flow, permeability, leukocyte infiltration, and tissue edema (2). If the stimulus persists, chronic endothelial activation accompanied of sustained inflammation may lead to vascular dysfunction, precipitating macrophage recruitment, angiogenesis, and subsequent loss of vascular homeostasis (3). Chronic activation and dysfunction of endothelial cells are common features and part of the underlying origin of myocardial infarction, diabetes, stroke, obesity, unstable angina, metabolic syndrome, and sudden cardiac death (4). Although diverse conditions are present during these diseases, including high blood glucose levels, insulin resistance, oxidative stress, and upregulated cytokine production (5), the full underlying mechanisms associated with endothelial activation and dysfunction are not fully understood.

In the last decade, several studies have established that hemichannels mediate the physiological release of different signaling molecules (e.g., ATP, glutamate, NAD^+, and PGE_2) that preserve the progression of multiple biological processes, including long-term synaptic transmission (6), vessel contractility (7), and glucose sensing (8), among others. Hemichannels result from the oligomerization of six connexin monomers around a central pore, which along with forming the building blocks of gap junction channels, also acts as a solitary or non-junctional channels in the plasma membrane (9). Hemichannels are permeable to ions and small molecules; constituting routes of exchange between intracellular and extracellular compartments (10). Under certain pathophysiological scenarios, rather than being beneficial, the prolonged opening of hemichannels contributes to disease progression by different ways, including the enhanced release of paracrine substances (e.g., ATP and glutamate), intracellular Ca^{2+} handling alterations, and ionic and osmotic imbalance (11). A cornerstone underlying this phenomenon rise from the overproduction of inflammatory mediators as result of impaired operation of the innate and adaptive immune system (12).

There are plenty of data pointing out the detrimental effects of inflammation on endothelial function (2) and hyperglycemia is one of the most emblematic pro-inflammatory condition during different cardiovascular diseases (13, 14). Indeed, animal and clinical studies have shown that hyperglycemia causes the systemic production of pro-inflammatory cytokines such as TNFα and IL-1β (15, 16), as well as endothelial dysfunction (5). Among other changes, high glucose concentration in concert with pro-inflammatory cytokines alters numerous intracellular signaling pathways in endothelial cells (17, 18), which consequently lead to reduced endothelial barrier function, compromised vascular tone regulation and insulin resistance (5). Although prior evidence has described that IL-1β/TNF-α or high glucose (25–45 mM) causes a prominent opening of hemichannels in diverse brain cell types (8, 19–23), whether high glucose concentration and/or pro-inflammatory cytokines can modulate hemichannel activity in endothelial cells remain poorly studied.

We hypothesize that high glucose concentration in combination IL-1β/TNF-α increase the hemichannel activity of endothelial cells, resulting in several cell alterations. Here, we show that high glucose concentration and IL-1β/TNF-α and increase the activity of endothelial connexin 43 (Cx43) hemichannels. Inhibition of these channels prevented the alterations of purinergic signaling, $[Ca^{2+}]_i$ signal dynamics, and nitric oxide (NO) production. Moreover, two endogenous cannabinoids (CBs): methanandamide (Meth) or 2-arachidonylglycerol (2-AG), as well as one synthetic CB: WIN 55,212-2 (WIN), prevent these events. In particular, they counteracted the persistent opening of endothelial Cx43 hemichannels mainly due to increase in the amount of Cx43 in the cell surface, which consequently prevented the manifestation of different endothelial alterations.

MATERIALS AND METHODS

Reagents and Antibodies

The mimetic peptides Gap19 (KQIEIKKFK, intracellular loop domain of Cx43), Tat-L2 (YGRKKRRQRRRDGANVDMHLK QIEIKKFKYGIEEHGK, second intracellular loop domain of Cx43), and ^{10}panx1 [WRQAAFVDSY, first extracellular loop domain of pannexin1 (Panx1)] were obtained from Genscript (NJ, USA). HEPES, water (W3500), Dulbecco's Modified Eagle Medium (DMEM), A74003, MRS2179, brilliant blue G (BBG), oxidized ATP (oATP), ns-398, sc-19220, indometacin, L-N6, SB203580, Lucifer yellow (LY), Meth and 2-AG, WIN-55,212-2 (WIN), Cx43 polyclonal antibody, ethidium (Etd) bromide, and probenecid (Prob) were purchased from Sigma-Aldrich (St. Louis, MO, USA). Fetal bovine serum (FBS) was obtained from Hyclone (Logan, UT, USA). Penicillin, streptomycin, FURA-2AM, DAF-FM diacetate, diamidino-2-phenylindole (DAPI), BAPTA-AM, goat anti-mouse Alexa Fluor 488 were obtained from Invitrogen (Carlsbad, CA, USA). The CB1 receptor antagonist (SR1): SR-141716A and the CB2 receptor antagonist (SR2): SR-144528 were kindly provided by Sanofi-Aventis Recherche (Bagneux, France). Normal goat serum (NGS) was purchased from Zymed (San Francisco, CA, USA). Anti-Cx43 monoclonal antibody (610061) was obtained from BD Biosciences (Franklin Lakes, NJ, USA). IL-1β and TNF-α were obtained from Roche Diagnostics (Indianapolis, MI, USA). Horseradish peroxidase (HRP)-conjugated anti-rabbit IgG, Sulfo-NHS-SS-biotin, and NeutrAvidin immobilized on agarose beads were purchased from Pierce (Rockford, IL, USA).

Cell Cultures

The human endothelial cell line EAhy 926 was kindly donated by Cora-Jean S. Edgell, University of North Carolina, Chapel Hill. ECs were seeded onto plastic dishes (Nunclon) or onto glass coverslips (Gassalem, Limeil-Brevannes, France) in DMEM, supplemented with penicillin (5 U/ml), streptomycin (5 μg/mL), and 10% FBS and kept at 37°C in a 5% CO_2/95% air atmosphere at nearly 100% relative humidity. Passaging was performed at ~90% confluence and cells were re-seeded at 1 × 10^4 cells/cm^2. Primary endothelial cells were isolated by collagenase (0.25 mg/mL) digestion from umbilical cord veins (HUVEC) from normal pregnancies and cultured (37°C, 5% CO_2) up to passage 2 in medium 199 (M199) containing 10% new born calf serum, 10% fetal calf serum, 3.2 mM L-glutamine, and 100 U/mL penicillin–streptomycin. Passaging was performed at ~90% confluence and cells were re-seeded at 1 × 10^4 cells/cm^2.

Treatments

Cells were treated for 1, 24, 48, or 72 h with a mixture of IL-1β and TNF-α (10 ng/mL of each) plus different concentrations of glucose (5, 25, or 45 mM). Mimetic peptides against Cx43 hemichannels (gap19 and Tat-L2, 100 μM) and Panx1 channels (^{10}panx1, 100 μM), as well as Prob (500 μM), were applied to cell cultures 15 min prior to and co-applied with Etd for time-lapse recordings (see below). CB agonists: WIN, Meth, and 2-AG were applied 1 h prior to and co-applied with the cytokines and glucose treatment. SR1 and SR2 antagonists were co-applied with the CB agonists. Similarly, in another set of experiments, SB203580 (p38 MAP kinase inhibitor), L-N6 [inducible NO synthase (iNOS) inhibitor], indomethacin (COX_1 and COX_2 inhibitor), sc-560 (COX_1 inhibitor), ns-398 (COX_2 inhibitor), sc-19220 (EP_1 receptor antagonist), BAPTA-AM (intracellular Ca^{2+} chelator), BBG (non-competitive $P2X_7$ antagonist), oATP ($P2X_7$ antagonist), MRS2179 ($P2Y_1$ antagonist), or A740003 ($P2X_7$ antagonist) were applied 1 h prior to and co-applied with IL-1β and TNF-α plus 25 mM glucose for 72 h.

siRNA Transfection

siRNA duplexes against mouse Cx43 or Panx1 were predesigned and obtained from Origene (Rockville, MD, USA). siRNA (10 nM) was transfected using Oligofectamine (Invitrogen) according to the Origene application guide for Trilencer-27 siRNA. Sequences for siRNAs against human Cx43 and Panx1 were siRNA-Cx43: rGrCrCrTrTrCrTrTrGrCrTrGrArTrCrCrArGrTrGrGrTrAr-CrATC and siRNA-Panx1: rGrArTrCrTrCrGrArTrTrGrGr-TrArCrArCrArGrArTrArArGrCTG, respectively. Transfection experiment was performed 24 h before treating cells with IL-1β and TNF-α plus 25 mM glucose for 72 h.

Dye Uptake and Time-Lapse Fluorescence Imaging

For time-lapse fluorescence imaging, cells plated on glass coverslips were washed twice in Hank's balanced salt solution. Then, cells were incubated with Locke's solution containing 5 μM Etd and mounted on the stage of an Olympus BX 51W1I upright microscope with a 40× water immersion objective for time-lapse imaging. Images were captured by a Retiga 1300I fast-cooled monochromatic digital camera (12-bit) (Qimaging, Burnaby, BC, Canada) controlled by imaging software Metafluor software (Universal Imaging, Downingtown, PA, USA) every 30 s (exposure time = 0.5 s; excitation and emission wavelengths were 528 and 598 nm, respectively). The fluorescence intensity recorded from 25 regions of interest (representing 25 cells per coverslip) was defined as the subtraction (F-F0) between the fluorescence (F) from respective cell (25 cells per field) and the background fluorescence (F0) measured where no labeled cells were detected. The mean slope of the relationship F-F0 over a given time interval (ΔF/ΔT; F0 remained constant along the recording time) represents the Etd uptake rate. To assess for changes in slope, regression lines were fitted to points before and after the various experimental conditions using Excel software, and mean values of slopes were compared using GraphPad Prism software and expressed as AU/min. At least four replicates (four sister coverslips) were measured in each independent experiment.

Western Blot Analysis

Cells were rinsed twice with PBS (pH 7.4) and harvested by scraping with a rubber policeman in ice-cold PBS containing 5 mM EDTA, Halt (78440), and M-PER protein extraction cocktail (78501) according to the manufacturer instructions (Pierce, Rockford, IL, USA). The cell suspension was sonicated on ice. Proteins were measured using the Bio-Rad Bradford assay. Aliquots of cell lysates (100 μg of protein) were resuspended in Laemmli's sample buffer, separated in an 8% sodium dodecyl sulfate polyacrylamide gel electrophoresis (SDS-PAGE) and electro-transferred to nitrocellulose sheets. Nonspecific protein binding was blocked by incubation of nitrocellulose sheets in PBS-BLOTTO (5% nonfat milk in PBS) for 30 min. Blots were then incubated with primary antibody at 4°C overnight, followed by four 15 min washes with PBS. Then, blots were incubated with HRP-conjugated goat anti-rabbit antibody at room temperature for 1 h and then rinsed four times with PBS for 15 min. Immunoreactivity was detected by enhanced chemiluminescence reaction using the SuperSignal kit (Pierce, Rockford, IL, USA) according to the manufacturer's instructions.

Cell Surface Biotinylation and Quantification

Cells cultured on 100-mm dishes were washed three times with ice-cold Hank's saline solution (pH 8.0), and 3 mL of sulfo-NHS-SS-biotin solution (0.5 mg/mL) was added followed by a 30 min incubation at 4°C. Then, cells were washed three times with ice-cold saline containing 15 mM glycine (pH 8.0) to block unreacted biotin. The cells were harvested and incubated with an excess of immobilized NeutrAvidin (1 mL of NeutrAvidin per 3 mg of biotinylated protein) for 1 h at 4°C after which 1 mL of wash buffer (saline solution, pH 7.2 containing 0.1% SDS and 1% Nonidet P-40) was added. The mixture was centrifuged for 2 min at 600 *g* at 4°C. The supernatant was removed and discarded, and the pellet was resuspended in 40 μL of saline solution, pH 2.8 containing 0.1 M glycine, to release the proteins from the biotin. After the mixture was centrifuged at 600 *g* at 4°C for 2 min, the supernatant was collected, and the pH was adjusted immediately by adding 10 μL of 1 M Tris, pH 7.5. Relative protein amount was measured using Western blot analysis as described above. Resulting immunoblot signals were scanned, and the densitometric analysis was performed with IMAGEJ software.

Dye Coupling

Cells plated on glass coverslips were bathed with recording medium (HCO_3^- free F-12 medium buffered with 10 mM HEPES, pH 7.2) and permeability mediated by gap junctions was tested by evaluating the transfer of LY to neighboring cells. Briefly, single ECs were iontophoretically microinjected with a glass micropipette filled with 75 mM LY (5% w/v in 150 mM LiCl) in recording medium containing 200 μM La^{3+} to avoid cell leakage of the microinjected dye *via* hemichannels, leading to underscore the extent of dye coupling. Fluorescent cells were observed using a Nikon inverted microscope equipped with epifluorescence illumination (Xenon arc lamp) and Nikon B filter to LY (excitation wavelength 450–490 nm; emission wavelength above 520 nm) and XF34 filter to DiI fluorescence (Omega Optical, Inc., Brattleboro, VT, USA). Photomicrographs were obtained using a CCD monochrome camera (CFW-1310M; Scion; Frederick, MD, USA). Three minutes after dye injection, cells were observed to determine whether dye transfer occurred. The incidence of dye coupling was scored as the percentage of injections that resulted in dye transfer from the injected cell to more than one neighboring cell. Three experiments were performed for every treatment and dye coupling was tested by microinjecting a minimum of 10 cells per experiment.

Immunofluorescence

Cells grown on glass coverslips were fixed at room temperature with 2% paraformaldehyde for 30 min and then washed three times with PBS. Then, cells were incubated three times for 5 min in 0.1 M PBS-glycine, followed by 30 min incubation with 0.1% PBS-Triton X-100 containing 10% NGS. The permeabilized cells were incubated with anti-β-tubulin monoclonal antibody (Sigma, 1:400) and anti-Cx43 polyclonal antibody (SIGMA, 1:400) diluted in 0.1% PBS-Triton X-100 with 2% NGS at 4°C overnight. After five rinses in 0.1% PBS-Triton X-100, cells were incubated with goat anti-mouse IgG Alexa Fluor 555 (1:1,000), goat anti-rabbit IgG Alexa Fluor 488 (1:1,000), or Alexa Fluor 488-phalloidin at room temperature for 50 min. After several rinses, coverslips were mounted in DAPI Fluoromount-G medium and examined with an Olympus BX 51W1I upright microscope with a 40× water immersion objective or a confocal laser-scanning microscope with a 63× objective (Olympus, Fluoview FV1000, Tokyo, Japan).

Intracellular Ca^{2+} and NO Imaging

Cells plated on glass coverslips were loaded with 5 μM Fura-2-AM or 5 μM DAF-FM diacetate in DMEM without serum at 37°C for 45 min and then washed three times in Locke's solution (154 mM NaCl, 5.4 mM KCl, 2.3 mM $CaCl_2$, 5 mM HEPES, pH 7.4) followed by de-esterification at 37°C for 15 min. The experimental protocol for Ca^{2+} signal and NO imaging involved data acquisition every 5 s (emission at 510 and 515 nm, respectively) at 340/380-nm and 495 excitation wavelengths, respectively, using an Olympus BX 51W1I upright microscope with a 40× water immersion objective. Changes were monitored using an imaging system equipped with a Retga 1300I fast-cooled monochromatic digital camera (12-bit) (Qimaging, Burnaby, BC, Canada), monochromator for fluorophore excitation, and METAFLUOR software (Universal Imaging, Downingtown, PA, USA) for image acquisition and analysis. Analysis involved determination of pixels assigned to each cell. The average pixel value allocated to each cell was obtained with excitation at each wavelength and corrected for background. Due to the low excitation intensity, no bleaching was observed even when cells were illuminated for a few minutes. The FURA-2 ratio was obtained after dividing the 340-nm by the 380-nm fluorescence image on a pixel-by-pixel base ($R = F_{340\,nm}/F_{380\,nm}$).

Measurement of Extracellular ATP Concentration

Cells were seeded (2×10^6 cells in 35 mm dishes) in DMEM containing 10% FBS and treated with IL-1β and TNF-α plus 25 mM glucose for 72 h. Supernatants were collected, filtered (0.22 μm), and stored at −20°C before used for experiments. Then, extracellular ATP was measured using a luciferin/luciferase bioluminescence assay kit (Sigma-Aldrich). The amount of ATP in each sample was inferred from standard curves and normalized for the protein concentration as determined by the BCA assay (Pierce).

Data Analysis and Statistics

For each data group, results were expressed as mean ± SEM; *n* refers to the number of independent experiments. Detailed statistical results were included in the figure legends. Statistical analyses were performed using GraphPad Prism (version 7, GraphPad Software, La Jolla, CA, USA). Normality and equal variances were assessed by the Shapiro–Wilk normality test and Brown–Forsythe test, respectively. Unless otherwise stated, data that passed these tests were analyzed by unpaired *t* test in case of comparing two groups, whereas in case of multiple comparisons, data were analyzed by one or two-way analysis of variance (ANOVA) followed, in case of significance, by a Tukey's *post hoc* test. A probability of $p < 0.05$ was considered statistically significant.

RESULTS

IL-1β/TNF-α Plus High Glucose Enhance the Activity of Cx43 Hemichannels in Endothelial Cells

Previous studies have revealed that stimulation with IL-1β/TNF-α or high glucose (25–45 mM) causes a prominent opening of hemichannels in diverse brain cell types (8, 19–22). Given that inflammatory mediators play crucial roles in the activation of endothelial cells and because hemichannels may contribute to this process as they do in other tissues (24, 25), we examined whether two pro-inflammatory cytokines and high glucose could modulate the activity of these channels in the human endothelial cell line EAhy 926. The functional state of hemichannels was evaluated by measuring the rate of ethidium (Etd) uptake. Etd only move across the plasma membrane in normal cells by permeating specific large-pore channels such as hemichannels (26). After its binding to RNA and DNA, Etd becomes fluorescent, revealing channel opening when appropriate blockers are employed.

After incubation with 45 mM but not 25 mM glucose, EAhy cells exhibited a significant twofold increment in Etd uptake compared with physiological glucose concentration (5 mM)

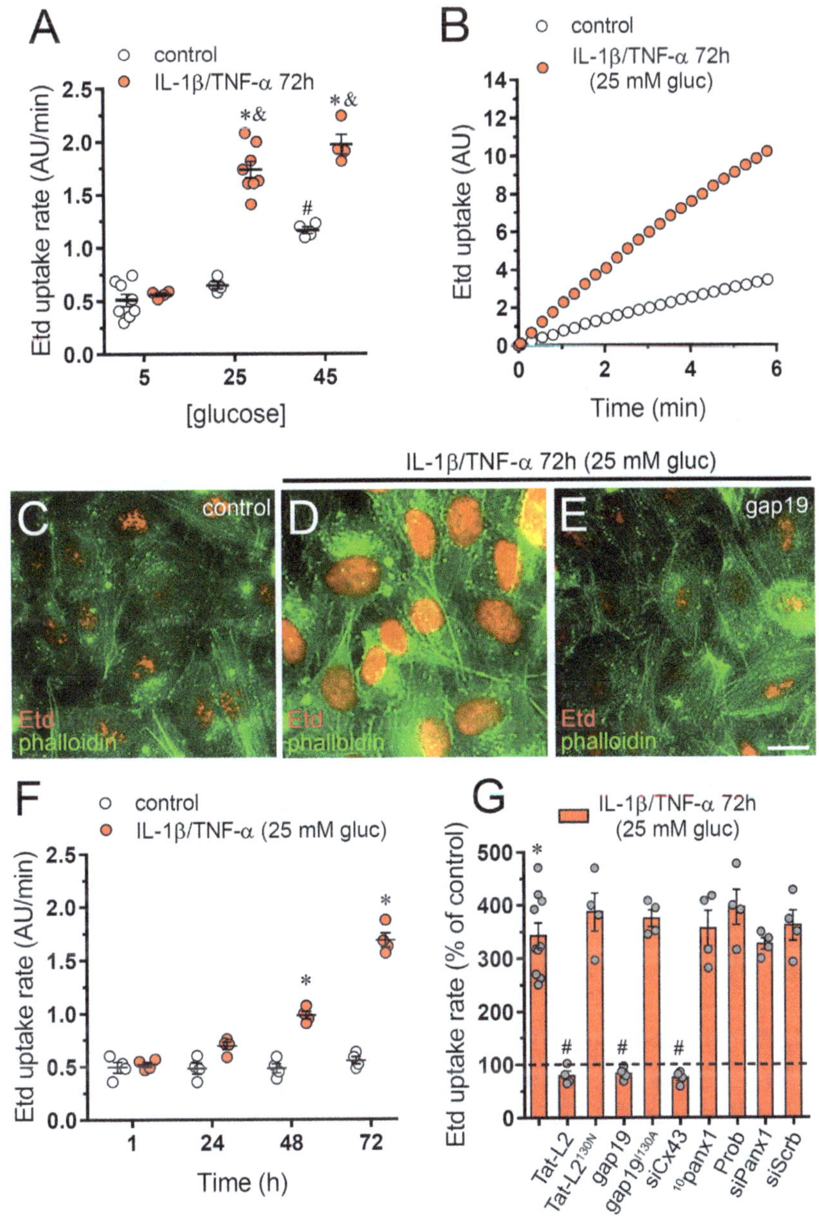

FIGURE 1 | High glucose and IL-1β plus TNF-α increase the activity of connexin 43 (Cx43) hemichannels in endothelial cells. **(A)** Averaged Etd uptake rate of EAhy cells treated for 72 h with different concentrations of glucose alone (control, white circles) or in combination with a mixture of IL-1β/TNF-α (red circles; 10 ng/mL for each). $^{\#}p < 0.05$, 45 mM glucose (control) compared to 5 mM glucose (control), $^{*}p < 0.05$, IL-1β/TNF-α compared to control; $^{\&}p < 0.05$, high glucose (IL-1β/TNF-α) compared to 5 mM glucose (IL-1β/TNF-α) [two-way analysis of variance (ANOVA) followed by Tukey's *post hoc* test]. **(B)** Time-lapse measurements of Etd uptake by EAhy cells treated for 72 h with 5 mM glucose (control, white circles) or 25 mM glucose and IL-1β/TNF-α (red circles). **(C–E)** Representative immunofluorescence images depicting phalloidin-actin (green) and Etd-nucleus (red) staining from dye uptake measurements (10 min exposure to dye) in EAhy cells treated for 72 h with 5 mM glucose [control **(C)**], 25 mM glucose and IL-1β/TNF-α **(D)** alone or plus 100 μM gap19. **(F)** Averaged Etd uptake rate by EAhy cells treated for several time periods with 5 mM glucose (control, white circles) or 25 mM glucose and IL-1β/TNF-α (red circles). $^{*}p < 0.05$, IL-1β/TNF-α and high glucose compared to control (two-way ANOVA followed by Tukey's *post hoc* test). **(G)** Averaged Etd uptake rate normalized with control condition (dashed line) by EAhy cells treated for 72 h with 25 mM glucose and IL-1β/TNF-α alone or in combination with the following blockers: 100 μM Tat-L2, 100 μM Tat-$L2^{H126K/I130N}$, 100 μM gap19, 100 μM $gap19^{I130A}$, $siRNA^{Cx43}$, 100 μM ^{10}panx1, 500 μM probenecid (Prob), $siRNA^{Panx1}$; and $siRNA^{scrb}$. $^{*}p < 0.05$, IL-1β/TNF-α and high glucose compared to control; $^{\#}p < 0.05$, effect of blockers compared IL-1β/TNF-α and high glucose (one-way ANOVA followed by Tukey's *post hoc* test). Data were obtained from at least three independent experiments (see scatter dot plot) with four repeats each one (≥35 cells analyzed for each repeat). Calibration bar = 20 μm.

(**Figure 1A**). Relevantly, a combination of IL-1β and TNF-α (10 ng/mL of each) enhanced the response evoked by 45 mM glucose (**Figure 1A**), whereas 25 mM glucose (hereinafter referred as to "high glucose") only increased Etd uptake when applied in combination with IL-1β/TNF-α (**Figures 1A–D**). Moreover, IL-1β/TNF-α and high glucose triggered a time-dependent proportional rise in Etd uptake, being 72 h of treatment the most significant as it evoked a 3.5-fold augment in relation to control treatment (**Figure 1F**). No changes in Etd uptake were observed upon treatment with IL-1β/TNF-α and plus high sucrose or high mannitol excluding the possibility of an osmolarity-mediated response (Figure S1A in Supplementary Material).

Endothelial cells express functional Cx43 hemichannels (27–29) and Panx1 channels (30, 31). Pannexins encompass a three-member protein family that constitute unopposed membrane channels referred as pannexons that—just like hemichannels—allow paracrine/autocrine communication in cellular tissues (32). The involvement of Cx43 hemichannels in IL-1β/TNF-α and high glucose-mediated Etd uptake was examined employing specific mimetic peptides (Tat-L2 and gap19) with sequences homologous to intracellular L2 loop domains of Cx43 (33, 34). Cells treated with IL-1β/TNF-α and high glucose for 72 h and incubated for 15 min of incubation with Tat-L2 (100 μM) or gap19 (100 μM) before and during the dye uptake evaluation showed an Etd uptake close to that of control cells (**Figures 1C,E,G**). In addition, a mutated TAT-L2 (200 μM TAT-L2$^{H126K/I130N}$), in which 2 aa crucial for interaction of L2 domain to the carboxyl tail of Cx43 are modified, was unsuccessful in trigger a comparable inhibition (**Figure 1G**). Likewise, we noticed that an inactive form of gap19 containing the I130A modification (gap19^{I130A}), did not inhibit the IL-1β/TNF-α and high glucose-induced Etd uptake in EAhy cells (**Figure 1G**). Consistent with these findings, knockdown of Cx43 with siRNA fully abolished the Etd uptake caused by IL-1β/TNF-α and high glucose (**Figure 1G**). Conversely, scrambled siRNA, siRNA for Panx1, the Panx1 mimetic peptide ^{10}panx1 (100 μM), or probenecid (200 μM) failed to cause a similar suppression (**Figure 1G**). These results strongly bring up that IL-1β/TNF-α and high glucose significantly increase the activity of Cx43 hemichannels, but not Panx1 channels in EAhy endothelial cells.

Endothelial Cx43 Hemichannel Activity Induced by IL-1β/TNF-α Plus High Glucose Depends on p38 MAP Kinase/iNOS/COX₂/EP₁ and Purinergic Pathways

During inflammatory conditions, endothelial cells display a strong stimulation of the iNOS and cyclooxygenase 2 (COX_2) (35, 36), two enzymes that generate byproducts (NO and prostaglandins, respectively) associated with Cx43 hemichannel activation (37–39). In addition, prior research has unveiled the participation of p38 MAP kinase (p38 MAPK) in both the opening of Cx43 hemichannels (20) and inflammatory activation of endothelial cells (40, 41). Accordingly, we examined the influence of p38 MAPK, iNOS, and COX_2 pathways on the IL-1β/TNF-α and high glucose-induced Etd uptake in EAhy cells. The Etd uptake triggered by IL-1β/TNF-α and high glucose treatment for 72 h was greatly reduced by blockade of p38 MAPK with SB202190 (10 μM) or inhibition of iNOS with L-N6 (5 μM) (**Figure 2A**). Notably, COX inhibition by indomethacin (15 μM) reduced the ~3.5-fold increase on Etd uptake evoked by IL-1β/TNF-α and high glucose to control conditions (**Figure 2A**). To investigate which COX was implicated in the above effect, we used sc-560 and ns-398, specific inhibitors for COX_1 and COX_2, respectively.

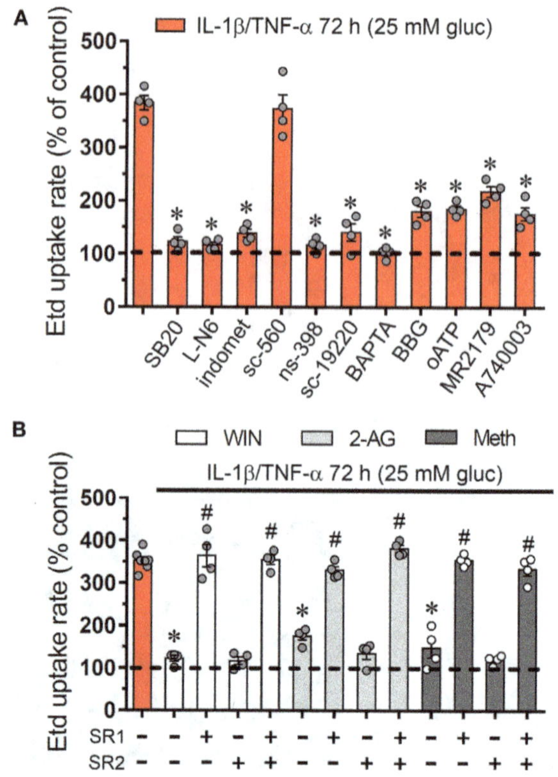

FIGURE 2 | Endothelial connexin 43 (Cx43) hemichannel opening evoked by high glucose and IL-1β/TNF-α depends on Ca^{2+} signaling and activation of p38 MAPK/inducible NO synthase/COX_2-dependent pathways and EP_1/P2 receptors: prevention by cannabinoids. **(A)** Averaged Etd uptake rate normalized with control conditions (5 mM glucose, dashed line) of EAhy cells treated for 72 h with 25 mM glucose and IL-1β/TNF-α alone or in combination with the following agents: 10 μM SB203580, 1 μM L-N6, 15 μM indometacin (indomet); 1 μM sc-560; 5 μM ns-398; 20 μM sc-19220, 10 μM BAPTA, 10 μM Brilliant blue G (BBG), 200 μM oxidized ATP (oATP), 10 μM MRS2179; and 10 μM A740003. $^{*}p < 0.05$, effect of blockers compared to IL-1β/TNF-α and high glucose [one-way analysis of variance (ANOVA) followed by Tukey's *post hoc* test]. **(B)** Averaged Etd uptake rate normalized with control conditions (5 mM glucose, dashed line) by EAhy cells treated for 72 h with 25 mM glucose and IL-1β/TNF-α (red bar) alone or in combination with the following cannabinoids: WIN (5 μM, white bars), 2-arachidonylglycerol (5 μM, light gray bars), and Meth (5 μM, dark gray bars). It is also shown the effect of the respective cannabinoid co-treatment with the CB_1 or CB_2 receptor antagonist, SR-141716A (5 μM) and/or SR-144528 (5 μM), respectively. $^{*}p < 0.05$, effect of each cannabinoid compared to the effect induced by 72 h treatment with IL-1β/TNF-α and high glucose; $^{\#}p < 0.05$, effect of each cannabinoid receptor antagonist compared to the effect of the respective cannabinoid (one-way ANOVA followed by Tukey's *post hoc* test). Data were obtained from at least three independent experiments (see scatter dot plot) with four repeats each one (≥35 cells analyzed for each repeat).

sc-560 (1 μM) failed in neutralizing the Etd uptake caused by IL-1β/TNF-α and high glucose, whereas ns-398 (5 μM) completely abolished it (**Figure 2A**).

Previous findings indicate that NO elevates COX_2 activity and prostaglandin E_2 (PEG_2) generation in macrophages (42) and a similar phenomenon seems to occur in inflamed endothelial cells (43). Given that activation of PEG_2 receptor 1 (EP_1) lead to increases in $[Ca^{2+}]_i$ (44) and the latter is a well-known mechanism that increase the open probability of Cx43 hemichannels (45), we examined if this signaling is involved in the IL-1β/TNF-α and high glucose-mediated Etd uptake in EAhy cells. Blockade of EP_1 receptor with sc-19220 (20 μM) was found to diminish the Etd uptake caused by IL-1β/TNF-α and high glucose, whereas 5 μM BAPTA-AM, a Ca^{2+} chelator, caused a similar inhibition (**Figure 2A**). The opening of Cx43 hemichannels has been correlated with $[Ca^{2+}]_i$-mediated purinergic signaling (46, 47), thereby, we tested if purinergic receptors participate in the IL-1β/TNF-α and high glucose-induced Etd uptake in EAhy cells. Remarkably, 200 μM oATP, a general P2X receptor blocker, or 10 μM A740003 and 10 μM BBG, both $P2X_7$ receptor inhibitors, partially antagonized the Etd uptake induced by IL-1β/TNF-α and high glucose (**Figure 2A**). Similarly, the blockade of $P2Y_1$ receptors with 10 μM MRS2179 evoked a partial but significant reduction in the IL-1β/TNF-α and high glucose-induced Etd uptake. All these data suggest that endothelial Cx43 hemichannel activity triggered by IL-1β/TNF-α and high glucose rely on the stimulation of p38 MAPK/iNOS/COX_2/EP_1–dependent pathway(s) and the $P2X_7$/$P2Y_1$ receptor-mediated changes in cytoplasmic Ca^{2+} signal.

CBs Counteract the Opening of Cx43 Hemichannels Induced by IL-1β/TNF-α Plus High Glucose in Endothelial Cells

An unresolved topic in the field of hemichannels is to recognize compounds that could prevent their increased opening during pathological conditions. Possible aspirants for this intent are CBs, as they successfully prevent the persistent Cx43 hemichannel opening triggered by different inflammatory conditions in glial cells (48–50). Whether plant-derived, synthetic, or endocannabinoids, CBs are biolipid molecules that activate at least two CB receptors: CB_1 and CB_2 (51). Because endothelial cells express CB_1/CB_2 receptors (52) and CBs elicit anti-inflammatory defense facing cytokine-dependent endothelial dysfunction (53), we examined whether CBs could ameliorate the increase in Cx43 hemichannel activity evoked by IL-1β/TNF-α and high glucose in EAhy cells.

To elucidate whether CBs could regulate the Cx43 hemichannel activity in EAhy cells, we pre-incubated the cells with synthetic and endogenous CBs for 1 h and then were co-applied for 72 h along with IL-1β/TNF-α and high glucose. WIN-55,212-2 (WIN; 5 μM), a synthetic agonist of CB_1/CB_2 receptors, completely blunted the IL-1β/TNF-α and high glucose-induced Etd uptake in EAhy cells since these cells showed an Etd uptake comparable to control values (**Figure 2B**). Furthermore, we used two endogenous CB_1/CB_2 receptor agonists: 2-AG and methanandamide (Meth), the latter being a synthetic analog of the endocannabinoid anandamide. We observed that 5 μM 2-AG and 5 μM Meth reduced the increase in Etd uptake rate of EAhy cells caused by the IL-1β/TNF-α and high glucose treatment to ~169 and ~146%, respectively (**Figure 2B**). CB_1 and CB_2 receptor antagonists, SR-141716 (SR1) and SR-144528 (SR2), respectively, were employed to characterize the sub-type of CB receptor implicated in the counteracting response on Etd uptake evoked by IL-1β/TNF-α and high glucose (**Figure 2B**). With the application of 10 μM SR1 antagonist, WIN, 2-AG, and Meth failed in preventing the IL-1β/TNF-α and high glucose-mediated Etd uptake in EAhy cells, whereas 10 μM SR2 was ineffective in evoke a comparable preventing effect (**Figure 2B**). These findings indicate that CB_1, but not CB_2 receptors are the major contributors to the WIN, 2-AG, and Meth counteracting responses of the IL-1β/TNF-α and high glucose-evoked Cx43 hemichannel activity in endothelial cells.

WIN Counteract the Increment in Cx43 Surface Amount and Gap Junctional Uncoupling Triggered by IL-1β/TNF-α Plus High Glucose in Endothelial Cells

Connexin 43 hemichannel activity could depend on increments in both the open probability per channel and/or the number of channels at the cell surface. Previous studies have correlated the hemichannel-dependent Etd uptake with elevated surface levels of Cx43 in different cell types (8, 39, 50) or increase in open probability without changes in the total amount of Cx43 in the cell surface (54). Here, we evaluated if the counteracting effect of CBs on IL-1β/TNF-α and high glucose-mediated hemichannel activity depend on changes in surface amount of Cx43. IL-1β/TNF-α and high glucose caused a slight but significant ~30% decrease in total Cx43 compared to control conditions, a response fully suppressed by 5 μM WIN (**Figures 3A,B**). Moreover, IL-1β/TNF-α and high glucose also evoked a ~1.7-fold rise in surface amount of Cx43 and experiments with WIN fully blunted this effect (**Figures 3A,B**). Therefore, the ameliorative effects of CBs on IL-1β/TNF-α and high glucose-induced Cx43 hemichannel

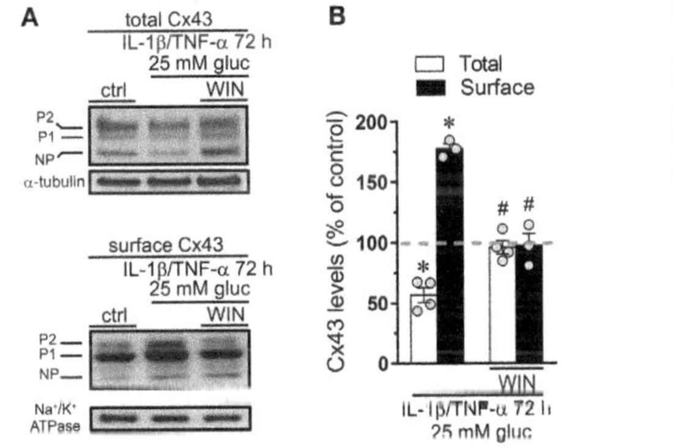

FIGURE 3 | WIN counteracts the increase in surface levels of connexin 43 (Cx43) induced by high glucose and IL-1β/TNF-α in endothelial cells. **(A)** Total (upper panel) and surface (bottom panel) levels of Cx43 by EAhy cells treated for 72 h with 5 mM glucose (control), 25 mM glucose, and IL-1β/TNF-α alone or in combination with 5 μM WIN. The Cx43 phosphorylated (P1–P2) and non-phosphorylated (NP) forms are indicated in the left. Total and surface amount of each analyzed band were normalized according to the amount of α-tubulin and Na^+/K^+ ATPase detected in each lane, respectively. **(B)** Quantification of total (white bars) and surface (black bars) amount of Cx43 normalized to control (dashed line) in EAhy cells harvested 72 h after treatment with 25 mM glucose and IL-1β/TNF-α alone or in combination with 5 μM WIN. $^*p < 0.05$, IL-1β/TNF-α and high glucose compared to control; $^{\#}p < 0.05$, effect of each cannabinoid compared to the effect induced by IL-1β/TNF-α and high glucose (two-tailed Student's unpaired *t*-test). Averaged data were obtained from at least three independent experiments (see scatter dot plot).

activity may take place because they interfere with the increment in surface amount of Cx43.

Endothelial-to-endothelial gap junctional communication is critical for the endothelium-derived hyperpolarization and concomitant vasodilation of the arteriolar smooth muscle (55). Given that increased Cx43 hemichannel opening induced by inflammatory conditions has been described to occur along with a rise in endothelial dye coupling (27), we evaluated if the endothelial gap junction coupling was altered upon treatment with IL-1β/TNF-α and high glucose. Under control conditions around ~80% of EAhy cells exhibited LY intercellular diffusion to neighboring cells (**Figures 4A,D,G**). Nonetheless, 72 h after treatment with IL-1β/TNF-α and high glucose intercellular dye transfer decreased by ~38% compared with control levels

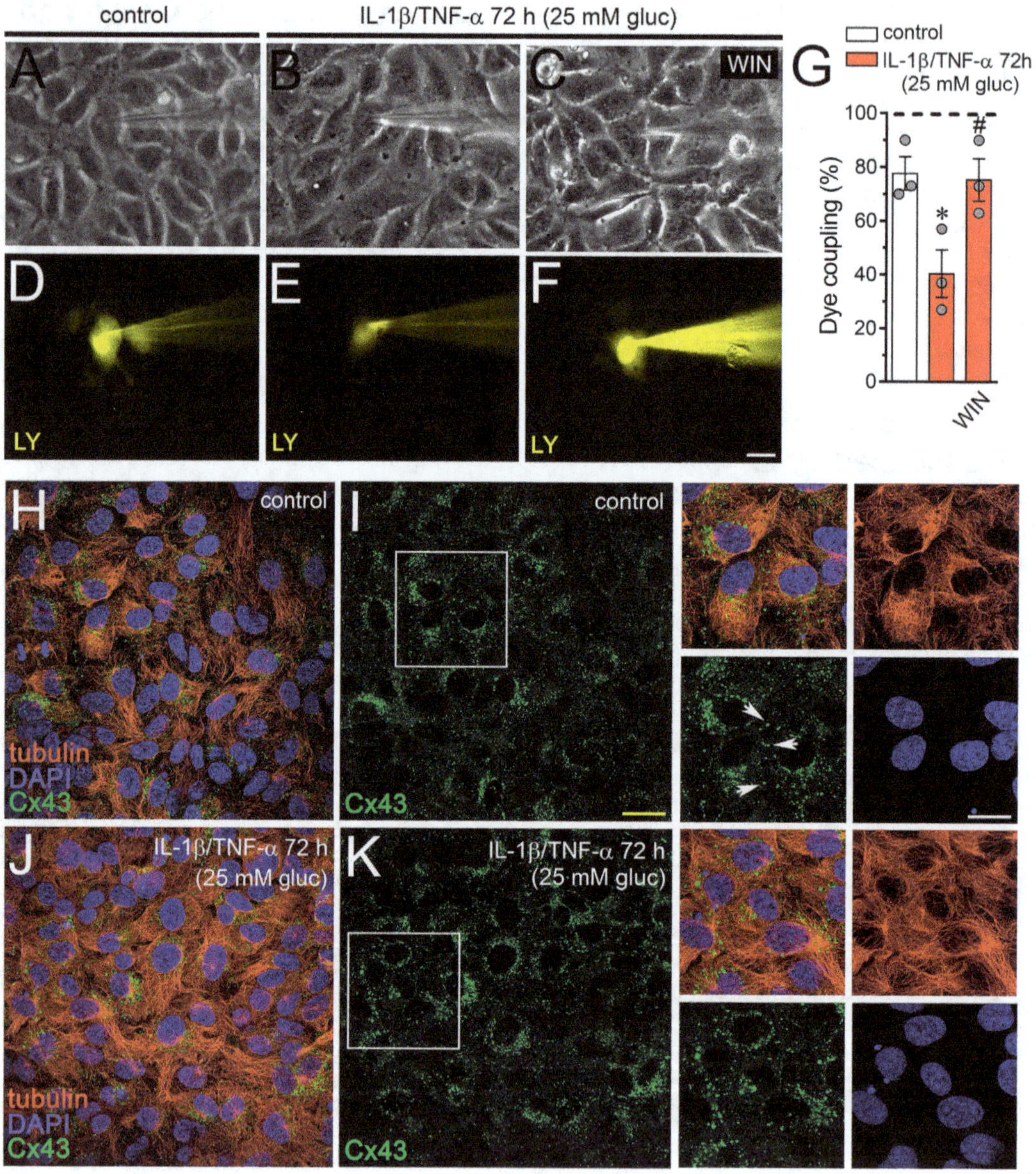

FIGURE 4 | WIN prevents the high glucose and IL-1β/TNF-α-induced decrease in endothelial coupling through a mechanism that does not involve changes in connexin 43 (Cx43) distribution. **(A–F)** Representative fluorescence and phase contrast micrographs of Lucifer yellow (LY) transfer by EAhy cells treated for 72 h with 5 mM glucose [control **(A,D)**], 25 mM glucose, and IL-1β/TNF-α **(B,E)** alone or in combination with 5 μM WIN **(C,F)**. **(G)** Averaged data of dye coupling (percentage of injections that resulted in LY transfer) of EAhy cells treated for 72 h with 5 mM glucose (control, white bar), 25 mM glucose, and IL-1β/TNF-α (red bars) alone or in combination with 5 μM WIN. *$p < 0.05$, IL-1β/TNF-α and high glucose compared to control; #$p < 0.05$, effect of each cannabinoid compared to the effect induced by IL-1β/TNF-α and high glucose (one-way analysis of variance followed by Dunnett's *post hoc* test). Data were obtained from at least three independent experiments (see scatter dot plot) with four repeats each one (≥10 cells analyzed for each repeat). **(H–K)** Representative fluorescence images depicting Cx43 (green), tubulin (red), and DAPI (blue) immunolabeling of EAhy cells treated for 72 h with 5 mM glucose [control **(H,I)**] and 25 mM glucose plus IL-1β/TNF-α **(J,K)**. Insets: 1.7× magnification of the indicated area of panels **(I,K)**. White arrows indicate Cx43 labeling in cell–cell interfaces. Calibration bars: white = 35 μm, yellow = 60 μm, and green = 25 μm.

(**Figures 4B,E,G**). Equivalently, to the counteracting influence on IL-1β/TNF-α and high glucose-evoked Etd uptake, WIN entirely prevented the reduction in endothelial cell–cell coupling induced by IL-1β/TNF-α and high glucose (**Figures 4C,F,G**). Given that endocytosis of gap junctions from the plasma membrane is a process that might cause cellular uncoupling, we explored if IL-1β/TNF-α and high glucose-induced endothelial uncoupling was correlated with alterations in the cellular distribution of Cx43. In control EAhy cells, Cx43 was observed as fine to large granules scattered at cellular interfaces and perinuclear regions (**Figures 4H,I**) and comparable features were detected in those treated with IL-1β/TNF-α and high glucose (**Figures 4J,K**) or plus 5 μM WIN (Figures S1B–D in Supplementary Material). These findings indicate that IL-1β/TNF-α and high glucose-induced cell-to-cell uncoupling may depend on a mechanism implicating the closure and/or decreased permeability of Cx43 gap junctions rather than withdrawal from the apposition membranes.

IL-1β/TNF-α Plus High Glucose Promotes the Cx43 Hemichannel-Induced Release of ATP From Endothelial Cells: Counteracting Action by WIN

Endothelial cells subjected to inflammatory conditions exhibit elevated release of ATP *via* the opening of Cx43 hemichannels (27, 56), a major signal involved in leukocyte recruitment and vascular inflammation (57). Given that $P2X_7$ and $P2Y_1$ receptors are involved in the Etd uptake evoked by IL-1β/TNF-α and high glucose in EAhy cells (**Figure 2A**), we evaluated whether this treatment could also impact the release of ATP *via* Cx43 hemichannels. IL-1β/TNF-α and high glucose strongly enhanced the release of ATP by ~6-folds compared to control conditions (**Figure 5**). Importantly, gap19 and Tat-L2, but not ^{10}panx1 or probenecid, prominently reduced to control values the extracellular ATP concentration of cells treated with IL-1β/TNF-α and high glucose-induced release of ATP (from ~68 to ~13 and ~12 pmol/10^6 cells, respectively) (**Figure 5**). These findings indicate that IL-1β/TNF-α and high glucose elevate the release of ATP in a Cx43 hemichannel-dependent form in EAhy endothelail cells. In this context, we tested the probable counteracting influence of WIN on this response. We observed that 1 h pretreatment and co-incubation with 5 μM WIN drastically reduced the IL-1β/TNF-α and high glucose-mediated release of ATP (from ~68 to ~11 pmol/10^6 cells) (**Figure 5**). Interestingly, WIN failed in decreasing the ATP release in EAhy cells pre-incubated with 10 μM SR1 antagonist. Altogether, these findings support that CB_1 receptors are the main contributors to the WIN-mediated inhibition of Cx43 hemichannel-dependent release of ATP evoked by IL-1β/TNF-α and high glucose in endothelial cells.

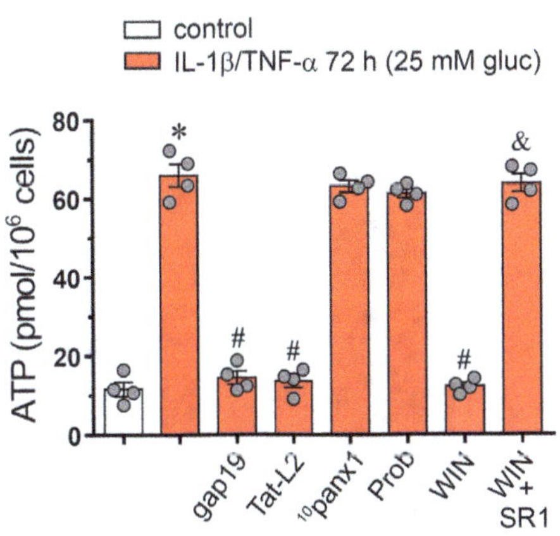

FIGURE 5 | WIN mitigates the connexin 43 (Cx43) hemichannel-dependent release of ATP evoked by high glucose and IL-1β/TNF-α in endothelial cells. Averaged data of ATP release from EAhy cells treated for 72 h with 5 mM glucose (control, white bar), 25 mM glucose, and IL-1β/TNF-α (black bars) alone or in combination with the following agents: 100 μM gap19, 100 μM Tat-L2, 100 μM ^{10}panx1, 500 μM probenecid (Prob), 5 μM, WIN and/or 5 μM SR-141716A (SR1). $^*p < 0.05$, IL-1β/TNF-α and high glucose compared to control; $^\#p < 0.05$, effect of each agent compared to the effect induced by IL-1β/TNF-α and high glucose; $^\&p < 0.05$, effect of each cannabinoid receptor antagonist compared to the effect of the respective cannabinoid (one-way analysis of variance followed by Tukey's *post hoc* test). Data were obtained from at least three independent experiments (see scatter dot plot) with four repeats each one.

IL-1β/TNF-α and High Glucose-Induced Changes in ATP-Dependent Ca^{2+} Dynamics Are Prevented by WIN in Endothelial Cells

Although cytoplasmic Ca^{2+} is crucial for proper endothelial barrier permeability and remodeling, its abnormal signaling during inflammatory conditions could lead to multiple vascular diseases (58, 59). Relevantly, both endothelial $[Ca^{2+}]$ signaling and hemichannel functional state are interdependent processes that may be enhanced during pathological conditions (60). In this context and because intracellular BAPTA greatly blunted IL-1β/TNF-α and high glucose-mediated Etd uptake (**Figure 1A**), we investigated if this condition could modulate the basal Ca^{2+} signal in EAhy cells. As indicated by the assessment of Fura-2 ratio (340/380), IL-1β/TNF-α and high glucose-stimulated EAhy cells showed basal Ca^{2+} signal that was similar to control conditions (**Figures 6A,C,K**). Despite that IL-1β/TNF-α and high glucose fail in modulate basal Ca^{2+} signal, these data do not rule out whether this condition affects the Ca^{2+} signal responses evoked by autocrine/paracrine signals, including ATP. With this in mind, we also studied the impact of IL-1β/TNF-α and high glucose on ATP-mediated Ca^{2+} signaling, as this transmitter can be released through Cx43 hemichannels from EAhy cells (**Figure 6**). Under control conditions, treatment with 500 μM ATP caused a rapid Ca^{2+} signal response with a small peak amplitude (**Figures 6A,B,E,L**). However, high glucose induced a sustained ATP-dependent Ca^{2+} signal response with a peak amplitude ~4-fold higher than that of control conditions (**Figures 6C,D,F,L**). This phenomenon was accompanied of a ~4- and ~4.5-fold increment in the integrated ATP-dependent Ca^{2+} signal response (**Figure 6M**) and the remaining difference between final and initial basal Ca^{2+} signal (**Figure 6N**), respectively.

In endothelial cells, ATP-mediated $[Ca^{2+}]_i$ responses involve different purinergic receptors, including $P2X_7$ and $P2Y_1$ receptors (61, 62), both being implicated in the hemichannel opening

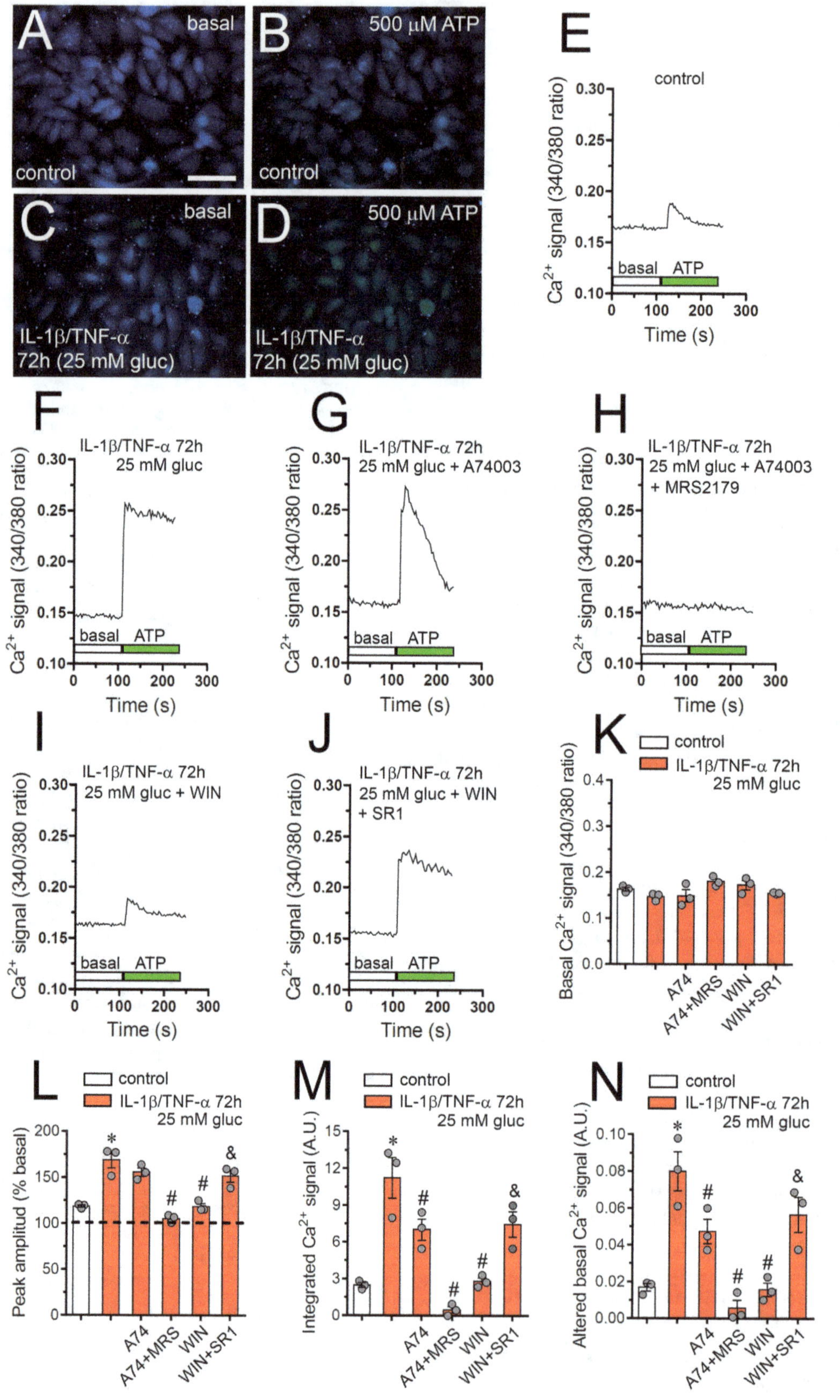

FIGURE 6 | Continued

FIGURE 6 | High glucose and IL-1β/TNF-α enhance ATP-dependent Ca^{2+} dynamics in endothelial cells: prevention by WIN. **(A–D)** Representative photomicrographs of basal **(A,C)** or 500 μM ATP-induced **(B,D)** Ca^{2+} signal denoted as Fura-2 ratio (340/380 nm excitation) of EAhy cells treated for 72 h with 5 mM glucose [control **(A,B)**] or 25 mM glucose and IL-1β/TNF-α **(C,D)**. Calibration bar: 180 μm. **(E–J)** Representative plots of relative changes in $[Ca^{2+}]_i$ signal over time induced by 500 μM ATP (gray vertical line) in EAhy cells treated for 72 h with 5 mM glucose [control **(E)**], 25 mM glucose, and IL-1β/TNF-α **(F)** alone or in combination with the following agents: 10 μM A740003 **(G)**, 10 μM A740003 plus 10 μM MRS2179 **(H)**, 5 μM, WIN **(I)** and 5 μM, WIN plus 5 μM SR-141716A [SR1 **(J)**]. **(K)** Averaged data of basal Fura-2 ratio by EAhy cells treated for 72 h with 5 mM glucose (control, white bar), 25 mM glucose, and IL-1β/TNF-α (red bars) alone or in combination with the following agents: 10 μM A740003 (A74), 10 μM A740003 plus 10 μM MRS2179 (A74 + MRS), 5 μM WIN (WIN) and 5 μM, WIN plus 5 μM SR-141716A (WIN + SR1). **(L–N)** Averaged data of ATP-induced peak amplitude normalized to basal Fura-2 ratio **(L)**, integrated ATP-induced Fura-2 ratio response **(M)**, and altered basal Fura-2 ratio **(N)** of EAhy cells treated for 72 h with 5 mM glucose (control, white bar), 25 mM glucose, and IL-1β/TNF-α (red bars) alone or in combination with the following agents: 10 μM A740003 (A74), 10 μM A740003 plus 10 μM MRS2179 (A74 + MRS), 5 μM WIN (WIN) and 5 μM, WIN plus 5 μM SR-141716A (WIN + SR1). $^*p < 0.05$, IL-1β/TNF-α and high glucose compared to control; $^{\#}p < 0.05$, effect of each pharmacological agent compared to the effect induced by IL-1β/TNF-α and high glucose; $^{\&}p < 0.05$, effect of each cannabinoid receptor antagonist compared to the effect of the respective cannabinoid (one-way analysis of variance followed by Tukey's *post hoc* test). Data were obtained from at least three independent experiments (see scatter dot plot) with four repeats each one (≥35 cells analyzed for each repeat).

triggered by IL-1β/TNF-α and high glucose (**Figure 2A**). Notably, blockade of $P2X_7$ receptors with 10 μM A740003 completely suppressed the sustained response pattern of ATP-mediated Ca^{2+} signal in IL-1β/TNF-α and high glucose-stimulated EAhy cells (**Figure 6G**). In addition, A740003 partially inhibited the integrated and remaining basal ATP-dependent Ca^{2+} signal responses (**Figures 6M,N**), but did not affect the peak amplitude induced by IL-1β/TNF-α and high glucose (**Figure 6L**). Notably, simultaneous inhibition of $P2X_7$ and $P2Y_1$ receptors with 10 μM A740003 and 10 μM MRS2179, respectively, completely blunted the ATP-dependent Ca^{2+} signal in IL-1β/TNF-α and high glucose-stimulated EAhy cells (**Figure 6H**). The latter was paralleled with a total suppression of the IL-1β/TNF-α and high glucose-induced increase of the Ca^{2+} signal evoked by ATP (**Figures 6L–N**). These findings indicate that upon ATP exposure, the transient peak in $[Ca^{2+}]_i$ signal recorded in IL-1β/TNF-α and high glucose-stimulated EAhy cells, likely came from Ca^{2+} released from intracellular stores due to stimulation of $P2Y_1$ and IP_3 receptors, whereas the following sustained Ca^{2+} signal could involve the participation of $P2X_7$ receptors. Interestingly, IL-1β/TNF-α and high glucose-stimulated EAhy cells showed ATP-mediated Ca^{2+} signals similar to those recorded in control conditions when they were pre-treated with 10 μM WIN (**Figures 6I,L–N**). Moreover, WIN-induced prevention of ATP-induced Ca^{2+} signal did not occur in IL-1β/TNF-α and high glucose-stimulated EAhy cells co-incubated with the CB_1 receptor antagonist SR1 (**Figures 6J,L–N**). The above data support that CB_1 receptors are responsible of the WIN-mediated prevention in the disturbing actions of IL-1β/TNF-α and high glucose on the dynamics of ATP-mediated Ca^{2+} signals in endothelial cells.

WIN and Blockers of Cx43 Hemichannels Prevent the NO Production of Endothelial Cells Treated With IL-1β/TNF-α and High Glucose

Altered iNOS-derived NO production has been involved in the beginning of acute and chronic inflammatory conditions associated with diverse diseases, including arthritis, sepsis, ischemia/reperfusion, diabetes, and atherosclerosis (63). Because LN-6, a specific iNOS blocker, strongly blunted the IL-1β/TNF-α and high glucose-mediated Etd uptake in EAhy cells (**Figure 2A**), we investigated whether Cx43 hemichannels also modulate NO production. DAF fluorescence experiments indicated that IL-1β/TNF-α and high glucose-treated EAhy cells exhibited a ~2-fold increase in basal NO amount compared with control values (**Figures 7A,B,G**). Interestingly, treatment with 5 μM WIN fully prevented the IL-1β/TNF-α and high glucose-induced increase in NO production, the latter response being dependent on CB_1 receptors as SR1 abolished the counteracting action of WIN (**Figures 7C,G**). Insulin is a well-known inducer of NO production in normal endothelial cells, however, under inflammatory conditions, the insulin-mediated production of NO is impaired (64). In this context, we evaluated whether IL-1β/TNF-α and high glucose could disturb the insulin-mediated production of NO. As expected, 30 min treatment with 1 μM insulin induced a ~75% increase in NO levels in control EAhy cells (**Figures 7D,G**). Remarkably, IL-1β/TNF-α and high glucose increased in ~1-fold the insulin-mediated production of NO (**Figures 7E,G**), a response that was completely prevented by 5 μM WIN (**Figures 7F,G**). Supporting the involvement of CB_1 receptors in the latter phenomenon, the counteracting influence of WIN on the insulin-mediated NO production did not occur in EAhy cells stimulated with IL-1β/TNF-α and high glucose plus co-incubation with SR1 (**Figure 7G**). Finally, we found that 100 μM gap19 or 100 μM Tat-L2 co-applied along with IL-1β/TNF-α and high glucose, fully suppressed the IL-1β/TNF-α and high glucose-mediated potentiation in NO production induced by insulin, turning NO levels to control values (**Figure 7G**). Altogether, these results support that Cx43 hemichannels serve as a crucial step in the modulatory actions evoked by IL-1β/TNF-α and high glucose on insulin-mediated production of NO in endothelial cells.

DISCUSSION

Here, we demonstrated for the first time that high glucose concentrations elevate the Cx43 hemichannel activity in cultured endothelial cells. A mixture of IL-1β and TNF-α, two pro-inflammatory cytokines that open hemichannels in different cell types (19, 20, 22), enhanced this phenomenon. Furthermore, IL-1β/TNF-α and high glucose-induced Cx43 hemichannel activity was associated with ATP release and activation of p38 MAPK, iNOS, COX_2, PGE_2 receptor EP_1, and $P2X_7/P2Y_1$ receptors. In addition,

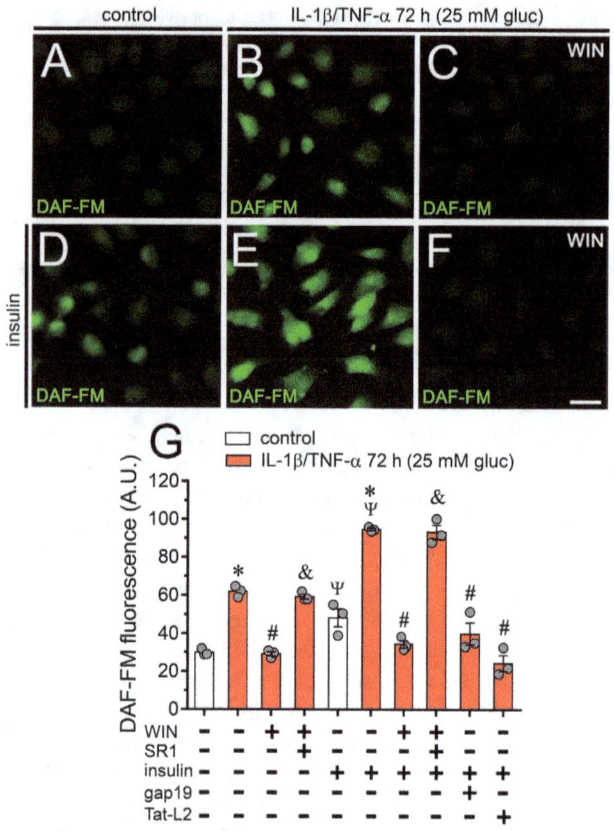

FIGURE 7 | High glucose and IL-1β/TNF-α increase basal and insulin-induced production of nitric oxide (NO) in endothelial cells: prevention by WIN and connexin 43 (Cx43) hemichannel blockers. **(A–F)** Representative fluorescence micrographs of basal **(A–C)** or 1 μM insulin-induced **(D–F)** production of NO (DAF-FM, green and pseudo-colored scale) of EAhy cells treated for 72 h with 5 mM glucose [control **(A,D)**], 25 mM glucose, and IL-1β/TNF-α **(B,E)** alone or in combination with 5 μM WIN **(C,F)**. **(G)** Average of DAF fluorescence by EAhy cells treated for 72 h with 5 mM glucose (control; white bars), 25 mM glucose and IL-1β/TNF-α (red bars) alone or with different combinations of the following compounds: 5 μM WIN (WIN), 5 μM SR-141716A (SR1), 1 μM insulin, 100 μM gap19, and 100 μM Tat-L2. *$p < 0.05$, IL-1β/TNF-α and high glucose compared to control; #$p < 0.05$, effect of each compound compared to the effect induced by IL-1β/TNF-α and high glucose; &$p < 0.05$, effect of each cannabinoid receptor antagonist compared to the effect of the respective cannabinoid; Ψ$p < 0.05$, effect of insulin compared to the respective control (one-way analysis of variance followed by Tukey's *post hoc* test). Data were obtained from at least three independent experiments (see scatter dot plot) with four repeats each one (≥35 cells analyzed for each repeat). Calibration bar = 40 μm.

we describe that a synthetic CB: WIN, and two endogenous CBs; 2-AG and Meth; counteract the IL-1β/TNF-α and high glucose-mediated Cx43 hemichannel opening and subsequent ATP release. These CBs also counteract diverse cell endothelial alterations evoked by IL-1β/TNF-α plus high glucose, including the increase in ATP-mediated Ca^{2+} signals and NO production.

As assayed by Etd uptake, we demonstrated that 45 mM glucose increments by itself the activity of Cx43 hemichannels in EAhy cells, whereas 25 mM glucose did it only in combination with the mixture of IL-1β and TNF-α. In fact, two specific mimetic peptides known to reduce Cx43 hemichannel opening (Tat-L2 and gap19), but not their inactive forms, significantly inhibited the IL-1β/TNF-α and high glucose-evoked Etd uptake. In addition, the latter effect did not occur in EAhy cells stimulated with siRNAs that downregulated Cx43. All these data indicate that IL-1β/TNF-α and high glucose specifically elevate the opening of Cx43 hemichannels in EAhy endothelial cells.

How do IL-1β/TNF-α and high glucose induce Cx43 hemichannel activity in EAhy endothelial cells? Prior research has determined that IL-1β and TNF-α or high glucose augment the functional state of Cx43 hemichannels *via* the p38 MAPK pathway and subsequent NO-mediated S-nitrosylation of Cx43 (20, 37, 39). Moreover, COX and PGE_2 receptor EP_1 stimulation is necessary for the long-lasting Cx43 hemichannel activity elicited during inflammatory conditions (38). Here, by using a battery of selective inhibitors, we have shown that the IL-1β/TNF-α and high glucose-induced Cx43 hemichannel opening comprises the activation of both p38 MAPK and iNOS, as well as the stimulation of PGE_2 receptor EP_1. In addition, IL-1β/TNF-α and high glucose raised the production of NO in EAhy cells (see below). These findings are consistent with the fact that NO stimulates COXs and the subsequent production of PGE_2 (42). The latter prostaglandin is essential for $[Ca^{2+}]_i$ elevations evoked by EP_1 receptors (44), which are highly expressed in endothelial cells (65).

Multiple studies argue that pro-inflammatory cytokines or high glucose may contribute to a chronic activation of endothelial cells and thereby a long-term production of key "danger" signals, such as ATP (66–68), which is involved with vascular inflammation (62). In this context, two findings reveal that ATP signaling is fundamental in the opening of endothelial Cx43 hemichannels evoked by IL-1β/TNF-α and high glucose. First, we detected that blockade of both $P2X_7$ and $P2Y_1$ receptors partially abrogated the IL-1β/TNF-α and high glucose-induced Cx43 hemichannel activity. Second, the activity of Cx43 hemichannels was linked to the release of ATP in IL-1β/TNF-α and high glucose-stimulated EAhy cells. In conformity with this study, recent findings have elucidated that ATP elicits its own release *via* hemichannels and further stimulation of purinergic receptors (8, 38, 39). Here, autocrine/paracrine release of ATP seems to govern Cx43 hemichannel activity as an alternative mechanism to that caused by p38 MAPK and NO production (**Figure 8**). The activity of Cx43 hemichannels could take place upon elevations in $[Ca^{2+}]_i$ caused by activation of $P2Y_1$ or $P2X_7$ receptors (8, 38, 39). Accordingly, prior evidence have described that a moderate rise in $[Ca^{2+}]_i$ (>500 nM) increase the open probability of Cx43 hemichannel opening (6, 34, 45). In agreement with this evidence, we detected that chelation of $[Ca^{2+}]_i$ with BAPTA totally blunted the IL-1β/TNF-α and high glucose-induced Etd uptake in EAhy cells. In this scenario, endothelial Cx43 hemichannels could participate directly in the release of ATP, as they are permeable to this compound (69). Alternatively, because these channels are conduits for Ca^{2+} (70), they indirectly may contribute to perpetuate $[Ca^{2+}]_i$-dependent pathways associated with ATP release (e.g., exocytosis) (**Figure 8**). The intensity of this response might impact the outcome of the inflammation. In that regard, it has been demonstrated that opening of Cx43 hemichannels could lead to preconditioning (71) as well as to cell death (21).

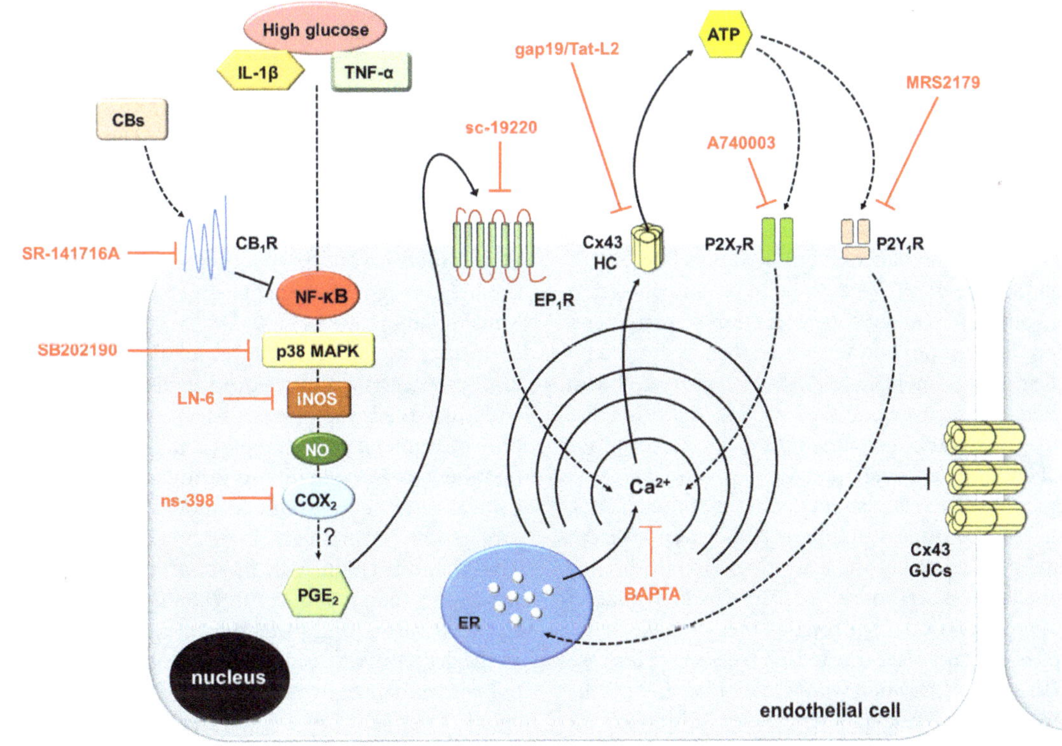

FIGURE 8 | Schematic diagram showing the possible pathways involved in the activation of connexin 43 (Cx43) hemichannels evoked by high glucose and IL-1β/TNF-α in endothelial cells. Upon stimulation with high glucose and IL-1β/TNF-α, endothelial cells respond with intracellular signal transduction that possibly involve NF-κβ signaling associated with p38 MAPK and inducible NO synthase (iNOS) activation, nitric oxide (NO) production, and further stimulation of COX_2. The latter likely induce the production of PGE_2, which acting on EP_1 metabotropic receptor promotes the release of Ca^{2+} from intracellular stores. Rise in $[Ca^{2+}]_i$ is a known condition that causes opening of Cx43 hemichannels enabling the release of ATP. ATP released *via* Cx43 hemichannels may activate $P2X_7$ receptors, and its degradation to ADP may stimulate $P2Y_1$ receptors. These events trigger the influx of extracellular Ca^{2+} and activation of IP_3 receptors and further release of Ca^{2+} stored in the endoplasmic reticulum. The later induces an unknown self-perpetuating mechanism (see Discussion), in which high levels of $[Ca^{2+}]_i$ could reactivate iNOS, COX_2, EP_1 metabotropic receptors, and Cx43 hemichannels (not depicted). On the other hand, cannabinoids (CBs) acting on CB_1Rs possibly counteract the NF-κβ-dependent activation of the above-mentioned pathways. This response results in the inhibition of p38 MAPK and NO production, as well as the consequent reduction ATP release through Cx43 hemichannels. In parallel, activation of CB_1Rs may neutralize the reduction in gap junction communication evoked by high glucose and IL-1β/TNF-α. Main inhibitors used throughout this study are shown in red.

Past research has established that plant-derived, synthetic, and endogenous CBs may provide protective actions against several cardiovascular pathologies, including ventricular arrhythmias (72) and cardiomyopathies (73). In fact, CBs diminish endothelial dysfunction by inhibiting the production of inflammatory mediators (e.g., free radical and cytokines) and their signaling pathways (e.g., NF-κβ) (53, 74). However, whether endothelial hemichannels are part of the targets involved in the anti-inflammatory actions of CBs remained unknown. Here, we observed that WIN, 2-AG, and Meth completely suppressed the Cx43 hemichannel-mediated Etd uptake induced by IL-1β/TNF-α and high glucose in EAhy cells. These preventive actions were completely neutralized by the CB_1 receptor antagonist SR1, which is in according with the participation of CB_1 receptors in Cx43 hemichannel opening (48, 50), as well as their demonstrated expression and function in endothelial cells (52, 75). Interestingly, WIN fully reduced not only the IL-1β/TNF-α and high glucose-induced Etd uptake but also significantly prevented the release of ATP triggered by these pro-inflammatory conditions. Similar inhibitory responses on Cx43 hemichannel-dependent ATP release have been observed for CBs in activated astrocytes (50). Other mechanism of hemichannel modulation different of that resulting from covalent modifications (e.g., phosphorylation and/or S-nitrosylation) is the trafficking of hemichannels to non-junctional membranes. In this study, we demonstrated that WIN fully abrogated the IL-1β/TNF-α and high glucose-induced augment in plasma membrane levels of Cx43, revealing that alterations in surface protein expression are possibly sufficient to account for the regulation of hemichannel activity triggered by IL-1β/TNF-α and high glucose or CBs in EAhy cells. It is important to mention that pharmacotherapy involving CBs is still under intense debate. The latter is mainly due to the negative side effects that CBs may exert on the nervous system and peripheral glucose metabolism (76, 77) most likely due to their low affinity to the molecular targets. Future studies will elucidate whether or not targeting specifically endothelial cells with CB receptor agonists could counteract endothelial dysfunction *in vivo*.

Multiple lines of work point out that hemichannels and gap junctions are contrarily modulated by inflammatory agents (78). In agreement with those observations, we noted that in addition to elevate endothelial Cx43 hemichannel activity, IL-1β/TNF-α and high glucose suppressed the cell-to-cell gap junctional communication in EAhy cells, as measured by intercellular LY diffusion. Relevantly, WIN fully prevented the IL-1β/TNF-α and high glucose-induced reduction in endothelial coupling *via* the activation of CB1 receptors. As deducted from western blot analysis, the modulation of dye coupling triggered by IL-1β/TNF-α and high glucose or WIN could be in part attributed to changes in Cx43 amount, namely, total reduction or increment, respectively. Moreover, immunofluorescence labeling showed no differences in the distribution of Cx43 in EAhy cells treated with IL-1β/TNF-α and high glucose alone or plus WIN, indicating that endocytosis or degradation of gap junctions do not account for the regulation of endothelial coupling.

Prior findings in diverse cell types, including endothelial cells, have revealed that ATP produces a biphasic $[Ca^{2+}]_i$ response: the release of stored Ca^{2+} (first spike) and Ca^{2+} influx from the extracellular medium (sustained response) (61, 79). The first spike in ATP-elicited $[Ca^{2+}]_i$ response depends on P2Y receptors, while the second sustained event take place due to P2X receptors. Here, we noticed that upon acute stimulation with ATP, control EAhy cells displayed a small Ca^{2+} signal peak that returned rapidly to control values. In contrast, IL-1β/TNF-α and high glucose-treated EAhy cells showed increased ATP-induced Ca^{2+} signals compared to control, particularly, in terms of peak amplitude, integrated area, and sustained signal. Notably, in these conditions the initial Ca^{2+} signal peak was inhibited by MRS2179, but not by $P2X_7$ receptor blockers, suggesting the implication of metabotropic $P2Y_1$ receptors. Given that ADP is the major ligand for $P2Y_1$ receptors, and because they participate in endothelial Ca^{2+} dynamics (80), in our studies, ADP produced from ATP conversion possibly generated the $P2Y_1$-mediated changes in $[Ca^{2+}]_i$ elicited by acute ATP application. On the other hand, the ATP-induced sustained Ca^{2+} signal detected in IL-1β/TNF-α and high glucose-stimulated EAhy cells was fully counteracted by blocking $P2X_7$ receptors, indicating that influx of Ca^{2+} is also necessary for ATP-induced Ca^{2+} signal in EAhy cells. Interestingly, the above Ca^{2+} response associated with $P2Y_1/P2X_7$ receptors was completely inhibited by WIN-dependent activation of CB1 receptors in IL-1β/TNF-α and high glucose-stimulated EAhy cells. These data denote that ATP-mediated Ca^{2+} dynamics depend on the inflammatory profile of endothelial cells and can be antagonized by the anti-inflammatory actions of CBs (**Figure 8**). ATP released from endothelial cells could activate distant cells in a paracrine form, resulting in Ca^{2+} responses that may rely on the endothelial inflammatory profile. In this scenario, stimulation of purinergic receptors may be shut down due to diffusion of ATP to far-off areas in conjunction with desensitization of $P2Y_1$ receptors and degradation of extracellular ATP *via* exonucleases.

In endothelial cells, NO can be produced from L-arginine in a reaction catalyzed by endothelial NO synthase (eNOS) and iNOS (36, 81). Yet despite both NOS isoforms catalyze the same biochemical reaction, eNOS and iNOS are very different enzymes, being the former involved in the constitutive NO production at nanomolar levels, whereas the latter generates micromolar amounts of NO only when stimulated (82). NO exerts important vasodilatory and protective effects on the vasculature (83). However, high NO production has been linked to the pathogenesis of chronic inflammatory diseases, including atherosclerosis (63). Relevant to this point, previous studies have revealed that pro-inflammatory conditions (e.g., high glucose) elicit the formation of endothelial NO (36, 84). In agreement with this information, we identify that IL-1β/TNF-α and high glucose clearly increase NO production in EAhy cells, which could be an alternative mechanism of hemichannel regulation through the S-nitrosylation of Cx43 (37).

Insulin is a direct-acting vasodilator in intact vessels (85) and has been described to induce the production of NO in normal endothelial cells (86). Nevertheless, endothelial cells subjected to pro-inflammatory conditions, such as high glucose and cytokine treatment, loss the ability to form NO (87, 88). As expected, in control EAhy cells, insulin promoted an evident augment in NO production. Surprisingly, in EAhy cells stimulated with IL-1β/TNF-α and high glucose, the insulin-mediated NO production was higher than that of control conditions, revealing that insulin sensitivity is not inhibited. This unexpected finding might occur by the degree of inflammation developed by EAhy cells under the pro-inflammatory treatment used. Perhaps the NO response to insulin treatment become reduced at later time points not analyzed in the present work or the application of more intense pro-inflammatory conditions is required to develop that outcome. As occurred with IL-1β/TNF-α and high glucose-induced changes in hemichannel opening, ATP release and $[Ca^{2+}]_i$ dynamics, the enhanced production of NO was greatly prevented by the activation of CB_1 receptors with WIN.

High glucose and IL-1β/TNF-α are well established conditions that disturb vascular homeostasis through different cellular and molecular mechanisms (5). Here, we identify the function of endothelial Cx43 hemichannels as a new pathway affected by inflammatory mediators, revealing their possible implication in the pathogenesis of multiple vascular diseases. Supporting this idea, the increased production of NO caused by IL-1β/TNF-α and high glucose was completely impeded by blockade of endothelial Cx43 hemichannels. Furthermore, this study demonstrated that intracellular Ca^{2+} associated with COX_2/EP_1 receptor signaling and purinergic receptor activation—likely *via* ATP release—are crucial to maintain persistent opening of Cx43 hemichannels and possibly for preserving the p38 MAPK-dependent NO production observed in IL-1β/TNF-α and high glucose-stimulated endothelial cells. The above may reproduce a self-perpetuating mechanism, in which both NO or high $[Ca^{2+}]_i$ levels could reactivate Cx43 hemichannels (**Figure 8**). This phenomenon likely may lead to cell death, either by Ca^{2+} overload or through the reaction of NO with the superoxide anion, which yield peroxynitrite, a potent oxidant that alters DNA, lipids and proteins. We propose that reduction of hemichannel activity by CB agonists or selective hemichannel blockers might represent a strategy against the activation of deleterious pathways that trigger endothelial dysfunction and possibly cell damage evoked by high glucose and pro-inflammatory cytokines. The latter should favor the generation and design of novel CB agonists that could preserve their positive role without having side effects in general physiology.

ETHICS STATEMENT

This study was carried out in accordance with the recommendations of the Animal Care Guidelines of the Research Ethic Committee from the Pontificia Universidad Católica de Chile. The protocol was approved by Research Ethic Committee from the Pontificia Universidad Católica de Chile.

AUTHOR CONTRIBUTIONS

Conceived, performed, and analyzed the experiments: JAO, JCS, VV, SC-D, GG, VL, CS, RG-G, BA, ED, and TM. Wrote and edited the manuscript: JAO, JCS, and VV. All authors read and approved the final manuscript.

ACKNOWLEDGMENTS

CONICYT, PIA, FONDECYT, ICM, and Pontificia Universidad Católica de Chile.

FUNDING

This work was supported by the Fondo Nacional de Desarrollo Científico y Tecnológico (FONDECYT) Grant 1160710 (to JAO), 1150291 (to JCS), the Comisión Nacional de Investigación Científica y Tecnológica (CONICYT) and Programa de Investigación Asociativa (PIA) Grant Anillo de Ciencia y Tecnología ACT1411 (to JAO), P09-022-F from ICM-ECONOMIA, Chile (to JCS).

SUPPLEMENTARY MATERIAL

FIGURE S1 | Etd uptake induced by high glucose and IL-1β/TNF-α is not related to osmolarity changes, whereas high glucose/IL-1β/TNF-α plus WIN do not affect connexin 43 (Cx43) distribution in endothelial cells. **(A)** Averaged Etd uptake rate normalized with respect to control condition (dashed line) of EAhy cells treated for 72 h with 5 mM glucose and IL-1β/TNF-α alone or in combination with 20 or 40 mM sucrose or 20 or 40 mM mannitol. Data were obtained from three independent experiments (see scatter dot plot) with two repeats each one (≥35 cells analyzed for each repeat). **(B,C)** Representative fluorescence images depicting Cx43 (green), tubulin (red), and DAPI (blue) immunolabeling of EAhy cells treated for 72 h with 25 mM glucose plus IL-1β/TNF-α and 5 μM WIN. Insets: 1.7× magnification of the indicated area of panels **(C)**. Calibration bars: white = 35 μm, yellow = 60 μm, and green = 25 μm.

FIGURE S2 | High glucose and IL-1β/TNF-α increase the activity of connexin 43 hemichannels and nitric oxide production in HUVEC endothelial cells. **(A)** Averaged Etd uptake rate normalized with control condition (dashed line) by HUVEC cells treated for 72 h with 25 mM glucose and IL-1β/TNF-α alone or in combination with the following blockers: 100 μM gap26, 100 μM ^{10}panx1, 10 μM WIN or 5 μM WIN plus 5 μM SR-141716A (SR1). $^{*}p < 0.05$, IL-1β/TNF-α and high glucose compared to control; $^{\#}p < 0.05$, effect of blockers compared IL-1β/TNF-α and high glucose. **(B)** Average of DAF fluorescence by HUVEC cells treated for 72 h with 5 mM glucose (control; white bars), 25 mM glucose and IL-1β/TNF-α (red bars) alone or with different combinations of the following compounds: 5 μM WIN (WIN), 5 μM SR-141716A (SR1), 1 μM insulin or 100 μM gap26. $^{*}p < 0.05$, IL-1β/TNF-α and high glucose compared to control; $^{\#}p < 0.05$, effect of each compound compared to the effect induced by IL-1β/TNF-α and high glucose; $^{\&}p < 0.05$, effect of each cannabinoid receptor antagonist compared to the effect of the respective cannabinoid; $^{\Psi}p < 0.05$, effect of insulin compared to the respective control (one-way analysis of variance followed by Tukey's *post hoc* test). Data were obtained from three independent experiments (see scatter dot plot) with three repeats each one (≥35 cells analyzed for each repeat).

REFERENCES

1. McCarron JG, Lee MD, Wilson C. The endothelium solves problems that endothelial cells do not know exist. *Trends Pharmacol Sci* (2017) 38:322–38. doi:10.1016/j.tips.2017.01.008
2. Pober JS, Sessa WC. Inflammation and the blood microvascular system. *Cold Spring Harb Perspect Biol* (2014) 7:a016345. doi:10.1101/cshperspect.a016345
3. Vestweber D. How leukocytes cross the vascular endothelium. *Nat Rev Immunol* (2015) 15:692–704. doi:10.1038/nri3908
4. Cahill PA, Redmond EM. Vascular endothelium – gatekeeper of vessel health. *Atherosclerosis* (2016) 248:97–109. doi:10.1016/j.atherosclerosis.2016.03.007
5. Hansen NW, Hansen AJ, Sams A. The endothelial border to health: mechanistic evidence of the hyperglycemic culprit of inflammatory disease acceleration. *IUBMB Life* (2017) 69:148–61. doi:10.1002/iub.1610
6. Meunier C, Wang N, Yi C, Dallerac G, Ezan P, Koulakoff A, et al. Contribution of astroglial Cx43 hemichannels to the modulation of glutamatergic currents by D-serine in the mouse prefrontal cortex. *J Neurosci* (2017) 37:9064–75. doi:10.1523/JNEUROSCI.2204-16.2017
7. Bol M, Wang N, De Bock M, Wacquier B, Decrock E, Gadicherla A, et al. At the cross-point of connexins, calcium, and ATP: blocking hemichannels inhibits vasoconstriction of rat small mesenteric arteries. *Cardiovasc Res* (2017) 113:195–206. doi:10.1093/cvr/cvw215
8. Orellana JA, Sáez PJ, Cortes-Campos C, Elizondo RJ, Shoji KF, Contreras-Duarte S, et al. Glucose increases intracellular free Ca(2+) in tanycytes via ATP released through connexin 43 hemichannels. *Glia* (2012) 60:53–68. doi:10.1002/glia.21246
9. Sáez JC, Leybaert L. Hunting for connexin hemichannels. *FEBS Lett* (2014) 588:1205–11. doi:10.1016/j.febslet.2014.03.004
10. Sáez JC, Berthoud VM, Branes MC, Martinez AD, Beyer EC. Plasma membrane channels formed by connexins: their regulation and functions. *Physiol Rev* (2003) 83:1359–400. doi:10.1152/physrev.00007.2003
11. Leybaert L, Lampe PD, Dhein S, Kwak BR, Ferdinandy P, Beyer EC, et al. Connexins in cardiovascular and neurovascular health and disease: pharmacological implications. *Pharmacol Rev* (2017) 69:396–478. doi:10.1124/pr.115.012062
12. Kim Y, Davidson JO, Gunn KC, Phillips AR, Green CR, Gunn AJ. Role of hemichannels in CNS inflammation and the inflammasome pathway. *Adv Protein Chem Struct Biol* (2016) 104:1–37. doi:10.1016/bs.apcsb.2015.12.001
13. Esposito K, Nappo F, Marfella R, Giugliano G, Giugliano F, Ciotola M, et al. Inflammatory cytokine concentrations are acutely increased by hyperglycemia in humans: role of oxidative stress. *Circulation* (2002) 106:2067–72. doi:10.1161/01.CIR.0000034509.14906.AE
14. Stentz FB, Umpierrez GE, Cuervo R, Kitabchi AE. Proinflammatory cytokines, markers of cardiovascular risks, oxidative stress, and lipid peroxidation in patients with hyperglycemic crises. *Diabetes* (2004) 53:2079–86. doi:10.2337/diabetes.53.8.2079
15. Ling PR, Mueller C, Smith RJ, Bistrian BR. Hyperglycemia induced by glucose infusion causes hepatic oxidative stress and systemic inflammation, but not STAT3 or MAP kinase activation in liver in rats. *Metabolism* (2003) 52:868–74. doi:10.1016/S0026-0495(03)00057-X
16. Li J, Huang M, Shen X. The association of oxidative stress and pro-inflammatory cytokines in diabetic patients with hyperglycemic crisis. *J Diabetes Complications* (2014) 28:662–6. doi:10.1016/j.jdiacomp.2014.06.008
17. Urata Y, Yamamoto H, Goto S, Tsushima H, Akazawa S, Yamashita S, et al. Long exposure to high glucose concentration impairs the responsive expression of gamma-glutamylcysteine synthetase by interleukin-1beta and tumor necrosis

factor-alpha in mouse endothelial cells. *J Biol Chem* (1996) 271:15146–52. doi:10.1074/jbc.271.25.15146

18. Nahomi RB, Palmer A, Green KM, Fort PE, Nagaraj RH. Pro-inflammatory cytokines downregulate Hsp27 and cause apoptosis of human retinal capillary endothelial cells. *Biochim Biophys Acta* (2014) 1842:164–74. doi:10.1016/j.bbadis.2013.11.011
19. Takeuchi H, Jin S, Wang J, Zhang G, Kawanokuchi J, Kuno R, et al. Tumor necrosis factor-alpha induces neurotoxicity via glutamate release from hemichannels of activated microglia in an autocrine manner. *J Biol Chem* (2006) 281(30):21362–8. doi:10.1074/jbc.M600504200
20. Retamal MA, Froger N, Palacios-Prado N, Ezan P, Sáez PJ, Sáez JC, et al. Cx43 hemichannels and gap junction channels in astrocytes are regulated oppositely by proinflammatory cytokines released from activated microglia. *J Neurosci* (2007) 27:13781–92. doi:10.1523/JNEUROSCI.2042-07.2007
21. Orellana JA, Hernandez DE, Ezan P, Velarde V, Bennett MV, Giaume C, et al. Hypoxia in high glucose followed by reoxygenation in normal glucose reduces the viability of cortical astrocytes through increased permeability of connexin 43 hemichannels. *Glia* (2010) 58:329–43. doi:10.1002/glia.20926
22. Abudara V, Roux L, Dallerac G, Matias I, Dulong J, Mothet JP, et al. Activated microglia impairs neuroglial interaction by opening Cx43 hemichannels in hippocampal astrocytes. *Glia* (2015) 63:795–811. doi:10.1002/glia.22785
23. Mugisho OO, Green CR, Kho DT, Zhang J, Graham ES, Acosta ML, et al. The inflammasome pathway is amplified and perpetuated in an autocrine manner through connexin43 hemichannel mediated ATP release. *Biochim Biophys Acta* (2018) 1862:385–93. doi:10.1016/j.bbagen.2017.11.015
24. Cea LA, Riquelme MA, Cisterna BA, Puebla C, Vega JL, Rovegno M, et al. Connexin- and pannexin-based channels in normal skeletal muscles and their possible role in muscle atrophy. *J Membr Biol* (2012) 245:423–36. doi:10.1007/s00232-012-9485-8
25. Hernandez-Salinas R, Vielma AZ, Arismendi MN, Boric MP, Sáez JC, Velarde V. Boldine prevents renal alterations in diabetic rats. *J Diabetes Res* (2013) 2013:593672. doi:10.1155/2013/593672
26. Johnson RG, Le HC, Evenson K, Loberg SW, Myslajek TM, Prabhu A, et al. Connexin hemichannels: methods for dye uptake and leakage. *J Membr Biol* (2016) 249:713–41. doi:10.1007/s00232-016-9925-y
27. Robertson J, Lang S, Lambert PA, Martin PE. Peptidoglycan derived from *Staphylococcus epidermidis* induces Connexin43 hemichannel activity with consequences on the innate immune response in endothelial cells. *Biochem J* (2010) 432:133–43. doi:10.1042/BJ20091753
28. Danesh-Meyer HV, Kerr NM, Zhang J, Eady EK, O'carroll SJ, Nicholson LF, et al. Connexin43 mimetic peptide reduces vascular leak and retinal ganglion cell death following retinal ischaemia. *Brain* (2012) 135:506–20. doi:10.1093/brain/awr338
29. D'Hondt C, Himpens B, Bultynck G. Mechanical stimulation-induced calcium wave propagation in cell monolayers: the example of bovine corneal endothelial cells. *J Vis Exp* (2013) 77:e50443. doi:10.3791/50443
30. Godecke S, Roderigo C, Rose CR, Rauch BH, Godecke A, Schrader J. Thrombin-induced ATP release from human umbilical vein endothelial cells. *Am J Physiol Cell Physiol* (2012) 302:C915–23. doi:10.1152/ajpcell.00283.2010
31. Kaneko Y, Tachikawa M, Akaogi R, Fujimoto K, Ishibashi M, Uchida Y, et al. Contribution of pannexin 1 and connexin 43 hemichannels to extracellular calcium-dependent transport dynamics in human blood-brain barrier endothelial cells. *J Pharmacol Exp Ther* (2015) 353:192–200. doi:10.1124/jpet.114.220210
32. Bond SR, Naus CC. The pannexins: past and present. *Front Physiol* (2014) 5:58. doi:10.3389/fphys.2014.00058
33. Ponsaerts R, De Vuyst E, Retamal M, D'hondt C, Vermeire D, Wang N, et al. Intramolecular loop/tail interactions are essential for connexin 43-hemichannel activity. *FASEB J* (2010) 24:4378–95. doi:10.1096/fj.09-153007
34. Wang N, De Bock M, Decrock E, Bola M, Gadicherla A, Bultynck G, et al. Connexin targeting peptides as inhibitors of voltage- and intracellular Ca2+-triggered Cx43 hemichannel opening. *Neuropharmacology* (2013) 75:506–16. doi:10.1016/j.neuropharm.2013.08.021
35. Kuwano T, Nakao S, Yamamoto H, Tsuneyoshi M, Yamamoto T, Kuwano M, et al. Cyclooxygenase 2 is a key enzyme for inflammatory cytokine-induced angiogenesis. *FASEB J* (2004) 18:300–10. doi:10.1096/fj.03-0473com
36. Cortese-Krott MM, Kulakov L, Oplander C, Kolb-Bachofen V, Kroncke KD, Suschek CV. Zinc regulates iNOS-derived nitric oxide formation in endothelial cells. *Redox Biol* (2014) 2:945–54. doi:10.1016/j.redox.2014.06.011
37. Retamal MA, Cortes CJ, Reuss L, Bennett MV, Sáez JC. S-nitrosylation and permeation through connexin 43 hemichannels in astrocytes: induction by oxidant stress and reversal by reducing agents. *Proc Natl Acad Sci U S A* (2006) 103:4475–80. doi:10.1073/pnas.0511118103
38. Orellana JA, Busso D, Ramirez G, Campos M, Rigotti A, Eugenin J, et al. Prenatal nicotine exposure enhances Cx43 and Panx1 unopposed channel activity in brain cells of adult offspring mice fed a high-fat/cholesterol diet. *Front Cell Neurosci* (2014) 8:403. doi:10.3389/fncel.2014.00403
39. Avendano BC, Montero TD, Chavez CE, Von Bernhardi R, Orellana JA. Prenatal exposure to inflammatory conditions increases Cx43 and Panx1 unopposed channel opening and activation of astrocytes in the offspring effect on neuronal survival. *Glia* (2015) 63(11):2058–72. doi:10.1002/glia.22877
40. Liu ZF, Zheng D, Fan GC, Peng T, Su L. Heat stress prevents lipopolysaccharide-induced apoptosis in pulmonary microvascular endothelial cells by blocking calpain/p38 MAPK signalling. *Apoptosis* (2016) 21:896–904. doi:10.1007/s10495-016-1263-0
41. Pan W, Yu H, Huang S, Zhu P. Resveratrol protects against TNF-alpha-induced injury in human umbilical endothelial cells through promoting sirtuin-1-induced repression of NF-KB and p38 MAPK. *PLoS One* (2016) 11:e0147034. doi:10.1371/journal.pone.0147034
42. Swierkosz TA, Mitchell JA, Warner TD, Botting RM, Vane JR. Co-induction of nitric oxide synthase and cyclo-oxygenase: interactions between nitric oxide and prostanoids. *Br J Pharmacol* (1995) 114:1335–42. doi:10.1111/j.1476-5381.1995.tb13353.x
43. Park S, Sung B, Jang EJ, Kim DH, Park CH, Choi YJ, et al. Inhibitory action of salicylideneamino-2-thiophenol on NF-kappaB signaling cascade and cyclooxygenase-2 in HNE-treated endothelial cells. *Arch Pharm Res* (2013) 36:880–9. doi:10.1007/s12272-013-0116-4
44. Woodward DF, Jones RL, Narumiya S. International Union of basic and clinical pharmacology. LXXXIII: classification of prostanoid receptors, updating 15 years of progress. *Pharmacol Rev* (2011) 63:471–538. doi:10.1124/pr.110.003517
45. De Bock M, Wang N, Bol M, Decrock E, Ponsaerts R, Bultynck G, et al. Connexin 43 hemichannels contribute to cytoplasmic Ca2+ oscillations by providing a bimodal Ca2+-dependent Ca2+ entry pathway. *J Biol Chem* (2012) 287:12250–66. doi:10.1074/jbc.M111.299610
46. Baroja-Mazo A, Barbera-Cremades M, Pelegrin P. The participation of plasma membrane hemichannels to purinergic signaling. *Biochim Biophys Acta* (2013) 1828:79–93. doi:10.1016/j.bbamem.2012.01.002
47. Chi Y, Gao K, Li K, Nakajima S, Kira S, Takeda M, et al. Purinergic control of AMPK activation by ATP released through connexin 43 hemichannels – pivotal roles in hemichannel-mediated cell injury. *J Cell Sci* (2014) 127:1487–99. doi:10.1242/jcs.139089
48. Froger N, Orellana JA, Cohen-Salmon M, Ezan P, Amigou E, Sáez JC, et al. Cannabinoids prevent the opposite regulation of astroglial connexin43 hemichannels and gap junction channels induced by pro-inflammatory treatments. *J Neurochem* (2009) 111:1383–97. doi:10.1111/j.1471-4159.2009.06407.x
49. Froger N, Orellana JA, Calvo CF, Amigou E, Kozoriz MG, Naus CC, et al. Inhibition of cytokine-induced connexin43 hemichannel activity in astrocytes is neuroprotective. *Mol Cell Neurosci* (2010) 45:37–46. doi:10.1016/j.mcn.2010.05.007
50. Gajardo-Gomez R, Labra VC, Maturana CJ, Shoji KF, Santibanez CA, Sáez JC, et al. Cannabinoids prevent the amyloid beta-induced activation of astroglial hemichannels: a neuroprotective mechanism. *Glia* (2017) 65:122–37. doi:10.1002/glia.23080
51. Piomelli D. The molecular logic of endocannabinoid signalling. *Nat Rev Neurosci* (2003) 4:873–84. doi:10.1038/nrn1247
52. Gasperi V, Evangelista D, Chiurchiu V, Florenzano F, Savini I, Oddi S, et al. 2-Arachidonoylglycerol modulates human endothelial cell/leukocyte interactions by controlling selectin expression through CB1 and CB2 receptors. *Int J Biochem Cell Biol* (2014) 51:79–88. doi:10.1016/j.biocel.2014.03.028
53. Wilhelmsen K, Khakpour S, Tran A, Sheehan K, Schumacher M, Xu F, et al. The endocannabinoid/endovanilloid N-arachidonoyl dopamine (NADA) and synthetic cannabinoid WIN55,212-2 abate the inflammatory activation of human endothelial cells. *J Biol Chem* (2014) 289:13079–100. doi:10.1074/jbc.M113.536953
54. Schalper KA, Palacios-Prado N, Retamal MA, Shoji KF, Martinez AD, Sáez JC. Connexin hemichannel composition determines the FGF-1-induced membrane permeability and free [Ca2+]i responses. *Mol Biol Cell* (2008) 19:3501–13. doi:10.1091/mbc.e07-12-1240

55. Figueroa XF, Duling BR. Gap junctions in the control of vascular function. *Antioxid Redox Signal* (2009) 11:251–66. doi:10.1089/ars.2008.2117
56. Kim Y, Griffin JM, Harris PWR, Chan SHC, Nicholson LFB, Brimble MA, et al. Characterizing the mode of action of extracellular connexin43 channel blocking mimetic peptides in an in vitro ischemia injury model. *Biochim Biophys Acta* (2017) 1861:68–78. doi:10.1016/j.bbagen.2016.11.001
57. McDonald B, Pittman K, Menezes GB, Hirota SA, Slaba I, Waterhouse CCM, et al. Intravascular danger signals guide neutrophils to sites of sterile inflammation. *Science* (2010) 330:362–6. doi:10.1126/science.1195491
58. Moccia F, Tanzi F, Munaron L. Endothelial remodelling and intracellular calcium machinery. *Curr Mol Med* (2014) 14:457–80. doi:10.2174/15665240 13666131118113410
59. Di A, Mehta D, Malik AB. ROS-activated calcium signaling mechanisms regulating endothelial barrier function. *Cell Calcium* (2016) 60:163–71. doi:10.1016/j.ceca.2016.02.002
60. De Bock M, Wang N, Decrock E, Bol M, Gadicherla AK, Culot M, et al. Endothelial calcium dynamics, connexin channels and blood-brain barrier function. *Prog Neurobiol* (2013) 108:1–20. doi:10.1016/j.pneurobio.2013.06.001
61. Lyubchenko T, Woodward H, Veo KD, Burns N, Nijmeh H, Liubchenko GA, et al. P2Y1 and P2Y13 purinergic receptors mediate Ca2+ signaling and proliferative responses in pulmonary artery vasa vasorum endothelial cells. *Am J Physiol Cell Physiol* (2011) 300:C266–75. doi:10.1152/ajpcell.00237.2010
62. Green JP, Souilhol C, Xanthis I, Martinez-Campesino L, Bowden NP, Evans PC, et al. Atheroprone flow activates inflammation via endothelial ATP-dependent P2X7-p38 signalling. *Cardiovasc Res* (2018) 114:324–35. doi:10.1093/cvr/cvx213
63. Lind M, Hayes A, Caprnda M, Petrovic D, Rodrigo L, Kruzliak P, et al. Inducible nitric oxide synthase: good or bad? *Biomed Pharmacother* (2017) 93:370–5. doi:10.1016/j.biopha.2017.06.036
64. Muniyappa R, Sowers JR. Role of insulin resistance in endothelial dysfunction. *Rev Endocr Metab Disord* (2013) 14:5–12. doi:10.1007/s11154-012-9229-1
65. Bundey RA, Insel PA. Adenylyl cyclase 6 overexpression decreases the permeability of endothelial monolayers via preferential enhancement of prostacyclin receptor function. *Mol Pharmacol* (2006) 70:1700–7. doi:10.1124/mol.106.028035
66. Vandamme W, Braet K, Cabooter L, Leybaert L. Tumour necrosis factor alpha inhibits purinergic calcium signalling in blood-brain barrier endothelial cells. *J Neurochem* (2004) 88:411–21. doi:10.1046/j.1471-4159.2003.02163.x
67. Lohman AW, Leskov IL, Butcher JT, Johnstone SR, Stokes TA, Begandt D, et al. Pannexin 1 channels regulate leukocyte emigration through the venous endothelium during acute inflammation. *Nat Commun* (2015) 6:7965. doi:10.1038/ncomms8965
68. Sathanoori R, Sward K, Olde B, Erlinge D. The ATP receptors P2X7 and P2X4 modulate high glucose and palmitate-induced inflammatory responses in endothelial cells. *PLoS One* (2015) 10:e0125111. doi:10.1371/journal.pone.0125111
69. Kang J, Kang N, Lovatt D, Torres A, Zhao Z, Lin J, et al. Connexin 43 hemichannels are permeable to ATP. *J Neurosci* (2008) 28:4702–11. doi:10.1523/JNEUROSCI.5048-07.2008
70. Schalper KA, Sanchez HA, Lee SC, Altenberg GA, Nathanson MH, Saez JC. Connexin 43 hemichannels mediate the Ca2+ influx induced by extracellular alkalinization. *Am J Physiol Cell Physiol* (2010) 299:C1504–15. doi:10.1152/ajpcell.00015.2010
71. Schulz R, Heusch G. Connexin 43 and ischemic preconditioning. *Cardiovasc Res* (2004) 62:335–44. doi:10.1016/j.cardiores.2003.12.017
72. Gonca E, Darici F. The effect of cannabidiol on ischemia/reperfusion-induced ventricular arrhythmias: the role of adenosine A1 receptors. *J Cardiovasc Pharmacol Ther* (2015) 20:76–83. doi:10.1177/1074248414532013
73. Hao E, Mukhopadhyay P, Cao Z, Erdelyi K, Holovac E, Liaudet L, et al. Cannabidiol protects against doxorubicin-induced cardiomyopathy by modulating mitochondrial function and biogenesis. *Mol Med* (2015) 21:38–45. doi:10.2119/molmed.2014.00261
74. Rajesh M, Mukhopadhyay P, Batkai S, Hasko G, Liaudet L, Huffman JW, et al. CB2-receptor stimulation attenuates TNF-alpha-induced human endothelial cell activation, transendothelial migration of monocytes, and monocyte-endothelial adhesion. *Am J Physiol Heart Circ Physiol* (2007) 293:H2210–8. doi:10.1152/ajpheart.00688.2007
75. Sanchez-Pastor E, Andrade F, Sanchez-Pastor JM, Elizalde A, Huerta M, Virgen-Ortiz A, et al. Cannabinoid receptor type 1 activation by arachidonylcyclopropylamide in rat aortic rings causes vasorelaxation involving calcium-activated potassium channel subunit alpha-1 and calcium channel, voltage-dependent, L type, alpha 1C subunit. *Eur J Pharmacol* (2014) 729:100–6. doi:10.1016/j.ejphar.2014.02.016
76. Gruden G, Barutta F, Kunos G, Pacher P. Role of the endocannabinoid system in diabetes and diabetic complications. *Br J Pharmacol* (2016) 173:1116–27. doi:10.1111/bph.13226
77. Cohen K, Weinstein AM. Synthetic and non-synthetic cannabinoid drugs and their adverse effects-a review from public health prospective. *Front Public Health* (2018) 6:162. doi:10.3389/fpubh.2018.00162
78. De Bock M, Decrock E, Wang N, Bol M, Vinken M, Bultynck G, et al. The dual face of connexin-based astroglial Ca(2+) communication: a key player in brain physiology and a prime target in pathology. *Biochim Biophys Acta* (2014) 1843:2211–32. doi:10.1016/j.bbamcr.2014.04.016
79. Choi J, Hammer LW, Hester RL. Calcium-dependent synthesis of prostacyclin in ATP-stimulated venous endothelial cells. *Hypertension* (2002) 39:581–5. doi:10.1161/hy0202.103289
80. Moccia F, Baruffi S, Spaggiari S, Coltrini D, Berra-Romani R, Signorelli S, et al. P2y1 and P2y2 receptor-operated Ca2+ signals in primary cultures of cardiac microvascular endothelial cells. *Microvasc Res* (2001) 61:240–52. doi:10.1006/mvre.2001.2306
81. Heiss C, Rodriguez-Mateos A, Kelm M. Central role of eNOS in the maintenance of endothelial homeostasis. *Antioxid Redox Signal* (2015) 22:1230–42. doi:10.1089/ars.2014.6158
82. Forstermann U, Sessa WC. Nitric oxide synthases: regulation and function. *Eur Heart J* (2012) 33:829–37, 837a–d. doi:10.1093/eurheartj/ehr304
83. Shu X, Keller TCT, Begandt D, Butcher JT, Biwer L, Keller AS, et al. Endothelial nitric oxide synthase in the microcirculation. *Cell Mol Life Sci* (2015) 72:4561–75. doi:10.1007/s00018-015-2021-0
84. Cosentino F, Hishikawa K, Katusic ZS, Luscher TF. High glucose increases nitric oxide synthase expression and superoxide anion generation in human aortic endothelial cells. *Circulation* (1997) 96:25–8. doi:10.1161/01.CIR.96.1.25
85. Scherrer U, Randin D, Vollenweider P, Vollenweider L, Nicod P. Nitric oxide release accounts for insulin's vascular effects in humans. *J Clin Invest* (1994) 94:2511–5. doi:10.1172/JCI117621
86. Zeng GY, Quon MJ. Insulin-stimulated production of nitric oxide is inhibited by wortmannin – direct measurement in vascular endothelial cells. *J Clin Invest* (1996) 98:894–8. doi:10.1172/JCI118871
87. Salt IP, Morrow VA, Brandie FM, Connell JM, Petrie JR. High glucose inhibits insulin-stimulated nitric oxide production without reducing endothelial nitric-oxide synthase Ser1177 phosphorylation in human aortic endothelial cells. *J Biol Chem* (2003) 278:18791–7. doi:10.1074/jbc.M210618200
88. Andreozzi F, Laratta E, Procopio C, Hribal ML, Sciacqua A, Perticone M, et al. Interleukin-6 impairs the insulin signaling pathway, promoting production of nitric oxide in human umbilical vein endothelial cells. *Mol Cell Biol* (2007) 27:2372–83. doi:10.1128/MCB.01340-06

11

Mast Cells in Cardiac Fibrosis: New Insights Suggest Opportunities for Intervention

Stephanie A. Legere[1], Ian D. Haidl[1], Jean-François Légaré[2,3] and Jean S. Marshall[1,2*]

[1] Departments of Microbiology and Immunology, Dalhousie University, Halifax, NS, Canada, [2] Department of Pathology, Dalhousie University, Halifax, NS, Canada, [3] Department of Surgery, Dalhousie Medicine New Brunswick, Saint John, NB, Canada

***Correspondence:**
Jean S. Marshall
jean.marshall@dal.ca

Mast cells (MC) are innate immune cells present in virtually all body tissues with key roles in allergic disease and host defense. MCs recognize damage-associated molecular patterns (DAMPs) through expression of multiple receptors including Toll-like receptors and the IL-33 receptor ST2. MCs can be activated to degranulate and release pre-formed mediators, to synthesize and secrete cytokines and chemokines without degranulation, and/or to produce lipid mediators. MC numbers are generally increased at sites of fibrosis. They are potent, resident, effector cells producing mediators that regulate the fibrotic process. The nature of the secretory products produced by MCs depend on micro-environmental signals and can be both pro- and anti-fibrotic. MCs have been repeatedly implicated in the pathogenesis of cardiac fibrosis and in angiogenic responses in hypoxic tissues, but these findings are controversial. Several rodent studies have indicated a protective role for MCs. MC-deficient mice have been reported to have poorer outcomes after coronary artery ligation and increased cardiac function upon MC reconstitution. In contrast, MCs have also been implicated as key drivers of fibrosis. MC stabilization during a hypertensive rat model and an atrial fibrillation mouse model rescued associated fibrosis. Discrepancies in the literature could be related to problems with mouse models of MC deficiency. To further complicate the issue, mice generally have a much lower density of MCs in their cardiac tissue than humans, and as such comparing MC deficient and MC containing mouse models is not necessarily reflective of the role of MCs in human disease. In this review, we will evaluate the literature regarding the role of MCs in cardiac fibrosis with an emphasis on what is known about MC biology, in this context. MCs have been well-studied in allergic disease and multiple pharmacological tools are available to regulate their function. We will identify potential opportunities to manipulate human MC function and the impact of their mediators with a view to preventing or reducing harmful fibrosis. Important therapeutic opportunities could arise from increased understanding of the impact of such potent, resident immune cells, with the ability to profoundly alter long term fibrotic processes.

Keywords: mast cell, cardiac fibrosis, inflammation, tissue remodeling, immunology

INTRODUCTION

Mast cells (MCs) are tissue-specific innate immune cells located in sites throughout the body, including the heart (1). After differentiation from hematopoietic stem cells along the myeloid pathway, committed MC precursors which can be identified by flow cytometry transiently travel through the blood and enter into tissues to differentiate into a terminal tissue-specific MC phenotype (2). Degranulated mast cells can be identified in most species by their expression of c-Kit, FCεRI and mast cell specific proteases. MCs are known as sentinel cells, surveying the microenvironment and responding to stimuli via expression of Pattern Recognition Receptors (PRRs) that detect Pathogen and Damage-Associated Molecular Patterns (PAMPs and DAMPs) (3, 4). MCs respond in several ways: (1) they can be activated to degranulate and release stores of pre-formed mediators from their characteristic granules, (2) they can synthesize and secrete mediators *de novo* without degranulation, or (3) a combination of degranulation and *de novo* synthesis can occur.

MC degranulation occurs not only in the context of allergy (5), but also in viral infection (6, 7), skin burns (8), fractures (9), and cardiac (10) and liver ischemia reperfusion injury (11, 12). MC degranulation is associated with pro-inflammatory effects, primarily due to release of histamine, tumor necrosis factor [TNF], and proteases. MC granules contain a plethora of mediators including, but not limited to: MC-specific and non-specific proteases (tryptase, chymase, cathepsin G), lysosomal enzymes (β-hexosaminidase), biogenic amines (histamine, serotonin, dopamine), cytokines (TNF, interleukin[IL]-4, IL-5), and growth factors (stem cell factor [SCF], basic fibroblast growth factor [bFGF]) (13). Overall, MC degranulation is an important contributor to inflammatory processes in injury and infection.

MCs are multi-functional cells capable of discrete as well as overwhelming responses and have ongoing immune regulatory and sentinel roles. They can selectively secrete numerous mediators that range from pro-inflammatory (IL-1β, IL-6, interferon[IFN]-γ) to anti-inflammatory (IL-10, IL-13), as well as pro-fibrotic (transforming growth factor-β1 [TGF-β1], bFGF) and anti-fibrotic (vascular endothelial growth factor [VEGF], IL-33, prostaglandin D_2 [PGD_2]) (14–17). Given the potential for MCs to produce pro- and anti-fibrotic mediators, their role in tissue remodeling is controversial. Local stimuli present after tissue injury and during wound healing can result in vastly different MC responses.

After myocardial infarction (MI), wound healing restores function to damaged tissue. Fibrosis is the deposition of a collagen-based scar mediated by fibroblasts, which differentiate upon activation into myofibroblasts for collagen deposition. Normally, fibrotic deposition is essential to restore proper function, but excessive remodeling decreases contractility and cardiac function leading to chronic heart failure (18–20). Cardiac tissue resident MCs respond to DAMPs after injury to influence the progression of cardiac remodeling. Yet the exact role of MCs in cardiac fibrosis is controversial, as numerous studies have ascribed detrimental, neutral and beneficial roles (**Table 1**). Achieving a better understanding of how the multifaceted MC response influences post-MI healing should increase the potential to harness their activities and provide opportunities for therapy.

MAST CELLS AS ENHANCERS IN CARDIAC FIBROSIS

MC degranulation products have important impacts on fibrosis (**Figure 1A**), though exact cardiac degranulation stimuli are not well-defined. MC chymase and tryptase generate the active pro-fibrotic form of TGF-β1 from latent forms released by MCs during degranulation, as well as what is present in the microenvironment (44–51). TGF-β1 is important in fibrosis through promotion of fibroblast activation, myofibroblast differentiation and collagen synthesis (18, 19). MC tryptase can directly induce these actions on fibroblasts independently of TGF-β1 (52–57). *In vitro*, MC chymase induces TGF-β1 production by rat cardiac fibroblasts (58). Angiotensin II (AngII) is a major mediator of fibrosis that activates fibroblasts to the myofibroblast phenotype for proliferation and collagen deposition (18, 19). MC chymase is an angiotensin converting enzyme (ACE)-independent generator of AngII in humans, dogs and mice (20, 47, 59–61). Studies employing ACE inhibition or reduction of AngII show decreased cardiac fibrosis (62–65).

In addition to tryptase and chymase, MCs store bFGF in their granules (3, 20, 45, 66), which, as its name suggests, is another enhancer of fibrosis. MCs also serve as sources of TNF, which is released during degranulation (13) and promotes cardiac fibrosis via induction of cardiomyocyte apoptosis, inflammation and MMP-9 production (67–70). Finally, MCs produce IL-1β during degranulation (14), which promotes fibrotic remodeling of the heart in a similar manner to TNF (70–74). Although mechanisms of action are not well-elucidated, Wang et al. found that blocking TNF and IL-1β reduced cardiac remodeling and cardiomyocyte apoptosis following AngII-induced fibrosis (70).

Numerous studies have attempted to understand MC roles in cardiac fibrosis *in vivo* (**Table 1**). Studies in rats, dogs and mice have shown that inhibition of MC degranulation or chymase activity reduces expression of fibrosis-associated genes and collagen deposition in models of dilated cardiomyopathy (DCM), ovariectomy-induced left ventricular diastolic dysfunction and MI (22–24, 26, 29). These studies are limited in their assessment of MC function exclusively through degranulation capacity, as they did not assess MC involvement in fibrosis through *de novo* mediator production. In a spontaneously hypertensive rat (SHR) model, degranulation inhibition increased MC number observed histologically, as well as myocardial IL-10 and IL-6 content, leading to improved outcomes and reduced fibrosis compared to untreated SHR (30). MCs are well-established sources of both IL-6 and IL-10 (14, 75). Therefore these results could suggest a potential role for MCs independent of degranulation.

Studies assessing MCs in cardiac fibrosis often analyze MC density changes that occur during remodeling, concluding a pro-fibrotic role. Studies in the mouse have demonstrated peak increases in mast cells at 7 days post-MI which result from increased infiltration of mast cell precursors identified as

TABLE 1 | The role of mast cells in animal models of cardiac fibrosis.

Study	Findings	Confounder?
PRO-FIBROTIC		
Zweifel et al. (21)	Rat cardiac allograft model, fibrosis correlated to mucosal MC density	Formaldehyde fixed tissue
Palaniyandi et al. (22)	Rat dilated cardiomyopathy, degranulation inhibitor reduced fibrosis and MC density	Formaldehyde fixed tissue, fibrosis associated with granulated MC density
Kanemitsu et al. (23)	Rat MI and left ventricular repair, chymase inhibition reduced fibrosis-associated gene expression	None
Wang et al. (24)	OVX rats, degranulation inhibition reduced collagen content and MC density	Formaldehyde fixed, fibrosis associated with granulated MC density
Somasundaram et al. (25)	Canine MI, MC density elevated 7–28 dpMI, associated with increased inflammatory infiltration	Fibrosis associated with granulated MC density
Matsumoto et al. (26)	Canine heart failure, chymase inhibition decreased type I and III collagen gene expression	None
Luitel et al. (27)	Murine pulmonary artery bypass, MC density, fibrosis, hypertrophy increased 21 days post overload	Formaldehyde fixed, fibrosis associated with granulated MC density
Liao et al. (28)	Murine transverse aortic constriction, disodium cromoglycate reduced atrial fibrillation and associated fibrosis, reconstitution of WT mice with *W/W^V^* bone marrow decreased collagen content	Use of Kit-dependent MC deficient mice, formaldehyde fixed, fibrosis associated with granulated MC density, improper use of disodium cromoglycate
Wei et al. (29)	Rat MI, chymase inhibition reduced hypertrophy, fibrosis, and infarct size	None
Levick et al. (30)	Spontaneously hypertensive rats, degranulation inhibition decreased collagen volume fraction and improved outcomes	Telly's fixative (contains formaldehyde and glacial acetic acid), degranulation inhibition increased MC density and improved outcome
Akgul et al. (31)	Human end stage cardiomyopathy, positive correlation between MC and collagen content pre-LVAD that did not persist post-LVAD	Formaldehyde fixed
Dilsizian et al. (32)	Human ischemic cardiomyopathy, MCs elevated in ischemic patients	Formaldehyde fixed, fibrosis associated with granulated MC density
Batlle et al. (33)	Human idiopathic dilated cardiomyopathy, positive correlation between MC density and collagen content	Formaldehyde fixed
Roldão et al. (34)	Human Chagas disease, MC chymase content positively correlated to collagen content	Autopsy samples, no indication of fixative used
ANTI-FIBROTIC		
Joseph et al. (35)	Rat homocysteine-induced hypertrophy, *Ws/Ws* MC deficient rats have increased fibrosis and collagen content	Kit-dependent MC deficiency, formaldehyde fixed
Shao et al. (36)	Murine ischemic injury, W/W^V MC deficient mice had impaired fractional shortening and increased scar size, MC transplantation into the myocardium increased cardiac function, capillary density and decreased scar size	Kit-dependent MC deficiency, no indication of fixative used
Kwon et al. (37)	Rat MI, administration of low doses of MC granule content increased capillary density and decreased fibrosis at infarct	No indication of fixative used
Nazari et al. (38)	Murine MI, MCs injected into hearts of mice promoted mesenchymal stem cell proliferation early after MI and reduced fibrosis	No indication of fixative used
NEUTRAL		
Briest et al. (39)	Rat norepinephrine cardiac fibrosis, degranulation inhibition did not impact collagen content or gene expression	None
Buckley et al. (40)	Murine transverse aortic constriction, Wsh MC deficient mice had no difference in fibrosis compared to WT	Kit-dependent MC deficiency, formaldehyde fixed (but didn't assess MC density)
Ngkelo et al. (41)	Murine MI, $Cpa3^{cre+/-}$ mice had no difference in fibrosis compared to WT	No indication of fixative used
Frangogiannis et al. (42)	Human chronic ischemic LV dysfunction in LV samples from CABG patients, no relationship between MC density and fibrosis	Formaldehyde fixed
Milei et al. (43)	Human Chagas disease, no relationship between MC density and fibrosis	No indication of fixative used nor of disease stage, controls were autopsy samples

$Lin^-CD45^+CD34^+\beta7$-integrin$^+Fc\gamma RII/III^+$ cells. Such mast cell increases were dependent on SCF (41), and are also associated with a degree of local mast cell precursor proliferation within the heart tissue. In canine MI and murine pulmonary artery bypass models, increases in MC density occurred alongside increases in inflammatory cell infiltration (25), fibrosis and cardiomyocyte hypertrophy (27), but no mechanistic relationships were found. Studies often only identify granulated MC populations. Common

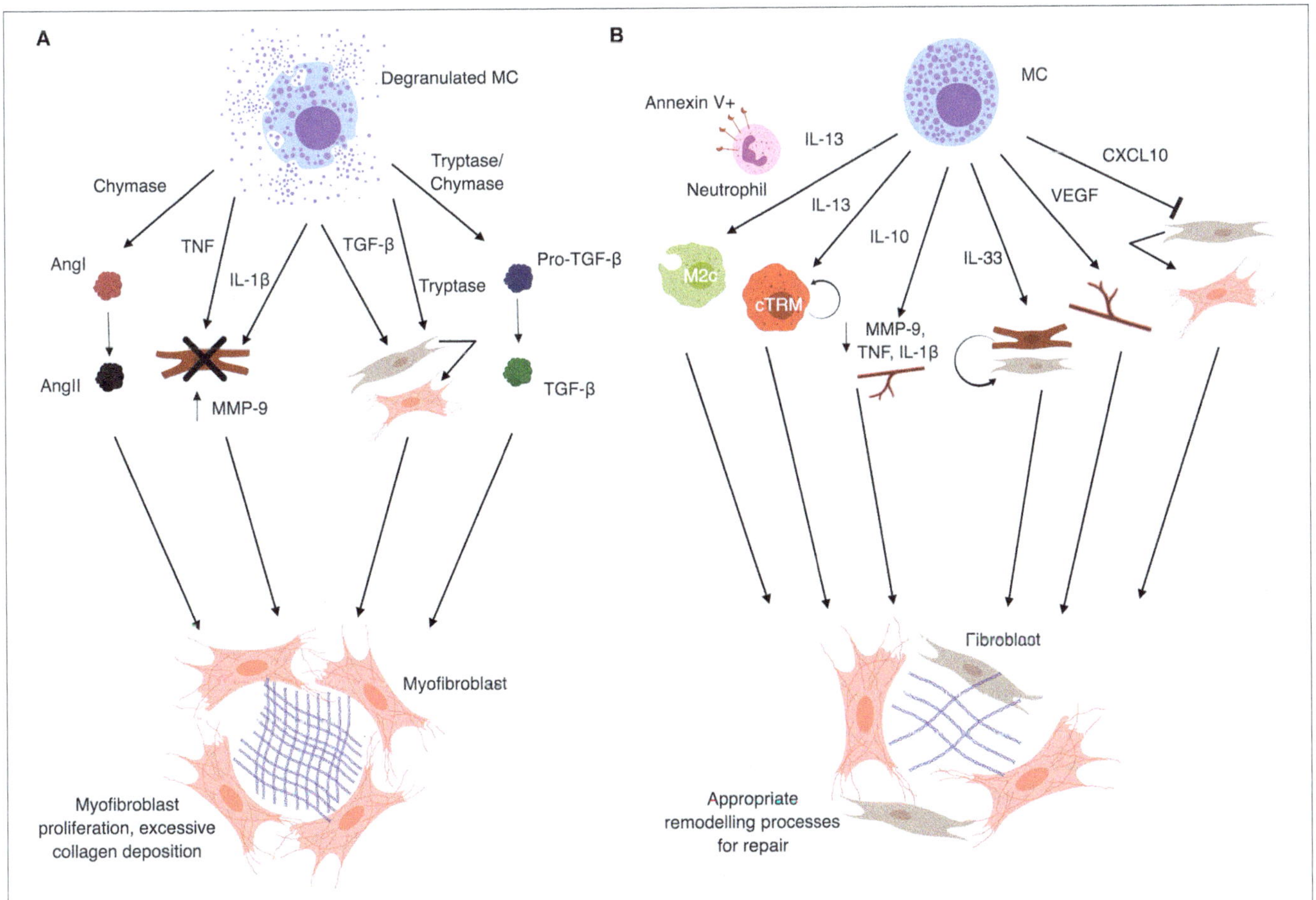

FIGURE 1 | (A) Mast cell granule products are typically associated with fibrosis. Mast cell chymase converts Angiotensin I (AngI) to AngII independently of ACE. AngII generation directly contributes to fibrosis by inducing differentiation of fibroblasts to myofibroblasts. Mast cell degranulation-derived TNF and IL-1β induce cardiomyocyte apoptosis, MMP-9 production and inflammatory cell recruitment that enhances tissue remodeling. Mast cell tryptase can act directly on fibroblasts to induce proliferation and differentiation to the myofibroblast phenotype. Tryptase and chymase both act on latent TGF-β to convert it to the active form, which also induces fibroblast differentiation to the myofibroblast phenotype and collagen deposition. Additionally, mast cells release TGF-β upon degranulation, further contributing to the activation and differentiation of fibroblasts. **(B)** Mast cell secretion products can protect against fibrosis. Mast cells can produce IL-13, which in the presence of apoptotic neutrophils can induce M2c phenotype macrophages. M2c macrophages are associated with decreased fibrosis. IL-13 can also induce proliferation of local cTRM via IL-4Rα signaling, which are known to be anti-fibrotic. Mast cells can also produce IL-10, which acts in the heart to decrease IL-1β and TNF levels, reduce MMP-9 expression and activity, and increase capillary density to reduce fibrotic remodeling. IL-33, which is released by stressed cardiomyocytes and fibroblasts, but can also be produced by mast cells, has been shown to protect cardiomyocytes and fibroblasts from death under hypoxic conditions. This results in decreased inflammation and reduction in fibrosis. VEGF, which promotes angiogenesis and recapillarization of the cardiac tissue, is associated with reduced fibrosis and is another mast cell product. Finally, CXCL10 has been shown to inhibit fibroblast migration into the myocardium and delay differentiation to the pro-fibrotic myofibroblast phenotype. Figure created in BioRender.

immunohistochemical (IHC) techniques for MCs identify granule-associated contents, ignoring populations of MCs that are not granulated, either due to immaturity or recent granule release. Additionally, MC degranulation releases SCF, a potent growth and chemotactic factor for MCs (13, 76), resulting in local proliferation (77) and recruitment (78). Therefore, increases in MC density may be due to activation of MCs from degranulation and not tissue damage.

In a transverse aortic constriction model (TAC), reconstitution of irradiated WT mice with bone marrow from W/W^{v} MC-deficient mice led to decreased collagen content compared to WT bone marrow recipients (28). MCs are radioresistant (79), therefore efficiency of MC removal after irradiation must be assessed, and was not in this paper. In a rat cardiac allograft model, fibrosis was positively correlated with certain subsets of "mucosal" MCs (MMC) but not "connective tissue"(CTMC) as defined by expression of mouse MCP-1 and MCP-2, respectively (21). This may reflect changes in the maturity of MC populations at this site and the presence of newly recruited cells. MC activation in atherosclerosis was associated with plaque progression and destabilization (80), which implicate MCs in promoting MI but does not directly link them to later fibrotic changes. Overall, MCs have the potential to promote cardiac fibrosis and increased numbers of granulated MCs are often associated with fibrosis in animal models, but mechanistic data is lacking. Care needs to be taken in experimental design to properly assess MC contribution.

MAST CELLS AS INHIBITORS OF CARDIAC FIBROSIS

MCs can synthesize and secrete a wide array of proteins without degranulating, allowing them to manipulate the cardiac microenvironment after ischemic damage or reperfusion injury in the heart (**Figure 1B**). MCs produce a wide array of pro-inflammatory cytokines and chemokines with proven roles in the recruitment of immune cells (13, 14). Conversely, MCs produce anti-inflammatory mediators such as IL-10 (75), IL-13, and CXCL10. IL-10 is known to prevent excessive cardiac remodeling via STAT3 activation and NF-κB suppression (81–83). CXCL10 acts in the damaged myocardium independently of CXCR3 to delay fibroblast migration and differentiation (84–87). While not classically considered part of the anti-fibrotic response, MCs can produce VEGF-A (13, 14), among other important angiogenic mediators, which can increase capillary density in damaged tissues and promote proper repair in cardiac and hepatic fibrosis (88–90).

IL-13 is produced by MC in response to several stimuli (14), including IL-33 (91). MCs express the IL-33 receptor ST2 abundantly on their cell surface (92–95). IL-33 is released by cardiomyocytes and fibroblasts after damage and also produced by MCs themselves (14). IL-33 is known to promote cardiomyocyte survival and reduces fibrosis after MI (96–98). Some of these actions may be via IL-13 induction. IL-13 acts on cardiac tissue resident macrophage (cTRM) populations, which are seeded embryonically in the heart and display M2-associated and anti-fibrotic phenotypes (99–102). cTRM self-renew and expand their populations in response to sterile inflammation and IL-4Rα signaling (103). Cardiac MC IL-13 production could expand the cTRM population locally. IL-13 also reduces expression of pro-inflammatory cytokines by infiltrating cells and may impact efferocytosis, the clearance of apoptotic cells from injured or inflamed tissues (104).

Anti-fibrotic roles of MCs have also been analyzed *in vivo* (**Table 1**). MC-deficient rats and mice had reduced collagen content compared to controls in models of homocysteine induced hypertrophy and coronary artery ligation (CAL) (35), while direct MC transplantation into the murine myocardium post-CAL increased cardiac function, and capillary density and decreased scar size (36). It is important to note that traditional MC-deficient models (rat and mouse) involve mutations in the gene for c-Kit (105), which encodes the SCF receptor, a growth factor critical for MCs. This mutation also reduces hematopoietic stem cells, germ cells and melanocytes, among other effects (105). MC reconstitution experiments should be performed to confirm observations are truly MC dependent, though it is not practical in all models. Several studies have focused on MC granule (MCG) contents in fibrosis. Administration MCGS isolated from rat peritoneal MCs to the myocardium during acute MI decreased fibrosis and increased capillary density. *In vitro* MCG treatment of cardiomyocytes promoted survival under hypoxic conditions (37). MCG treatment of mesenchymal stem cells (MSC) *in vitro* prevented TGF-β1 mediated transition of MSCs to myofibroblasts in an alternative fibrotic pathway (38), even though individual MC granule products chymase and tryptase are pro-fibrotic. While there is limited evidence showing MCs are protective during cardiac fibrosis, these studies indicate that MC can have an anti-fibrotic role and could potentially be targeted therapeutically.

MAST CELLS AS BYSTANDERS IN CARDIAC FIBROSIS

Several studies suggest MCs do not influence cardiac fibrosis (**Table 1**). In a norepinephrine model, rats treated with degranulation inhibitor disodium cromoglycate had comparable collagen and *Col1* mRNA content compared to untreated rats, therefore MCs were thought to be irrelevant (39). However, degranulation inhibition would have little impact on MC production of fibrosis regulating mediators. TAC of Wsh MC-deficient mice, another Kit-dependent deficiency model, resulted in hypertrophy and impaired cardiac function, but equivalent fibrosis compared to WT mice (40). Ngkelo et al. compared a newly developed MC-deficient mouse strain to a classical c-Kit mutation-dependent model. W/W^v mice and WT mice treated with disodium cromoglycate underwent MI, resulting in increased fibrosis and infarct size. Upon utilization of MC-deficient $Cpa3^{Cre/+}$ mouse model, a more MC-specific deficiency, no difference in fibrosis was observed. Rather, MCs were important in myofilament Ca^{2+} sensitization and cardiac contractility (41). It remains problematic that animal models for cardiac fibrosis are limited in their ability to mimic chronic fibrotic changes seen clinically. Several potential factors in experimental design may also contribute to discrepancies in animal models that will be discussed herein.

RELEVANCE OF RESEARCH IN HUMAN CARDIAC FIBROSIS

Similar to animal models, data on MC involvement in human cardiac fibrosis is inconsistent (**Table 1**). Several human studies of cardiovascular disease have equated increases in MC density to a detrimental role in fibrotic remodeling without a clear functional relationship between the two variables (31, 32, 106). Positive correlations were observed between MC density and collagen content in human idiopathic dilated cardiomyopathy (33), end stage cardiomyopathy (31), and Chagas disease (34). It remains unclear whether this is a protective response, epiphenomenon or pathological process. Studies also indicate that MCs have no role in human cardiac fibrosis in data from patients with ischemic LV dysfunction (42) and Chagas disease (43). Overall, data varies as to the role of MCs in human cardiac fibrosis.

Human cardiac tissue is difficult to obtain and usually received as a biopsy or autopsy sample. Biopsy samples are limited in their location and tissue volume, while autopsy samples are often delayed in being treated appropriately to preserve MC. Normal control tissues are even more difficult to obtain than diseased. Future human cardiac fibrosis studies should aim to better characterize the role of MCs in disease and expand analysis beyond histological characteristics to gain mechanistic insights necessary to design new therapeutic strategies.

CONFOUNDING FACTORS IN MAST CELL CARDIAC FIBROSIS RESEARCH

The role of MCs in cardiac fibrosis is contentious, although it is clear they have the potential to modify fibrotic responses and tissue repair. There are several potential reasons for observed discrepancies. First, mice are not an ideal model to study cardiac MCs. Unlike rats and dogs, mice have low heart MC content. Dogs on average have 6.8 $\pm$ 1.6 cardiac MCs/mm^2, while C57BL/6 mice have 0.6 $\pm$ 0.2 cardiac MCs/mm^2 (107). Data shows that MC density increases in murine hearts after damage (22, 28, 30, 33, 76, 108, 109), but it is unclear if statistically significant increases in MC content have physiological relevance, or that murine cardiac MC responses mirror those in humans. Recent evidence suggests that the distribution of mast cells in the hearts of mice also differs considerably from that in humans (110).

Second, there is widespread improper use of MC stabilizing agents. Disodium cromoglycate is used to inhibit MC degranulation in mice and rats. However, while disodium cromoglycate can inhibit IgE-dependent MC degranulation in rats, it does not inhibit this response in mice at similar or higher doses (111). This calls into question the validity of studies in which disodium cromoglycate has been used to treat mice. MC stabilization drugs only prevent calcium-dependent MC degranulation, but MC secretion of mediators independently of degranulation is not impeded.

Third, mouse models of MC deficiency involving mutations in c-Kit result in a lack of hematopoietic stem cells, germ cells, and melanocytes, among others (105). The advent of several Kit-independent models of MC deficiency have allowed researchers to determine if lack of MCs impacts the pathogenesis of various diseases, or if differences are due to deficiencies in other areas. Preferable models include Cpa3$^{Cre/+}$ and Cpa3-Cre; Mcl-1$^{fl/fl}$ mice. Discrepancies are already starting to appear (41, 112, 113), suggesting that increases or decreases in density of numerous cell types in Kit-dependent models contribute more to disease than lacking MCs. Reconstitution experiments help in this respect, but only if appropriate reconstitution can be achieved, which is not always possible.

Finally, tissue fixation for MC staining greatly impacts the ability to visualize MCs. The aldehyde tissue fixation does not allow for proper visualization of MCs, but reduces detection of MCs by 57–49% depending on the IHC method. Proper identification of MCs via IHC requires fixation with Carnoy's fixative to fully visualize MCs in tissue (114). Care needs to be taken in designing studies of MCs in cardiac fibrosis, with consideration given to the variety of actions of these cells and the difficulty of their experimental manipulation.

THERAPEUTIC APPROACHES

There are discrepancies as to the exact role of MCs in cardiac fibrosis, but it is clear that these cells have the potential to promote or protect against remodeling in the myocardium. MCs have been reported in numerous studies to be increased at sites of fibrosis (21, 25, 27, 33, 41, 76) and are a rich source of selectively induced regulatory mediators, making them a powerful target for manipulation of the remodeling myocardium. Stem cell therapies are an emerging area of research to promote cardiac regeneration after damage. Adenoviral gene transfer of SCF into pig and mouse myocardium increased c-Kit$^+$ cells following MI, and reduced fibrosis (115, 116). Direct myocardial injection of SCF following MI increased recruitment of Lin$^-$/c-Kit$^+$ cells to the heart and promoted wound healing (117). SCF is thought to recruit and induce proliferation of cardiac cells (CSC), c-Kit$^+$ bone marrow cells that regenerate damaged tissue (118, 119).

However, few efforts have been made to differentiate CSCs from MCs in cardiac tissue, often only identifying Lin$^-$/c-Kit$^+$ cells and assessing CD45 expression (116). Recent evidence suggests that in human hearts, the vast majority of c-Kit$^+$ cells are tryptase$^+$ with weak/low CD45$^+$ (120), indicating these are MCs, not CSCs. Benefits conferred by SCF expansion of c-Kit$^+$ cells could therefore be due to expansion of MC populations instead.

MC degranulation products are pro-fibrotic through several pathways (44–49, 52–57) (**Figure 1A**). Inhibiting MC degranulation or actions of MC-associated proteases promotes proper wound healing after myocardial damage (23, 26, 29, 30). MC stabilizing drugs, such as ketotifen and disodium cromoglycate, have been used in human subjects (121–125). MCs express a wide array of receptors that can be targeted for activation and secretion of chemokines, growth factors, and cytokines (13, 14) without degranulation (3, 4, 126). MC activation with IL-33 via ST2 results in production of several cytokines that may protect against remodeling (91). Examples include the aforementioned beneficial roles of IL-13 and VEGF-A. Additionally, MCs could be targeted to produce IL-33, which is known to be present in the injured myocardium and is associated with improved outcomes post MI (96–98, 127). Induction of MC IL-10 production in combination with degranulation inhibition could limit excessive production of AngII and TGF-β1 while dampening excessive remodeling processes through IL-10 inhibition of NF-κB and activation of STAT3 (81, 83). Given that MCs respond to DAMPs (e.g., IL-33) by producing mediators that are beneficial in fibrosis, blocking degranulation alone could allow them to exert beneficial effects without further stimulation that has the potential to be off target. Future studies should focus on elucidating mechanisms by which cardiac MC respond to DAMPs *in situ*, as well as the potential of a dual function therapy that blocks MC degranulation and promotes beneficial mediator production to fully harness the power of these cells.

CONCLUSION

Overall, the role of MCs in cardiac fibrosis is still not well-understood. Discrepancies exist within and between animal models, and *in vitro* data indicates a potential for pro- and anti-fibrotic activity. Future studies into the role of MCs in cardiac fibrosis should be carefully designed to use animal models with appropriate MC content and accurate MC deficiencies with confirmation by MC reconstitution. MC stabilizing drugs should also be employed with appropriate species activity. Effort should be made wherever possible to expand on the current breadth of knowledge in human patient samples, as cardiac tissue is underused but potentially valuable. Human *in vitro* models could also be employed more effectively since primary human MCs can be readily generated. MCs are situated in cardiac tissue in close proximity to the remodeling myocardium and represent a valuable target for therapeutic manipulation following cardiac damage when we have the necessary information to more reliably predict the impact of such interventions in the human cardiac setting. A better understanding of their role and activities is urgently needed to move forward in this field.

AUTHOR CONTRIBUTIONS

SL contributed to drafting and organizing the manuscript. IH provided input on the molecular and immunological aspects of the manuscript and edited the manuscript. J-FL provided input on the clinical aspects of the manuscript, assisted with writing and edited the manuscript. JM conceptualized the review, re-wrote sections of the manuscript, and edited the manuscript. All authors provided critical appraisal and approval.

FUNDING

This work was supported by the Canadian Institutes of Health research (CIHR) THC-135230, and also by Dalhousie Medical Research Foundation. SL—CIHR 394140, NS Heart and Stroke foundation Bright Red award, Killam Laureate.

ACKNOWLEDGMENTS

We would like to acknowledge funding from Canadian Institutes of Health Research, Dalhousie Medical Research Foundation, and The Nova Scotia Heart and Stroke Foundation. Additionally, we would like to thank Drs. Liliana Portales-Cervantes and Dihia Meghnem for editing assistance.

REFERENCES

1. Sperr WR, Bankl HC, Mundigler G, Klappacher G, Grossschmidt K, Agis H, et al. The human cardiac mast cell: localization, isolation, phenotype, and functional characterization. *Blood.* (1994) 84:3876–84.
2. Hallgren J, Gurish MF. Mast cell progenitor trafficking and maturation. *Adv Exp Med Biol.* (2011) 716:14–28. doi: 10.1007/978-1-4419-9533-9_2
3. Redegeld FA, Yu Y, Kumari S, Charles N, Blank U. Non-IgE mediated mast cell activation. *Immunol Rev.* (2018) 282:87–113. doi: 10.1111/imr.12629
4. Halova I, Rönnberg E, Draberova L, Vliagoftis H, Nilsson GP, Draber P. Changing the threshold—Signals and mechanisms of mast cell priming. *Immunol Rev.* (2018) 282:73–86. doi: 10.1111/imr.12625
5. Amin K. The role of mast cells in allergic inflammation. *Respir Med.* (2012) 106:9–14. doi: 10.1016/j.rmed.2011.09.007
6. Syenina A, Jagaraj CJ, Aman SA, Sridharan A, St John AL. Dengue vascular leakage is augmented by mast cell degranulation mediated by immunoglobulin Fcγ receptors. *Elife.* (2015) 4:1–16. doi: 10.7554/eLife.05291
7. Shirato K, Taguchi F. Mast cell degranulation is induced by A549 airway epithelial cell infected with respiratory syncytial virus. *Virology.* (2009) 386:88–93. doi: 10.1016/j.virol.2009.01.011
8. Bankova LG, Lezcano C, Pejler G, Stevens RL, Murphy GF, Austen KF, et al. Mouse mast cell proteases 4 and 5 mediate epidermal injury through disruption of tight junctions. *J Immunol.* (2014) 192:2812–20. doi: 10.4049/jimmunol.1301794
9. Li WW, Guo TZ, Liang D, Sun Y, Kingery WS, Clark JD. Substance P signaling controls mast cell activation, degranulation, and nociceptive sensitization in a rat fracture model of complex regional pain syndrome. *Anesthesiology.* (2012) 116:882–95. doi: 10.1097/ALN.0b013e31824bb303
10. Zheng J, Wei CC, Hase N, Shi K, Killingsworth CR, Litovsky SH, et al. Chymase mediates injury and mitochondrial damage in cardiomyocytes during acute ischemia/reperfusion in the dog. *PLoS ONE.* (2014) 9:e94732. doi: 10.1371/journal.pone.0094732
11. El-Shitany N, El-desoky K. Cromoglycate, not ketotifen, ameliorated the injured effect of warm ischemia/reperfusion in rat liver: role of mast cell degranulation, oxidative stress, proinflammatory cytokine, and inducible nitric oxide synthase. *Drug Des Devel Ther.* (2015) 9:5237–46. doi: 10.2147/DDDT.S88337
12. Yang M, Ma Y, Tao S, Ding J, Rao L, Jiang H, et al. Mast cell degranulation promotes ischemia-reperfusion injury in rat liver. *J Surg Res.* (2014) 186:170–8. doi: 10.1016/j.jss.2013.08.021
13. Wernersson S, Pejler G. Mast cell secretory granules: armed for battle. *Nat Rev Immunol.* (2014) 14:478–94. doi: 10.1038/nri3690
14. Mukai K, Tsai M, Saito H, Galli SJ. Mast cells as sources of cytokines, chemokines, and growth factors. *Immunol Rev.* (2018) 282:121–50. doi: 10.1111/imr.12634
15. Lefrancais E, Duval A, Mirey E, Roga S, Espinosa E, Cayrol C, et al. Central domain of IL-33 is cleaved by mast cell proteases for potent activation of group-2 innate lymphoid cells. *Proc Natl Acad Sci USA.* (2014) 111:15502–7. doi: 10.1073/pnas.1410700111
16. Janicki JS, Brower GL, Levick SP. Chapter 8 - The emerging prominence of the cardiac mast cell as a potent mediator of adverse myocardial remodeling. In: Hughes MR, McNagny KM, editors. *Mast Cells: Methods and Protocols.* New York, NY: Springer Science+Business Media (2015). p. 121–39.
17. Overed-Sayer C, Rapley L, Mustelin T, Clarke DL. Are mast cells instrumental for fibrotic diseases? *Front Pharmacol.* (2014) 4:174. doi: 10.3389/fphar.2013.00174
18. Kong P, Christia P, Frangogiannis NG. The pathogenesis of cardiac fibrosis. *Cell Mol Life Sci.* (2014) 71:549–74. doi: 10.1007/s00018-013-1349-6
19. Prabhu SD, Frangogiannis NG. The biological basis for cardiac repair after myocardial infarction. *Circ Res.* (2016) 119:91–112. doi: 10.1161/CIRCRESAHA.116.303577
20. Bradding P, Pejler G. The controversial role of mast cells in fibrosis. *Immunol Rev.* (2018) 282:198–231. doi: 10.1111/imr.12626
21. Zweifel M, Matozan K, Dahinden C, Schaffner T, Mohacsi P. Eotaxin/CCL11 levels correlate with myocardial fibrosis and mast cell density in native and transplanted rat hearts. *Transplant Proc.* (2010) 42:2763–6. doi: 10.1016/j.transproceed.2010.05.152
22. Palaniyandi SS, Inagaki K, Mochly-Rosen D. Mast cells and εPKC: a role in cardiac remodeling in hypertension-induced heart failure. *J Mol Cell Cardiol.* (2008) 45:779–86. doi: 10.1016/j.yjmcc.2008.08.009
23. Kanemitsu H, Takai S, Tsuneyoshi H, Yoshikawa E, Nishina T, Miyazaki M, et al. Chronic chymase inhibition preserves cardiac function after left ventricular repair in rats. *Eur J Cardio Thoracic Surg.* (2008) 33:25–31. doi: 10.1016/j.ejcts.2007.09.040
24. Wang H, Da Silva J, Alencar A, Zapata-Sudo G, Lin MR, Sun X, et al. Mast cell inhibition attenuates cardiac remodeling and diastolic dysfunction in

middle-aged, ovariectomized fischer 344 × brown Norway rats. *J Cardiovasc Pharmacol.* (2016) 68:49–57. doi: 10.1097/FJC.0000000000000385

25. Somasundaram P, Ren G, Nagar H, Kraemer D, Mendoza L, Michael LH, et al. Mast cell tryptase may modulate endothelial cell phenotype in healing myocardial infarcts. *J Pathol.* (2005) 205:102–11. doi: 10.1002/path.1690
26. Matsumoto T, Wada A, Tsutamoto T, Ohnishi M, Isono T, Kinoshita M. Chymase inhibition prevents cardiac fibrosis and improves diastolic dysfunction in the progression of heart failure. *Circulation.* (2003) 107:2555–8. doi: 10.1161/01.CIR.0000074041.81728.79
27. Luitel H, Sydykov A, Schymura Y, Mamazhakypov A, Janssen W, Pradhan K, et al. Pressure overload leads to an increased accumulation and activity of mast cells in the right ventricle. *Physiol Rep.* (2017) 5:1–14. doi: 10.14814/phy2.13146
28. Liao C, Akazawa H, Tamagawa M, Ito K, Yasuda N, Kudo Y, et al. Cardiac mast cells cause atrial fibrillation through PDGF-A-mediated fibrosis in pressure-overloaded mouse hearts. *J Clin Invest.* (2010) 120:242–53. doi: 10.1172/JCI39942
29. Wei CC, Hase N, Inoue Y, Bradley EW, Yahiro E, Li M, et al. Mast cell chymase limits the cardiac efficacy of Ang I-converting enzyme inhibitor therapy in rodents. *J Clin Invest.* (2010) 120:1229–39. doi: 10.1172/JCI39345
30. Levick SP, McLarty JL, Murray DB, Freeman RM, Carver WE, Brower GL. Cardiac mast cells mediate left ventricular fibrosis in the hypertensive rat heart. *Hypertension.* (2009) 53:1041–7. doi: 10.1161/HYPERTENSIONAHA.108.123158
31. Akgul A, Youker KA, Noon GP, Loebe M. Quantitative changes in mast cell populations after left ventricular assist device implantation. *ASAIO J.* (2005) 51:275–80. doi: 10.1097/01.MAT.0000150507.61120.00
32. Dilsizian V, Eckelman WC, Loredo ML, Jagoda EM, Shirani J. Evidence for tissue angiotensin-converting enzyme in explanted hearts of ischemic cardiomyopathy using targeted radiotracer technique. *J Nucl Med.* (2007) 48:182–7.
33. Batlle M, Pérez-Villa F, Lázaro A, Garcia-Pras E, Ramirez J, Ortiz J, et al. Correlation between mast cell density and myocardial fibrosis in congestive heart failure patients. *Transplant Proc.* (2007) 39:2347–9. doi: 10.1016/j.transproceed.2007.06.047
34. Roldão JA, Beghini M, Ramalho LS, Porto CS, Rodrigues DBR, Teixeira VPA, et al. Comparison between the collagen intensity and mast cell density in the lingual muscles and myocardium of autopsied chronic chagasic and nonchagasic patients. *Parasitol Res.* (2012) 111:647–54. doi: 10.1007/s00436-012-2882-1
35. Joseph J, Kennedy RH, Devi S, Wang J, Joseph L, Hauer-jensen M, et al. Protective role of mast cells in homocysteine-induced cardiac remodeling. *Am J Physiol Heart Circ Physiol.* (2005) 2132:2541–5. doi: 10.1152/ajpheart.00806.2004
36. Shao Z, Nazari M, Guo L, Li SH, Sun J, Liu SM, et al. The cardiac repair benefits of inflammation do not persist: Evidence from mast cell implantation. *J Cell Mol Med.* (2015) 19:2751–62. doi: 10.1111/jcmm.12703
37. Kwon JS, Kim YS, Cho AS, Cho HH, Kim JS, Hong MH, et al. The novel role of mast cells in the microenvironment of acute myocardial infarction. *J Mol Cell Cardiol.* (2011) 50:814–25. doi: 10.1016/j.yjmcc.2011.01.019
38. Nazari M, Ni NC, Lüdke A, Li SH, Guo J, Weisel RD, et al. Mast cells promote proliferation and migration and inhibit differentiation of mesenchymal stem cells through PDGF. *J Mol Cell Cardiol.* (2016) 94:32–42. doi: 10.1016/j.yjmcc.2016.03.007
39. Briest W, Rabler B, Deten A, Zimmer HG. Norepinephrine-induced cardiac hypertrophy and fibrosis are not due to mast cell degranulation article. *Mol Cell Biochem.* (2003) 252:229–37. doi: 10.1023/A:1025596404975
40. Buckley CL, Stokes AJ. Corin-deficient W-sh mice poorly tolerate increased cardiac afterload. *Regul Pept.* (2011) 172:44–50. doi: 10.1016/j.regpep.2011.08.006
41. Ngkelo A, Richart A, Kirk JA, Bonnin P, Vilar J, Lemitre M, et al. Mast cells regulate myofilament calcium sensitization and heart function after myocardial infarction. *J Exp Med.* (2016) 213:1353–74. doi: 10.1084/jem.20160081
42. Frangogiannis NG, Shimoni S, Chang SM, Ren G, Shan K, Aggeli C, et al. Evidence for an active inflammatory process in the hibernating human myocardium. *Am J Pathol.* (2002) 160:1425–33. doi: 10.1016/S0002-9440(10)62568-0
43. Milei J, Fernández Alonso G, Vanzulli S, Storino R, Matturri L, Rossi L. Myocardial inflammatory infiltrate in human chronic chagasic cardiomyopathy: Immunohistochemical findings. *Cardiovasc Pathol.* (1996) 5:209–19.
44. Saarinen J, Kalkkinen N, Welgus HG, Kovanen PT. Activation of human interstitial procollagenase through direct cleavage of the Leu83-Thr84bond by mast cell chymase. *J Biol Chem.* (1994) 269:18134–40.
45. Kanbe N, Kurosawa M, Nagata H, Yamashita T, Kurimoto F, Miyachi Y. Production of fibrogenic cytokines by cord blood-derived cultured human mast cells. *J Allergy Clin Immunol.* (2000) 106:S85–90. doi: 10.1067/mai.2000.106777
46. Kanbe N, Kurosawa M, Nagata H, Saitoh H, Miyachi Y. Cord blood-derived human cultured mast cells produce transforming growth factor beta1. *Clin Exp Allergy.* (1999) 29:105–13. doi: 10.1046/j.1365-2222.1999.00459.x
47. Miyazaki M, Takai S, Jin D, Muramatsu M. Pathological roles of angiotensin II produced by mast cell chymase and the effects of chymase inhibition in animal models. *Pharmacol Ther.* (2006) 112:668–76. doi: 10.1016/j.pharmthera.2006.05.008
48. Cho SH, Lee SH, Kato A, Takabayashi T, Kulka M, Shin SC, et al. Cross-talk between human mast cells and bronchial epithelial cells in plasminogen activator inhibitor-1 production via transforming growth factor-β1. *Am J Respir Cell Mol Biol.* (2015) 52:88–95. doi: 10.1165/rcmb.2013-0399OC
49. Takai S, Jin D, Sakaguchi M, Katayama S, Muramatsu M, Sakaguchi M, et al. A novel chymase inhibitor, 4-[1-([bis-(4-methyl-phenyl)-methyl]-carbamoyl)3-(2-ethoxy-benzyl)-4-oxo-azetidine-2-yloxy]-benzoic acid (BCEAB), suppressed cardiac fibrosis in cardiomyopathic hamsters. *J Pharmacol Exp Ther.* (2003) 305:17–23. doi: 10.1124/jpet.102.045179
50. Lindstedt KA, Wang Y, Shiota N, Saarinen J, Hyytiäinen M, Kokkonen JO, et al. Activation of paracrine TGF-β1 signaling upon stimulation and degranulation of rat serosal mast cells: a novel function for chymase. *FASEB J.* (2001) 15:1377–88. doi: 10.1096/fj.00-0273com
51. Tatler AL, Porte J, Knox A, Jenkins G, Pang L. Tryptase activates TGFβ in human airway smooth muscle cells via direct proteolysis. *Biochem Biophys Res Commun.* (2008) 370:239–42. doi: 10.1016/j.bbrc.2008.03.064
52. Akers IA, Parsons M, Hill MR, Hollenberg MD, Sanjar S, Laurent GJ, et al. Mast cell tryptase stimulates human lung fibroblast proliferation via protease-activated receptor-2. *Am J Physiol Cell Mol Physiol.* (2000) 278:L193–201. doi: 10.1152/ajplung.2000.278.1.L193
53. Abe M, Kurosawa M, Ishikawa O, Miyachi Y, Kido H. Mast cell tryptase stimulates both human dermal fibroblast proliferation and type I collagen production. *Clin Exp. Allergy.* (1998) 28:1509–17. doi: 10.1046/j.1365-2222.1998.00360.x
54. Garbuzenko E, Nagler A, Pickholtz D, Gillery P, Reich R, Maquart FX, et al. Human mast cells stimulate fibroblast proliferation, collagen synthesis and lattice contraction: a direct role for mast cells in skin fibrosis. *Clin Exp Allergy.* (2002) 32:237–46. doi: 10.1046/j.1365-2222.2002.01293.x
55. Gruber BL, Kew RR, Jelaska A, Marchese MJ, Garlick J, Ren S, et al. Human mast cells activate fibroblasts: tryptase is a fibrogenic factor stimulating collagen messenger ribonucleic acid synthesis and fibroblast chemotaxis. *J Immunol.* (1997) 158:2310–7.
56. Cairns JA, Walls AF. Mast cell tryptase stimulates the synthesis of type I collagen in human lung fibroblasts. *J Clin Invest.* (1997) 99:1313–21. doi: 10.1172/JCI119290
57. Gailit J, Marchese MJ, Kew RR, Gruber BL. The Differentiation and function of myofibroblasts is regulated by mast cell mediators. *J Invest Dermatol.* (2001) 117:1113–19. doi: 10.1046/j.1523-1747.2001.15211.x
58. Zhao XY, Zhao LY, Zheng QS, Su JL, Guan H, Shang FJ, et al. Chymase induces profibrotic response via transforming growth factor-β1/Smad activation in rat cardiac fibroblasts. *Mol Cell Biochem.* (2008) 310:159–66. doi: 10.1007/s11010-007-9676-2
59. Caughey GH, Raymond WW, Wolters PJ. Angiotensin II generation by mast cell alpha- and beta-chymases. *Biochim Biophys Acta.* (2000) 1480:245–57. doi: 10.1016/S0167-4838(00)00076-5
60. Li M, Liu K, Michalicek J, Angus JA, Hunt JE, Dell'Italia LJ, et al. Involvement of chymase-mediated angiotensin II generation in blood pressure regulation. *J Clin Invest.* (2004) 114:112–20. doi: 10.1172/JCI20805
61. Takai S, Jin D, Sakaguchi M, Miyazaki M. A single treatment with a specific chymase inhibitor, TY-51184, prevents vascular proliferation in

canine grafted veins. *J Pharmacol Sci.* (2004) 94:443–8. doi: 10.1254/jphs.94.443
62. Hale TM, Robertson SJ, Burns KD, deBlois D. Short-term ACE inhibition confers long-term protection against target organ damage. *Hypertens Res.* (2012) 35:604–10. doi: 10.1038/hr.2012.2
63. D'Souza KM, Biwer LA, Madhavpeddi L, Ramaiah P, Shahid W, Hale TM. Persistent change in cardiac fibroblast physiology after transient ACE inhibition. *Am J Physiol Circ Physiol.* (2015) 309:H1346–53. doi: 10.1152/ajpheart.00615.2015
64. Liang B, Leenen FHH. Prevention of salt induced hypertension and fibrosis by angiotensin converting enzyme inhibitors in Dahl S rats. *Br J Pharmacol.* (2007) 152:903–14. doi: 10.1038/sj.bjp.0707472
65. Gut N, Piecha G, Aldebssi F, Schaefer S, Bekeredjian R, Schirmacher P, et al. Erythropoietin combined with ACE inhibitor prevents heart remodeling in 5/6 nephrectomized rats independently of blood pressure and kidney function. *Am J Nephrol.* (2013) 38:124–35. doi: 10.1159/000353106
66. Koskinen PK, Kovanen PT, Lindstedt KA, Lemström KB. Mast cells in acute and chronic rejection of rat cardiac allografts - a major source of basic fibroblast growth factor. *Transplantation.* (2001) 71:1741–7. doi: 10.1097/00007890-200106270-00007
67. Sun M, Chen M, Dawood F, Zurawska U, Li JY, Parker T, et al. Tumor necrosis factor- mediates cardiac remodeling and ventricular dysfunction after pressure overload state. *Circulation.* (2007) 115:1398–407. doi: 10.1161/CIRCULATIONAHA.106.643585
68. Kleinbongard P, Schulz R, Heusch G. TNFα in myocardial ischemia/reperfusion, remodeling and heart failure. *Heart Fail Rev.* (2011) 16:49–69. doi: 10.1007/s10741-010-9180-8
69. Duerrschmid C, Crawford JR, Reineke E, Taffet GE, Trial J, Entman ML, et al. TNF receptor 1 signaling is critically involved in mediating angiotensin-II-induced cardiac fibrosis. *J Mol Cell Cardiol.* (2013) 57:59–67. doi: 10.1016/j.yjmcc.2013.01.006
70. Wang Y, Li Y, Wu Y, Jia L, Wang J, Xie B, et al. 5TNF-α and IL-1β neutralization ameliorates angiotensin II-induced cardiac damage in male mice. *Endocrinology.* (2014) 155:2677–87. doi: 10.1210/en.2013-2065
71. Wang Y, Wu Y, Chen J, Zhao S, Li H. Pirfenidone attenuates cardiac fibrosis in a mouse model of TAC-induced left ventricular remodeling by suppressing NLRP3 inflammasome formation. *Cardiology.* (2013) 126:1–11. doi: 10.1159/000351179
72. Fairweather DL, Frisancho-Kiss S, Yusung SA, Barrett MA, Davis SE, Gatewood SJL, et al. Interferon-γ protects against chronic viral myocarditis by reducing mast cell degranulation, fibrosis, and the profibrotic cytokines transforming growth factor-β1, interleukin-1β, and interleukin-4 in the heart. *Am J Pathol.* (2004) 165:1883–94. doi: 10.1016/S0002-9440(10)63241-5
73. Coronado MJ, Brandt JE, Kim E, Bucek A, Bedja D, Abston ED, et al. Testosterone and interleukin-1β increase cardiac remodeling during coxsackievirus B3 myocarditis via serpin A 3n. *Am J Physiol Circ Physiol.* (2012) 302:H1726–36. doi: 10.1152/ajpheart.00783.2011
74. Frangogiannis NG. Interleukin-1 in cardiac injury, repair, and remodeling: pathophysiologic and translational concepts. *Discov.* (2015) 3:1–14. doi: 10.15190/d.2015.33
75. Lin TJ, Befus AD. Differential regulation of mast cell function by IL-10 and stem cell factor. *J. Immunol.* (1997) 159:4015–23.
76. Li J, Lu H, Plante E, Meléndez GC, Levick SP, Janicki JS. Stem cell factor is responsible for the rapid response in mature mast cell density in the acutely stressed heart. *J Mol Cell Cardiol.* (2012) 53:469–74. doi: 10.1016/j.yjmcc.2012.07.011
77. Ito T, Smrz D, Jung MY, Bandara G, Desai A, Smrzova S, et al. Stem cell factor programs the mast cell activation phenotype. *J Immunol.* (2012) 188:5428–37. doi: 10.4049/jimmunol.1103366
78. Faber TW, Pullen NA, Fernando JFA, Kolawole EM, McLeod JJA, Taruselli M, et al. ADAM10 is required for SCF-induced mast cell migration. *Cell Immunol.* (2014) 290:80–8. doi: 10.1016/j.cellimm.2014.05.005
79. Oldford SA, Haidl ID, Howatt MA, Leiva CA, Johnston B, Marshall JS. A critical role for mast cells and mast cell-derived IL-6 in TLR2-mediated inhibition of tumor growth. *J Immunol.* (2010) 185:7067–76. doi: 10.4049/jimmunol.1001137
80. Bot I, Shi GP, Kovanen PT. Mast cells as effectors in atherosclerosis. *Arterioscler Thromb Vasc Biol.* (2015) 35:265–71. doi: 10.1161/ATVBAHA.114.303570
81. Verma SK, Garikipati VNS, Krishnamurthy P, Schumacher SM, Grisanti LA, Cimini M, et al. Interleukin-10 inhibits bone marrow fibroblast progenitor cell-mediated cardiac fibrosis in pressure-overloaded myocardium. *Circulation.* (2017) 136:940–53. doi: 10.1161/CIRCULATIONAHA.117.027889
82. Verma SK, Krishnamurthy P, Barefield D, Singh N, Gupta R, Lambers E, et al. Interleukin-10 treatment attenuates pressure overload-induced hypertrophic remodeling and improves heart function via signal transducers and activators of transcription 3-dependent inhibition of nuclear factor- B. *Circulation.* (2012) 126:418–29. doi: 10.1161/CIRCULATIONAHA.112.112185
83. Krishnamurthy P, Rajasingh J, Lambers E, Qin G, Losordo DW, Kishore R. IL-10 inhibits inflammation and attenuates left ventricular remodeling after myocardial infarction via activation of STAT3 and suppression of HuR. *Circ Res.* (2009) 104:9–19. doi: 10.1161/CIRCRESAHA.108.188243
84. Bujak M, Dobaczewski M, Gonzalez-Quesada C, Xia Y, Leucker T, Zymek P, et al. Induction of the CXC chemokine interferon-γ-inducible protein 10 regulates the reparative response following myocardial infarction. *Circ Res.* (2009) 105:973–83. doi: 10.1161/CIRCRESAHA.109.199471
85. Saxena A, Bujak M, Frunza O, Dobaczewski M, Gonzalez-Quesada C, Lu B, et al. CXCR3-independent actions of the CXC chemokine CXCL10 in the infarcted myocardium and in isolated cardiac fibroblasts are mediated through proteoglycans. *Cardiovasc Res.* (2014) 103:217–27. doi: 10.1093/cvr/cvu138
86. Shiraha H, Glading A, Gupta K, Wells A. IP-10 inhibits epidermal growth factor-induced motility by decreasing epidermal growth factor receptor-mediated calpain activity. *J Cell Biol.* (1999) 146:243–54.
87. Tager AM, Kradin RL, LaCamera P, Bercury SD, Campanella GSV, Leary CP, et al. Inhibition of pulmonary fibrosis by the chemokine IP-10/CXCL10. *Am J Respir Cell Mol Biol.* (2004) 31:395–404. doi: 10.1165/rcmb.2004-0175OC
88. Nako H, Kataoka K, Koibuchi N, Dong YF, Toyama K, Yamamoto E, et al. Novel mechanism of angiotensin II-induced cardiac injury in hypertensive rats: the critical role of ASK1 and VEGF. *Hypertens Res.* (2012) 35:194–200. doi: 10.1038/hr.2011.175
89. Tang JM, Luo B, Xiao JH, Lv YX, Li XL, Zhao JH, et al. VEGF-A promotes cardiac stem cell engraftment and myocardial repair in the infarcted heart. *Int J Cardiol.* (2015) 183:221–31. doi: 10.1016/j.ijcard.2015.01.050
90. Yang L, Kwon J, Popov Y, Gajdos GB, Ordog T, Brekken RA, et al. Vascular endothelial growth factor promotes fibrosis resolution and repair in mice. *Gastroenterology.* (2014) 146:1339–50.e1. doi: 10.1053/j.gastro.2014.01.061
91. Allakhverdi Z, Smith DE, Comeau MR, Delespesse G. Cutting edge: The ST2 ligand IL-33 potently activates and drives maturation of human mast cells. *J Immunol.* (2007) 179:2051–4. doi: 10.4049/jimmunol.179.4.2051
92. Saluja R, Khan M, Church MK, Maurer M. The role of IL-33 and mast cells in allergy and inflammation. *Clin Transl Allergy.* (2015) 5:1–8. doi: 10.1186/s13601-015-0076-5
93. Saluja R, Zoltowska A, Ketelaar ME, Nilsson G. IL-33 and thymic stromal lymphopoietin in mast cell functions. *Eur J Pharmacol.* (2016) 778:68–76. doi: 10.1016/j.ejphar.2015.04.047
94. Motakis E, Guhl S, Ishizu Y, Itoh M, Kawaji H, Hoon MD, et al. Redefinition of the human mast cell transcriptome by deep-CAGE sequencing. *Blood.* (2014) 123:e58–67. doi: 10.1182/blood-2013-02-483792
95. Bandara G, Beaven MA, Olivera A, Gilfillan AM, Metcalfe DD. Activated mast cells synthesize and release soluble ST2-a decoy receptor for IL-33. *Eur J Immunol.* (2015) 45:3034–44. doi: 10.1002/eji.201545501
96. Yin H, Li P, Hu F, Wang Y, Chai X, Zhang Y. IL-33 attenuates cardiac remodeling following myocardial infarction via inhibition of the p38 MAPK and NF-κB pathways. *Mol Med Rep.* (2014) 9:1834–8. doi: 10.3892/mmr.2014.2051
97. Ruisong M, Xiaorong H, Gangying H, Chunfeng Y, Changjiang Z, Xuefei L, et al. The protective role of interleukin-33 in myocardial ischemia and reperfusion is associated with decreased HMGB1 expression and up-regulation of the P38 MAPK signaling pathway. *PLoS ONE.* (2015) 10:e0143064. doi: 10.1371/journal.pone.0143064

98. Rui T, Zhang J, Xu X, Yao Y, Kao R, Martin CM. Reduction in IL-33 expression exaggerates ischaemia/reperfusion-induced myocardial injury in mice with diabetes mellitus. *Cardiovasc Res.* (2012) 94:370–8. doi: 10.1093/cvr/cvs015
99. Lavine KJ, Epelman S, Uchida K, Weber KJ, Nichols CG, Schilling JD, et al. Distinct macrophage lineages contribute to disparate patterns of cardiac recovery and remodeling in the neonatal and adult heart. *Proc Natl Acad Sci USA.* (2016) 113:E1414. doi: 10.1073/pnas.1602039113
100. Gomez Perdiguero E, Klapproth K, Schulz C, Busch K, Azzoni E, Crozet L, et al. Tissue-resident macrophages originate from yolk-sac-derived erythro-myeloid progenitors. *Nature.* (2015) 518:547–51. doi: 10.1038/nature13989
101. Molawi K, Wolf Y, Kandalla PK, Favret J, Hagemeyer N, Frenzel K, et al. Progressive replacement of embryo-derived cardiac macrophages with age. *J Exp Med.* (2014) 211:2151–8. doi: 10.1084/jem.20140639
102. Falkenham A, De Antueno R, Rosin N, Betsch D, Lee TDG, Duncan R, et al. Nonclassical resident macrophages are important determinants in the development of myocardial fibrosis. *Am J Pathol.* (2015) 185:927–42. doi: 10.1016/j.ajpath.2014.11.027
103. Jenkins SJ, Ruckerl D, Thomas GD, Hewitson JP, Duncan S, Brombacher F, et al. IL-4 directly signals tissue-resident macrophages to proliferate beyond homeostatic levels controlled by CSF-1. *J Exp Med.* (2013) 210:2477–91. doi: 10.1084/jem.20121999
104. Bosurgi L, Cao YGG, Cabeza-Cabrerizo M, Tucci A, Hughes LD, Kong Y, et al. Macrophage function in tissue repair and remodeling requires IL-4 or IL-13 with apoptotic cells. *Science.* (2017) 356:1072–6. doi: 10.1126/science.aai8132
105. Reber LL, Marichal T, Galli SJ. New models for analyzing mast cell functions *in vivo. Trends Immunol.* (2012) 33:613–25. doi: 10.1016/j.it.2012.09.008
106. Petrovic D, Zorc M, Zorc-Pleskovic R, Vraspir-Porenta O. Morphometrical and stereological analysis of myocardial mast cells in myocarditis and dilated cardiomyopathy. *Folia Biol.* (1999) 45:63–6.
107. Gersch C, Dewald O, Zoerlein M, Michael LH, Entman ML, Frangogiannis NG. Mast cells and macrophages in normal C57/BL/6 mice. *Histochem. Cell Biol.* (2002) 118:41–9. doi: 10.1007/s00418-002-0425-z
108. Huang ZG, Jin Q, Fan M, Cong XL, Han SF, Gao H, et al. Myocardial remodeling in diabetic cardiomyopathy associated with cardiac mast cell activation. *PLoS ONE.* (2013) 8:22–4. doi: 10.1371/journal.pone.0060827
109. Zhang W, Chancey AL, Tzeng HP, Zhou Z, Lavine KJ, Gao F, et al. The development of myocardial fibrosis in transgenic mice with targeted overexpression of tumor necrosis factor requires mast cell-fibroblast interactions. *Circulation.* (2011) 124:2106–16. doi: 10.1161/CIRCULATIONAHA.111.052399
110. Ingason AB, Mechmet F, Atacho DAM, Steingrímsson E, Petersen PH. Distribution of mast cells within the mouse heart and its dependency on Mitf. *Mol Immunol.* (2019) 105:9–15. doi: 10.1016/j.molimm.2018.11.009
111. Oka T, Kalesnikoff J, Starkl P, Tsai M, Galli SJ. Evidence questioning cromolyn's effectiveness and selectivity as a mast cell stabilizer in mice. *Lab Invest.* (2012) 92:1472–82. doi: 10.1038/labinvest.2012.116
112. Reber LL, Daubeuf F, Pejler G, Abrink M, Frossard N. Mast cells contribute to bleomycin-induced lung inflammation and injury in mice through a chymase/mast cell protease 4-dependent mechanism. *J Immunol.* (2014) 192:1847–54. doi: 10.4049/jimmunol.1300875
113. Gutierrez DA, Muralidhar S, Feyerabend TB, Herzig S, Rodewald HR. Hematopoietic kit deficiency, rather than lack of mast cells, protects mice from obesity and insulin resistance. *Cell Metab.* (2015) 21:678–91. doi: 10.1016/j.cmet.2015.04.013
114. Marshall JS, Ford GP, Bell EB. Formalin sensitivity and differential staining of mast cells in human dermis. *Br J Dermatol.* (1987) 117:29–36. doi: 10.1111/j.1365-2133.1987.tb04087.x
115. Ishikawa K, Fish K, Aguero J, Yaniz-Galende E, Jeong D, Kho C, et al. Stem cell factor gene transfer improves cardiac function after myocardial infarction in swine. *Circ Hear Fail.* (2015) 8:167–74. doi: 10.1161/CIRCHEARTFAILURE.114.001711
116. Yaniz-Galende E, Chen J, Chemaly E, Liang L, Hulot JS, McCollum L, et al. Stem cell factor gene transfer promotes cardiac repair after myocardial infarction via in situ recruitment and expansion of c-kit+ cells. *Circ Res.* (2012) 111:1434–45. doi: 10.1161/CIRCRESAHA.111.263830
117. Lutz M, Rosenberg M, Kiessling F, Eckstein V, Heger T, Krebs J, et al. Local injection of stem cell factor (SCF) improves myocardial homing of systemically delivered c-kit + bone marrow-derived stem cells. *Cardiovasc Res.* (2008) 77:143–50. doi: 10.1093/cvr/cvm027
118. Reinecke H, Minami E, Zhu WZ, Laflamme MA. Cardiogenic differentiation and transdifferentiation of progenitor cells. *Circ Res.* (2008) 103:1058–71. doi: 10.1161/CIRCRESAHA.108.180588
119. Martin-Puig S, Wang Z, Chien KR. Lives of a heart cell: tracing the origins of cardiac progenitors. *Cell Stem Cell.* (2008) 2:320–31. doi: 10.1016/j.stem.2008.03.010
120. Zhou Y, Pan P, Yao L, Su M, He P, Niu N, et al. CD117-positive cells of the heart: progenitor cells or mast cells? *J. Histochem. Cytochem.* (2010) 58:309–16. doi: 10.1369/jhc.2009.955146
121. Klooker TK, Braak B, Koopman KE, Welting O, Wouters MM, van der Heide S, et al. The mast cell stabiliser ketotifen decreases visceral hypersensitivity and improves intestinal symptoms in patients with irritable bowel syndrome. *Gut.* (2010) 59:1213–21. doi: 10.1136/gut.2010.213108
122. Okayama Y, Benyon RC, Rees PH, Lowman MA, Hillier K, Church MK. Inhibition profiles of sodium cromoglycate and nedocromil sodium on mediator release from mast cells of human skin, lung, tonsil, adenoid and intestine. *Clin. Exp. Allergy.* (1992) 22:401–9. doi: 10.1111/j.1365-2222.1992.tb03102.x
123. Church MK, Hiroi J. Inhibition of IgE-dependent histamine release from human dispersed lung mast cells by anti-allergic drugs and salbutamol. *Br J Pharmacol.* (1987) 90:421–9. doi: 10.1111/j.1476-5381.1987.tb08972.x
124. Okayama Y, Church MK. Comparison of the modulatory effect of ketotifen, sodium cromoglycate, procaterol and salbutamol in human skin, lung and tonsil mast cells. *Int Arch Allergy Immunol.* (1992) 97:216–25. doi: 10.1159/000236122
125. Brannan JD, Gulliksson M, Anderson SD, Chew N, Seale JP, Kumlin M. Inhibition of mast cell PGD2 release protects against mannitol-induced airway narrowing. *Eur Respir J.* (2006) 27:944–50. doi: 10.1183/09031936.06.00078205
126. Draber P, Halova I, Polakovicova I, Kawakami T. Signal transduction and chemotaxis in mast cells. *Eur J Pharmacol.* (2016) 778:11–23. doi: 10.1016/j.ejphar.2015.02.057
127. Seki K, Sanada S, Kudinova AY, Steinhauser ML, Handa V, Gannon J, et al. Interleukin-33 prevents apoptosis and improves survival after experimental myocardial infarction through ST2 signaling. *Circ Hear Fail.* (2009) 2:684–91. doi: 10.1161/CIRCHEARTFAILURE.109.873240

12

Trimetazidine Attenuates Cardiac Dysfunction in Endotoxemia and Sepsis by Promoting Neutrophil Migration

Jing Chen[1,2†], Bei Wang[1,2,3†], Jinsheng Lai[1,2], Zachary Braunstein[4], Mengying He[1,2], Guoran Ruan[1,2], Zhongwei Yin[1,2], Jin Wang[1,2], Katherine Cianflone[5], Qin Ning[6], Chen Chen[1,2] and Dao Wen Wang[1,2*]*

[1] Division of Cardiology, Department of Internal Medicine, Tongji Hospital, Tongji Medical College, Huazhong University of Science and Technology, Wuhan, China, [2] Hubei Key Laboratory of Genetics and Molecular Mechanisms of Cardiological Disorders, Wuhan, China, [3] Department of Rheumatology and Immunology, Tongji Hospital, Tongji Medical College, Huazhong University of Science and Technology, Wuhan, China, [4] Department of Internal Medicine, The Ohio State University, Columbus, OH, United States, [5] Centre de Recherche de l'Institut Universitaire de Cardiologie & Pneumologie de Québec, Université Laval, Québec, QC, Canada, [6] Department of Infectious Disease, Institute of Infectious Disease, Tongji Hospital, Tongji Medical College, Huazhong University of Science and Technology, Wuhan, China

***Correspondence:**
Chen Chen
chenchen@tjh.tjmu.edu.cn
Dao Wen Wang
dwwang@tjh.tjmu.edu.cn*

†These authors have contributed equally to this work

Aims: Cardiac dysfunction can be a fatal complication during severe sepsis. The migration of neutrophils is significantly impaired during severe sepsis. We sought to determine the role of trimetazidine (TMZ) in regulation of neutrophil migration to the heart in a mouse model of sepsis and endotoxemia, and to identify the mechanism whereby TMZ confers a survival advantage.

Methods and Results: C57/BL6 mice were (1) injected with LPS followed by 24-h TMZ administration, or (2) treated with TMZ (20 mg/kg/day) for 1 week post cecal ligation and puncture (CLP) operation. Echocardiography and Millar system detection showed that TMZ alleviated cardiac dysfunction and histological staining showed the failure of neutrophils migration to heart in both LPS- and CLP-induced mice. Bone marrow transplantation revealed that TMZ-pretreated bone marrow cells improved LPS- and CLP-induced myocardial dysfunction and enhanced neutrophil recruitment in heart. In CXCL2-mediated chemotaxis assays, TMZ increased neutrophils migration via AMPK/Nrf2-dependent up-regulation of CXCR2 and inhibition of GRK2. Furthermore, using luciferase reporter gene and chromatin immunoprecipitation assays, we found that TMZ promoted the binding of the Nrf2 and CXCR2 promoter regions directly. Application of CXCR2 inhibitor completely reversed the protective effects of TMZ *in vivo*. Co-culture of neutrophils and cardiomyocytes further validated that TMZ decreased LPS-induced cardiomyocyte pyroptosis by targeting neutrophils.

Conclusion: Our findings suggested TMZ as a potential therapeutic agent for septic or endotoxemia associated cardiac dysfunction in mice.

STUDY HIGHLIGHTS

What is the current knowledge on the topic?

Migration of neutrophils is significantly impaired during severe sepsis, but the underlying mechanisms remain unknown.

What question did this study address?
The effects of TMZ on cardiac dysfunction via neutrophils migration.

What this study adds to our knowledge
TMZ attenuated LPS-induced cardiomyocyte pyroptosis and cardiac dysfunction by promoting neutrophils recruitment to the heart tissues via CXCR2.

How this might change clinical pharmacology or translational science
Our findings suggested TMZ as a potential therapeutic agent for septic cardiac dysfunction.

Keywords: pyroptosis, trimetazidine, septic cardiac dysfunction, neutrophil, AMPK-Nrf2-CXCR2 axis

KEY POINTS

1. TMZ attenuates cardiac dysfunction via neutrophils migration
2. TMZ decreases cardiomyocyte pyroptosis by targeting neutrophils

INTRODUCTION

Sepsis is a life-threatening organ dysfunction caused by a dysregulated host response to infection, and is one of the most common causes of death in hospitalized patients (1). So far, the therapeutic options for sepsis are nonspecific and are limited to support of organ function. In addition, there are still no approved drugs that specifically target sepsis (2). One of the major complications of sepsis, myocardial dysfunction, contributes significantly to increased mortality (3). However, the precise mechanisms that cause myocardial dysfunction during sepsis remain incompletely understood (3). Thus, elucidation of the pathophysiologic processes of sepsis-induced myocardial dysfunction, and seeking new specific drugs, may develop more effective therapies to treat it.

Neutrophil migration into infection sites constitutes the first line of defense against infection (4). The failure of neutrophil migration to the infection site is associated with increased severity of illness and multi-organ dysfunction during septic shock (5, 6). Neutrophil recruitment to the infection site is dependent on the CXC chemokines (7). In murine, CXC chemokines regulate the recruitment of neutrophils via a specific seven-transmembrane type G protein-coupled receptor, CXCR2, while in humans it is dependent on both CXCR1 and CXCR2 (8). However, in some pathological conditions, phosphorylation of CXCR2 by the G protein-coupled receptor kinase 2 (GRK2) triggered receptor desensitization and internalization, resulting in reduced expression of CXCR2 on the surface of neutrophils (9). Previous studies have revealed that the decreased expression of CXCR2 impaired neutrophil recruitment to the infection site and played a major role in the poor outcome secondary to the sepsis (10). Hence, it is necessary to investigate the regulation of neutrophil recruitment during sepsis-induced myocardial dysfunction.

AMPK, 5′ adenosine monophosphate-activated protein kinase, is a crucial regulator of cellular energy homeostasis (11). A recent study has reported that activated AMPK enhanced the abilities of neutrophil chemotaxis and bacterial killing in sepsis (12). Nuclear factor erythroid-2-related factor-2 (Nrf2), which is one of the downstream signals of AMPK, is a critical transcriptional factor for antioxidation. We, and others, have found that activation of Nrf2, via AMPK, inhibited LPS-induced inflammatory response (13, 14). Upon activation, Nrf2 dissociates from Kelch-like ECH-associated protein 1 (Keap1), and in turn, translocates into the nucleus to bind to the antioxidant responsive element (ARE) in gene promoters (15). Nrf2 was found to regulate the expression of many antioxidant enzymes and proteins, such as NADPH quinineoxidoreductase-1 (NQO-1), heme oxygenase-1 (HO-1), and glutathione S-transferase (GST). Recently, it has been indicated that Nrf2 also transcriptionally regulates inflammation-related genes (16).

Trimetazidine (TMZ) is a clinically effective anti-anginal agent due to the inhibition of long-chain 3 ketoacyl coenzyme A thiolase activity, which leads to decreased fatty acid oxidation and increased glucose oxidation (17). Previous studies have indicated the protective effects of TMZ on heart failure (18), oxidative stress damage (19), cell apoptosis (14), and endothelial function (20). Our recent study has demonstrated that TMZ improves LPS-induced cardiac dysfunction by regulating the function of macrophages (14). Given the pivotal function of neutrophils in inflammatory response, the detailed role of TMZ in regulating neutrophils function during septic cardiac dysfunction need to be explored.

Pyroptosis is a form of inflammatory programmed cell death (PCD). Unlike apoptosis or necrosis, pyroptosis features pore formation of the plasma membrane, cell swelling, and membrane rupture, causing leakage of cytosolic contents (21). During LPS-induced pyroptosis, caspase-11 is first activated by directly binding to LPS (22). Subsequently, activated caspase-11 processes interleukin (IL)-1β/IL-18 into their active forms (23). Pyroptosis

Abbreviations: NADPH, nicotinamide adenine dinucleotide phosphate; EF, ejection fraction; FS, fraction shortening; LVAW, left ventricle anterior wall; LVPW, left ventricle posterior wall; dP/dt max, peak instantaneous rate of left ventricular pressure increase; dP/dt min, peak instantaneous rate of left ventricular pressure decline; LPS, lipopolysaccharide; MPO, myeloperoxidase. TMZ, trimetazidine.

was initially defined as an antimicrobial reaction in immune cells (24). However, few studies have focused on cardiomyocyte pyroptosis in septic cardiac dysfunction.

In this study, we demonstrated that TMZ ameliorated LPS- and cecal ligation and puncture (CLP)-induced cardiac dysfunction and cardiomyocyte pyroptosis by promoting CXCR2-dependent neutrophil migration to cardiac tissue.

MATERIALS AND METHODS

Reagents

LPS, SB225002, Percoll, and Compound C (CC) were from Sigma-Aldrich (St. Louis, MO). TMZ was from Servier (Tianjin, China). RPMI1640 medium was from Thermo Fisher Scientific (Walham, MA). Nrf2 siRNA was from RiboBio (Guangzhou, China). CXCL2 was from R&D Systems (Minneapolis, MN). DAPI and IL-1β ELISA kit were from Boster (Wuhan, China). Myeloperoxidase (MPO) assay kit and lacate dehydrogenase (LDH) assay kit were from Nanjing Jiancheng Bioengineering Institute (Nanjing, China). Lipofectamine 2000 was from Invitrogen (Waltham, MA). Protein A/G agroase, anti-Nrf2, and anti-CXCR2 were from Santa Cruz Biotechnology (Dallas, TX). Anti-Ly6G, anti-MPO, anti-GRK2, and isotype antibody were from Abcam (Cambridge, MA). Anti-AMPK and anti-phospho-AMPK were from Cell Signaling Technology (Danvers, MA). Anti-caspase-11 was from Novus Biologicals (Littleton, CO). FITC-CD11b and Percp/Cy5.5-Ly6G were from eBioscience (San Diego, CA). PE-CXCR2 was from BD Biosciences (San Jose, CA). Lysis buffer and BCA protein assay were from Beyotime (Shanghai, China).

Animals

All experiments were performed with the approval of the Animal Research Committee of Tongji Medical College, and in accordance with ARRIVE and NIH guidelines for animal welfare. Male C57BL/6 mice at the age of 8–10 week-olds were purchased from the Institutional Animal Research Committee of Tongji Medical College, housed at a temperature of 23–25°C and a humidity of 55 ± 5% with free access to food and water. (1) Model of LPS-induced endotoxemia: Mice were randomly divided into 4 groups ($n = 8$), and received saline, single TMZ, single LPS, or LPS and TMZ combination interventions, respectively. In LPS and TMZ combination interventions, mice were first injected with LPS (15 mg/kg) in 100 μl of sterile saline by intraperitoneal injection, then 6 h later, TMZ (20 mg/kg) was administrated intragastrically (i.g.) every 6 h for a total of three times. In the 6-group animal experiments, the CXCR2 antagonist SB225002 (10 mg/kg) was injected intraperitoneally 30 min before LPS injection (10). (2) Model of CLP sepsis: The mice ($n = 10$ in each group) were first pre-treated with TMZ for 1 day. Then the CLP model of sepsis of moderate severity was performed in accordance with the original protocol developed by Chaudry's lab, with additional modifications (25). In brief, mice were anesthetized with i.p. injection of sodium pentobarbital (Sigma-Aldrich) with a dose of 30 mg/kg. A midline incision was made, and after externalization, the cecum was ligated (1 cm from the apex) and punctured twice (through-through) with a 27-G needle. Next, a small amount of fecal mass from the punctured cecum was gently squeezed out to ensure patency of punctures, cecum was relocated, and 4/0 sutures were used to close the peritoneum and skin. Sham-operated mice underwent only incision and cecum exteriorization. After the sham or CLP operations, the mice were then treated with TMZ (20 mg/kg/day) for 6 consecutive days. The survival rate was determined daily for 7 days after CLP. Cardiac function of mice was assessed by echocardiography and Millar catheter, and then the mice were sacrificed. Part of heart tissue was kept in 10% formalin, dissected and cut into slices. The remaining portions of heart tissue was immediately snap-frozen and stored at −80°C for western blotting examination.

Bone Marrow Transplantation

We performed bone marrow transplantation in TMZ or vehicle treated-wild type (WT) C57BL/6 mice using previously established methods (26). Briefly, 10-week-old WT C57BL/6 donor mice were pre-treated using TMZ (20 mg/kg in saline solution for 3 days) or equal amount of solvent (saline solution) as vehicle (TMZ BM and Vehicle BM groups in donor mice), meanwhile, the recipient mice were also pre-treated using TMZ (20 mg/kg in saline solution for 3 days) or equal amount of solvent (saline solution) as vehicle (TMZ and Vehicle groups in recipient mice). Then before the BM transplantation, the recipient mice received 850 rads of γ-irradiation and were administered with the antibiotic, Baytril. The next day, fresh bone marrow cells were isolated from a separate cohort of saline pre-treated C57BL/6 vehicle mice and nonirradiated TMZ pre-treated mice (n = 5 mice/group and pooled), respectively, and were injected into irradiated mice (6×10^6) in 200 μL volume through the tail vein. Twenty-four hours after bone marrow transplantation, the mice were subjected to LPS injection (15 mg/kg) or CLP surgery. Six hours after LPS administration and 1 day after CLP, mice hearts were harvested for immunohistochemistry Ly6G, MPO staining, and other tests.

Echocardiography and Haemodynamic Analyses

Transthoracic echocardiography (Vevo3100, Visual Sonics, Canada) was performed under anesthesia (2% isoflurane) (27). For the haemodynamic analyses, a Millar Cather Transducer (Millar Instruments, Houston), connected to a pressure transducer (Millar Instruments), was inserted through the right carotid artery into the left ventricle cavity, and stable-state haemodynamic parameters were recorded and analyzed with LabChart software (ADInstruments, Colorado Springs, CO).

Bone Marrow Derived Neutrophil (BMDN) Isolation and Chemotaxis Assay

BMDNs were isolated by Percoll gradient method as described previously (6). The purity of BMDNs was > 95% and was identified by Wright-Giemsa staining and Gr-1^+ expression using flow cytometry, respectively.

Isolated BMDNs were re-suspended in RPMI1640 medium and pretreated with AMPK inhibitor CC (2 μM) or Nrf2 siRNA. BMDNs were then treated with LPS (5 μg/ml) for 1 h, followed with TMZ (20 μM) treatment for 2 h. After that, BMDN chemotaxis was assessed toward CXCL2 (30 ng/ml) or medium alone in a 24-well Boyden chamber using a 5-μm-pore membrane. Two hours later, the membrane was removed. The images of migrated BMDNs were captured under an optical microscope, and numbers of BMDNs were counted in at least five random fields per well.

Immunofluorescent Assay of CXCR2

Isolated BMDNs were pretreated with LPS (5 μg/ml) for 1 h, and then treated with TMZ (20 μM) for 2 h. After that, BMDNs were affixed on glass slides and incubated with anti-CXCR2 as described previously (8). BMDN nuclei were stained with DAPI. Fluorescent images were captured using fluorescence microscope (Nikon, Japan).

Flow Cytometry Analysis

To determine the expression of CXCR2 on cell surface, BMDNs were stained with antibodies against FITC-CD11b, Percp/Cy5.5-Ly6G and PE-CXCR2. The expression of CXCR2 levels were analyzed by FACS Calibur flow cytometer (BD Biosciences, San Jose, CA) in the cell population of $CD11b^{+}Ly6G^{+}$.

Transfection With siRNA

For the transfection, BMDNs were seeded in 6-well plate in optium-medium, then transfected using Lipofectamine 2,000 according to manufacturer's instruction.

Luciferase Reporter Assays

Promoter fragments (−3011/+254, −2319/+254, and −1408/+254) of mouse CXCR2 were subcloned into the MluI/XhoII sites of PGL3 vector (Promega, Madison, WI). The primers are shown in **Supplemental Table 2**. The construct of mutant CXCR2 was introduced by site-directed mutagenesis (Stratagene, La Jolla, CA). Mouse Nrf2 expression vector was purchased from Genecopoeia (EX-Mm04093-M03, Rockville, MD). All plasmids were sequenced in order to ensure sequence accuracy. Cells were transfected with CXCR2 promoter constructs and Nrf2 expressing plasmid using Lipofectamine 2000. pRL-TK (Promega, Madison, WI) was co-transfected as an internal control in each group. Forty-eight hours after transfection, cells were harvested for the Dual-Luciferase reporter assay (Promega, Madison, WI).

Chromatin Immunoprecipitation (ChIP) Assays

HEK293T cells were cultured in 100-mm plates and transfected with empty or Nrf2 vector. Cells were incubated with 1% formaldehyde to cross-link protein-DNA complexes at 48 h after transfection. Cells were then lysed and sonicated to shear the chromatin to fragments. Sheared chromatin was then immunoprecipitated with anti-Nrf2 or normal IgG overnight at 4°C. Chromatin-antibody complexes were recovered by Protein A/G agroase. The immunoprecipitated DNA was analyzed by PCR to amplify CXCR2 promoter sequences. PCR products were analyzed by 1% agarose gel.

Co-culture of BMDNS and Cardiomyocytes

Primary adult cardiomyocytes were isolated as described previously (28). BMDNs seeded in 6-well plates were first administrated with SB225002 (1 μM), then stimulated with LPS (5 μg/ml) for 1 h, and finally with TMZ (20 μM) treatment for 2 h. After that, BMDNs were collected, washed, and seeded onto the transwell insert (0.4 μm pore size) above cardiomyocytes. Cardiomyocytes were harvested for 24 h at 37°C and then used for further analysis.

Western Blotting Analysis

Cell lysates were generated by lysis buffer containing protease and phosphatase inhibitors. Equal amounts of protein were separated by 10% SDS-polyacyral-amide gels and transferred to PVDF membranes. Membranes were blocked with blocking buffer containing 5% BSA in TBST for 2 h at room temperature. Incubation of specific primary antibodies at 1:1000 dilutions was followed by appropriate second antibody. Then, immunoreactive bands were detected using ECL and analyzed by Quantity One software (Bio-Rad Laboratories, Philadelphia, PA).

Statistical Analysis

All animal data are presented as mean ± SEM and *in-vitro* data are presented as mean ± SD. One-way ANOVA with Bonferroni *post hoc* test was used for comparison among multiple groups using SPSS 17.0 software, and sample distribution was determined by the Shapiro–Wilk normality test (W test). Differences with $P < 0.05$ were considered statistically significant.

RESULTS

TMZ Protected Against LPS- and CLP-Induced Cardiac Dysfunction and Promoted Neutrophil Migration to Heart Tissue

An LPS-induced endotoxemia model and a CLP-induced sepsis model were both taken in C57BL/6 mice. In the endotoxemia model, mice were injected intraperitoneally with LPS, and then either TMZ or saline (**Figure 1A**) was administered. In the sepsis model, mice were treated with TMZ (20 mg/kg/day) for 7 consecutive days post CLP or sham operations (**Figure 1B**). Consistent with our previous observations, echocardiographic parameters showed that LPS stimulation induced significant cardiac dysfunction, as indicated by decreased EF%, FS%, LVAW;s and LVPW;s, and increased LVID;s (**Figures 1C–E**). Similarly, haemodynamic analyses revealed that LPS injection led to decreased values of heart rate, P_{max}, dp/dt_{max} and dp/dt_{min} (**Figures 1F–I**). However, TMZ administration reversed the impairments of LPS-induced cardiac functions. In addition, TMZ treatment exerted similar cardioprotective effects 1 day and 7 days post CLP surgery, including increased EF%, FS%, without affecting heart rates of mice (**Figure 1K**, **Supplemental Figures 1A–D**). Moreover, the 7-day survival rate was increased from 20.74 to 70.00% after TMZ treatment compared with CLP-induced septic mice,

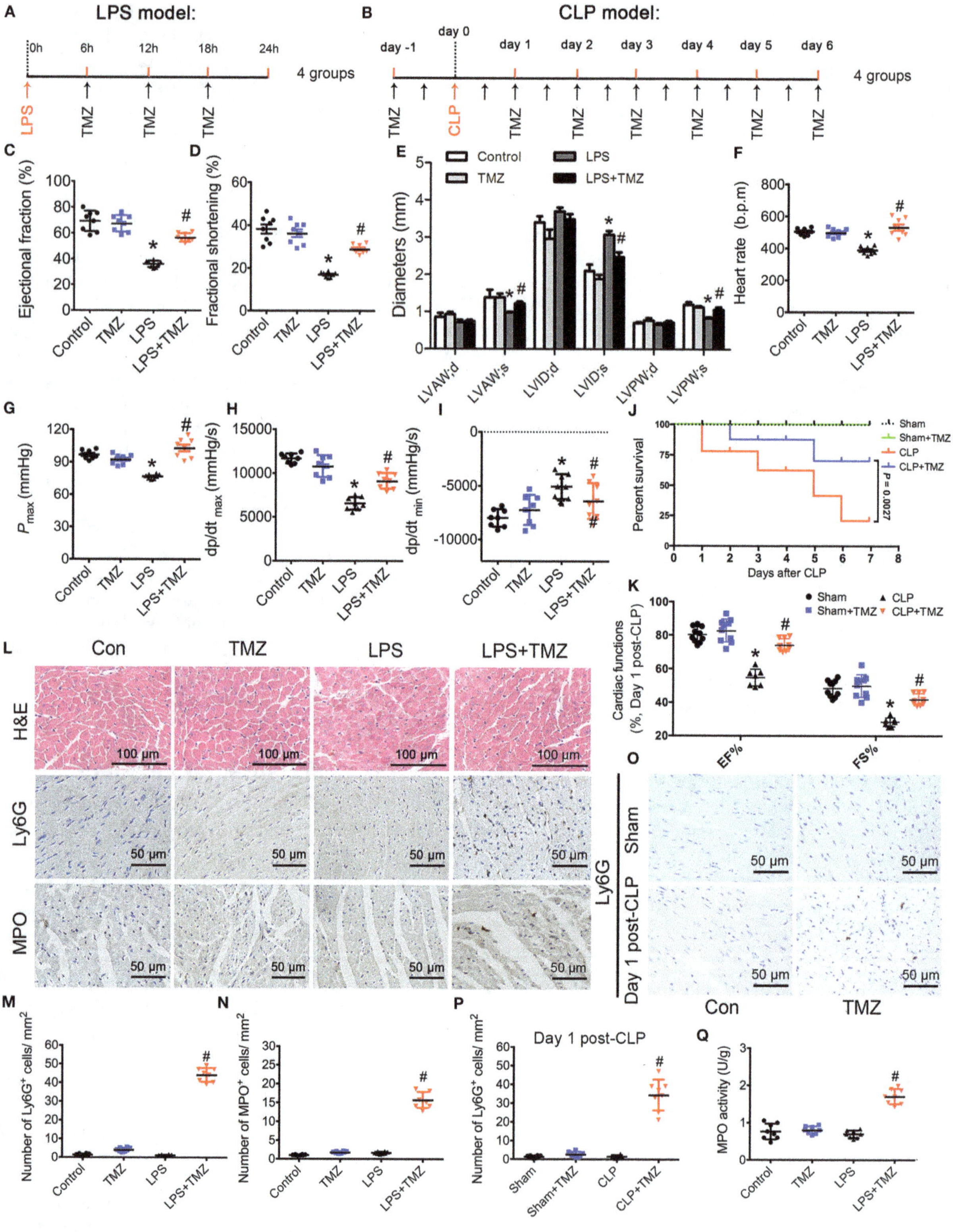

FIGURE 1 | TMZ improved LPS- and CLP-induced myocardial dysfunction and increased neutrophil migration to heart tissue. **(A)** Schematic drawing of experimental schedule for the endotoxemia mice study ($n = 8$ mice per group). Mice were first injected with LPS (15 mg/kg) in 100 μl of sterile saline by i.p. Then TMZ (20 mg/kg) was administrated by i.g. every 6 h for three times at 6 h after LPS injection. 24 h after injection with LPS or saline, cardiac function of the mice was assessed by echocardiography and Millar catheter. **(B)** Schematic drawing of experimental schedule for the septic mice study ($n = 10$ mice per group). Mice were treated with TMZ

(Continued)

FIGURE 1 | (20 mg/kg/day) for 7 consecutive days post CLP or sham operations, 1 and 7 days post CLP, cardiac function of mice was assessed by echocardiography; **(C–E)** Left ventricular ejection fraction (LVEF), left ventricular fractional shortening (LVFS) and left ventricular diameters were measured by two-dimensional echocardiography. **(F–I)** Heart rate, P_{max}, dp/dt_{max}, and dp/dt_{min} were assessed by cardiac catheterization. **(J)** Survival rates of wild-type (WT) ($n = 10$ per group) undergoing severe sepsis (cecal ligation and puncture [CLP] operation). **(K)** LVEF and LVFS in CLP model were measured by two-dimensional echocardiography. **(L)** Representative histological cardiac tissues stained with H&E, Ly6G, and MPO as the indicated groups at 24 h after LPS injection. **(M)** Quantification of Ly6G positive cells in 1 mm^2 after LPS stimulation; **(N)** Quantification of MPO positive cells in 1 mm^2. **(O)** Representative images of heart tissues immunostained with Ly6G on day 1 post CLP. Scale bar: 50 μm. **(P)** Quantification of Ly6G positive cells in 1 mm^2 post CLP. **(Q)** MPO activity assay in heart tissues was performed at 24 h after LPS injection. Data is presented as mean ± SEM of three independent experiments. $^*P < 0.05$ vs. Con group in LPS-induced model or Sham group in CLP-induced model; $^{\#}P < 0.05$ vs. LPS-treated group or CLP-induced group. LVAW;d, left ventricular anterior wall in diastole; LVAW;s, left ventricular anterior in systole; LVID;d, left ventricular internal diameter in diastole; LVID;s, left ventricular internal diameter in diastole; P_{max}, peak systolic pressure.

accompanied by reduced peritoneal bacterial load (**Figure 1J** and **Supplemental Figure 1E**), indicating the improved cardiac function after TMZ treatment confers a survival advantage in sepsis.

In histological studies, H&E staining of heart tissue in the control and TMZ group represented normal distribution of cardiomyocyte and myocardial structures (**Figure 1L**). Meanwhile, the LPS-induced cardiac structural disarray and interstitial edema was reversed by TMZ (**Figure 1L**). Ly6G and MPO staining (markers of infiltrating neutrophils) showed that the numbers of Ly6G and MPO positive cells in heart tissue was negligible in both the saline and TMZ groups, as well as in LPS- and CLP-induced mice heart. Interestingly, the number of neutrophils in heart tissue was significantly increased in the LPS+TMZ group when compared with LPS group (**Figures 1L–N**, **Supplemental Figure 2**). TMZ treatment also increased the number of neutrophils in heart tissue post CLP surgery (**Figures 1N–P**, **Supplemental Figure 2**). Meanwhile, the MPO activity in LPS+TMZ group was markedly higher than in the LPS group 24 h after LPS injection (**Figure 1Q**). Collectively, these results suggest that TMZ ameliorates LPS- and CLP-induced cardiac dysfunction in endotoxemia and sepsis, accompanied by increasing neutrophils recruitment into heart tissues.

TMZ-Pretreated Bone Marrow Cells Ameliorated LPS- and CLP-Induced Myocardial Dysfunction and Enhanced Neutrophil Recruitment to the Heart

To detect whether the effects of TMZ on neutrophil recruitment was dependent on resident cells or bone marrow (BM) derived cells, we performed BM transplantation experiments. Compared with mice that received vehicle BM cells, mice receiving TMZ pretreated BM cells showed improvement of cardiac function, reflected by increased values of EF%, FS%, LVAW;s, LVPW;s, heart rate, P_{max}, dp/dt_{max} and dp/dt_{min}, as well as decreased values of LVID;d and LVID;s (**Figures 2A–G**) post LPS stimulation. In the CLP-induced sepsis model, mice receiving TMZ pretreated BM cells showed similar improvement of cardiac function as observed in the post LPS-induced endotoxemia model (**Figure 2H**). Furthermore, H&E staining revealed that compared with vehicle pretreated BM cells, the TMZ pretreated BM cells that injected in recipient mice attenuated the myocardial injury, indicated by reduced irregular arrangement of cardiomyocyte and interstitial edema (**Figure 2I**). Moreover, in both LPS-induced endotoxemia and CLP-induced sepsis models, the Ly6G and MPO staining showed that the number of neutrophils recruited into heart tissue was significantly increased in TMZ BM > vehicle mice compared with vehicle BM > vehicle mice, and TMZ BM > TMZ mice compared with TMZ BM > vehicle mice, respectively, (**Figures 2I–M**). Consistently, the MPO activities in TMZ BM > vehicle and TMZ BM > TMZ groups were remarkably higher compared with vehicle BM > vehicle and TMZ BM > vehicle groups (**Figure 2N**). Taken together, this data indicates that TMZ-pretreated bone marrow cells attenuate LPS- and CLP-induced myocardial depression, and enhance the migration of neutrophils into heart tissue.

TMZ Enhanced Neutrophil Migration by Regulating CXCR2 Expression Through AMPK Pathway

To examine whether TMZ had a direct effect on neutrophil migration, we isolated bone marrow derived neutrophils (BMDNs) from differentially treated mice, and assessed the migration ability of BMDNs. As shown in **Figures 3A,B**, BMDNs isolated from LPS-induced mice showed a marked impaired chemotactic response toward CXCL2, when compared with the control group (29). However, TMZ treatment remarkably rescued declined BMDN migration by LPS stimulation.

Next, isolated BMDNs from C57BL/6 mice were pretreated with TMZ or LPS *in vitro*. Consistently, TMZ significantly ameliorated LPS-induced failure of BMDN migration toward CXCL2 (**Figures 3C,D**). Additionally, both the untreated and TMZ-treated BMDNs exhibited normal and homogeneous expression of CXCR2 in the CXCR2 fluorescent staining. However, LPS significantly reduced expression of CXCR2 in BMDNs, which was reversed by TMZ treatment (**Figures 3E–F**).

Next, we found that TMZ reversed LPS-reduced phosphorylation of AMPK in BMDNs (**Figure 3G**). Consistently, pretreatment with the AMPK specific inhibitor, CC, significantly prevented TMZ-enhanced BMDNs migration (**Figures 3H–I**). In addition, flow cytometry analyses showed that TMZ elevated the expression of CXCR2 on the membrane in LPS-induced BMDNs, which was reversed by CC (**Figures 3J–K**). Thus, the TMZ regulated CXCR2 expression in an AMPK-dependent manner, which in turn enhanced neutrophil migration.

TMZ Improved Neutrophil Migration by Decreasing GRK2 and Increasing CXCR2 Expression in an AMPK/Nrf2 Dependent Manner

As shown in **Figures 4A,B**, we found that TMZ markedly reversed the reduced Nrf2 expression in the nucleus of

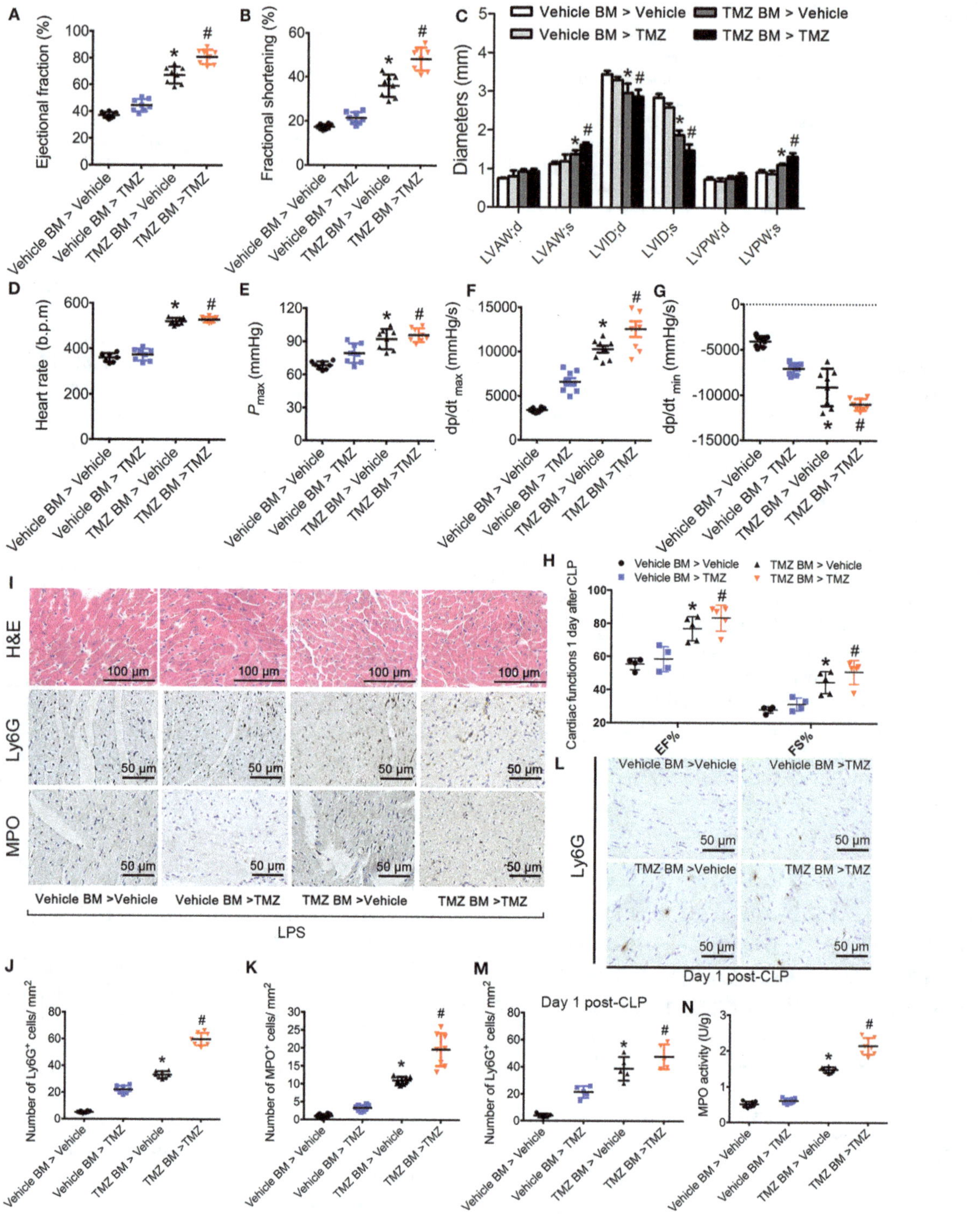

FIGURE 2 | TMZ-pretreated bone marrow cells ameliorated LPS- and CLP-induced myocardial dysfunction and promoted neutrophils recruitment to heart tissues. Irradiated TMZ pretreated (20 mg/kg, i.g., Tid, for 3 days) and vehicle pretreated wild-type (WT) mice received either vehicle or TMZ pretreated bone marrow subjected to LPS challenge (15 mg/kg, i.p.) or CLP surgery, respectively. 6 h after LPS injection and 1 day post-CLP, mice were subjected to echocardiography and haemodynamic analyses. Mice were then sacrificed and heart tissues were stained with H&E and immunochemistry staining. **(A–C)** Statistical analysis of echocardiographic results after LPS challenge. **(D–G)** Statistical analysis of haemodynamic results after LPS challenge. **(H)** Statistical analysis of echocardiographic results post-CLP. **(I)** Representative histological H&E, Ly6G, and MPO staining of heart sections as the indicated groups. **(J)** Quantitative analysis of Ly6G-positive cells in 1 mm^2 after LPS challenge. **(K)** Quantitative analysis of MPO-positive cells in 1 mm^2 after LPS challenge. **(L)** Representative Ly6G staining of heart sections as the indicated groups in CLP-induced sepsis. **(M)** Quantitative analysis of Ly6G-positive cells in 1 mm^2 post CLP; **(N)** MPO activity assay in heart tissues was performed at 6 h after LPS injection. Data is presented as mean ± SEM of three independent experiments. $^*P < 0.05$ vs. vehicle BM > vehicle mice; $^\#P < 0.05$ vs. vehicle BM > TMZ mice, $n = 8$ mice per group after LPS challenge, and $n = 5$ mice per group post CLP.

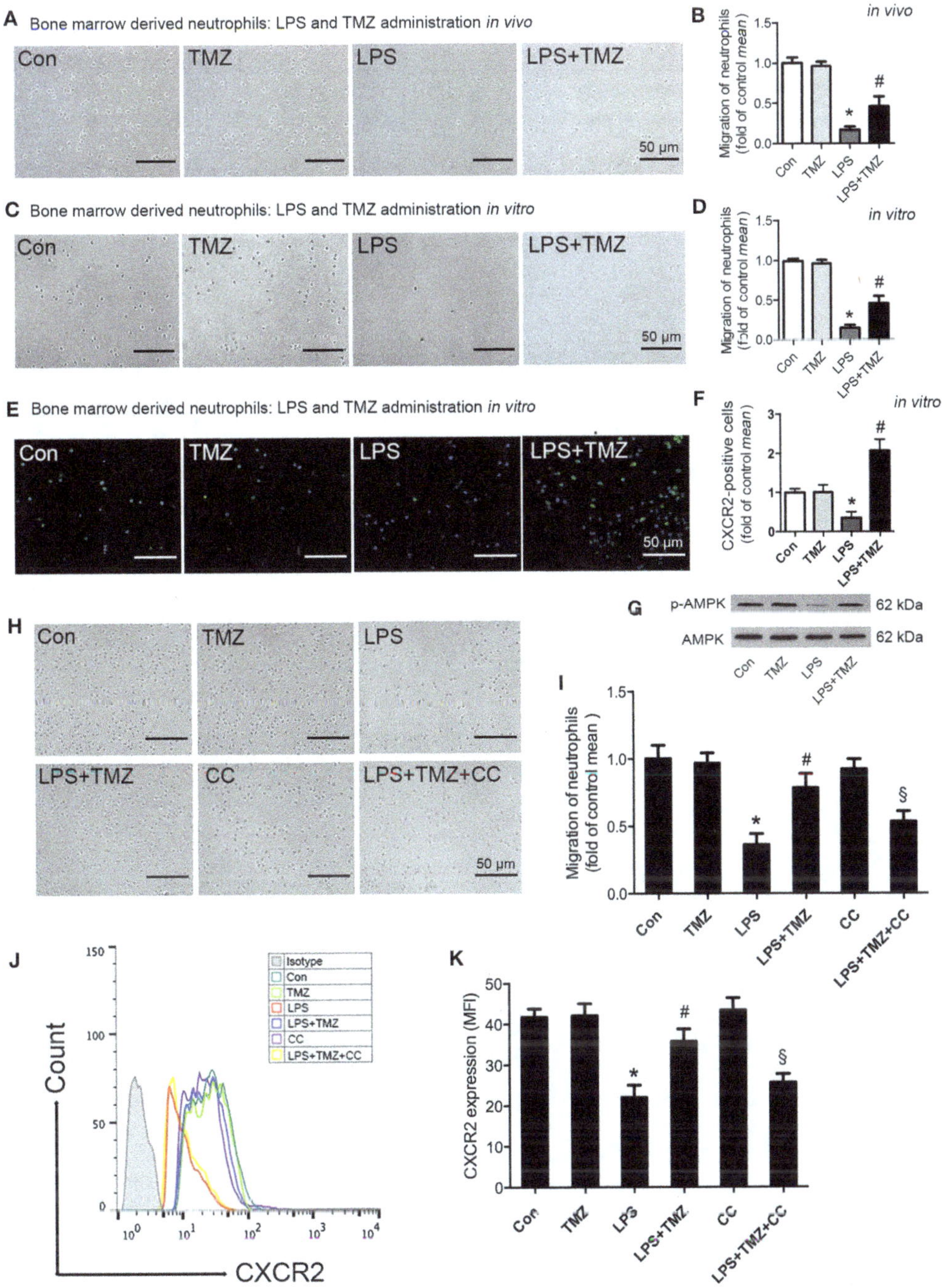

FIGURE 3 | TMZ enhanced neutrophil migration by regulating CXCR2 expression through AMPK pathway. **(A)** 8–10 week-old C57BL/6 male mice were first injected with LPS (15 mg/kg), then TMZ (20 mg/kg) was administrated by gavage every 6 h for 3 times after LPS injection for 6 h. Representative images of migrated BMDNs by transwell assay. **(B)** Relative quantitative assay of migrating BMDNs under optical microscopy. **(C)** Neutrophils isolated from non-simulated mice bone marrow, then BMDNs were subjected to LPS stimulation (5 μg/ml) for 1 h and subsequently treated with TMZ (20 μM) for 2 h. Representative images of migrated BMDNs by transwell assay. **(D)** Relative quantitative assay of migrating BMDNs under optical microscopy. **(E)** Representative images of BMDN immunofluorescent CXCR2 (green) staining. Nuclei were stained by DAPI (blue). **(F)** Quantitative of CXCR2 expression by measuring fluorescence intensity. **(G)** Phosphorylation of AMPK in BMDNs was examined by western blotting. **(H)** BMDNs were first treated with AMPK inhibitor CC (CC) (1 μM) for 1 h, then subjected to LPS stimulation (5 μg/ml) for 1 h, subsequently treated with TMZ (20 μM) for 2 h *in vitro*. Representative images of migrated BMDNs by transwell assay. **(I)** Relative quantitative assay of migrating BMDNs under optical microscopy. **(J)** Flow cytometry was performed to examine the expression of CXCR2 on the membrane of neutrophils. **(K)** Quantitative of CXCR2 expression by FACS. Data were presented as mean ± SEM *in vivo* and mean ± SD *in vitro* of three independent experiments. Scale bar: 50 μm. $^{*}P < 0.05$ vs. Con group; $^{\#}P < 0.05$ vs. LPS group; $^{\S}P < 0.05$ vs. LPS+TMZ group, $n = 8$ mice per group.

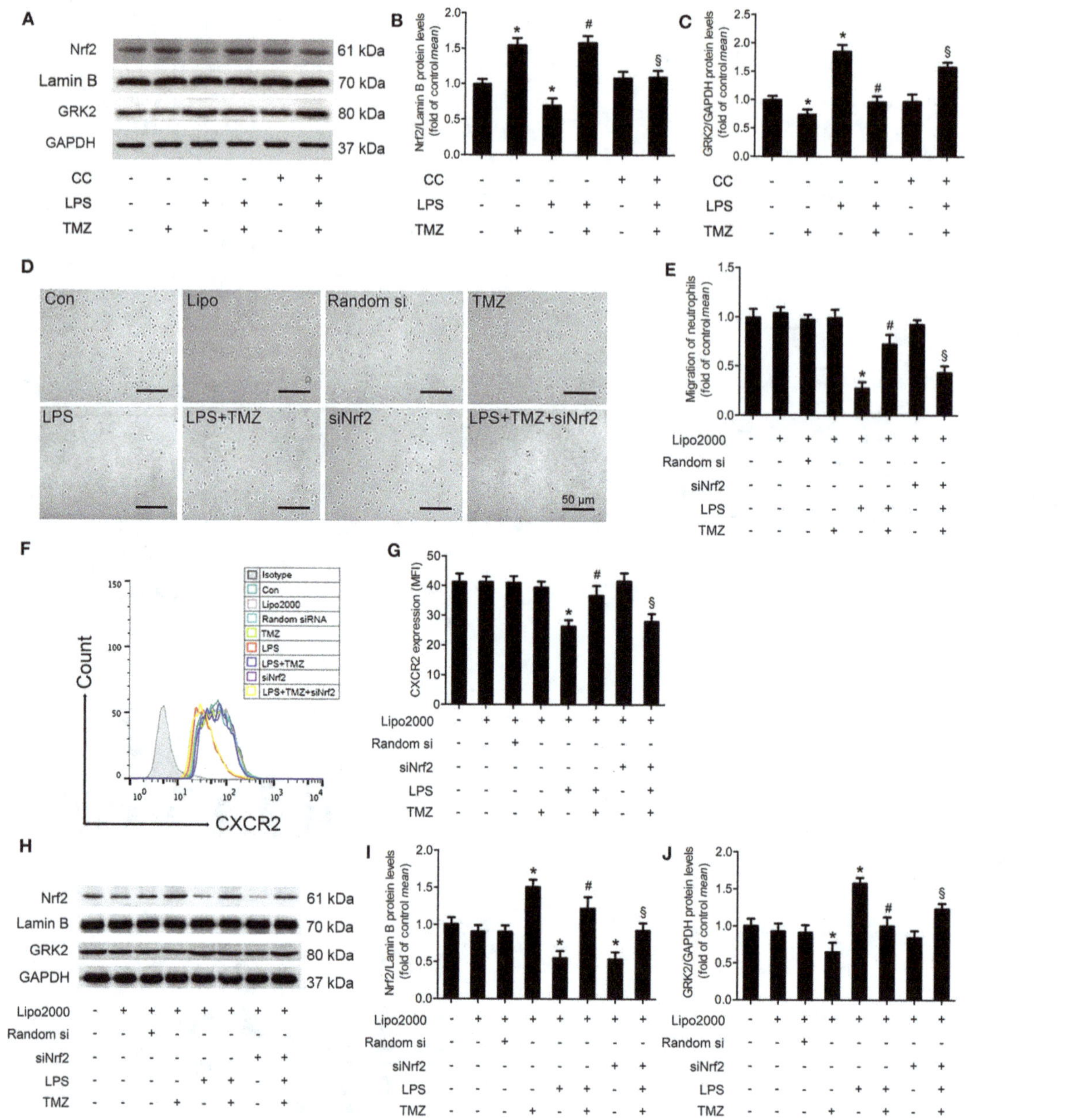

FIGURE 4 | TMZ promoted neutrophil migration by decreasing GRK2 and increasing CXCR2 expression in an AMPK/Nrf2 dependent manner. **(A)** BMDNs were first treated with CC (1 μM) for 1 h, then subjected to LPS stimulation (5 μg/ml) for 1 h, subsequently treated with TMZ (20 μM) for 2 h. Western blotting analysis of nuclear Nrf2 and total GRK2 in response to different stimulations. Lamin B and GAPDH were used as loading controls, respectively. **(B,C)** Quantification of Nrf2/Lamin B and GRK2/GAPDH was performed from the western blotting and expressed as fold induction. **(D)** BMDNs were first transfected with si-Nrf2 for 24 h, then subjected to LPS stimulation (5 μg/ml) for 1 h, subsequently treated with TMZ (20 μM) for 2 h. Representative images of transwell assays for BMDNs under optical microscope. Scale bar: 50 μm. **(E)** Relative quantitative assay of migrating BMDNs under optical microscopy. **(F)** Flow cytometry was performed to examine the expression of CXCR2 on the membrane of BMDNs. **(G)** Quantitative assay of CXCR2 expression by FACS. **(H)** Western blotting analysis of nuclear Nrf2 and total GRK2 in response to different stimulations after transfection. Lamin B and GAPDH were used as loading controls, respectively. **(I,J)** Quantification of Nrf2/Lamin B and GRK2/GAPDH was performed from the western blotting and expressed as fold induction. Data is presented as mean ± SEM *in vivo* and mean ± SD *in vitro* of three independent experiments. $^{*}P < 0.05$ vs. Con group; $^{\#}P < 0.05$ vs. LPS group; $^{\S}P < 0.05$ vs. LPS+TMZ group.

LPS-treated BMDNs, whereas CC abrogated this influence of TMZ. On the other hand, by Western blotting analyses, we found that TMZ treatment significantly inhibited LPS-induced GRK2 over-expression, which was attenuated by CC, indicating that TMZ negatively affected GRK2 expression via AMPK activation (**Figures 4A,C**). To verify whether Nrf2 regulates BMDN migration, BMDNs were transfected with Nrf2 siRNA. In LPS-treated BMDNs, Nrf2 silence significantly prevented the effects of TMZ on enhancing neutrophil migration (**Figures 4D,E**), downregulating CXCR2 membrane expression (**Figures 4F,G**), inhibiting Nrf2 expression (**Figures 4H,I**), and increasing GRK2 expression (**Figures 4H,J**).

CXCR2 Is Transcriptionally Regulated by TMZ via Nrf2 in LPS-Induced Cardiac Dysfunction

To understand how Nrf2 affects the expression of CXCR2, we performed *in silico* promoter analyses on mouse CXCR2 gene. Bioinformatic analyses revealed a CXCR2 potential ARE (antioxidant responsive element) binding sequence upstream of the CXCR2 translational initiation site (−919/−909). Subsequently, three fragments (−3011/+254, −2319/+254, −1408/+254) of promoter sequence of CXCR2 and an ARE mutant fragment of −1408/+254 were inserted into the luciferase reporter plasmid (**Figures 5A,B**). Luciferase reporter gene assays revealed that Nrf2 increased the luciferase activity of all three fragments, but not in the mutant fragment (**Figure 5B**), indicating that Nrf2 affected the transcriptional activity of CXCR2 via binding to the potential ARE sequence. To confirm this binding, we performed chromatin immunoprecipitation assays. In agreement with the results of luciferase reporter gene assays, the CXCR2 proximal promoter (−919/−909) was present in Nrf2 immunoprecipitates from cells expressing Nrf2, but not cells expressing the empty vector control. In contrast, distal promoter sequences (−2727/−2717) could not be amplified in Nrf2 immunoprecipitates (**Figure 5C**). Moreover, TMZ increased transcriptional activity of CXCR2 in the proximal promoter sequence from −1408 to +254 compared with LPS, and this effect was dependent on the expression of Nrf2 (**Figure 5D**). Together, this data demonstrates that CXCR2 is transcriptionally regulated by TMZ through the transcription factor Nrf2.

To test whether the expression of CXCR2 in neutrophils contributes to the protective effects of TMZ against LPS-induced cardiac dysfunction, a specific CXCR2 antagonist, SB225002, was introduced to inhibit the expression of CXCR2 *in vivo* (**Figure 5E**). Results showed that TMZ significantly ameliorated LPS-induced cardiac dysfunction, whereas CXCR2 antagonist almost completely abrogated the protective effects of TMZ in LPS-induced mice (**Figures 5F–H** and **Supplemental Table 1**). These results indicate that TMZ prevents LPS-induced cardiac depression via up-regulating the expression of neutrophil's CXCR2.

TMZ Decreased LPS-Induced Cardiomyocyte Pyroptosis by Targeting Neutrophils

Inflammatory response in some pathological conditions can induce cardiac cell death, subsequently leading to heart failure, which is associated with pyroptosis (13). Activation of caspase-11 (cleaved caspase-11) and marked increase of IL-1β and LDH were served as biomarkers of pyroptosis (22, 30). In this study, Western blotting showed that the expression of cardiac cleaved caspase-11 was remarkably increased in the LPS group (**Figures 6A,B**), and similar changes in IL-1β and LDH were consistently observed (**Figures 6C,D**). Increased caspase-11 in the LPS stimulated heart was also detectable by fluorescence staining (**Figures 6E,F**). These results indicated an induction of cardiomyocyte pyroptosis in LPS stimulated septic mice. As expected, TMZ treatment effectively reduced LPS-induced cardiomyocyte pyroptosis (**Figures 6A–F**). On the other hand, the specific CXCR2 antagonist, SB225002, attenuated the protective effects of TMZ on LPS-induced cardiomyocyte pyroptosis (**Figures 6A–F**). Moreover, the protective effects of TMZ on LPS-induced cardiac pyroptosis were associated with increased neutrophils in heart tissue (**Figures 6G,H**). Consistently, in *in-vitro* experiments, cardiomyocytes co-cultured with LPS-stimulated neutrophils exhibited significant pyroptosis, reflected by increased levels of cleaved caspase-11, IL-1β, and LDH (**Figures 6I–L**). Conversely, TMZ-pretreated BMDNs decreased cardiomyocyte pyroptosis induced by LPS, indicating a protective effect of TMZ on cardiomyocyte pyroptosis mediated by neutrophils (**Figures 6I–L**). After adding the CXCR2 specific inhibitor SB225002, the protective effects of TMZ on LPS-induced cardiomyocyte pyroptosis were blocked (**Figures 6I–L**). This data suggests that TMZ attenuates LPS-induced cardiomyocyte pyroptosis via neutrophils mediated by CXCR2 *in vivo* and *in vitro*.

DISCUSSION

In the current study, we found that the anti-anginal agent TMZ significantly attenuated LPS- and CLP-induced myocardial dysfunction in mice, by increasing neutrophilic migration to heart tissue (**Figure 6M**), via promoting neutrophil recruitment to the heart. Mechanistically, we found that TMZ promoted neutrophils through an AMPK/Nrf2/CXCR2 dependent manner secondary to LPS stimulation. CXCR2 was transcriptionally regulated by TMZ via Nrf2, which directly bound to the CXCR2 promoter sequence. Finally, TMZ reduced LPS-induced cardiomyocyte pyroptosis via neutrophils.

Sepsis and endotoxemia are both systemic inflammatory responses to infection and can lead to tissue injury and multiple organ failure (31–33). The cardiovascular system is one of the most frequently affected organ systems in sepsis and endotoxemia (33, 34). Septic patients with secondary cardiac dysfunction had a 50-70% increase in mortality when compared to those without cardiac dysfunction (3). The myocardial contractile dysfunction is driven by several factors, such as cardiodepressant mediators, mitochondrial dysfunction and/or apoptosis (35, 36). During sepsis-induced cardiac dysfunction, various cell types and factors involved in the up-regulation of inflammatory gene transcription and initiation of innate immunity in heart (3). Our previous study demonstrated the protective role of TMZ against LPS-induced cardiac dysfunction, by targeting the macrophage mediated pro-inflammatory response, especially through activating macrophages in bone marrow (14). In this study, we found that the myocardial beneficial effects of TMZ were associated with increased neutrophil recruitment after LPS challenge. Furthermore, in

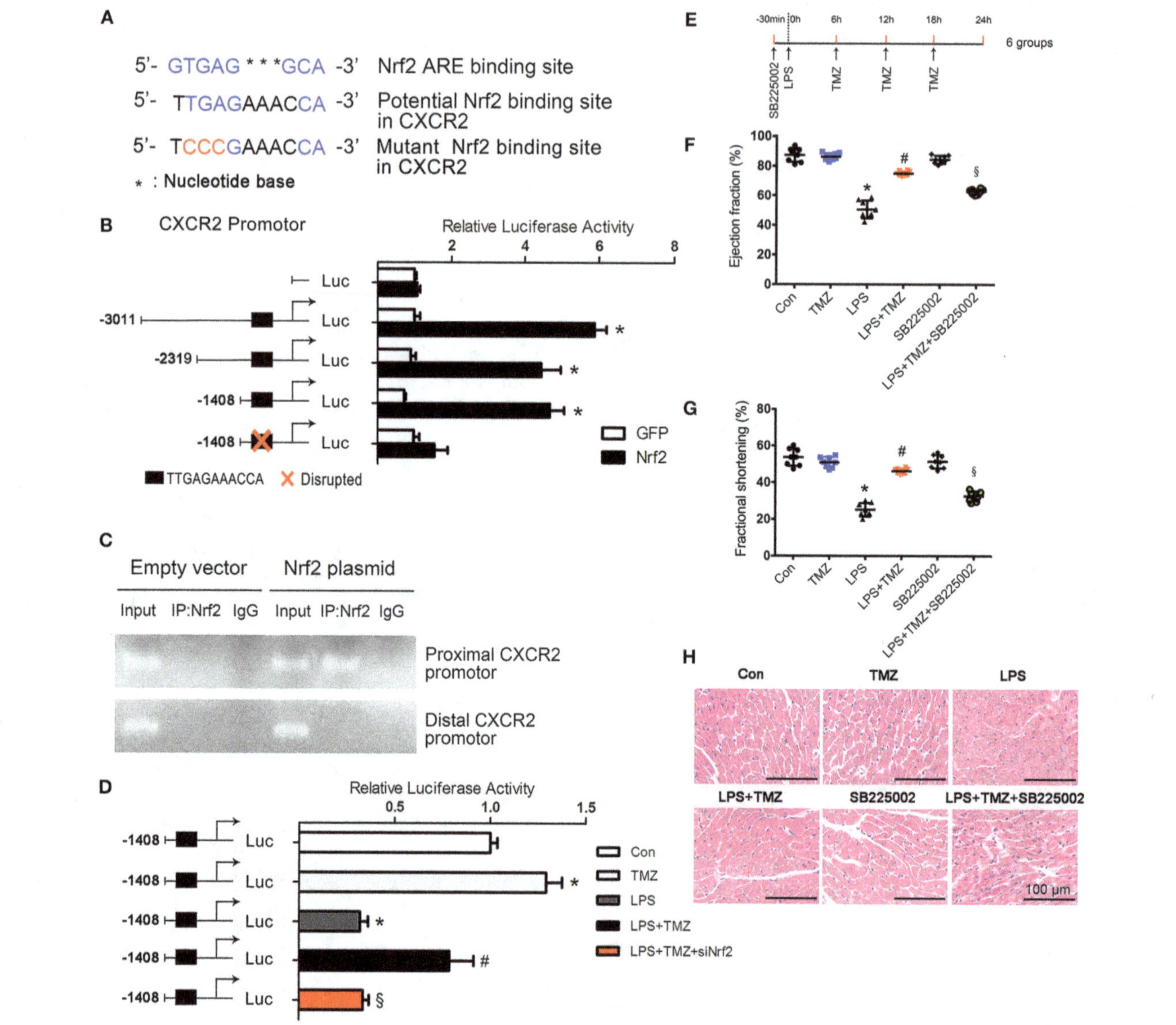

FIGURE 5 | CXCR2 is transcriptionally regulated by TMZ via Nrf2 in LPS-induced cardiac dysfunction. **(A)** Nrf2 ARE consensus binding site, potential Nrf2 binding site and the mutant Nrf2 binding site relative to potential Nrf2 binding site on mouse CXCR2. Blue indicates binding site, red indicates mutated base. **(B)** Luciferase activity of the constructs transfected into HEK293T cells. The first base before ATG represents−1. **(C)** Nrf2 chromatin immunoprecipitation. HEK293T cells were transfected with an empty plasmid or plasmid expressing Nrf2. PCR assays on input and IP fractions amplified the CXCR2 promoter containing the putative Nrf2 site (−919/−909, top panel) or a distal region of the Nrf2 promoter (−2727/−2717, bottom panel). **(D)**−1408/+254 CXCR2 promoter constructs and si-Nrf2 were transfected into HEK293T cells, and then subjected to TMZ (20 μM), LPS (5 μg/ml) or combination stimulations. Relative luciferase activity of−1408/+254 CXCR2 promoter construct after stimulations. **(E)** Schematic drawing of experimental schedule for the mice study. 8–10 week-old C57BL/6 male mice were first intraperitoneally injected with the CXCR2 inhibitor SB225002 (10 mg/kg) and LPS (15 mg/kg), then TMZ was administrated by gavage every 6 h for 3 times after LPS injection for 6 h. **(F,G)** Ejection fraction and fractional shortening was measured by two-dimensional echocardiography. **(H)** Representative images of left ventricular myocardium H&E staining. Scale bars: 100 μm. Data is presented as mean ± SEM *in vivo* and mean ± SD *in vitro* of three independent experiments. $^{*}P < 0.05$ vs. corresponding Control group or GFP control; $^{\#}P < 0.05$ vs. LPS group; $^{\S}P < 0.05$ vs. LPS+TMZ group. $n = 8$ mice per group.

bone marrow transplantation experiments, we identified that TMZ pre-treated bone marrow cells, other than resident cells, prevented LPS-induced cardiac dysfunction and promoted neutrophil recruitment into the heart. Even though TMZ was pre-treated in the group vehicle BM > TMZ, vehicle pre-treated bone marrow cells did not prevent LPS- or CLP-induced cardiac dysfunction and failed to promote neutrophil recruitment into the heart. Given that CXCR2 plays an important role in the retention and release of neutrophils in bone marrow (37), we speculate that the role of TMZ is different in bone marrow versus peripheral tissue (heart), and TMZ mainly acts in bone marrow.

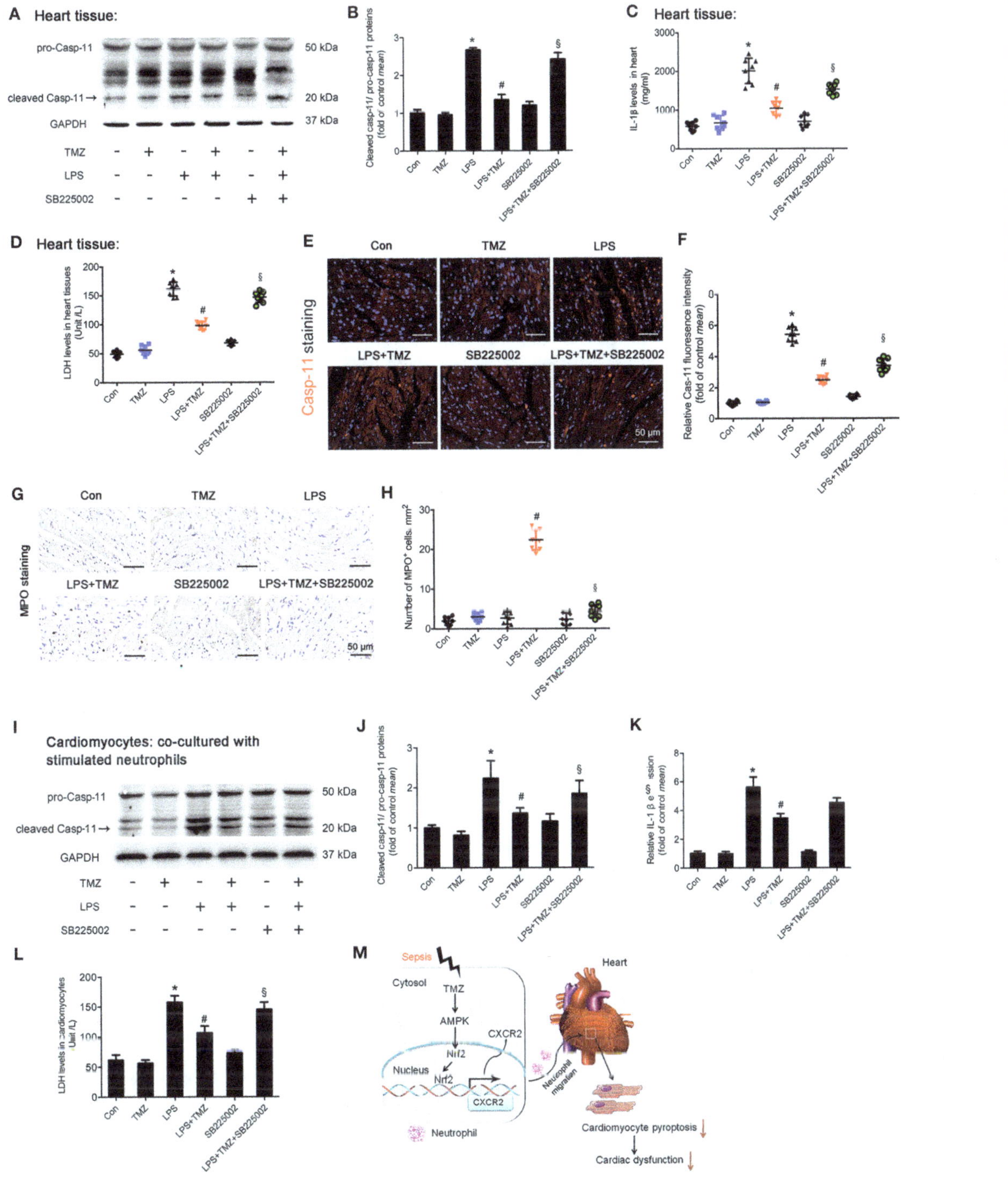

FIGURE 6 | TMZ decreased LPS-induced cardiomyocyte pyroptosis by targeting neutrophils. **(A)** 8–10 week-old C57BL/6 male mice were first injected with the CXCR2 inhibitor SB225002 (10 mg/kg) and LPS (15 mg/kg), then TMZ was administrated by gavage every 6 h for 3 times after LPS injection for 6 h. Cleaved caspase-11 (marked by arrow) expression in heart tissue was measured by western blotting. **(B)** Quantification of cleaved Casp-11/ pro-Casp-11 was performed from the western blotting analysis and expressed as fold induction. **(C)** IL-1β levels in heart tissues were measured by ELISA. **(D)** LDH levels in heart tissue. **(E)** Representative images of left ventricular myocardium caspase-11 (red) fluorescent staining. Blue indicates DAPI staining. Scale bar: 50 μm. **(F)** Relative caspase-11 fluorescent intensity. **(G)** Representative images of left ventricular myocardium MPO staining. Scale bar: 50 μm. **(H)** Quantification of MPO-positive cells in 1 mm^2. **(I)** BMDNs were first administrated with SB225002 (1 μM), then stimulated with LPS (5 μg/ml) for 1 h, and finally with TMZ (20 μM) treatment. Primary cardiomyocytes of adult mice were co-cultured with stimulated BMDNs by transwell. Cardiomyocytes were seeded in the bottom chamber and BMDNs into the upper chamber. Western blotting analysis of Casp-11 in cardiomyocyte and GAPDH used as loading control. **(J)** Quantification of cleaved Casp-11/ pro-Casp-11 was performed from the western blotting analysis and expressed as fold induction. **(K)** Relative expression of IL-1β mRNA in cardiomyocyte (normalized to GAPDH mRNA). **(L)** LDH levels in cardiomyocytes. **(M)** The proposed model for this study was summarized. Data is presented as mean ± SEM *in vivo* and mean ± SD *in vitro* of three independent experiments. $^{*}P < 0.05$ vs. corresponding Control group; $^{\#}P < 0.05$ vs. LPS group; $^{\S}P < 0.05$ vs. LPS+TMZ group.

To elucidate the functions of increased neutrophils in heart tissue, we assessed the ability of neutrophil migration. Migration of neutrophils was regulated by corresponding chemokines via binding to the specific chemokine receptors, which belong to the G protein-coupled receptor family (38). CXCR2 plays an important role in mice neutrophil recruitment into the infected site (39). The failure of neutrophil migration was associated with CXCR2 depression (8). GRK2 is a serine/threonine proteins kinase and its activation increased the internalization of the chemokine receptor CXCR2 (9). However, the detailed mechanism underlying the direct regulation of CXCR2 expression on the membrane of neutrophils during sepsis has been poorly investigated. Previous studies have reported that AMPK activation enhances neutrophil chemotaxis and bacterial killing (12). The present study demonstrates that TMZ promoted LPS-inhibited BMDN migration *in vitro* is accompanied by an increase in CXCR2 membrane expression, which was significantly prevented by the AMPK inhibitor CC. Moreover, TMZ induced accumulation of Nrf2 in the nucleus in BMDNs contributed to the increased CXCR2 membrane expression. Additionally, the suppression of GRK2 induced by TMZ also reduced the rapid internalization of CXCR2.

When cells were exposed to oxidative or electrophilic stress, Nrf2 disassociated from Keap1 and translocated into the nucleus, where it was able to regulate the transcription of its target genes by binding to the anti-oxidative response element (ARE) located in the promoter area (13). Nrf2 regulates antioxidant genes, resulting in elimination of reactive oxygen species (ROS) and decreased inflammation (40). Recently, Nrf2 has been evidenced to bind to the pro-inflammatory genes IL-6 and IL-1, blocking their transcriptions in macrophages (41). Moreover, Nrf2 activation protected cardiac tissue from injury caused by diabetic cardiomyopathy (42). In this study, for the first time, we provided evidences that Nrf2 directly binds to a new site located in the CXCR2 promoter sequence, resulting in higher expression of CXCR2 on the membrane and increased neutrophil migration. Furthermore, TMZ significantly enhanced the LPS-inhibited transcriptional activity of CXCR2, while blockage of Nrf2 abrogated the effects of TMZ. In addition, blockage of CXCR2 *in vivo* inhibited the cardiac protective effects of TMZ in LPS-stimulated mice.

Sepsis is the systemic inflammatory response to infection and the inflammatory process contributed to the occurrence of pyroptosis (1). Whether or not cardiomyocyte pyroptosis is involved in sepsis-induced cardiac dysfunction still needs to be elucidated. Pyroptosis is a highly pro-inflammatory form of programmed cell death that occurs in response to diverse organism insults. Pyroptosis occurs when canonical inflammasomes, including NLRP1, NLRP3, NLRC4, and AIM2 activates caspase- 1. On the other hand, activation of noncanonical inflammasomes is triggered by intracellular LPS directly binding to the murine caspase-11 and its human counterparts, caspase-4 and caspase-5 (22). Inhibition of caspase-1 protected against inflammation and cardiac dysfunction that results from myocardial infarction (MI) (43). Recent studies have revealed that attenuation of cardiomyocyte pyroptosis effectively ameliorates diabetic cardiomyopathy (13). Our results showed the involvement of pyroptosis in the heart of LPS-treated mice, indicated by activation of caspase-11, IL-1β release, and LDH release. Interestingly, TMZ significantly suppressed LPS-induced pyroptosis, which was reversed by the CXCR2 antagonist, SB225002. Combined with MPO staining, these results suggest that increased neutrophil recruitment is associated with decreased cardiomyocyte pyroptosis. The direct recruitment of neutrophils to the injured tissue is essential to eliminate the pathogen. However, in some specific condition (just like pyroptosis, a form of inflammatory programmed cell death), the neutrophils were pronounced accumulated in heart to help opsonization of pore-induced intracellular traps (PITs). The PIT initiated a robust and coordinated innate immune response involving multiple mediators that attracted neutrophils to efferocytose the PIT (44, 45). The enhanced neutrophils recruitment would effectively contribute to the attenuation of pyroptosis via efferocytosing the PIT. TMZ may reduce pyroptosis via efferocytosing the PIT, which is mediated by the enhanced neutrophils. Considering the complex inflammatory environment during lytic cell death, we reasoned that additional signals likely contributed to neutrophil recruitment. Indeed, besides inducing pyroptosis, caspase-1 also induces secretion of IL-1β and IL-18. IL1β$^{-/-}$IL18$^{-/-}$ mice had significantly reduced neutrophil recruitment after the induction of pyroptosis in the tissue (44, 46). Thus, the normal caspase-1 induced pyroptosis led to secretion of IL-1β and IL-18, which could increase neutrophil recruitment. Besides inflammatory cytokines, the CXCL2 and CXCR2 signaling pathway also contributed to the neutrophil recruitment. In our current study, we mainly focused on the CXCR2 signaling pathway and investigated the role of TMZ during sepsis. We speculate that neutrophil mediated efferocytose of the PITs would play a corresponding role during LPS-induced cardiomyocyte pyroptosis.

In conclusion, our results showed that TMZ attenuated LPS-induced cardiomyocyte pyroptosis and cardiac dysfunction by promoting neutrophil recruitment to cardiac tissue via CXCR2. This suggests that TMZ may be a potential drug for the treatment of septic cardiac dysfunction.

AUTHOR CONTRIBUTIONS

CC and DWW: conception and design. JC and BW: experiments, analysis, and draft writing. JL, MH, GR, ZY, and JW: part experiments. ZB, KC, and QN: English editing.

FUNDING

This work was supported by grant from the National Natural Science Foundation of China [91439203, 81630010 and 81790624 to DWW, 31771264 to CC and 81700333 to JC] and Changjiang Scholars and Innovative Research Team in University [IRT_14R20 to QN]. The funders had no role in study design, data collection and analysis, decision to publish, or preparation of the manuscript.

ACKNOWLEDGMENTS

We would like to thank our colleagues in Dr. Wang's group for various technical help and stimulating discussion during the course of this investigation.

REFERENCES

1. Singer M, Deutschman CS, Seymour CW, Shankar-Hari M, Annane D, Bauer M, et al. The third international consensus definitions for sepsis and septic shock (Sepsis-3). *JAMA* (2016) 315:801–10. doi: 10.1001/jama.2016.0287
2. Deutschman CS, Tracey KJ. Sepsis: current dogma and new perspectives. *Immunity* (2014) 40:463–75. doi: 10.1016/j.immuni.2014.04.001
3. Merx MW, Weber C. Sepsis and the heart. *Circulation* (2007) 116:793–802. doi: 10.1161/CIRCULATIONAHA.106.678359
4. Brown KA, Brain SD, Pearson JD, Edgeworth JD, Lewis SM, Treacher DF. Neutrophils in development of multiple organ failure in sepsis. *Lancet* (2006) 368:157–69. doi: 10.1016/S0140-6736(06)69005-3
5. Alves-Filho JC, Sonego F, Souto FO, Freitas A, Verri WAJr, Auxiliadora-Martins M, et al. Interleukin-33 attenuates sepsis by enhancing neutrophil influx to the site of infection. *Nat Med.* (2010) 16:708–12. doi: 10.1038/nm.2156
6. Spiller F, Costa C, Souto FO, Vinchi F, Mestriner FL, Laure HJ, et al. Inhibition of neutrophil migration by hemopexin leads to increased mortality due to sepsis in mice. *Am J Respir Crit Care Med.* (2011) 183:922–31. doi: 10.1164/rccm.201002-0223OC
7. Chishti AD, Shenton BK, Kirby JA, Baudouin SV. Neutrophil chemotaxis and receptor expression in clinical septic shock. *Intensive Care Med.* (2004) 30:605–11. doi: 10.1007/s00134-004-2175-y
8. Rios-Santos F, Alves-Filho JC, Souto FO, Spiller F, Freitas A, Lotufo CM, et al. Down-regulation of CXCR2 on neutrophils in severe sepsis is mediated by inducible nitric oxide synthase-derived nitric oxide. *Am J Respir Crit Care Med.* (2007) 175:490–7. doi: 10.1164/rccm.200601-103OC
9. Arraes SM, Freitas MS, da Silva SV, de Paula Neto HA, Alves-Filho JC, Auxiliadora Martins M, et al. Impaired neutrophil chemotaxis in sepsis associates with GRK expression and inhibition of actin assembly and tyrosine phosphorylation. *Blood* (2006) 108:2906–13. doi: 10.1182/blood-2006-05-024638
10. Tancevski I, Nairz M, Duwensee K, Auer K, Schroll A, Heim C, et al. Fibrates ameliorate the course of bacterial sepsis by promoting neutrophil recruitment via CXCR2. *EMBO Mol Med.* (2014) 6:810–20. doi: 10.1002/emmm.201303415
11. Long YC, Zierath JR. AMP-activated protein kinase signaling in metabolic regulation. *J Clin Invest.* (2006) 116:1776–83. doi: 10.1172/JCI29044
12. Park DW, Jiang S, Tadie JM, Stigler WS, Gao Y, Deshane J, et al. Activation of AMPK enhances neutrophil chemotaxis and bacterial killing. *Mol Med.* (2013) 19:387–98. doi: 10.2119/molmed.2013.00065
13. Mo C, Wang L, Zhang J, Numazawa S, Tang H, Tang X, et al. The crosstalk between Nrf2 and AMPK signal pathways is important for the anti-inflammatory effect of berberine in LPS-stimulated macrophages and endotoxin-shocked mice. *Antioxid Redox Signal.* (2014) 20:574–88. doi: 10.1089/ars.2012.5116
14. Chen J, Lai J, Yang L, Ruan G, Chaugai S, Ning Q, et al. Trimetazidine prevents macrophage-mediated septic myocardial dysfunction via activation of the histone deacetylase sirtuin 1. *Br J Pharmacol.* (2016) 173:545–61. doi: 10.1111/bph.13386
15. Ganan-Gomez I, Wei Y, Yang H, Boyano-Adanez MC, Garcia-Manero G. Oncogenic functions of the transcription factor Nrf2. *Free Radic Biol Med.* (2013) 65:750–61. doi: 10.1016/j.freeradbiomed.2013.06.041
16. Kobayashi E, Suzuki T, Yamamoto M. Roles nrf2 plays in myeloid cells and related disorders. *Oxid Med Cell Longev.* (2013) 2013:529219. doi: 10.1155/2013/529219
17. Kantor PF, Lucien A, Kozak R, Lopaschuk GD. The antianginal drug trimetazidine shifts cardiac energy metabolism from fatty acid oxidation to glucose oxidation by inhibiting mitochondrial long-chain 3-ketoacyl coenzyme A thiolase. *Circ Res.* (2000) 86:580–8. doi: 10.1161/01.RES.86.5.580
18. Tuunanen H, Engblom E, Naum A, Nagren K, Scheinin M, Hesse B, et al. Trimetazidine, a metabolic modulator, has cardiac and extracardiac benefits in idiopathic dilated cardiomyopathy. *Circulation* (2008) 118:1250–8. doi: 10.1161/CIRCULATIONAHA.108.778019
19. Zhou X, Li C, Xu W, Chen J. Trimetazidine protects against smoking-induced left ventricular remodeling via attenuating oxidative stress, apoptosis, and inflammation. *PLoS ONE* (2012) 7:e40424. doi: 10.1371/journal.pone.0040424
20. Monti LD, Setola E, Fragasso G, Camisasca RP, Lucotti P, Galluccio E, et al. Metabolic and endothelial effects of trimetazidine on forearm skeletal muscle in patients with type 2 diabetes and ischemic cardiomyopathy. *Am J Physiol Endocrinol Metab.* (2006) 290:E54–E59. doi: 10.1152/ajpendo.00083.2005
21. Shi J, Zhao Y, Wang K, Shi X, Wang Y, Huang H, et al. Cleavage of GSDMD by inflammatory caspases determines pyroptotic cell death. *Nature* (2015) 526:660–5. doi: 10.1038/nature15514
22. Shi J, Zhao Y, Wang Y, Gao W, Ding J, Li P, et al. Inflammatory caspases are innate immune receptors for intracellular LPS. *Nature* (2014) 514:187–92. doi: 10.1038/nature13683
23. Yang D, He Y, Munoz-Planillo R, Liu Q, Nunez G. Caspase-11 requires the pannexin-1 channel and the purinergic P2X7 pore to mediate pyroptosis and endotoxic shock. *Immunity* (2015) 43:923–32. doi: 10.1016/j.immuni.2015.10.009
24. Jorgensen I, Miao EA. Pyroptotic cell death defends against intracellular pathogens. *Immunol Rev.* (2015) 265:130–42. doi: 10.1111/imr.12287
25. Rittirsch D, Huber-Lang MS, Flierl MA, Ward PA. Immunodesign of experimental sepsis by cecal ligation and puncture. *Nat Protoc.* (2009) 4:31–6. doi: 10.1038/nprot.2008.214
26. Zhang L, Freedman NJ, Brian L, Peppel K. Graft-extrinsic cells predominate in vein graft arterialization. *Arterioscler Thromb Vasc Biol.* (2004) 24:470–6. doi: 10.1161/01.ATV.0000116865.98067.31
27. Manning WJ, Wei JY, Katz SE, Litwin SE, Douglas PS. *In vivo* assessment of LV mass in mice using high-frequency cardiac ultrasound: necropsy validation. *Am J Physiol.* (1994) 266:H1672–5. doi: 10.1152/ajpheart.1994.266.4.H1672
28. Louch WE, Sheehan KA, Wolska BM. Methods in cardiomyocyte isolation, culture, and gene transfer. *J Mol Cell Cardiol.* (2011) 51:288–98. doi: 10.1016/j.yjmcc.2011.06.012
29. Cavaillon JM, Adib-Conquy M. Bench-to-bedside review: endotoxin tolerance as a model of leukocyte reprogramming in sepsis. *Crit Care* (2006) 10:233. doi: 10.1186/cc5055
30. Kayagaki N, Warming S, Lamkanfi M, Vande Walle L, Louie S, Dong J, et al. Non-canonical inflammasome activation targets caspase-11. *Nature* (2011) 479:117–21. doi: 10.1038/nature10558
31. Barrientos-Vega R, Mar Sanchez-Soria M, Morales-Garcia C, Robas-Gomez A, Cuena-Boy R, Ayensa-Rincon A. Prolonged sedation of critically ill patients with midazolam or propofol: impact on weaning and costs. *Crit Care Med.* (1997) 25:33–40. doi: 10.1097/00003246-199701000-00009
32. Jia P, Wu X, Dai Y, Teng J, Fang Y, Hu J, et al. MicroRNA-21 is required for local and remote ischemic preconditioning in multiple organ protection against sepsis. *Crit Care Med.* (2017) 45:e703–10. doi: 10.1097/CCM.0000000000002363
33. Jin H, Fujita T, Jin M, Kurotani R, Namekata I, Hamaguchi S, et al. Cardiac overexpression of Epac1 in transgenic mice rescues lipopolysaccharide-induced cardiac dysfunction and inhibits Jak-STAT pathway. *J Mol Cell Cardiol.* (2017) 108:170–80. doi: 10.1016/j.yjmcc.2017.05.014
34. Martin GS, Mannino DM, Eaton S, Moss M. The epidemiology of sepsis in the United States from 1979 through 2000. *N Engl J Med.* (2003) 348:1546–54. doi: 10.1056/NEJMoa022139

35. Flierl MA, Rittirsch D, Huber-Lang MS, Sarma JV, Ward PA. Molecular events in the cardiomyopathy of sepsis. *Mol Med.* (2008) 14:327–36. doi: 10.2119/2007-00130
36. Makara MA, Hoang KV, Ganesan LP, Crouser ED, Gunn JS, Turner J, et al. Cardiac electrical and structural changes during bacterial infection: an instructive model to study cardiac dysfunction in sepsis. *J Am Heart Assoc.* (2016) 5:e003820. doi: 10.1161/JAHA.116.003820
37. Borregaard N. Neutrophils, from marrow to microbes. *Immunity* (2010) 33:657–70. doi: 10.1016/j.immuni.2010.11.011
38. Ley K, Laudanna C, Cybulsky MI, Nourshargh S. Getting to the site of inflammation: the leukocyte adhesion cascade updated. *Nat Rev Immunol.* (2007) 7:678–89. doi: 10.1038/nri2156
39. Reutershan J, Morris MA, Burcin TL, Smith DF, Chang D, Saprito MS, et al. Critical role of endothelial CXCR2 in LPS-induced neutrophil migration into the lung. *J Clin Invest.* (2006) 116:695–702. doi: 10.1172/JCI 27009
40. Kong X, Thimmulappa R, Kombairaju P, Biswal S. NADPH oxidase-dependent reactive oxygen species mediate amplified TLR4 signaling and sepsis-induced mortality in Nrf2-deficient mice. *J Immunol.* (2010) 185:569–77. doi: 10.4049/jimmunol.0902315
41. Kobayashi EH, Suzuki T, Funayama R, Nagashima T, Hayashi M, Sekine H, et al. Nrf2 suppresses macrophage inflammatory response by blocking proinflammatory cytokine transcription. *Nat Commun.* (2016) 7:11624. doi: 10.1038/ncomms11624
42. Li H, Yao W, Irwin MG, Wang T, Wang S, Zhang L, et al. Adiponectin ameliorates hyperglycemia-induced cardiac hypertrophy and dysfunction by concomitantly activating Nrf2 and Brg1. *Free Radic Biol Med.* (2015) 84:311–21. doi: 10.1016/j.freeradbiomed.2015.03.007
43. Frantz S, Ducharme A, Sawyer D, Rohde LE, Kobzik L, Fukazawa R, et al. Targeted deletion of caspase-1 reduces early mortality and left ventricular dilatation following myocardial infarction. *J Mol Cell Cardiol.* (2003) 35:685–94. doi: 10.1016/S0022-2828(03)00113-5
44. Jorgensen I, Lopez JP, Laufer SA, Miao EA. IL-1beta, IL-18, and eicosanoids promote neutrophil recruitment to pore-induced intracellular traps following pyroptosis. *Eur J Immunol.* (2016) 46:2761–6. doi: 10.1002/eji.201646647
45. Jorgensen I, Zhang Y, Krantz BA, Miao EA. Pyroptosis triggers pore-induced intracellular traps (PITs) that capture bacteria and lead to their clearance by efferocytosis. *J Exp Med.* (2016) 213:2113–28. doi: 10.1084/jem.20151613
46. Ross R. Atherosclerosis–an inflammatory disease. *N Engl J Med.* (1999) 340:115–26. doi: 10.1056/NEJM199901143400207

13

Cardio-Immunology of Myocarditis: Focus on Immune Mechanisms and Treatment Options

*Bernhard Maisch**

Faculty of Medicine, and Heart and Vessel Center, Philipps-University, Marburg, Germany

***Correspondence:**
Bernhard Maisch
bermaisch@gmail.com

Myocarditis and inflammatory cardiomyopathy are syndromes, not aetiological disease entities. From animal models of cardiac inflammation we have detailed insight of the strain specific immune reactions based on the genetic background of the animal and the infectiosity of the virus. Innate and adaptive immunity also react in man. An aetiological diagnosis of a viral vs. a non-viral cause is possible by endomyocardial biopsy with histology, immunohistology and PCR for microbial agents. This review deals with the different etiologies of myocarditis and inflammatory cardiomyopathy on the basis of the genetic background and the predisposition for inflammation. It analyses tho opidemiologic shift in cardiotropic viral agents in the last 30 years. Based on the understanding of the interaction between infection and the players of the innate and adaptive immune system it summarizes pathogenetic phases and clinical faces of myocarditis. It gives an up-to-date information on specific treatment options beyond symptomatic heart failure and antiarrhythmic therapy. Although inflammation can resolve spontaneously, specific treatment directed to the causative etiology is often required. For fulminant, acute, and chronic autoreactive myocarditis without viral persistence immunosuppressive treatment can be life-saving, for viral inflammatory cardiomyopathy ivIg treatment can resolve inflammation and often eradicate the virus.

Keywords: myocarditis, endomyocardial biopsy, immunohistology, PCR of cardiotropic viruses, immunopathogenesis, ivIg, immunosuppressive therapy

INTRODUCTION

More than a century ago, when coronary artery disease was neglectable, inflammation of the heart (=myocarditis) was thought to be the dominant cause of any cardiac disease (1). It has been known for decades that the heart is target of immunological effector organs, the T- and B-cells, their products such as circulating antibodies, mediators and cytokines (2). Nowadays, the heart is also considered an immunological organ reacting to damage and stress (3) and even with an antibody response to stress proteins (4). This occurs on the basis of a genetic background (5) and also epigenetic mechanisms (6), which led to the distinction between familial and non-familial cardiomyopathies in the latest classification of cardiomyopathies (7) and clarification of terms in the recent position statement of the working group on myocardial and pericardial diseases (8). Further insight in treatment options has been given in 2012 (9) and recently updated in 2018 (10).

The term cardiomyopathies is much younger than myocarditis and was first used by Hickie and Hall 1960 (11). The WHO/ISFC (World Health Organization/ International Society and Federation of Cardiology) Task Force defined it as "heart muscle diseases of unknown cause"

(12). In 1996 the term cardiomyopathies was applied to all heart muscle diseases, which lead to functional impairment of the heart (13). Dilated cardiomyopathy (DCM) was one of 3 main clinical phenotypes (dilated, hypertrophic, restrictive cardiomyopathy). Remarkably, the 1996 task force included inflammatory heart muscle diseases (myocarditis, perimyocarditis), hypertensive, and ischemic cardiomyopathies and other forms of heart failure of known origin in the group of secondary cardiomyopathies. Inflammatory cardiomyopathy was then defined as inflamed myocardium assessed histologically as myocarditis in association with cardiac dysfunction. The pathohistological criteria at that time were the Dallas criteria (14), which distinguished active, recurrent, healing and borderline myocarditis. The etiology was assumed to be either Infectious, toxic or autoimmune. Non inflammatory viral cardiomyopathy was defined as viral persistence in a dilated heart without ongoing inflammation. Inflammatory cardiomyopathy was further specified in a World Heart Federation consensus meeting in 1999 by quantitative immunohistological criteria for inflammation (> 14 infiltrating cells/mm^2) (15, 16) and referred to it in the consensus document 2013 (8). These infiltrating cells in the myocardium could be T- and B lymphocytes, their activated forms and up to 4 monocytes or macrophages/mm^2. The underlying microbial agent had to be assessed or excluded by molecular biological methods, e.g., polymerase chain reaction (PCR) or *in situ* hybridization (17).

LESSONS LEARNED FROM ANIMAL STUDIES

Animal studies have contributed much to our understanding of the role of the immune system in cardiac homeostasis and disease (18):

1) In *healthy mice hearts* all major leukocyte classes including mononuclear phagocytes, neutrophils, B and T cells are present. They can be resident or from circulating blood. The normal mouse heart also contains resident cardiac dendritic cells and mast cells.
2) Between individual cardiomyocytes a network of resident macrophages exists, which are heterogeneous and ontogenetically diverse.
3) Leukocyte distribution is not uniform but the cells adhere to niches: Embryonically derived macrophages are adjacent to coronary vasculature, fetally derived monocytes are close to endocardial trabeculae, the aortic valve is rich in dendritic cells, the AV node contains a relatively high concentration of macrophages.
4) Immune cells and macrophages in particular also participate in organ development and steady-state physiology of tissue such as housekeeping tasks for maintaining cardiac function, cell and matrix turnover, and angiogenesis.
5) Macrophages interact with the conduction system. Depletion of macrophages in mice hearts may lead to conduction abnormalities (19).
6) The pericardial adipose tissue can readily supply leukocytes during myocardial injury. Mast cells accumulate preferably in white adipose tissue.
7) It has been shown that in *injured hearts* of mice and men resident and circulating leukocytes can be activated any form of injury such as in infarction (20) or after cardiac surgery (21).
8) Genetic studies indicated that susceptibility to Coxsackievirus (CV) B3 depended on the strain of mice used for infection. Virological studies revealed that different strains of CVB developed different magnitudes of cardiac organ involvement from very active forms of myocarditis to no inflammation at all. Also organ specificity for either heart and/or pancreas depended on the susceptibility of the mice. But also infectiosity of different CVB strains was important. More recently CVB3 strains were isolated with 5-terminal deletions in genomic RNAs from a patient with idiopathic dilated cardiomyopathy. These deletions lacked portions of the 5′stem-loop I, which is a RNA secondary structure required for viral RNA replication. These findings suggest that even mutant viruses can be responsible for persistent infection. And in this changed structure they may also escape conventional PCR detection (22).
9) In the beginning of myocarditis viral infection of the heart is recognized by pattern recognition receptors (PRRs) such as toll like receptors (TLR) 2, 3, 4, 7, and 8. The downstream effects of each TLR activation may be different to each TLR, but all share a common a pro-inflammatory response. For instance after TLR2 stimulation by a damaged self-protein such as cardiac myosin monocytes produced pro-inflammatory cytokines such as IL-6, IL-8, and TNF-α. Cardiac myosin has often been used as antigen for immunization and initiation of experimental autoimmune myocarditis models. Viral murine myocarditis has focused on CVB3 infection. Signaling of the adaptor protein Myd88 downstream of TLR4 led to activation of NF-κB, which decreased survival. In contrast signaling of adaptor protein TRIF up-regulates the antiviral IFN-β response and improves survival.
10) In mice strains susceptible to infection with CVB3 myocardial disease occurs in 3 pathogenetic phases (infection, autoimmune reaction, dilated cardiomyopathy) with 3 symptomatic faces (malaise, inflammation, heart failure) (23, 24). In *phase 1* CVB3 enters the myocardial cells via the coxsackie/adenoviral receptor (CAR) hereby initiating first the innate and later the adaptive immune responses. Mast cells as early responders produce proinflammatory cytokines (TNF, IL-1ß, IL-r). Neutrophils and monocytes produce additional mediators such as IL-12. An increased production of interleukin-1b (IL-1b) and tumor necrosis factor-alpha during the early innate response to viral infection is a prerequisite for the induction of heart-specific autoimmune myocarditis. Its severity is determined by the number of T helper 1 (Th1) and Th2 cytokines. The Th1 pathway by interleukin-12 (IL-12) and gamma interferon (IFNgamma) is in principle proinflammatory and can lead to myocardial infiltration of the heart. It can also be down regulated by INFgamma production. The prototype Th2 cytokine is IL-4. It is frequent in severe forms of autoimmune myocarditis where eosinophils are prominent.

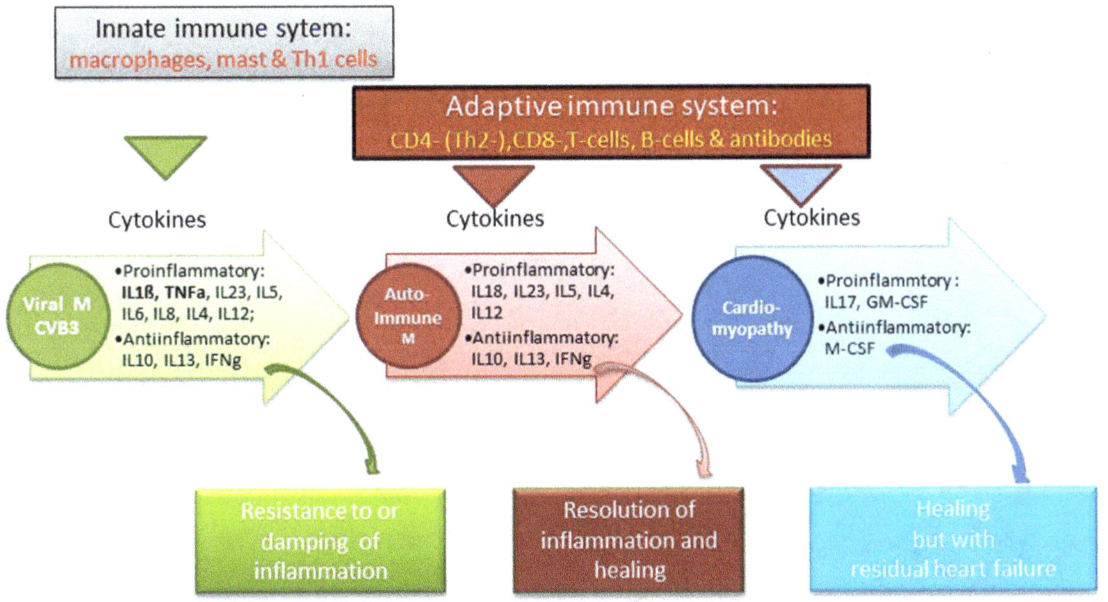

FIGURE 1 | Immune system and cytokine pattern in various susceptical and resistant mouse myocarditis models [Balbc, A/J mice, after CVB3 infection with a consecutive autoimmune reaction to cardiac myosi (25)].

Since it can go along with an IFNgamma increase, the disease is limited. IL-13, another Th2 cytokine, protects from infection, and reduces inflammation. Th17 cytokines also contribute to disease. The signature cytokine IL-17A is not essential for cardiac inflammation, but it is needed for the progression to heart failure (**Figure 1**) (25).

Myeloid differentiation primary response protein 88(MYD88) and IL-1 receptor-associated kinase 4(IRAK4) enhance myocardial inflammation by activating TNF receptor-associated factor 6(TRAF6) and nuclear factor-kappa b (NFKB). This decreases the production of antiviral type I interferons in the affected host. In *phase 2* after presentation by dendritic cells the antigen-specific T-cells are the key players of cardiac damage. They may be counteracted by Treg cells. Inflammation may thus be ended or go on chronically as autoimmune reaction. T helper cells promote the development of cardiac dilatation by stimulating cardiac fibroblasts (phase 3). The autoimmune reactivity develops because coxsackievirus shares epitopes with cardiac myosin (23, 26), which as endogenous antigen contributes to this chronic inflammation.

Cardiac myosin as antigen has been used as a prototype protein in experimental autoimmune myocarditis (EAM), as well as many others antigens, e.g., Troponin I. They all can be prototypes of a B-cell driven myocarditis.

In these animal models *phase 1*, the infection phase, was followed by an antiviral and an autoimmune reaction (*phase 2*) (23, 26). This 2nd phase can be followed by lethal cardiac decompensation in a fibrotic heart with severe myocyte loss (*phase 3*) or by the resolution of the inflammation.

In man a similar triphasic pathogenetic process was assumed. The corresponding clinical correlates are malaise, inflammation and heart failure.

11) Our understanding of the pathogenetic processes following viral infection or myocyte destruction has been widened particularly by analyzing the steps leading to the activation of the innate immune system. The innate immune system is triggered by pathogen-associated molecular patterns (PAMP) and damage-associated molecular patterns (DAMP via Toll-like (TLR) and Nod-like receptors (NLR). These receptors are assembled in the inflammasome, which is a multiprotein intracellular complex located predominantly in macrophages. It activates proinflammatory cytokines such as interleukin-1b and IL-18 after detecting infective microbial agents or sterile stressors. Inflammasomes can also induce pyroptosis, a form of programmed cell death. They can induce the adaptive immune system consequently (27). A dysregulation of inflammasomes can be associated with autoimmune syndromes such as an autoreactive myocarditis (**Figure 2**).

CLINICAL DIAGNOSIS IN HUMAN MYOCARDITIS

According to the position statement of the European Society of Cardiology Working Group on Myocardial and Pericardial Diseases (8) the appropriate clinical work-up includes careful patient assessment for symptoms, auscultation, EKG for a new left bundle branch block (LBB) or severe recent rhythm disturbances at rest or exercise. Laboratory investigations

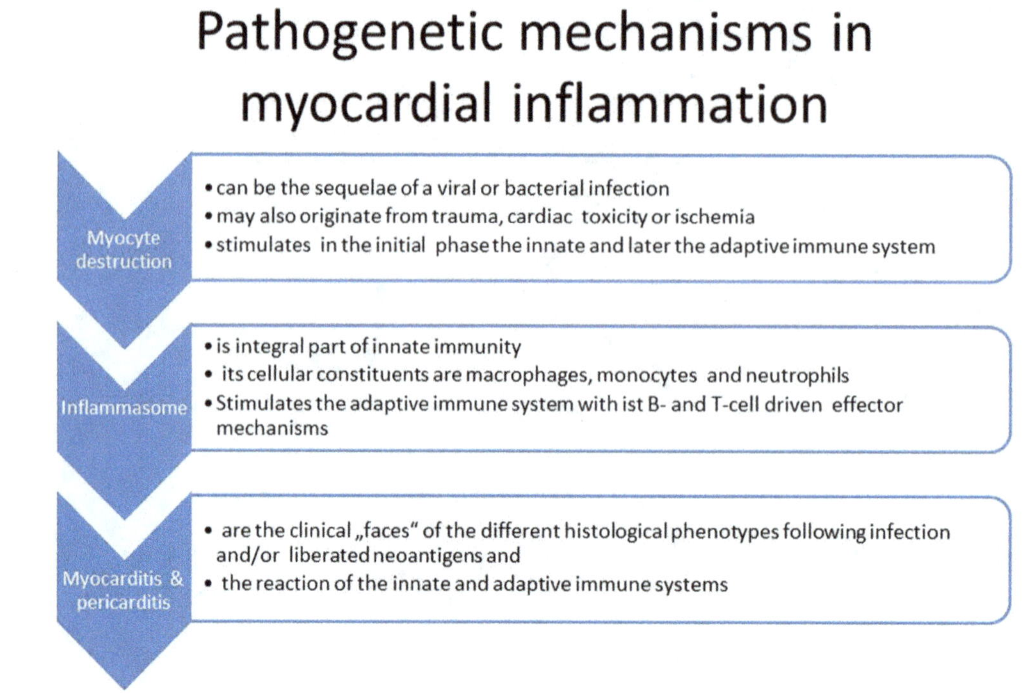

FIGURE 2 | Sequence of events in myocardial inflammation.

should include cardiac biomarkers such as nt-pro BNP for the assessment of heart failure, troponin I or T for myocyte necrosis and c-reactive protein (CRP) for inflammation. Among the non-invasive imaging techniques echocardiography can indicate cardiac inflammation, when in a symptomatic patient exhibits segmental or global wall motion abnormality and coronary artery disease or left bundle branch block (LBB) are not present. A small pericardial effusion in this context may also lead the way. Cardiac MRI is very helpful by establishing cardiac inflammation or postmyocarditic lesions in a follow-up investigation by early or late gadolinium enhancement (LGE). In principle the Lake Louise MRI protocol should be followed. But no noninvasive diagnostic method can substitute endomyocardial biopsy to reach a final aetiological diagnosis, when histology, immunhistology and PCR for microbial agents are evaluated together.

Clinical symptoms can be diverse, from to life-threating cardiogenic shock and lethal ventricular rhythm disturbances, acute or chronic heart failure or an acute chest wall syndrome. In some cases they might even allow a suspicion of the underlying pathogenetic process (**Table 1**).

Our understanding of the underlying aetiopathogenesis in man started some 35 years ago with the analysis of the antibody response to cardiac antigens in patients with suspected myocardial inflammation.

TABLE 1 | From symptoms to aetiological diagnoses.

Clinical phenotype	Symptoms and features	Aetiological diagnoses
Acute life-threating heart failure, severe rhythm disturbance	Shock, NYHA III-IV, elevated Troponin I/T, elevated Nt-proBNP	Fulminant myocarditis, e.g., giant cell or eosinophilia or toxic myocarditis, borreliosis
Acute heart failure(AHF)	Dyspnoe, edema, reduce EF, but also diastolic AHF, variable EKG, intermittent Troponin I/T-and Nt-proBNP elevations	Viral or autoreactive myocarditis order inflammatory cardiomyopathy (DCMi)
Chronic heart failure(CHF)	CHF symptoms, no CAD, EKG, with LSB, RSB, AV-Block, variable ST-/T-alterations, some troponin I/T and Nt-proBNP elevations	Viral or autoreactive focal myocarditis or DCMi or borderline myocarditis
Acute chest wall syndrome	Angina like symptoms, but no CAD, variable ST-/T-alterations, in EKG, some Troponin I/T and Nt-proBNP elevations	Parvovirus B19 or other virus with or without pericarditis

AUTOANTIBODY—MEDIATED IMMUNE RESPONSE IN HUMAN MYOCARDITIS

The humoral immune response was at that time assessed by the indirect immunoflourescence test or Elisa against cardiac proteins together with testing for antibodies against cardiotropic viruses. At that time we have focused on antibodies cross-reacting between enteroviral epitopes with cardiac myolemma and sarcolemma (28–31). We also examined the prevalence and possible pathogenicity against laminin (32), fibrils, intermediate filaments (33), and against mitochondria

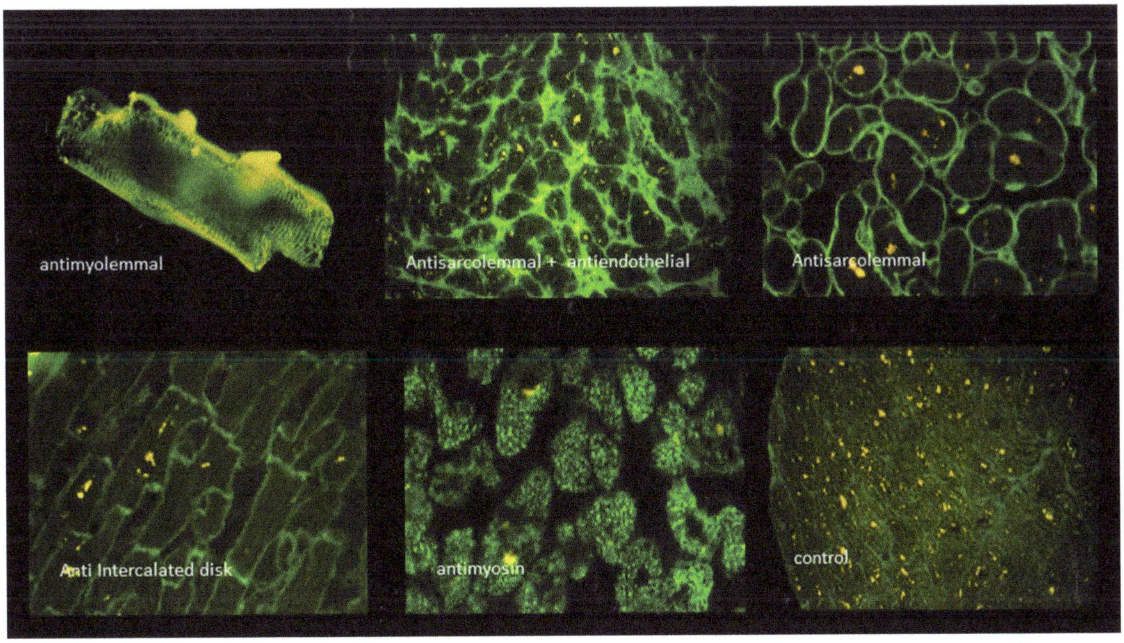

FIGURE 3 | A selection of circulating anticardiac antibodies.

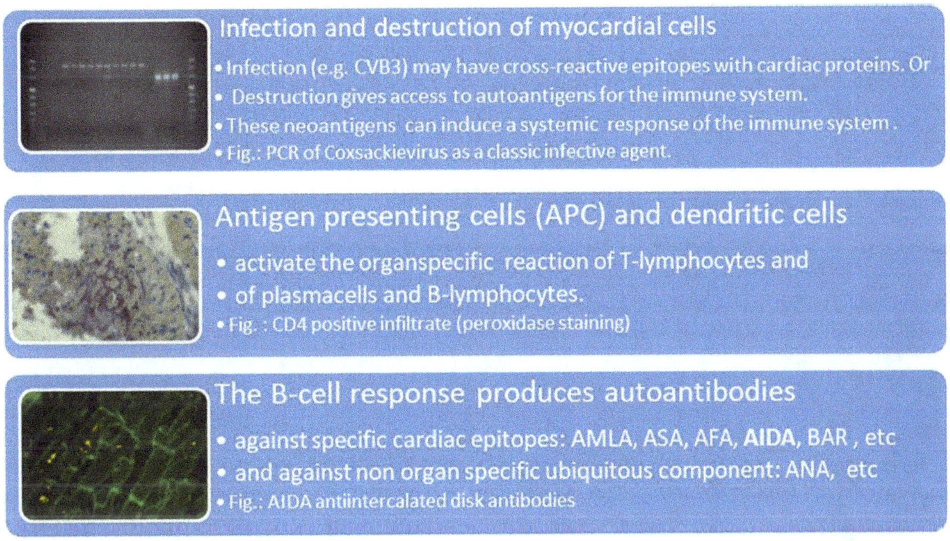

FIGURE 4 | Viral infection, antigen presentation, response by the adaptive immune system. AMLA, antimyolemmal antibodies(ab); ASA, antisarcolemmal ab; AFA, antifibrillary ab; AIDA, antiintercalated disk ab(fig.); BAR, betarecepator ab; ANA, antinuclear ab.

(34, 35). Antibodies directed against myofibrillar proteins (36), troponins were in the focus of other investigators (37). Of particular interest was also the antibody response to the beta-receptor in the sera of patients with myocarditis and dilated cardiomyopathy (38, 39) and the muscarinic acetylcholine receptor (40). Of note, also the cardiac conduction tissue was addressed by the humoral immune response to the sinus and atrioventricular nodes and Purkinje fibers (41, 42) (**Figures 3, 4, Table 2**).

IMMUNE COMPLEXES

Since anticardiac antibodies may find their corresponding targets in the circulating blood, in serous body fluids or the targeted tissue itself immune complexes may also play a role in the pathogenetic process (54).

The most important question still is, which of these antibodies were only diagnostic markers of former myocyte destruction similar to the antibodies after a vaccination or which antibodies

TABLE 2 | Anticardiac antibodies.

Antigen	Antibody	Cross-reactivity	Pathomechanism	References
Actin	Anti-actin	Unknown	Unknown	(43)
Acetylcholin-receptor	Anti-Ach	Unknown	Bradycardia	(44)
Aconitate hydratase	Anti-AH,	Unknown	Impaired metabolism	(31)
Adenin nucleotide translocator	Anti-ANT	Enterovirus	Impaired metabolism	(45)
Beta1-receptor	Anti-β1	Enterovirus	Pos. chronotropic	(38)
Beta1-receptor	Anti-β1		Neg. inotropic	(46, 47)
Creatine kinase	Anti-CK	Unknown	Impaired metabolism	(31)
Conduction system	Anti-sinus node Anti-AV node Anti-Purkinje	Unknown	Bradycardia AV-Block Conduction defect	(41, 42)
Desmin	Anti-desmin	Unknown	Unknown	(33)
Dihydrolipoamide dehydrogenase	Anti-DLD,	Unknown	Impaired metabolism	(31)
Extracted Nuclear Antigens (ENA, SSA, SSB)	ENA, ANCA Anti-SSA Anti-SSB	Unknown	Neutrophil degranulation, Congenital AV-Block	(48)
Hsp60, hsp70, Vimentin	Anti-hsp60, Anti-hsp70, Anti-vimentin	Multiple	Unknown	(4)
Laminin	Anti-laminin	Unknown	Unknown	(32, 49)
Mitochondria /Microsomes	AMA	Multiple	Inhibition of sarcosin dehydrogenase	(31, 34, 50)
Myolemma	AMLA	Enterovirus	Lytic ab	(2, 28, 29)
Myosin	Anti-myosin	Enterovirus	Neg. inotropic	(51, 52)
Nicotinamideadenine-dinucleotide dehydro-genase	Anti-NADD	Unknown	Impaired metabolism	(31)
Nuclear Antigens	ANA	Unknown	Immune complex – mediated	(4)
Pyruvate kinase	Anti-PK	Unknown	Impaired metabolism	(31)
Troponin I (& T)	Anti-Troponin I	Unknown	Negative inotropic	(53)
Ubiquinol-cyto-chrome-c-reductase	Anti-UCR	Unknown	Impaired metabolism	(31)
Sarcolemma	ASA	Enterovirus	Lytic	(3, 24, 26)

Ab, antibody; ASA, antisarcolemmal antibody; AMA, antimytochondrial antibody; AMLA, antimyolemmal antibody; Ach, acetylcholin; ANT, adenine nucleotide translocator; AH, aconitate hydratase; PK, pyruvate kinase; DLD, dihydrolipoamide dehydrogenase; CK, creatine kinase; NADD, nicotinamideadeninedinucleotide dehydrogenase; UCR, ubiquinol-cytochrome-c reductase; hsp, heat shock protein; ANA, antinuclear antigen; ANCA, anti-neutrophil cytoplasmic antigen; SR-Ca-ATPase, sarcoplasmatic reticulum calcium ATP-ase.

are pathogenetically truly harmful. Pathogenetic relevance was therefore attributed to those antibodies which were fixed to autologous cardiac tissue in the endomyocardial biopsy sample *in vivo* und proved cytolytic or protective in *in vitro* assays.

IMPROVEMENTS IN HISTOLOGY, IMMUNOHISTOLOGY AND MOLECULAR BIOLOGY METHODS

Endomyocardial biopsy (EMB) is the appropriate standard to diagnose myocarditis. It should be performed early in the course of the disease to optimize diagnostic accuracy and reduce the sampling error especially in focal myocarditis. Standard histology and immunohistology can be characteristic for certain types of inflammation (e.g., giant cell, eosinophilic myocarditis, sarcoidosis, lymphocytic). Immunohistology confirms the pathogenetic relevance of the autoantibodies, when they are fixed to the appropriate cardiac target protein. Polymerase chain reaction (PCR) identifies the underlying viral etiology or excludes it. This implies different treatment algorithms (13–17, 43, 55–59). Therefore, multiple specimens should be taken and immediately fixed in 10% buffered formalin. Additional samples should be snap frozen in liquid nitrogen for immunohistochemistry and stored at −80°C. And 1–2 samples should be stored in special tubes at room temperature for viral PCR (8, 15, 17, 60). To increase the diagnostic sensitivity of immunohistochemistry, the use of a large panel of monoclonal and polyclonal antibodies including anti-CD3, anti-CD4, anti-CD8, anti-CD68, and anti HLA-DR is mandatory for the identification and characterization of the inflammatory infiltrate (8, 15, 17). Quantitative immunohistochemistry should be performed for infiltrating cells. Specific binding of these antibodies indicating an inflammatory reaction is demonstrated by peroxidase double staining procedure.

TABLE 3 | Comparison of qualitative Dallas (14) and quantitative World Heart Federation (WHF) criteria (15, 16).

Biopsy diagnosis	Dallas criteria	WHF criteria histology*	WHF criteria viral etiology
1st EMB: Active myocarditis	Infiltrate (>5 per hpf or nests), myocytolysis, edema (only H&E staining)	>50/mm^2 =fulminant m. >14/mm^2 =active m.	(Quantitative) PCR on viruses If positive: viral m. or DCMi; If negative: autoreactive m.
Borderline myocarditis	Infiltrate (>5 per hpf or nests), (only H&E staining)	Not applicable	Not applicable
No myocarditis	No infiltrate	<14/mm^2	If negative: DCM If positive: viral DCM
2nd EMB: Ongoing myocarditis	Infiltrate (>5 per hpf or nests), myocytolysis, edema (only H&E staining)	>14/mm^2	(Quantitative) PCR on viruses, If positive: viral m. or DCMi; If negative: autoreactive m.
Healed/resolved myocarditis	No infiltrate, but focal fibrosis	<14/mm^2	If negative: DCM If positive: viral DCM

** The infiltrate should be classified according the leukocyte markers used by peroxidase staining of CD3, CD4, CD8, CH45R0, CD68 positive cells. MHC class I and class II activation can be assessed.*
DCMi, dilated cardiomyopathy with inflammation; EMB, endomyocardial biopsy; H&E, hematoxilin and eosin staining; hpf, high power field; m, myocarditis.

Inflammation in endomyocardial biopsies is diagnosed by the WHF-criteria, which means a presence of ≥14 leucocytes/mm^2 (8, 15) in European centers, whereas the qualitative Dallas criteria of active or borderline myocarditis in the first, and ongoing or resolving or resolved myocarditis in a subsequent biopsy are still applied in many American publications (**Table 3**).

An equally important diagnostic contribution of EMB comes from the molecular analysis with DNA-RNA extraction and RT-PCR amplification of suspected viral genomes (15–17, 61), which is also part of the WHF criteria (**Table 3**). In order to exclude systemic infection, peripheral blood should be investigated in parallel with the biopsies (15, 17). Quantification of virus load and determination of virus replication may add diagnostic value (61). For detection of cardiotropic viruses total DNA and RNA should be extracted from the biopsy samples. Primer pairs specific for Coxsackievirus B (CVB), parvovirus B19 (PVB19), cytomegalovirus (CMV), adenovirus type 2, influenza virus A, human herpes virus 6 (HHV6) and Epstein–Barr virus (EBV) should be used to perform polymerase chain reaction (PCR) and in case of PVB19 quantitative real-time PCR to determine viral load.

HISTOLOGICAL PHENOTYPES AND CLINICAL MANIFESTATIONS

The association of the clinical phenotypes such as cardiogenic shock with fulminant myocarditis, acute heart failure with active lymphocytic or other forms of viral and non-viral myocarditis and chronic heart failure with borderline myocarditis can be derived from **Table 1** and **Figure 5**. The biopsy findings in these patients fit into these histopathological categories. The inflammasome is a platform in cells of the innate immune system allowing transition from the innate to the adaptive anticardiac immune response directed against myocardial and pericardial targets (11, 46, 62). The proinflammatory cascade in inflammasomes can be terminated intrinsicly, for example by Caspase-1 self-cleavage (63).

EPIDEMIOLOGICAL INSIGHT BY HISTOLOGY AND PCR BASED ETIOLOGIES IN PATIENTS WITH SUSPECTED MYOCARDITIS

The last WHO report on the epidemiology of inflammatory heart diseases, which explicitly listed viral causes of myocarditis dates back to the year 1981. It filed the following incidences of viral myocarditis per 1000: Coxsackie- B 36, Influenza- B 18, Influenza A- 12, Coxsackie A- 10, Cytomegalo- 9, Echo- 7, Adeno- 5 und Epstein Barr Virus 4,5. Meanwhile epidemiological data show a wide divergence in different parts of the world with new endemics or epidemics. To follow epidemiological trends one can assess the incidence of aetiological factors in changing frequencies as assessed by endomyocardial biopsies in tertial referral centers. Their data have limits by the sample size of all biopsied patients per year as the denominator. The region or sometimes the continent could be another selection bias. Registries can show longitudinal trends, however. Our registry of suspected myocarditis / inflammatory dilated cardiomyopathy was started 1987. The histological diagnosis of myocarditis was based on the Dallas criteria in the first years 10 years. Later on we used the quantitative WHF-criteria and refined the PCR for cardiotropic microbial agents as part of a common consensus. By a longitudinal comparison an epidemiological shift from entero- and adenoviruses to Parvovirus B19 becomes apparent (**Figure 6A**).

A retrospective analysis of 3,345 patients' biopsies in the Marburg registry (60) revealed (**Figure 6B**):

- Only one third of the patients who underwent endomyocardial biopsy with the suspected diagnosis myocarditis or dilated cardiomyopathy showed inflammation in their biopsy.
- The greatest proportion of the patients was virus-negative, however. This applied to the patients with dilated cardiomyopathy with no inflammation. Such patients with an EF between 45 and 55% (3rd column) made up 71.5%, those with an EF <45% were virus-negative in

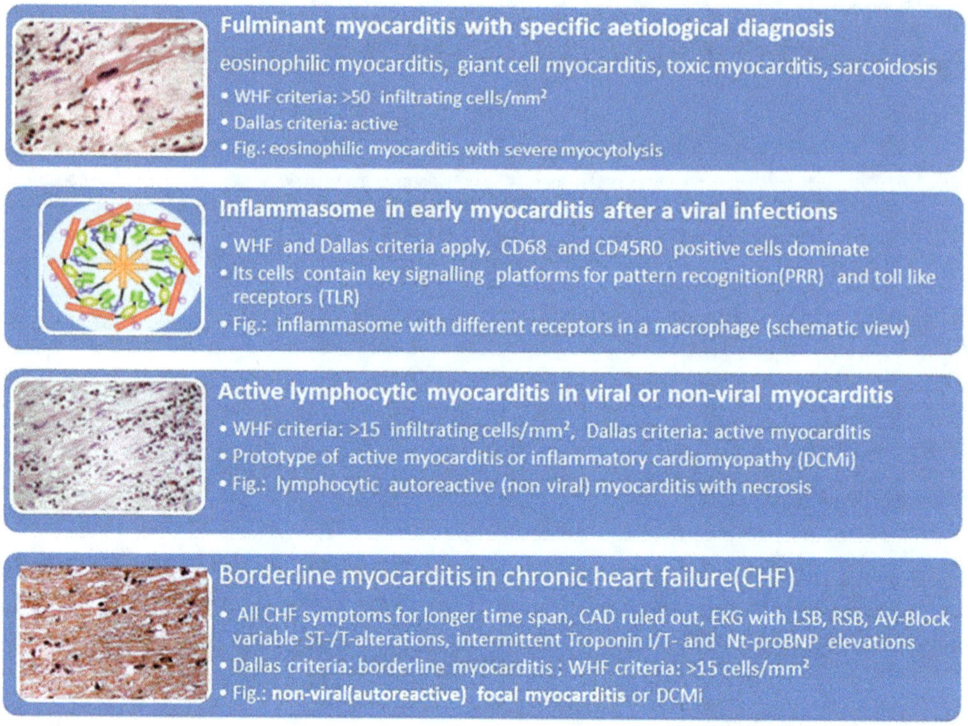

FIGURE 5 | Histological phenotypes and components of myocarditis and inflammatory cardiomyopathy can correlate with clinical manifestations (faces).

79.8%. These groups are identical with heart failure of unknown origin.

- Parvovirus B 19 became by far the leading viral aetiological factor across all 4 groups of cardiomyopathies with or without inflammation. It ranged between 17.6% in non-inflammatory but viral cardiomyopathy (=viral heart disease) and 33.3% in inflammatory Parvovirus B19 positive cardiomyopathy with an EF <45%.

FUTURE SEROLOGIC DIAGNOSTIC MARKERS

Distinct patterns of microRNAs are well described in coronary artery disease and myocardial infarction but not yet in inflammatory cardiomyopathies. De Rosa et al recently showed different gradients of microRNA expression in ischemic and non-ischemic forms of heart failure (64).

Treatment

Current recommendations and guidelines for the treatment of heart failure also apply to inflammatory cardiomyopathy. "Unloading the heart" is the principle of chronic heart failure of any cause. This has been successfully demonstrated in many heart failure trials on ACE-inhibition and angiotensin receptor blockade. Details and a comprehensive bibliography were summarized previously (9). Waagstein et al. demonstrated first a positive trend for betablockade in congestive cardiomyopathy (65).

Antiphlogistic treatment with non-steroidal anti-inflammatory drugs (NSAIDs) such as ibuprofen or indomethacin or IL-antagonists such as anakinra should be reserved for patients with additional pericardial involvement. NSAIDs should be used only for short term application (66, 67), since in murine Coxsackie B3 myocarditis it was shown that NSAIDs can be detrimental (68). NSAIDs are cyclooxigenase inhibitors. Anakinra blocks the cytokine activity of IL-1. In peri (myo)carditis first line treatment with colchicine is now recommended not only in recurrent forms but also for the first attack of pericarditis (67). **Figure 7** shows that colchicine is an inhibitor of the mitosis of tubulin in macrophages and neutrophiles. Its application inhibits primarily the innate immune system.

Antiarrhythmic treatment and device therapy also follows current heart failure guidelines [see Maisch and Pankuweit (9) for references].

Stem Cell Transplantation

Virtually no data on stem cell transplantation in myocarditis with heart failure and only scarce uncontrolled data in patients with dilated cardiomyopathy are available (9).

SPECIFIC TREATMENT ALGORITHMS

Figure 8 reflects diagnostic and therapeutic algorithms in different forms of myocarditis. They are also the basis of the double-blind randomized European Study on Epidemiology and Treatment of Inflammatory Myocardial Disease (ESETCID) (70).

A

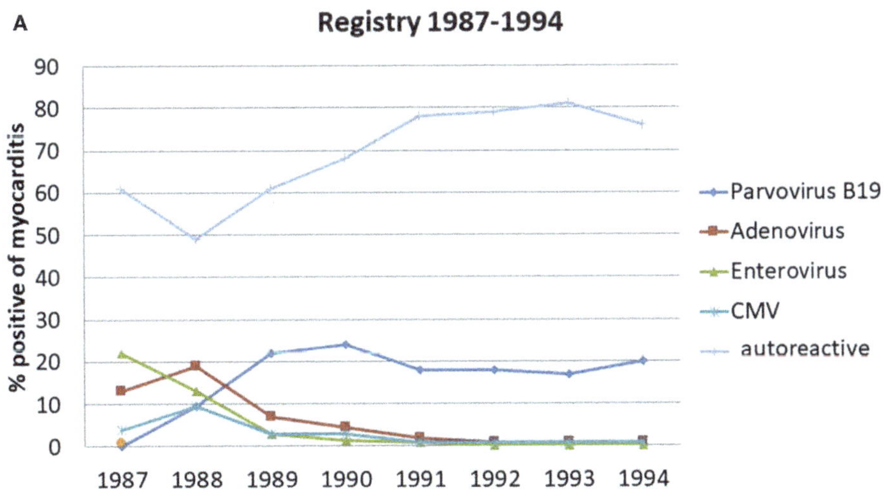

B

	Inflammation ($n = 1098$)		No inflammation ($n = 2247$)	
	(1) EF > 45%	(2) EF < 45%	(3) EF > 45%	(4) EF < 45%
$N =$	816	282	1663	584
LVEDD (mm)	54 ± 10	65 ± 7	51 ± 9	66 ± 11
VIRUS POSITIVE (%)				
Influenza A	1.3	0	0	0.1
PVB 19	20.4*	33.3**	23.9*	17.6
EV	1.5	2.8	1.1	0.5
ADV	1.5	2.1	1.4	1.2
CMV	3.1	3.9	2.0*	0.8
Borrel. Burgd.	0	0	0.1	0
Virus negative	72.2	57.9	71.5	79.8

*$p < 0.05$ (group1 vs. 2 or group 3)
**$p < 0.05$ (group 2 vs. 4).
Pankuweit et al. (60).

FIGURE 6 | (A) Epidemiological shift in the Myocarditis Registry from entero-(green line) and adenoviruses (brown line) to Parvovirus B 19 (dark blue line) in the late 1980-ties. The number of patients with nonviral myocarditis (light blue line) varied from 50 to 80% in the same time span. **(B)** PCR-based etiology of viral and autoreactive myocarditis and dilated cardiomyopathy without inflammation (4th column) [modified from Pankuweit et al. (60)]. PCR-Based etiology of myocarditis and dilated cardiomyopathy. Investigation of endomyocardial biopsies from 3345 patients (1997–2003).

Immunosuppressive Treatment

Idiopathic Giant Cell Myocarditis

Giant cells in addition to a lymphocytic infiltrate are the histological hall-mark of this very rare, fulminant and often lethal disease. If suspected, it is a clear biopsy indication. Its prevalence in Marburg registry 1989–2012 is 3 in 10,000 biopsied patients. The etiology is considered autoimmune based on a genetic predisposition. It resembles experimental giant cell myocarditis in Lewis rats after immunization with myosin (71). When compared to an isolated cardiac sarcoid the histological differential diagnosis is sometimes difficult (72). If untreated the natural course is lethal. The giant cell myocarditis treatment trial proposed treatment with 5 mg monoclonal anti CD3-antibodies given i.v. for 10 days. Cyclosporin should be started with 25 mg bid and increased daily by 25 mg to achieve a target serum level of 200 ng/ml. This serum level should be kept for 1 year. Methylprednisolone should be started with 10 mg/kg i.v. for 3 days and then be tapered after 3 weeks to a final dose of 5 mg for the rest of the year (73, 74). The study was stopped for lack of patients (**Table 4**).

Cardiac Sarcoidosis

In cardiac sarcoidosis the giant cells are only found in the non caseous granuloma (94, 95). In our registry it is 6-times more frequent with 19 in 10,000 biopsied patients than giant cell myocarditis. Granuloma are often located in the midmyocardial layer, which is not accessible to endomyocardial biopsy. So the diagnosis of cardiac sarcoidosis can be suspected in patients with systemic sarcoidosis and a biopsy just showing myocarditis. Early cardiac symptoms can be AV-block or severe ventricular arrhythmias leading to sudden death or severe heart failure. The etiology of sarcoidosis remains obscure, although recently a variant in the *btnl2* gene and the *btnl2* risk allele were described as risk factors (9, 96, 97). The treatment is either corticoid treatment

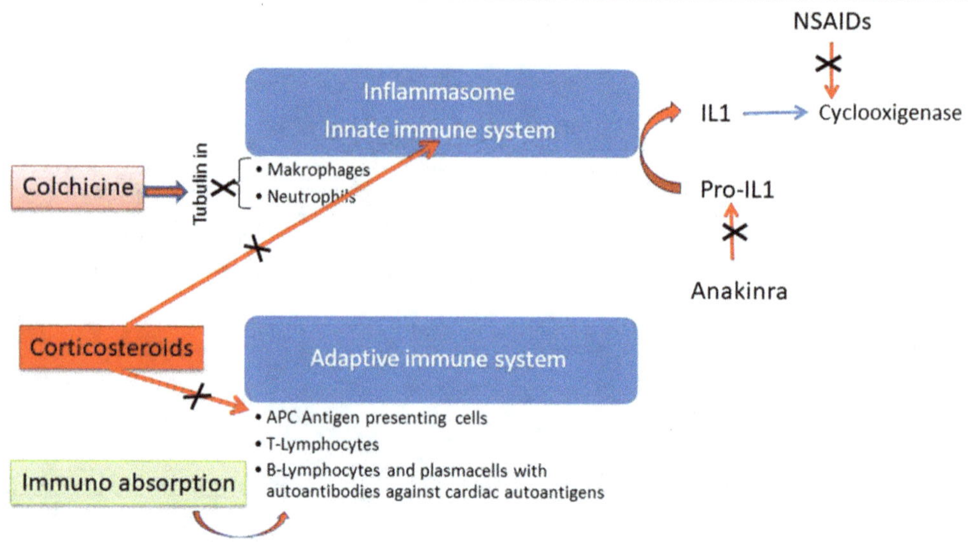

FIGURE 7 | Antininflammatory action of different modes of therapy in perimyocarditis.

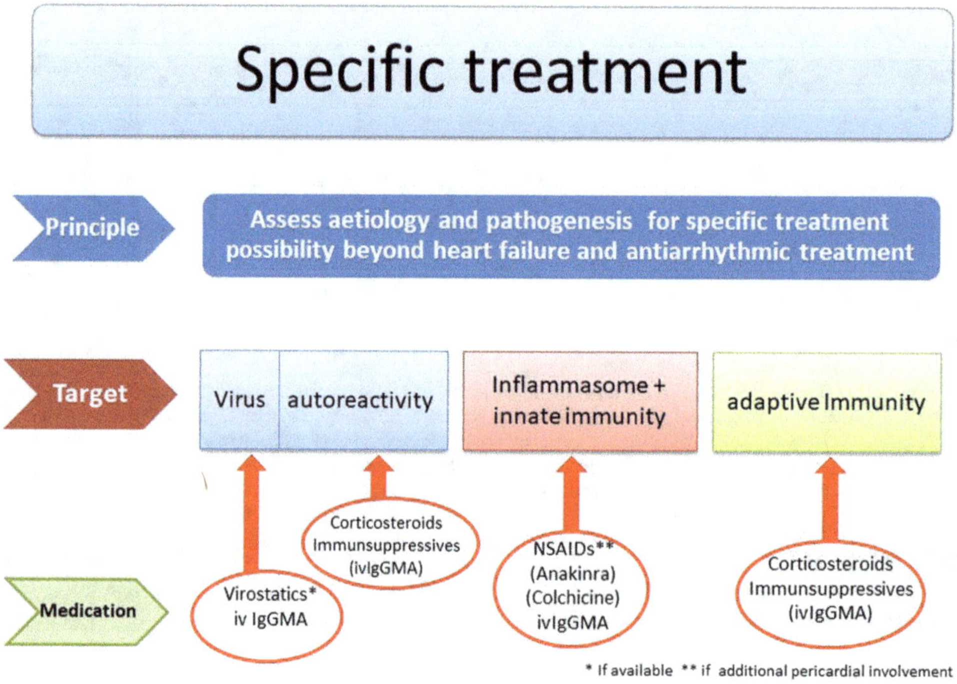

FIGURE 8 | Etiology driven treatment in myocarditis and inflammatory cardiomyopathy.

alone or in combination with other immunosuppressive drugs e.g., azathioprine or cyclosporine (98).

Eosinophilic Heart Disease

Eosinophilic heart disease (EHD) and endstage endomyocardial fibrosis are rare diseases. The Marburg Registry has collected 10 cases over 23 years. Its common pathogenetic denominator is the excessive production of cytotoxic eosinophils, which could damage the heart in different ways (9, 99, 100):

a) In the course of an allergic reaction,
b) As an autoimmune disease,
c) As malignant eosinophilic leukemia,
d) Following a parasitic or protozoal infection (tropical form),
e) As Churg-Strauss-syndrome or

TABLE 4 | Trials for immunosuppressive treatment in myocarditis.

References	Treatment	No pts/ Controls	Treated pts improved	Treated pts Unch/deter.	Controls improved	Controls unch/deter.	Endpoint/Comments
A. OBSERVATIONAL STUDIES AND SMALL TRIALS WITH IMMUNOSUPPRESSION							
Fenoglio et al. (75)	P, A & P	18/4	7 (39%)	11 (61%)	2 (50%)	2 (50%)	EF/observational, no PCR
Hosenpud et al. (76)	A & P	6/0	0 (0%)	6 (100%)			EF/No co, no PCR, no co biopsy
Anderson et al. (77)	A & P	10/7	3 (30%)	7 (70%)	2 (28,5%)	5 (71,5%)	Prospective, open label, randomized
Marboe and Fenoglio (78)	P, A & P	16/18	9 (56%)	7 (44%)	7 (39%)	11 (61%)	P, A & P mixed
Latham et al., (79)	P	26/26	Majority	Minority	nd	nd	EF/No viral PCR, no biopsy
Maisch et al. (80)	A & P	21/21 all virus negative	10 (47%)	11 (53%)	3 (14%)	18 (86%)	EF (6 mo)/RCT pilot
Kühl et al. (81)	P	31/0	20 (54%)	11 (46%)	nd	nd	EF; observational/ No co EMB
Camargo et al. (82)	P	68/0	Majority	Minority	nd	nd	EF/observational, No viral PCR
Liu Dezue et al. (83)	D	128/0	Favorable, but no data	nd	nd	nd	Observational/No EMB, CM
Sun (84)	D	32/0	Majority	Minority	nd	nd	EF/observational, EKG only, no PCR, CM
Wu and Chen (85)	D & P	31/0	Majority	Minority	nd	nd	Observational/ No EMB, CM,
Frustaci et al. (86)	A & P	41/0	21 (51%)	20 (49%)	nd	nd	EF/RCT, virus negative pts improved
Escher et al. (87)	A & P	114	Majority	Minority	nd	nd	EF 6 mo/observational, no co biopsy

References	No pts/Co	Treatment	Endpoints	Treated pts improved	Treated pts Unch/deter.	Controls improved	Controls unch/deter.	Comments
B. DOUBLE BLIND, RANDOMIZED, AND CONTROLLED TREATMENT TRIALS (RCT) WITH IMMUNOSUPPRESSIVE DRUGS IN MYOCARDITIS								
Parillo et al. (88)	51 /51	P vs. Pl	EF after 3 mo, mortality	53% No difference	47% No difference	27% No difference	73% No difference	RCT, no PCR
Mason et al. (89) MTT	64/47	A/C & P vs. Pl	EF/function +Mortality	No difference No difference	No difference No difference	No difference No difference	No difference No difference	RCT, no PCR (90)
Wojnicz et al. (91)	41/43	A & P vs. Pl	EF/function	In majority	In minority	Minority with spontaneous improvement	Majority	No PCR, HLA as criterium of inflammation
Cooper et al. (74), Maisch et al. (69, 70)	11/?	Cyclo+P vs. Pl	Mortality 12 mo	Improved	nd	nd	nd	RCT, stopped for lack of pts
Frustaci et al. (92) TIMIC	43/42	A & P vs. Pl	EF (6 mo) Mortality	88,3 nd	11,7 nd	0 nd	100 nd	WHF, RCT, virus negative pts only
Maisch et al. (93) ESETCID	54/47	Tx arms with A& P vs. Pl	EF/function MACE	EF+MACE improved after 6 month		Some spontaneous improvement		WHF, RCT, intermediate results

A, Azathioprin; co, controls; CM, Chinese medicine; Cyclo, Cyclosporine; D, Dexamethason; DC, dilated cardiomyopathy; deter, deteriorated; EF, Ejection fraction; EMB, endomyocardial biopsy, mo, months; nd, no data; P, prednisone; Pl, placebo; PCR, polymerase chain reaction for viral RNA and DNA in EMB; pts, patients; RCT, randomized controlled trial; unch, unchanged; WHF, quantitative World Heart Federation biopsy criteria.

f) As idiopathic form.

Classic Löffler's endocarditis develops in 3 stages:

1) *Eosinophilic endomyocarditis*, in which mature eosinophils infiltrate the endocardium and myocardium and damage with their products such as the cationic protein or by IL-5, which has also been discussed as a late mediator of fibrosis.
2) *Thrombotic endocardial disease*, in which apical obliteration and valve involvement occur.
3) *Endomyocardial fibrosis* as terminal stage, in which restrictive cardiomyopathy prevails.

The 3 stages can be identified noninvasively by colorflow Doppler echocardiography, cardiac MRI, and by EMB. In the peripheral blood the eosinophils can sometimes be degranulated. They are diagnosed as neutrophils, which obviously impairs the diagnosis of eosinophilia. The definite diagnosis should be established by endomyocardial biopsy. The causative therapy of the tropical form is the treatment of the underlying helminthic or protozoal infection. In all other forms immunosuppression has been recommended either by prednisone, interferon or the tyrosinekinase inhibitors imatinib or mepolizumab. As a humanized monoclonal antibody mepolizumab binds to and inhibits interleukin-5 (IL-5). In the Marburg registry longterm prednisone and azathioprine gave a survival rate of 9 out 10 patients over a mean period of 8.4 years (9).

Rheumatic Diseases and Collagen Disorders With Cardiac Manifestations

Cardiac symptoms may be "behind the curtain" of the clinical manifestations in rheumatic diseases. The diagnosis relies on clinical manifestation, echocardiography, cardiac MRI, and sometimes on endomyocardial biopsy and/or pericardiocentesis. The management includes pain relief with NSAIDs, immunosuppression as systemic therapy, and in patients with larger pericardial effusions undergoing pericardiocentesis with intrapericardial instillation of triamcinolone acetate. Longterm, oral colchicine (2–3 tablets per day with 0.5mg) is recommended (9).

Autoreactive Myocarditis

It is common belief that an infection with cardiotropic viruses may cause sequestration of myocardial cells. This can trigger in predisposed patients an autoreactive cellular and humoral immune reaction which in turn leads to further myocardial damage.

With this hypothesis in mind immunosuppressive treatment either by prednisone alone or in combination with azathioprin or cyclosporin was initiated. However, most studies listed in **Table 4A** were carried out before quantitative immunohistochemistry for the assessment of the infiltrate and PCR for cardiotropic viruses were available. So it remained unclear, if prednisone and immunosuppression were started when virus particles were still present. According to a current dogma, in such a situation immunosuppression is contraindicated.

Our controlled pilot study on immunosuppression (80) before the initiation of ESETCID (93) excluded patients with a viral genome in the myocardium and was therefore directed to autoreactive, virus-negative myocarditis cases. It demonstrated improvement of cardiac function (EF >5% after 6 months) in 47% of patients treated with verum, but also in 14% in the placebo group, which could be interpreted as spontaneous recovery.

In a *post-hoc* stratification of myocarditis patients treated with prednisone and azathioprine Frustaci et al. (86) also found that improvement with immunosuppression was demonstrable only in the virus-negative cases.

The first randomized controlled trial on prednisone in patients with idiopathic dilated cardiomyopathy with biopsies taken was carried out by Parillo et al (88), who randomly assigned 102 DCM patients to treatment with 60 mg/d for 3 months or without prednisone. 53% of the patients who received prednisone showed improvement of ejection fraction by >5%, but only 27% of the controls improved spontaneously ($p = 0.005$).

The Myocarditis Treatment Trial (MTT) by Mason et al. (89) showed neither benefit nor harm. Mortality after 6 months of treatment with cyclosporin A or azathioprine and prednisone showed an insignificant trend when compared to placebo. The study was underpowered and did not distinguish viral from non-viral disease as pointed out later (90). Wojnicz et al. (91) randomized 84 patients with dilated heart muscle disease and suspected myocarditis when an increased HLA MHC expression was found in EMB. Treatment of azathioprine and prednisone was compared with placebo after 3 months. In the treatment group ejection fraction improved, survival remained comparable, however, between verum and placebo groups.

In the TIMIC study the ejection fraction in the treatment group of 43 patients increased from 26.5% at baseline to 45.6% after 6 months ($p < 0.001$). Accordingly left ventricular enddiastolic volume, left ventricular enddiastolic diameter, and New York Heart Association class decreased significantly (92).

The ESETCID (European Study on the Epidemiology and Treatment of Cardiac Inflammatory Disease) is a double blind, randomized, placebo controlled three-armed trial with prednisolone and azathioprine for autoreactive (virus negative) inflammatory dilated cardiomyopathy in patients with an ejection fraction <45% at baseline. Its intermediate results from the immunosuppressive treatment arm demonstrated a positive trend in EF and MACE after 6 months of treatment and a significant benefit after 1 year of follow-up (93). For the initial and steady state dosages of prednisolone and azthioprine see Maisch et al. (93). The control group without immunosuppressive treatment also showed some spontaneous resolution of the infiltrate.

INTRAVENOUS IMMUNOGLOBULIN

Intravenous immunoglobulins (ivIg) interact widely with the host immune system. They can stimulate anti-inflammatory cytokines, develop anti-idiotypic activities, increase FCgamma receptor saturation and the expression of the inhibitory FCgRIIB. Inhibitory actions comprise the suppression of proinflammatory cytokines, the interruption of the complement cascade, the inhibition of dendritic cells, of leukocyte adhesion, of apoptosis and of metalloproteinases. They can bind microbial particles, contribute to the self-antigen sequestration and interfere with B and T cell regulation (9). Anthony et al have shown that the anti-inflammatory activity of monomeric IgG depends on the sialysation of the N-linked glycan of the IgG Fc fragment (101). Their beneficial effect has also been reported in different clinical settings of autoimmune disease including acute and chronic myocarditis, in dilated cardiomyopathy, in experimental enteroviral myocarditis (102) and in Parvovirus B19 associated heart disease (103). IgM and IgA enriched immunoglobulins appear to be effective in lower doses (104).

Table 5 gives an overview on the ivIg studies. Many, but not all studies reported hemodynamic benefit or clinical improvement. The IMAC, a randomized controlled trial, demonstrated improvement in both, the treatment and placebo

TABLE 5 | Iv-Immunoglobulin treatment in myocarditis and inflammatory dilated cardiomyopathy.

References	Design	*n*	EMB	Viral PCR	Ivlg dose	Outcome
Drucker et al. (105)	Retrospective, historic control	46 children	Partly	nd	2 g/kg single dose	Reduced LVEDD
McNamara et al. (106)	Uncontrolled	10 adults	Partly	nd	2 g/kg	Improvement of EF after 12 months
Takeda et al. (107)	Case report	1	Myocarditis	EBV	2 g/kg for 2 days	Improvement
Nigro et al. (108)	Case reports	3 children	Myocarditis	Parvo B19	2 g/kg over 5 days	Improved
Tsai et al. (109)	Case report	1 child	nd	Mycoplasma peumoniae (serology)	2 g/kg over 2 days	Improved
McNamara et al. (110) IMAC	RCT	62	Only ten active and 3 borderline myocarditis	nd	2 g/kg, single shot vs. controls	Not improved
Alter et al. (111)	Case report	1	Myocarditis	Varicella	2 g/kg over 2 days	Normalized
Shioji et al. (112)	Case report	1	Fulminant myocarditis	nd, negative serology	2 g/kg	Improved
Tedeschi et al. (113)	Case report	1	nd	nd, negative serology	2 g/kg	Improved
Kishimoto et al. (114)	Case series	9 adults	4 myocarditis only	nd	1-2 g/kg	Improved NYHA, EF & SF
Wang et al. (115)	Case report	1 child	Fulminant myocarditis	Coxsackie A 16	1/kg for 2 days	Patient died
Dennert et al. (116)	Uncontrolled	25	post mortem myocarditis	Parvo B19	2 g/kg	Decrease in viral load and improved EF after 6 months
Maisch et al. (117)	Controlled	18 (ivlg) vs. 17(controls)	CMV myocarditis	CMV by PCR or ISH	14 days, multiple doses	Improved and eradicated CMV

CMV, Cytomegalovirus; DC, dilated cardiomyopathy; deter, deteriorated; EBV, Epstein Barr virus; EF, Ejection fraction; EMB, endomyocardial biopsy; ISH, in situ hybridization; LVEDD, left ventricular enddiastolic diameter; NYHA, New York Heart Association classification; mo, months; n, number of pts; nd, no data; PCR, polymerase chain reaction for viral RNA and DNA in EMB; RCT, randomized controlled trial; SF, shortening fraction; unch, unchanged.

arms (110), so that in a multi-institutional analysis the benefit in a pediatric myocarditis or cardiomyopathy population was questioned (118).

In CMV-myocarditis one controlled trial of 18 patients showed the eradication of inflammation and the elimination of the virus (117). The patients had received 2 ml/kg i.v. cytomegalovirus hyperimmunoglobulin (CMVhIg) for 3 days and 1 ml/kg for 2 additional 2 days.

In a case of varicella myocarditis high-dose immunoglobulins demonstrated clinical improvement and the resolution of inflammation (111).

In the Marburg Registry 20 g i.v. pentaglobin (ivIgGAM) given in adenoviral myocarditis resulted in clinical improvement by the eradication of the inflammatory infiltrate and the virus. In Parvo B19 myocarditis clinical improvement and elimination of inflammation in the biopsy is noted, whereas the virus may still persist although the viral load may decrease.

IMMUNOADSORPTION

The therapeutical concept of immunoadsorption follows a different concept: the elimination of cardiotoxic autoantibodies together with proinflammatory cytokines. The positive result of a pilot study of patients with idiopathic dilated cardiomyopathy needs further confirmation in a larger endpoint study (119, 120).

ANTIVIRAL TREATMENT

Interferon-Beta

Interferons belong to the natural defense system against many viral infections. In entero- and adenoviral myocarditis interferon-beta has eliminated the viral genome and decreased inflammation in a phase 2 study, when applying dosages of 2 to 6 × 10^6 IU every 2nd day (121). The response to interferon-beta in Parvovirus B19 and human herpes virus 6 myocarditis has been less impressive as shown by the BICC study (122).

PERSPECTIVE AND CONCLUSION

Although we have learned much about inflammatory heart disease from various animal models of viral or autoimmune myocarditis, we are aware that animal models cannot be translated one to one to myocarditis in patients. Enteroviral myocarditis in man has almost completely disappeared in Europe. Parvovirus B 19 as infective agent has emerged instead but its pathogenesis is still poorly understood and animal models for this virus are still missing. Separation of myocarditis in 3 phases is an auxiliary construction. But myocardial inflammation in man is continuum. Personalized treatment should be tailored within the time frame from infection to innate and adaptive response. There is still much work to be done.

AUTHOR CONTRIBUTIONS

The author confirms being the sole contributor of this work and has approved it for publication.

REFERENCES

1. Kerr WW. Myocarditis. *Cal State J Med.* (1904) 2:369–71.
2. Maisch B, Trostel-Soeder R, Stechemesser E, Berg PA, Kochsiek K. Diagnostic relevance of humoral and cell-mediated immune reactions in patients with acute viral myocarditis. *Clin Exp Immunol.* (1982) 48:533–45.
3. Linde A, Mosier D, Blecha F, Melgarejo T. Innate immunity and inflammation— new frontiers in comparative cardiovascular pathology. *Cardiovasc Res.* (2007) 73:26–36. doi: 10.1016/j.cardiores.2006.08.009
4. Portig I, Pankuweit S, Maisch B. Antibodies against stress proteins in the sera of patients with dilated cardiomyopathy. *J Mol Cell Cardiol.* (1997) 29:2245–51. doi: 10.1006/jmcc.1997.0463
5. Wicks EC, Elliott PM. Genetics and metabolic cardiomyopathies. *Herz.* (2012) 37:598–611. doi: 10.1007/s00059-012-3659-0
6. Kloos W, Katus HA, Meder B. Genetic cardiomyopathies. Lessons learned from humans, mice, and zebrafish. *Herz.* (2012) 37:612–8. doi: 10.1007/s00059-012-3651-8
7. Elliott P, Andersson B, Arbustini E, Bilinska Z, Cecchi F, Charron P, et al. Classification of the cardiomyopathies: a position statement from the European Society of Cardiology working group on myocardial and pericardial disease. *Eur Heart J.* (2007) 29:270–6. doi: 10.1093/eurheartj/ehm342
8. Caforio A, Pankuweit S, Charron P, et al. Current state of knowledge on aetiology, diagnosis, management and therapy of myocarditis: a position statement of the European Society of Cardiology Working Group on Myocardial and Pericardial Diseases. *Eur Heart J.* (2013) 34:2636–48. doi: 10.1093/eurheartj/eht210
9. Maisch B, Pankuweit S. Current treatment options in (peri)myocarditis and inflammatory cardiomyopathy. *Herz.* (2012) 37:644–56. doi: 10.1007/s00059-012-3679-9
10. Maisch B, Alter P. Treatment options in myocarditis and inflammatory cardiomyopathy. Focus on i.v. immunoglobulins. *Herz.* (2018) 43:423–30. doi: 10.1007/s00059-018-4719-x
11. Hickie JB, Hall GV. The cardiomyopathies: a report of fifty cases. *Australas Ann Med.* (1960) 9:258–70. doi: 10.1111/imj.1960.9.4.258
12. Anonymous. Report of the WHO/ISFC Task Force on the definition and classification of cardiomyopathies. *Br Heart J.* (1980) 44:672–74. doi: 10.1136/hrt.44.6.672
13. Richardson P, McKenna W, Bristow M, Maisch B, Mautner B, O'Connell J, et al. Report of the 1995 World Health Organization/International Society and Federation of Cardiology Task Force on the definition and classification of cardiomyopathies. *Circulation.* (1996) 93:841–2. doi: 10.1161/01.CIR.93.5.841
14. Aretz HT. Myocarditis: the Dallas criteria. *Hum Pathol.* (1987) 18:619–24. doi: 10.1016/S0046-8177(87)80363-5
15. Maisch B, Bültmann B, Factor S, Groene HJ, Hufnagel G, Kawarmura K, et al. World Heart Federation consensus conferences's definition of inflammatory cardiomyopathy (myocarditis): report from two expert committees on histology and viral cardiomyopathy. *Heartbeat.* (1999) 4:3–4.
16. Maisch B, Portig I, Ristic A, Hufnagel G, Pankuweit S. Definition of inflammatory cardiomyopathy (myocarditis): on the way to consensus. *Herz.* (2000) 25:200–9. doi: 10.1007/s000590050007
17. Pankuweit S, Portig I, Eckhardt H, Crombach M, Hufnagel G, Maisch B. Prevalence of viral genome in endomyocardial biopsies from patients with inflammatory heart muscle disease. *Herz.* (2000) 25:221–6. doi: 10.1007/s000590050010
18. Swirski FK, Nahrendorf M. Cardioimmunology: the immune system in cardiac homeostasis and disease. *Nat Rev Immunol.* (2018) 18:733–44. doi: 10.1038/s41577-018-0065-8
19. Hulsmans M, Clauss S, Xiao L, Aguirre AD, King KR, Hanley A, et al. Macrophages facilitate electrical conduction in the heart. *Cell.* (2017) 169:510–22. doi: 10.1016/j.cell.2017.03.050
20. Horckmans M, Bianchini M, Santovito D, Megens RTA, Springael JY, Negri I, et al. Pericardial adipose tissue regulates granulopoiesis, fibrosis, and cardiac function after myocardial infarction. *Circulation.* (2018) 137:948–60. doi: 10.1161/CIRCULATIONAHA.117.028833
21. Butts B, Lee A. Goeddel LA, George DJ, Steele C, Davies JE, et al. Increased inflammation in pericardial fluid persists 48 hours after cardiac surgery. *Circulation.* (2017) 136:2284–6. doi: 10.1161/CIRCULATIONAHA.117.029589
22. Lévêque N, Garcia M, Bouin A, Nguyen JHC, Tran GP, Andreoletti L, et al. Functional consequences of RNA 5=-terminal deletions on coxsackievirus B3 RNA replication and ribonucleoprotein complex formation. *J Virol.* (2017) 91:e00423-17. doi: 10.1128/JVI.00423-17
23. Huber SA, Lodge PA. Coxsackievirus B-3 myocarditis in BALB/c mice: evidence for autoimmunity to myocyte antigens. *J Pathol.* (1984) 116:21–9.
24. Rose NR, Wolfgram LJ, Herskowitz A, Beisel KW. Postinfectious autoimmunity: two distinct phases of Coxsackievirus B3-induced myocarditis. *Ann N Y Acad Sci.* (1986) 475:146–56. doi: 10.1111/j.1749-6632.1986.tb20864.x
25. Rose NR. Critical cytokine pathways to cardiac inflammation. *J Interferon Cytok Res.* (2011) 31:705–9. doi: 10.1089/jir.2011.0057
26. Huber S, Ramsingh AI. Coxsackievirus-induced pancreatitis. *Viral Immunol.* (2004) 17: 358–69. doi: 10.1089/vim.2004.17.358
27. Latz E, Xiao TS, Stutz A. Activation and regulation of the inflammasomes. *Nat Rev Immunol.* (2013) 13:397–411. doi: 10.1038/nri3452
28. Maisch B, Deeg P, Liebau G, Kochsiek K. Diagnostic relevance of humoral and cytotoxic immune reactions in primary and secondary dilated cardiomyopathy. *Am J Cardiol.* (1983) 52:1072–8. doi: 10.1016/0002-9149(83)90535-0
29. Maisch B, Bauer E, Cirsi M, Kochsiek K. Cytolytic cross-reactive antibodies directed against the cardiac membrane and viral proteins in coxsackievirus B3 and B4 myocarditis. Characterization and pathogenetic relevance. *Circulation.* (1993) 87:49–65.
30. Maisch B. The sarcolemma as antigen in the secondary immunopathogenesis of myopericarditis. *Eur Heart J.* (1987) 8(Suppl J):155–65. doi: 10.1093/eurheartj/8.suppl_J.155
31. Pankuweit S, Portig I, Lottspeich F, Maisch B. Autoantibodies in sera of patients with myocarditis: characterization of the corresponding proteins by isoelectric focusing and N-terminal sequence analysis. *J Mol Cell Cardiol.* (1997) 29:77–84. doi: 10.1006/jmcc.1996.0253
32. Maisch B, Wedeking U, Kochsiek K. Quantitative assessment of antilaminin antibodies in myocarditis and perimyocarditis. *Eur Heart J.* (1987) 8(Suppl J):223–35. doi: 10.1093/eurheartj/8.suppl_J.233
33. Obermayer U, Scheidler J, Maisch B. Antibodies against micro- and intermediate filaments in carditis and dilated cardiomyopathy - are they a diagnostic marker? *Eur Heart J.* (1987) 8(Suppl. J):181–6. doi: 10.1093/eurheartj/8.suppl_J.181
34. Klein R, Maisch B, Kochsiek K, Berg PA. Demonstration of organ specific antibodies against heart mitochondria (anti M7) in sera from patients with some forms of heart diseases. *J Clin Exp Immunol.* (1984) 58:283–92.
35. Pohlner K, Portig I, Pankuweit S, Lottspeich F, Maisch B. Identification of mitochondrial antigens recognized by the antibodies in sera of patients with dilated cardiomyopathy by two-dimensional gel electrophoresis and protein sequencing. *Am J Cardiol.* (1997) 80:1040–5. doi: 10.1016/S0002-9149(97)00600-0

36. Caforio AL, Tona F, Bottaro S, Vinci A, Dequal G, Daliento L, et al. Clinical implications of anti-heart autoantibodies in myocarditis and dilated cardiomyopathy. *Autoimmunity.* (2008) 41:35–45. doi: 10.1080/08916930701619235
37. Kaya Z, Leib C, Katus HA. Autoantibodies in heart failure and cardiac dysfunction. *Circ Res.* (2012) 110:145–58. doi: 10.1161/CIRCRESAHA.111.243360
38. Wallukat G, Wollenberg A, Morwinski R, Pitschner HF. Anti-beta1-adrenoceptor autoantibodies with chronotropic activity from the serum of patients with dilated cardiomyopathy: mapping of epitopes in the first and second extracellular loops. *J Mol Cell Cardiol.* (1995) 27:3977–4006. doi: 10.1016/S0022-2828(08)80036-3
39. Jahns R, Boivin V, Siegmund C, Inselmann G, Lohse MJ, Boege F, et al. Autoantibodies activating human beta 1-adrenergic receptors are associated with reduced cardiac function in chronic heart failure. *Circulation.* (1999) 99:649–54. doi: 10.1161/01.CIR.99.5.649
40. Fu LX, Magnusson Y, Bergh CH, Liljeqvist JA, Waagstein F, Hjalmarson A, et al. Localization of a functional autoimmune epitope on the second extracellular loop of the human muscarinic acetylcholin receptor 2 in patients with idiopathic dilated cardiomyopathy. *J Clin Invest.* (1993) 91:1964–8. doi: 10.1172/JCI116416
41. Maisch B, Lotze U, Schneider J, Kochsiek K. Antibodies to human sinus node in sick-sinus syndrome. *Pacing Clin Electrophysiol.* (1986) 9:1101–9. doi: 10.1111/j.1540-8159.1986.tb06677.x
42. Lotze U, Maisch B. Humoral immune response to cardiac conducting tissue. *Springer Semin Immunopathol.* (1989) 11:409–22. doi: 10.1007/BF00201879
43. Maisch B. Autoreactivity to the cardiac myocyte, connective tissue and the extracellular matrix in heart disease and postcardiac injury. *Springer Semin Immunopathol.* (1989) 11:369–95. doi: 10.1007/BF00201877
44. Goin JC, Borda ES, Auger S, Storino R, Sterin-Borda L. Cardiac M(2) muscarinic cholinoceptor activation by human chagasic autoantibodies: association with bradycardia. *Heart.* (1999) 82:273–8. doi: 10.1136/hrt.82.3.273
45. Schultheiss HP, Bolte HD. Immunological analysis of autoantibodies against the adenine nucleotide translocator in dilated cardiomyopathy. *J Mol Cell Cardiol.* (1988) 17:603–17. doi: 10.1016/S0022-2828(85)80029-8
46. Limas CJ, Limas C, Kubo SH, Olivari MT. Anti-β-receptor antibodies in human dilated cardiomyopathy and correlation with HLA-DR antigens. *Am J Cardiol.* (1990) 65:483–7. doi: 10.1016/0002-9149(90)90815-I
47. Jahns R, Bolvin V, Hein L, Triebel S, Angermann CE, Ertl G, et al. Direct evidence for a ß1-adrenergic receptor-directed autoimmune attack as a cause of idiopathic dilated cardiomyopathy. *J Clin Invest.* (2004) 113:1419–29. doi: 10.1172/JCI200420149
48. Naparstek Y, Plotz PH. The role of autoantibodies in autoimmune disease. *Ann Rev Immunol.* (1993) 11:79–104. doi: 10.1146/annurev.iy.11.040193.000455
49. Wolff PG, Kühl U, Schultheiss HP. Laminin distribution and autoantibodies to laminin in dilated cardiomyopathy and myocarditis. *Am Heart J.* (1989) 117:1303–9
50. Ansari AA, Wang YC, Danner DJ, Gravanis MB, Mayne A, Neckelmann N, et al. Abnormal expression of histocompatibility and mitochondrial antigens by cardiac tissue from patients with myocarditis and dilated cardiomyopathy. *Am J Pathol.* (1991) 139:337–54.
51. Wittner B, Maisch B, Kochsiek K. Quantification of antimyosin antibodies in experimental myocarditis by a new solid-phase fluorometric assay. *J Immunol Methods.* (1983) 64:239–47. doi: 10.1016/0022-1759(83)90402-7
52. Caforio AL, Goldman JH, Haven AJ, Baig KM, McKenna WJ. Evidence for autoimmunity to myosin and other heart-specific autoantigens in patients with dilated cardiomyopathy and their relatives. *Int J Cardiol.* (1996) 54:157–63. doi: 10.1016/0167-5273(96)02593-4
53. Göser S, Andrassy M, Buss S, Leuschner F, Volz CH, Ottl R, et al. Cardiac troponin I but not cardiac troponin T induces severe autoimmune inflammation in the myocardium. *Circulation.* (2006) 114:1693–702. doi: 10.1161/CIRCULATIONAHA.106.635664
54. Herzum M, Maisch B, Kochsiek K. Circulating immune complexes in perimyocarditis and infective endocarditis. *Eur Heart J.* (1987) 8(Suppl. J):323–6. doi: 10.1093/eurheartj/8.suppl_J.323
55. Leone O, Veinot JP, Angelini A, Baandrup UT, Basso C, Berry G, et al. 2011 Consensus statement on endomyocardial biopsy from the Association for European Cardiovascular Pathology and the Society for Cardiovascular Pathology. *Cardiovasc Pathol.* (2012) 21:245–74. doi: 10.1016/j.carpath.2011.10.001
56. Kindermann I, Barth C, Mahfoud F, Ukena C, Lenski M, Yilmaz A, et al. Update on myocarditis. *J Am Coll Cardiol.* (2012) 59:779–92. doi: 10.1016/j.jacc.2011.09.074
57. Sagar S, Liu PP, Cooper LT. Myocarditis. *Lancet.* (2012) 379:738–47. doi: 10.1016/S0140-6736(11)60648-X
58. Maisch B, Richter A, Sandmöller A, Portig I, Pankuweit S, BMBF-Heart Failure Network. Inflammatory dilated cardiomyopathy (DCMI). *Herz.* (2005) 30:535–44. doi: 10.1007/s00059-005-2730-5
59. Dennert R, Crijns HJ, Heymans S. Acute viral myocarditis. *Eur Heart J.* (2008) 29:2073 82. doi: 10.1093/eurheartj/ehn296
60. Pankuweit S, Moll R, Baandrup U, Portig I, Hufnagel G, Maisch B. Prevalence of the parvovirus B19 genome in endomyocardial biopsy specimens. *Hum Pathol.* (2003) 34:497–503. doi: 10.1016/S0046-8177(03)00078-9
61. Bock CT, Klingel K, Kandolf R. Human parvovirus B19-associated myocarditis. *N Engl J Med.* (2010) 362:1248–9. doi: 10.1056/NEJMc0911362
62. Maisch B. Effusive-constrictive pericarditis: current perspectives. *J Cardiovasc Diagn Interv.* (2018) 6:7–14. doi: 10.2147/JVD.S125950
63. Boucher D, Monteleone M, Coll RC, Chen KW, Ross CM, Teo JL, et al. Caspase-1 self-cleavage is an intrinsic mechanism to terminate inflammasome activity. *J Exp Med.* (2018) 215:827–40. doi: 10.1084/jem.20172222
64. De Rosa S, Eposito F, Carella C, Strangio A, Ammirati G, Sabatino J, et al. Transcoronary concentration gradients of circulating microRNAs in heart failure. *Eur J Heart Fail.* (2018) 20:1000 10. doi: 10.1002/ejhf.1119
65. Waagstein F, Hjalmarson A, Varnauskas E, Walentin L. Effect of beta-adrenergic receptor blockade in congestive cardiomyoapthy. *Br Heart J.* (1975) 37:1022–36. doi: 10.1136/hrt.37.10.1022
66. Maisch B, Seferović PM, Ristić AD, Erbel R, Rienmüller R, Adler Y, et al. Guidelines on the diagnosis and management of pericardial diseases, executive summary; The Task force on the diagnosis and management of pericardial diseases of the European society of cardiology. *Eur Heart J.* (2004) 25:587–610. doi: 10.1016/j.ehj.2004.02.002
67. Adler Y, Charron P, Imazio M, Badano L, Barón-Esquivias G, Bogaert J, et al. 2015 ESC guidelines for the diagnosis and management of pericardial diseases. *Eur Heart J.* (2015) 36:2921–61. doi: 10.1093/eurheartj/ehv318
68. Costanzo-Nordin MR, Reap EA, O'Connell JB, Robinson JA, Scanlon PJ. A nonsteroid anti-inflammatory drug exacerbates Coxsackie B3 murine myocarditis. *J Am Coll Cardiol.* (1985) 6:1078–82. doi: 10.1016/S0735-1097(85)80312-0
69. Maisch B. Management von Perikarditis und Perikarderguss, konstriktiver und effusiv-konstriktiver Perikarditis. *Herz.* (2018) 43:663–78.
70. Maisch B, Hufnagel G, Schönian U, Hengstenberg C. The European Study of Epidemiology and Treatment of Cardiac Inflammatory Disease (ESETCID). *Eur Heart J.* (1995) 16:173–5.
71. Kodama M, Matsumoto Y, Fujiwara M, Masani F, Izumi T, Shibata A. A novel experimental model of giant cell myocarditis induced in rats by immunization with cardiac myosin fraction. *Clin Immunol Immunopathol.* (1990) 57:250–62. doi: 10.1016/0090-1229(90)90039-S
72. Cooper LT, Berry GHJ, Shabetai R. Giant cell myocarditis: distinctions from lymphocytic myocarditis and cardiac sarcoidosis. *J Heart Fail.* (1997) 4:227230.
73. Cooper LT, Okura Y. Idiopathic giant cell myocarditis. Current treatment options. *Cardiovasc Med.* (2001) 3:463–7. doi: 10.1007/s11936-001-0020-y
74. Cooper LT, Berry GJ, Shabetai R. Idiopathic giant cell myocarditis - natural history and treatment. *N Engl J Med.* (1997) 336:1860–6. doi: 10.1056/NEJM199706263362603
75. Fenoglio JJ, Ursell PC, Kellogg CF, Drusin RE, Weiss MB. Diagnosis and classification of myocarditis by endomyocardial biopsy. *N Engl J Med.* (1983) 308:12–18. doi: 10.1056/NEJM198301063080103

76. Hosenpud JD, McAnulty JH, Niles NR. Lack of objective improvement in ventricular systolic function in patients with myocarditis treated with azathioprine and prednisone. *J Am Coll Cardiol.* (1985) 6:797–801. doi: 10.1016/S0735-1097(85)80485-X
77. Anderson JL, Fowles RE, Unverferth DV, Mason JW. Immunosuppressive therapy of myocardial inflammatory disease. Initial experience and future trials to define indications for therapy. *Eur Heart J.* (1987) 8(Suppl J):263–6.
78. Marboe CC, Fenoglio JJ. Pathology and natural history of human myocarditis. *Pathol Immunopathol Res.* (1988) 7:226–39.
79. Latham RD, Mulrow JP, Virmani R, Robinowitz M, Moody JM. Recently diagnosed idiopathic dilated cardiomyopathy: incidence of myocarditis and efficacy of prednisone therapy. *Am Heart J.* (1989) 117:876–82. doi: 10.1016/0002-8703(89)90626-1
80. Maisch B, Schoenian U, Hengstenberg C, Herzum M, Hufnagel G, Bethge C, et al. Immunosuppressive therapy in autoreactive myocarditis: results from a controlled trial. *Postgrad Med J.* (1994) 70(Suppl. 1):S29–34.
81. Jühl U, Strauer BE, Schultheiss HP. Methylprednisolone in chronic myocarditis. *Postgrad Med J.* (1994) 70(Suppl. 1):S35–42.
82. Camargo PR, Snitcowsky R, da Luz PL, Mazzieri R, Higuchi ML, Rati M, et al. Favorable effects of immunosuppressive therapy in children with dilated cardiomyopathy and active myocarditis. *Pediatr Cardiol.* (1995) 16:61–8. doi: 10.1007/BF00796819
83. Liu D, Lei Y, Haixia J. Clinical search of Sheng Mai injection combined with corticosteroids for acute viral myocarditis in children. *J Sichuan Tradit Chin Med.* (2003) 21:59–60.
84. Sun D. Corticosteroid treatment effects in 36 cases diagnose with viral myocarditis with ventricle premature beats. *J Zhenjiang Med Coll.* (1999) 9:211–14.
85. Wu Y-Z, Chen B-W. Observation on curative effects of astragalus injection combined with glucocorticoids on acutely severe viral myocarditis. *Zhongguo Zhong Xe Yi Jie He Ji Jui Za Zhi.* (1999) 6:350–2.
86. Frustaci A, Chimenti C, Calabrese F, Pieroni M, Thiene G, Maseri A. Immunosuppressive therapy for active lymphocytic myocarditis: virological and immunologic profile for responders versus nonresponders. *Circulation.* (2003) 107:857–63. doi: 10.1161/01.CIR.0000048147.15962.31
87. Escher F, Kühl U, Lassner D, Poller W, Westermann D, Pieske B, et al. Long-term outcome of patients with virus negative chronic myocarditis or inflammatory cadiomyopathy after immunosuppressive therapy. *Clin Res Cardiol.* (2016) 105:1011–20. doi: 10.1007/s00392-016-1011-z
88. Parillo JE, Cunnion RE, Epstein SE, Parker MM, Suffredini AF, Brenner M, et al. A prospective, randomized, controlled trial of prednisone for dilated cardiomyopathy. *N Engl J Med.* (1989) 321:1061–8. doi: 10.1056/NEJM198910193211601
89. Mason JW, O'Connel JB, Hershkowitz A, Rose NR, McManus BM, Billingham ME, et al. A clinical trial of immunosuppressive therapy for myocarditis. The myocarditis treatment trial investigators. *N Engl J Med.* (1995) 33:269–75.
90. Maisch B, Camerini F, Schultheiss H-P. Immunosuppressive therapy for myocarditis (letter). *N Engl J Med.* (1995) 333:1713.
91. Wojnicz R, Nowalany-Kozielska E, Wojciechowska C, Glanowska G, Wilczewski P, Niklewski T, et al. Randomized, placebo-controlled study for immunosuppressive treatment of inflammatory dilated cardiomyopathy. Two-year follow-up results. *Circulation.* (2001) 104:39–45.
92. Frustaci A, Russo MA, Chimenti C. Randomized study on the efficacy of immunosuppressive therapy in patients with virus-negative inflammatory cardiomyopathy: the TIMIC study. *Eur Heart J.* (2009) 30:1995–2002. doi: 10.1093/eurheartj/ehp249
93. Maisch B, Kölsch S, Hufnagel G, et al. for the ESETCID Investigators. Orlando 2011, AHA Congress. *Circulation.* (2011) Suppl (Abstract).
94. Hufnagel G, Maisch B, Pfeiffer U. Immunhistologic investigations in suspected cardiac sarcoidosis. *Eur Heart J.* (1987) 8(Suppl. J):59–62. doi: 10.1093/eurheartj/8.suppl_J.59
95. Schoppet M, Pankuweit S, Moll R, Baandrup U, Maisch B. Images in cardiovascular medicine. Phenotype of infiltrating T lymphocytes in cardiac sarcoidosis. *Circulation.* (2002) 105:e67–8.
96. Valentonye R, Hampe J, Huse K, Rosenstiel P, Albrecht M, Stenzel A, et al. Sarcoidosis is associated with a truncating splice mutant in BTNL2. *Nat Genet.* (2005) 37:357–64. doi: 10.1038/ng1519
97. Meyer T, Lauschke J, Ruppert V, Richter A, Pankuweit S, Maisch B. Isolated cardiac sarcoidosis associated with the expression of a splice variant coding for a truncated BTNL2 protein. *Cardiology.* (2008) 109:117121. doi: 10.1159/000105552
98. Bargout R, Kelly RF. Sarcoid heart disease. Clinical course and treatment. *Int J Cardiol.* (2004) 97:173–82. doi: 10.1016/j.ijcard.2003.07.024
99. Spry CJ, Tai PC, Davies J. The cardiotoxicity of eosinophils. *Postgrad Med J.* (1983) 59:147–55. doi: 10.1136/pgmj.59.689.147
100. Tai PC, Ackerman SJ, Spry CJ, Dunnette S, Olsen EG, Gleich GJ. Deposits of eosinophil granule proteins in cardiac tissues of patients with eosinophilic endomyocardial disease. *Lancet.* (1987) 21:643–47. doi: 10.1016/S0140-6736(87)90412-0
101. Anthony RM, Nimmerjahn F, Ashline DJ, Reinhold VN, Paulson JC, Ravetch JV, et al. Recapitulation of IVIG anti-inflammatory activity with a recombinant Ig Fc. *Science.* (2008) 320:373–376. doi: 10.1126/science.1154315
102. Takada H, Kishimoto C, Hiraoka Y. Therapy with immunoglobulin suppresses myocarditis in a murine coxsackievirus B3 model–antiviral and anti-inflammatory effects. *Circulation.* (1995) 92:1604–11. doi: 10.1161/01.CIR.92.6.1604
103. Selbing A, Josefsson A, Dahle LO, Lindgren R. Parvovirus B19 infection during pregnancy treated with high-dose intravenous gammaglobulin. *Lancet.* (1995) 345:660–1. doi: 10.1016/S0140-6736(95)90569-3
104. Walpen AJ, Laumonier T, Aebi C, Mohacsi PJ, Rieben R. IgM enriched intravenous immunoglobulin inhibits classical pathway complement activation, but not bacterial killing by human serum. *Xenotransplantation.* (2004) 11:141–8. doi: 10.1046/j.1399-3089.2003.00098.x
105. Drucker NA, Colan SD, Lewis AB, Beiser AS, Wessel DL, Takahashi M, et al. Gamma-globulin treatment of acute myocarditis in the pediatric population. *Circulation.* (1994) 89:252–7. doi: 10.1161/01.CIR.89.1.252
106. McNamara DM, Rosenblum WD, Janosko KM, Trost MK, Villaneuva FS, Demetris AJ, et al. Intravenous immune gobulin in the therapy of myocarditis and acute cardiomyopathy. *Circulation.* (1997) 95:2476–8.
107. Takeda Y, Yasuda S, Miyazaki S, Daikoku S, Nakatani S, Nonogi H. High-dose immunoglobulin G therapy for fulminant myocarditis. *Jap Circ J.* (1998) 62:871–2. doi: 10.1253/jcj.62.871
108. Nigro G, Bastianon V, Colloridi V, Ventriglia F, Gallo P, D'Amati G, et al. Human parvovirus B19 infection in infancy associated with acute and chronic lymphocytic myocarditis and high cytokine levels: report of 3 cases and review. *Clin Infect Dis.* (2000) 31:65–9. doi: 10.1086/313929
109. Tsai YG, Ou TY, Wang CC, Tsai MC, Yuh YS, Hwang B. Intravenous gamma-globulin therapy in myocarditis complicated with complete heart block: report of one case. *Chung-Hua Min Kuo Hsiao Erh Ko I Hsueh Hui Ts Chih.* (2001) 42:311–3.
110. McNamara DM, Holubkov R, Starling RC, Dec GW, Loh E, Torre-Amione G, et al. Controlled trial of intravenous immune globuline in recent-onset dilated cardiomyopathy. *Circulation.* (2001) 103:2254–549. doi: 10.1161/01.CIR.103.18.2254
111. Alter P, Grimm W, Maisch B. Varicella myocarditis in an adult. *Heart.* (2001) 85:E2. doi: 10.1136/heart.85.1.e2
112. Shioji K, Kishimoto C, Sasyama S. Immunoglobulin therapy for acute myocarditis. *Resp Circul.* (2000) 48:1133–9. doi: 10.1161/01.CIR.95.11.2476
113. Tedeschi A, Airaghi L, Giannini S, Ciceri L, Massari FM. High-dose intravenous immunoglobulin in the treatment of acute myocarditis. A case report and review of the literature. *J Intern Med.* (2002) 251:169–73.
114. Kishimoto C, Fujita M, Kinoshita M, Iwase T, Tamaki S, Fujii M, et al. Immunglobulin therapy for myocarditis an acute dilated cardiomyopathy. *Circulation.* (2001) 103:220–5.
115. Wang CY, Li Lu F, Wu MH, Lee CY, Huang LM. Fatal coxsackievirus A16 infection. *Pediatr Infect Dis J.* (2004) 23:275–6. doi: 10.1097/01.inf.0000115950.63906.78
116. Dennert R, Velthuis S, Schalla S, Eurlings L, van Suylen RJ, van Paassen P, et al. Intravenous immunoglobulin therapy for patients with idiopathic cardiomyopathy and endomyocardial biopsy-proven high PVB19 viral load. *Antiviral Ther.* (2010) 15:193–201. doi: 10.3851/IMP1516
117. Maisch B, Pankuweit S, Funck R, Koelsch S. Effective CMV hyperimmunoglobulin treatment in CMV myocarditis – A

controled treatment trial. *Eur Heart J.* (2004) 25(Suppl.):114. doi: 10.1016/S0735-1097(16)31348-1
118. Klugman D, Berger JT, Sable CA, He J, Khandelwal SG, Slonim AD. Pediatric patients hospitalized with myocarditis: a multi-institutional analysis. *Pediatr Cardiol.* (2009) 31:222–8. doi: 10.1007/s00246-009-9589-9
119. Müller J, Wallukat G, Dandel M, Bieda H, Brandes K, Spiegelsberger S, et al. Immunoglobulin adsorption in patients with idiopathic dilated cardiomyopathy. *Circulation.* (2000) 101:385–91.
120. Wallukat G, Müller J, Hetzer R. Specific removal of beta1-adrenergic autoantibodies from patients with idiopathic dilated cardiomyopathy. *N Engl J Med.* (2002) 347:1806. doi: 10.1056/NEJM200211283472220
121. Kühl U, Pauschinger M, Schwimmbeck PL, Seeberg B, Lober C, Noutsias M, et al. Interferon-beta treatment eliminates cardiotropic viruses and improves left ventriclar function in patients with myocardial persistence of viral genomes and left ventricular dysfunction. *Circulation.* (2003) 107:2793–8. doi: 10.1161/01.CIR.0000072766.67150.51
122. Schultheiss HP, Piper C, Sowade O, Waagstein F, Kapp JF, Wegscheider K, et al. Betaferon in chronic viral cardiomyopathy (BICC) trial: effects of interferon-β treatment in patients with chronic viral cardiomyopathy. *Clin Res Cardiol.* (2016) 105:763–3. doi: 10.1007/s00392-016-0986-9

14

HIV Proteins and Endothelial Dysfunction: Implications in Cardiovascular Disease

Appakkudal R. Anand[1,2*], *Gladys Rachel*[2] *and Durgadevi Parthasarathy*[1]

[1] *L&T Microbiology Research Centre, Vision Research Foundation, Sankara Nethralaya, Chennai, India,* [2] *Department of HIV/AIDS, National Institute for Research in Tuberculosis, Chennai, India*

Correspondence:
Appakkudal R. Anand
aranand@gmail.com

With the success of antiretroviral therapy (ART), a dramatic decrease in viral burden and opportunistic infections and an increase in life expectancy has been observed in human immunodeficiency virus (HIV) infected individuals. However, it is now clear that HIV- infected individuals have enhanced susceptibility to non-AIDS (Acquired immunodeficiency syndrome)-related complications such as cardiovascular disease (CVD). CVDs such as atherosclerosis have become a significant cause of morbidity and mortality in individuals with HIV infection. Though studies indicate that ART itself may increase the risk to develop CVD, recent studies suggest a more important role for HIV infection in contributing to CVD independently of the traditional risk factors. Endothelial dysfunction triggered by HIV infection has been identified as a critical link between infection, inflammation/immune activation, and atherosclerosis. Considering the inability of HIV to actively replicate in endothelial cells, endothelial dysfunction depends on both HIV-encoded proteins as well as inflammatory mediators released in the microenvironment by HIV-infected cells. Indeed, the HIV proteins, gp120 (envelope glycoprotein) and Tat (transactivator of transcription), are actively secreted into the endothelial cell micro-environment during HIV infection, while Nef can be actively transferred onto endothelial cells during HIV infection. These proteins can have significant direct effects on the endothelium. These include a range of responses that contribute to endothelial dysfunction, including enhanced adhesiveness, permeability, cell proliferation, apoptosis, oxidative stress as well as activation of cytokine secretion. This review summarizes the current understanding of the interactions of HIV, specifically its proteins with endothelial cells and its implications in cardiovascular disease. We analyze recent *in vitro* and *in vivo* studies examining endothelial dysfunction in response to HIV proteins. Furthermore, we discuss the multiple mechanisms by which these viral proteins damage the vascular endothelium in HIV patients. A better understanding of the molecular mechanisms of HIV protein associated endothelial dysfunction leading to cardiovascular disease is likely to be pivotal in devising new strategies to treat and prevent cardiovascular disease in HIV-infected patients.

Keywords: HIV proteins, endothelial dysfunction, cardiovascular disease, gp120, Nef, Tat, atherosclerosis

INTRODUCTION

The introduction of highly active antiretroviral therapy has lead to a drastic reduction in viral burden and opportunistic infections, resulting in a remarkable improvement in the life expectancy of HIV-infected individuals. However, it is now evident that HIV-infected individuals have an enhanced susceptibility to non-AIDS (Acquired Immunodeficiency syndrome)-related comorbidities such as cardio-vascular diseases (CVDs), which have emerged as prominent causes of morbidity and mortality in this population (1–9). Atherosclerotic CVD rates and risk of myocardial infarction are significantly elevated in HIV-infected individuals than the general population (1, 10, 11). Studies further indicate that both clinical cardiovascular events such as coronary heart disease (11–13), peripheral artery disease (14), as well as subclinical cardiovascular damage such as elevation of intima-media thickness (15, 16), coronary calcification (17), abnormal ankle-brachial index (18) and silent myocardial ischemia (19) are much higher in HIV-infected individuals (20).

ETIOPATHOGENESIS OF CARDIOVASCULAR DISEASE IN PATIENTS WITH HIV INFECTION

The increased cardiovascular risk in HIV-infected individuals is attributable to a combination of multiple factors, including higher prevalence of traditional risk factors, inherent effects of the HIV infection, effects of antiretroviral therapy and the presence of other co-morbidities seen frequently in HIV-positive patients (such as hepatitis C virus and herpes family virus co-infections). Though initial studies indicated a predominance of traditional CVD risk factors (21, 22) and effect of ART (23) as major causes for CVD among HIV-positive individuals (10, 24, 25), evidence from experimental and observational studies (26, 27) in recent years have redirected attention more toward the consequences of HIV infection itself. Hsue et al demonstrated a correlation between HIV infection and premature atherosclerosis even in the absence of detectable viremia, immunodeficiency, and ART exposure, with the atherosclerosis being independent of traditional cardiovascular risk factors (28).

Among multiple pathogenic effects that contribute to atherosclerosis and ultimately CVD, HIV-induced endothelial dysfunction is now established as a major contributing factor. Higher plasma HIV RNA levels have been shown to correlate with endothelial dysfunction in HIV-infected patients (29). A transgenic mouse model expressing HIV viral proteins env, tat, nef, vpu, vpr, and rev demonstrated aortic endothelial dysfunction and increased arterial stiffness (30). HIV-infected patients had significantly impaired endothelial function, as demonstrated by reduced flow-mediated dilation, a measure of endothelial vasomotor function in comparison to the HIV-negative group (31).

ENDOTHELIAL DYSFUNCTION AND CARDIOVASCULAR DISEASE

Endothelial dysfunction as a precursor of atherosclerosis and future cardiovascular events has been demonstrated in multiple population studies (32, 33). The development of atherosclerosis resulting from dysfunctional endothelium is highly complex and regulated by several factors. Endothelial dysfunction is characterized by decreased anti-oxidant, anti-inflammatory and anti-thrombotic properties (due to reduced NO bioavailability) and increased endothelial permeability, pro-inflammatory cytokine levels, and adhesion molecule expression. Leukocyte recruitment and adhesion represent the initial events in development of atherosclerosis. Leukocyte recruitment is mediated by several chemoattractants such as IL-6, IL-8, and MCP-1 and adherence of leukocytes to the endothelium is mediated by cell adhesion molecules (CAM). Leukocytes, especially monocytes traverse the endothelium, and migrate into the intima (34). Transmigration of leukocytes, as well as infiltration of plasma contents into the vascular wall is facilitated by an increase in endothelial permeability. These infiltrated plasma contents such as modified low-density lipoprotein (LDL), along with substances produced by infiltrated leukocytes, such as cytokines and chemokines, alter smooth muscle function and contribute to the development of atherosclerosis (35). Further, in the intima, the monocytes differentiate into macrophages, expressing receptors that facilitate lipid uptake. On lipid uptake and accumulation, macrophages transform into foam cells. These foam cells initiate atherosclerotic lesions, which are later characterized by plaque formation (34). Studies suggest that HIV impairs several of these processes that maintain vascular homeostasis, potentially leading to atherosclerosis (**Table 1**). Several mechanisms have been suggested to explain how HIV infection induces endothelial dysfunction leading to CVD, including direct HIV infection of endothelial cells (ECs), inflammation and effect of HIV proteins HIV proteins released in the endothelial microenvironment or directly transferred to ECs by HIV and HIV-infected cells represent critical mediators of endothelial dysfunction. This article reviews the current understanding of the mechanisms by which HIV, in particular, the different HIV proteins drive EC dysregulation, potentially leading to CVD.

HIV ENCODED PROTEINS AND ENDOTHELIAL DYSFUNCTION

HIV is a retrovirus with a glycoprotein-rich envelope surrounding a nucleocapsid. The HIV structural and regulatory/accessory proteins are designed for the virus to adapt efficiently to the human host, thereby promoting its replication and transmission. The HIV viral genome contains 9 principal genes, gag, pol, env, tat, rev, vpu, vpr, vif, and nef. The Gag-Pol precursor protein undergoes proteolytic cleavage to generate the matrix p17, capsid p24, nucleocapsids p9 and p6, reverse transcriptase, protease, and integrase, all of which are major structural components of the viral core. The

TABLE 1 | Summary of the potential mechanisms by which HIV protein-induced endothelial dysfunction contribute directly or indirectly to the development of atherosclerosis and CVD.

HIV protein	Endothelial dysfunction[a]	Association with cardiovascular disease
Gp120 Tat Nef	↑Apoptosis (36–43)	Promotes atherosclerotic plaque formation and plaque instability
Gp120 Tat Nef	↑IL-6 (44–46)	Increases intima media thickness Monocyte/macrophage recruitment Stimulates synthesis of acute phase proteins (CRP)
Gp120	↑IL-8 (47)	Leukocyte recruitment Mediates release of MCP-1
Tat	↑IL-1β (48)	Induces macrophage/foam cell apoptosis, Increased expression of pro-inflammatory cytokines Increased expression of adhesion molecules Migration of vascular smooth muscle cells and ECs
Tat Nef	↑MCP-1 (49, 50)	Increases monocyte recruitment
Gp120	↑ET-1 (51)	Increased smooth muscle proliferation and migration
Gp120 Tat Nef	↑ICAM-1 (52–54)	Adherence and transmigration of leukocytes into the vessel wall
Tat	↑VCAM-1 (48, 55)	Adherence and transmigration of leukocytes into the vessel wall
Tat	↑E-selectin (48)	Initial rolling of leukocytes on ECs
Gp120 Tat	↑ Endothelial permeability (47, 51, 56–59)	Facilitates infiltration of leukocytes and plasma contents into vessel wall
Gp120	↑ MMP-2, ↑ MMP-9 (60)	Facilitates endothelial damage leading to unstable plaque formation
Gp120	↓ NO levels (61, 62)	Abnormal vascular tone regulation and enhanced platelet adhesion and aggregation
Gp120 Tat	↑ROS (55, 56, 63, 64)	Increased foam cell formation leading to plaque growth

[a] *References are in parenthesis.*

Env undergoes proteolytic cleavage to generate the envelope glycoproteins gp120 and gp41. Tat and Rev are the regulatory proteins, while Vpu, Vpr, Vif, and Nef are the accessory proteins (65). Among these viral proteins, gp120, Tat and Nef play a major role in the pathogenesis of endothelial dysfunction. The experimental evidence supporting a functional role for the HIV viral proteins in the disruption of EC cell biology is outlined in the following sections.

HIV gp120

HIV envelope glycoprotein is synthesized as a precursor glycoprotein, gp160, which is then processed into an amino terminus subunit, gp120, and a carboxyl transmembrane subunit, gp41. The envelope glycoprotein, gp120 is expressed on the outer layer of the virus, as well as on the surface of infected cells. Gp120 is critical for virus infection, as the protein is necessary for binding to specific cell surface receptors on target cells and facilitating virus entry. The primary receptor for gp120 is the CD4 receptor, while the main co-receptors are CXCR4 and CCR5. Gp120 is found both in the free form in the body fluids of HIV-positive patients (66, 67) and bound form on the surface of apoptotic CD4 positive T-cells (68). In fact, gp120 has been shown in the germinal center of lymph nodes in HIV-infected individuals under ART with no detectable viral replication (69). Multiple studies have confirmed that gp120, both in soluble and surface bound form, has an important role in viral pathogenesis on diverse uninfected bystander cells (70–74), including ECs.

Gp120 is associated with apoptosis, adhesion molecule expression, pro-inflammatory cytokine production and EC permeability. Gp120 present either on viral particles, surface of infected cells, or as free soluble protein causes endothelial apoptosis predominantly by direct interaction with the co-receptor, CXCR4. Gp120 induces apoptosis in human coronary ECs (36), human umbilical vein ECs (HUVECs) (37, 38), lung microvascular ECs (LMVECs) (39), and brain microvascular ECs (BMVECs) (40, 41). EC apoptosis is an important process, initially in atherosclerotic plaque formation, and later in the progression to an advanced stage of atherosclerosis, when the plaques become vulnerable to rupture (42, 75, 76). The molecular mechanism by which gp120 exerts its endothelial toxicity, may involve caspase-3 activation (38), Bax upregulation (38), protein kinase C (PKC) activation (77) and p38 mitogen-activated protein (MAP) kinase signaling (41). Gp120 also induces an increase in reactive oxygen species (ROS), signaling oxidative stress to the ECs (56, 63). Oxidative stress induced by generation of excess reactive oxygen species is a critical process in the development of atherosclerosis (78). HIV-induced ROS likely contributes to endothelial dysfunction through direct effects on the endothelium and/or indirectly through monocytes /macrophages contacting the vessel wall. The viral glycoptotein is also able to increase endothelin-1 (ET-1) secretion (51) and promote surface expression of Endothelial monocyte activating polypeptide II (EMAPII) (79). ET-1 mediates the reduction of vascular nitric oxide production by ECs, leading to the smooth muscle proliferation and migration, which in turn leads to arterial vasoconstriction (80), whereas EMAPII is released in response to stress such as hypoxia, mechanical strain and apoptosis (81) and acts as a pro-apoptotic factor. In addition, a recent study has shown that HIV gp120 (X4 and R5) promotes EC senescence and impairs the regulation of senescence-associated microRNAs (82). Senescent ECs develop a dysfunctional phenotype acquiring pro-inflammatory, pro-oxidant, vasoconstrictor, and prothrombotic properties (83).

Gp120 is directly involved in upregulation of pro-inflammatory cytokines such as IL-6 and IL-8 in primary ECs (44). IL-6 and IL-8 play a major role in recruitment of leukocytes, especially of the monocyte/macrophage and neutrophil lineage, respectively. IL-6 can also actively promote atherogenesis, both directly by inducing vascular endothelial dysfunction, extracellular matrix degradation and indirectly by stimulating hepatocytes synthesis of acute phase proteins involved in inflammation, such as C-reactive protein (84). Gp120 also facilitates monocyte (52) and T cell adherence (85) to the vascular endothelium through upregulation of CAMs. Among the CAMs, E-selectin is involved in the initial rolling of leukocytes on the endothelial cells, while ICAM-1 and VCAM-1 induce firm adhesion and transmigration of leukocytes across the endothelium (86). Gp120 augments expression of ICAM-1, but not VCAM-1 or E-selectin, in ECs of multiple origins, including human coronary artery, lung, brain, umbilical vein, and dermal microvascular ECs (52).

Gp120 also increases endothelial permeability by various mechanisms including cytoskeletal rearrangement (56), down-regulation of tight junction proteins (51) and PKC activation (47). An increase in endothelial permeability was observed in brain endothelial cultures of HIV gp120 transgenic mice (87), compared to non-transgenic mice. Gp120 also induces expression of the matrix metalloproteases (MMPs), MMP-2 and MMP-9, that mediate endothelial damage with the formation of an unstable atherosclerotic plaque morphology (60). Additionally, gp120 reduces the EC-derived nitric oxide (NO) synthesized by the NO synthase, thus affecting endothelium-dependent vasorelaxation and enhancing platelet adhesion and aggregation (61, 62).

HIV Tat

HIV Tat (trans-activator of transcription) is a regulatory protein encoded by the tat gene that enhances viral transcription (88). Tat has been detected in the sera of HIV patients (89), even during complete ART (cART) (90). Tat is secreted into the extracellular microenvironment by HIV-infected T-cells and monocyte/macrophages (89, 91). In the circulation, Tat is suggested to act as a proto-cytokine, modulating the functions of several cells including ECs (92). Thus, Tat is involved in the pathogenesis of several HIV-associated disease conditions ranging from pulmonary hypertension to cognitive abnormalities (36, 48, 93–95). Tat protein possesses both transcription promotion and membrane transduction properties. Tat has five discrete domains, the N-terminal, cysteine-rich, core, basic, and C-terminal domain. Tat interacts with three known receptors to trigger endothelial dysfunction. The C-terminal domain, containing an Arg-Gly-Asp (RGD) sequence, binds with high affinity to the integrins alphaVbeta1 and alphaVbeta3 receptors (96). The basic domain binds to the integrin alphaVbeta5 receptor (97) as well as the Flk-1/KDR receptor (98). Tat activates these receptors to initiate endothelial signaling pathways that affect diverse processes such as endothelial permeability (57, 58), cytokine production (59), adhesion (48), angiogenesis (99–102), and apoptosis (43).

Tat exhibits a dual function with regard to survival regulation, exhibiting either EC proliferation or apoptosis, depending on the micro-environment conditions (103). One of the prominent properties of Tat is that of a direct angiogenic factor (92). Endothelial proliferation is enhanced by factors such as FGF-2 (fibroblast growth factor) (104). Tat activates Rac1 through a signaling cascade involving RhoA, Ras, and extracellular signal-regulated kinase (ERK), which in turn, induces EC proliferation and survival (105). Tat mediates Rac1 activation through PAK-1, phosphorylates c-Jun N-terminal kinase (JNK), activates endothelial NADPH oxidase and regulates actin cytoskeletal dynamics (106). Tat has been suggested to play a role in HIV-related Kaposi sarcoma by promoting EC proliferation and tumor angiogenesis, where Tat binds specifically and activates the Flk-1/kinase insert domain receptor (Flk- 1/KDR), a VEGF-A tyrosine kinase receptor, and promotes angiogenesis (98). Contrary to its role in angiogenesis, Tat also induces the apoptosis of primary microvascular ECs via either TNF-alpha secretion or through activation of the Fas-dependent pathway (43). Fiala et al.

(36) analyzed the pathogenesis of HIV-related cardiomyopathy, and found that exogenous Tat protein was capable of activating apoptosis of both ECs or cardiomyocytes. A recent report indicates that HIV Tat along with morphine induces autophagy in pulmonary ECs, suggesting a role for Tat in HIV-related pulmonary arterial hypertension in the presence of opioids (107). In addition, Tat also promotes EC senescence and dysregulation of senescence-associated microRNAs (82).

Tat stimulates the release of pro-inflammatory cytokines and induces expression of CAMs (45, 48, 55, 108, 109) in ECs of diverse origin (i.e., pulmonary artery, umbilical vein, aorta, and brain). In human vascular ECs (HUVECs), Tat stimulates the upregulation of inflammatory mediators, including IL-1β, MCP-1, VCAM-1 and E-selectin through nuclear factor-kappa B (NF-κB) (48, 108). IL-1β can induce macrophage and foam cell apoptosis, causing the release of their lipid content into the intima of the artery and contributing toward the lipid core in the plaque (110). IL-1β can also induce the expression of cytokines, adhesion molecules and the migration and mitogenesis of vascular smooth muscle and endothelial cells (111). MCP-1 is a major chemokine involved in monocyte recruitment during atherosclerosis development (35). Expression of IL-6 and MCP-1 is dependent upon the activity of the kinases, PKC (45) and cAMP-dependent protein kinase A (49). Tat stimulated ICAM-1 expression in HUVECs by suppressing miR-221/-222 via an NF-κB-dependent pathway (53), while Tat stimulated VCAM-1 expression through p38 MAP kinase and NF-kB activation (55). Upregulation of these adhesion molecules resulted in monocyte (45, 108, 112) and T-cell (113) adhesion to the endothelium. Furthermore, Matzen et al showed that Tat in combination with TNF-alpha, a cytokine increased in sera and tissues of HIV-infected patients, acts synergistically to increase the adhesion of leukocytes to ECs, suggesting that both these proteins act in co-operation to contribute to the vascular damage during HIV infection (113). Finally, Tat induces endothelial oxidative stress through activation of NADPH oxidase and through decreased antioxidant capacity. Tat-induced MAPK signaling requires upstream superoxide production by various NADPH oxidase subunits. Moreover, Tat-induced ROS activates the NF-kB pathway (55) and decreases GSH levels (64). Tat also attenuates the expression of the mitochondrial superoxide scavenger, Manganese-superoxide dismutase (Mn-SOD) (46, 114).

HIV Nef

HIV Nef is a 27-kD, n-myristoylated accessory protein that lacks enzymatic activity. It is an adaptor molecule containing multiple domains essential for interaction with host cell signaling molecules (115, 116). Nef is involved in modulation of several intracellular functions that include regulation of protein trafficking and cell signaling pathways, attenuation of antibody maturation in B cells (117), and increase in HIV infectivity (118). The presence of Nef has been shown in the endothelium of coronary and pulmonary arteries of SIV-HIV-Nef-infected macaques (50). Sowinski et al (119) demonstrated that Nef induces the formation of conduit-like nanotubes, connecting HIV-positive cells to bystander cells. Further, Wang et al. (50) showed that Nef transfer from HIV-infected cells to ECs promotes endothelial dysfunction (50, 120). Nef is also delivered to bystander cells through exosomes (121). ECs, especially those present in developing atherosclerotic plaques, would therefore be in a prime physical position to receive Nef transfer from circulating monocytes and T cells. Transgenic mice that express CD4-promoter-driven Nef develop multiple pathologies including vasospasm in the heart (122). Studies show that Rhesus macaques demonstrate pulmonary hypertension (PH)-like pulmonary vascular remodeling, when infected with chimeric SHIVnef virions, but not with SIV, indicating a role of HIV-Nef in PH, with certain Nef gene variants showing a higher propensity to develop PH (123, 124).

Similar to gp120 and Tat, Nef has been associated with several aspects of HIV-induced endothelial dysfunction. Acheampong et al. (42) showed that Nef, when expressed both extracellularly and endogenously, induces apoptosis in primary human brain microvascular ECs (HB-MVECs) by activation of caspases. A microarray analysis of apoptosis genes in Nef-transduced HB-MVECs demonstrated that the up-regulated genes belong to both mitochondrial and Fas/FasL apoptotic pathways, indicating that Nef may utilize multiple pathways to induce apoptosis in ECs. In contrast, in the context of Kaposi's sarcoma, Nef and KSHV oncogene K1 synergistically promote angiogenesis by inducing cellular miR-718 to regulate the PTEN/AKT/mTOR signaling pathway. However, in Kaposi's sarcoma, Nef in combination with KSHV oncogene K1 synergistically induces cellular miR-718 to regulate the PTEN/AKT/mTOR signaling pathway and thus promotes angiogenesis. This pathway is an important factor in aberrant neovascularization caused by KS-associated herpesvirus (KSHV) (125).

Nef-expressing T cells demonstrate enhanced adherence to ECs as observed by their impaired diapedesis and migration into the subendothelial space (126). Fan et al have shown ERK kinase-mediated ICAM-1 upregulation in vascular ECs stably expressing Nef (54). Furthermore, Nef increases endothelial MCP-1 production through activation of the NF-kB signaling pathway (50). In a recent study, Nef was shown to be involved in the alteration of EC cholesterol homeostasis through phosphorylation of Caveolin-1 (Cav-1), leading to Cav-1 redistribution and impairment of HDL-mediated cholesterol efflux in ECs (127). In addition to its direct effects on ECs, Nef activates macrophages and produces foam cells (128). The interactions of these foam cells with ECs could also contribute to EC dysfunction, and potentially facilitate the development of atherosclerosis.

CONCLUSION AND FUTURE PERSPECTIVES

In summary, the present review underscores the role of HIV-encoded proteins, specifically Gp120, Tat and Nef, in the pathogenesis of endothelial dysfunction, a precursor for the development of CVD (**Figure 1**). Our understanding of the complex interaction of traditional factors, inflammation and immune activation, cART and HIV in the progression of CVD

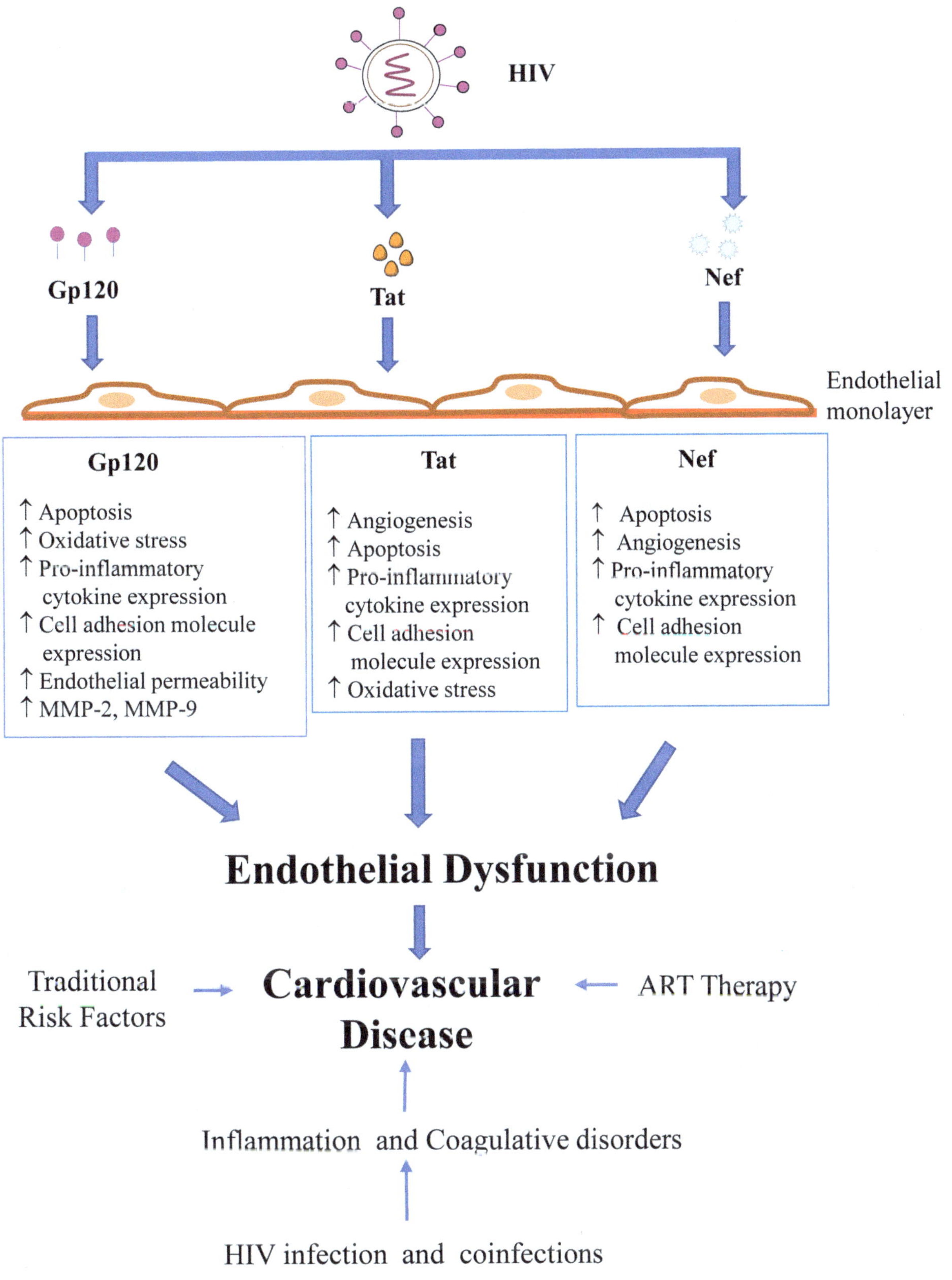

FIGURE 1 | HIV proteins and their effects on endothelial dysfunction.

has grown rapidly over the past decade. However, a more detailed exploration into the mechanisms of HIV-induced endothelial dysfunction is needed to formulate targeted approaches to prevent and treat HIV-related vascular diseases. Presently, large prospective studies such as REPRIEVE (NCT02344290), a randomized trial to prevent vascular events in HIV, are being carried out that will provide valuable data on the relation between inflammation, CVD and HIV infection (129). Research efforts will also need to focus on identifying HIV-specific markers that could predict the risk of developing CVD and facilitate the early detection of CVD in HIV patients. An accurate assessment of patients based on such biomarkers could be incorporated in guidelines such as the European AIDS Clinical Society guidelines (130) on the joint management and prevention of CVD in HIV patients, thereby providing vital information to guide clinicians on the most appropriate approach to prevent and treat CVD in this high-risk population.

AUTHOR CONTRIBUTIONS

GR and DP wrote the manuscript. AA wrote and revised the manuscript.

FUNDING

This work was supported by the DBT-Ramalingaswami re-entry fellowship grant (BT/RLF/10/2013) from the Department of Biotechnology, Ministry of Science & Technology, Government of India to AA.

ACKNOWLEDGMENTS

We would like to acknowledge Department of Biotechnology, New Delhi, India for financial support to GR.

REFERENCES

1. Palella FJ Jr, Baker RK, Moorman AC, Chmiel JS, Wood KC, Brooks JT, et al. Mortality in the highly active antiretroviral therapy era: changing causes of death and disease in the HIV outpatient study. *J Acquir Immune Defic Syndr.* (2006) 43:27–34. doi: 10.1097/01.qai.0000233310.90484.16
2. Crum NF, Riffenburgh RH, Wegner S, Agan BK, Tasker SA, Spooner KM, et al. Comparisons of causes of death and mortality rates among HIV-infected persons: analysis of the pre-, early, and late HAART (highly active antiretroviral therapy) eras. *J Acquir Immune Defic Syndr.* (2006) 41:194–200. doi: 10.1097/01.qai.0000179459.31562.16
3. Grinspoon SK, Grunfeld C, Kotler DP, Currier JS, Lundgren JD, Dube MP, et al. State of the science conference: initiative to decrease cardiovascular risk and increase quality of care for patients living with HIV/AIDS: executive summary. *Circulation* (2008) 118:198–210. doi: 10.1161/CIRCULATIONAHA.107.189622
4. Kamin DS, Grinspoon SK. Cardiovascular disease in HIV-positive patients. *AIDS* (2005) 19:641–52. doi: 10.1097/01.aids.0000166087.08822.bc
5. Sackoff JE, Hanna DB, Pfeiffer MR, Torian LV. Causes of death among persons with AIDS in the era of highly active antiretroviral therapy: New York City. *Ann Inter Med.* (2006) 145:397–406. doi: 10.7326/0003-4819-145-6-200609190-00003
6. Mateen FJ, Shinohara RT, Carone M, Miller EN, McArthur JC, Jacobson LP, et al. Neurologic disorders incidence in HIV+ vs HIV- men: multicenter AIDS cohort study, 1996-2011. *Neurology* (2012) 79:1873–80. doi: 10.1212/WNL.0b013e318271f7b8
7. Morlat P, Roussillon C, Henard S, Salmon D, Bonnet F, Cacoub P, et al. Causes of death among HIV-infected patients in France in 2010 (national survey): trends since 2000. *AIDS* (2014) 28:1181–91. doi: 10.1097/QAD.0000000000000222
8. French AL, Gawel SH, Hershow R, Benning L, Hessol NA, Levine AM, et al. Trends in mortality and causes of death among women with HIV in the United States: a 10-year study. *J Acquir Immune Defic Syndr.* (2009) 51:399–406. doi: 10.1097/QAI.0b013e3181acb4e5
9. Mocroft A, Reiss P, Gasiorowski J, Ledergerber B, Kowalska J, Chiesi A, et al. Serious fatal and nonfatal non-AIDS-defining illnesses in Europe. *J Acquir Immune Defic Syndr.* (2010) 55:262–70. doi: 10.1097/QAI.0b013e3181e9be6b
10. Currier JS, Lundgren JD, Carr A, Klein D, Sabin CA, Sax PE, et al. Epidemiological evidence for cardiovascular disease in HIV-infected patients and relationship to highly active antiretroviral therapy. *Circulation* (2008) 118:e29–35. doi: 10.1161/CIRCULATIONAHA.107.189624
11. Triant VA, Lee H, Hadigan C, Grinspoon SK. Increased acute myocardial infarction rates and cardiovascular risk factors among patients with human immunodeficiency virus disease. *J Clin Endocrinol Metabol.* (2007) 92:2506–12. doi: 10.1210/jc.2006-2190
12. Islam FM, Wu J, Jansson J, Wilson DP. Relative risk of cardiovascular disease among people living with HIV: a systematic review and meta-analysis. *HIV Med.* (2012) 13:453–68. doi: 10.1111/j.1468-1293.2012.00996.x
13. Currier JS, Taylor A, Boyd F, Dezii CM, Kawabata H, Burtcel B, et al. Coronary heart disease in HIV-infected individuals. *J Acquir Immune Defic Syndr.* (2003) 33:506–12. doi: 10.1097/00126334-200308010-00012
14. Palacios R, Alonso I, Hidalgo A, Aguilar I, Sanchez MA, Valdivielso P, et al. Peripheral arterial disease in HIV patients older than 50 years of age. *AIDS Res Hum Retroviruses* (2008) 24:1043–6. doi: 10.1089/aid.2008.0001
15. Lorenz MW, Stephan C, Harmjanz A, Staszewski S, Buehler A, Bickel M, et al. Both long-term HIV infection and highly active antiretroviral therapy are independent risk factors for early carotid atherosclerosis. *Atherosclerosis* (2008) 196:720–6. doi: 10.1016/j.atherosclerosis.2006.12.022
16. Jeong SJ, Kim HW, Ku NS, Han SH, Kim CO, Choi JY, et al. Clinical factors associated with carotid plaque and intima-medial thickness in HIV-infected patients. *Yonsei Med J.* (2013) 54:990–8. doi: 10.3349/ymj.2013.54.4.990
17. Kingsley LA, Cuervo-Rojas J, Munoz A, Palella FJ, Post W, Witt MD, et al. Subclinical coronary atherosclerosis, HIV infection and antiretroviral therapy: multicenter AIDS cohort study. *AIDS* (2008) 22:1589–99. doi: 10.1097/QAD.0b013e328306a6c5
18. Periard D, Cavassini M, Taffe P, Chevalley M, Senn L, Chapuis-Taillard C, et al. High prevalence of peripheral arterial disease in HIV-infected persons. *Clin Infect Dis.* (2008) 46:761–7. doi: 10.1086/527564
19. Carr A, Grund B, Neuhaus J, El-Sadr WM, Grandits G, Gibert C, et al. Asymptomatic myocardial ischaemia in HIV-infected adults. *AIDS* (2008) 22:257–67. doi: 10.1097/QAD.0b013e3282f20a77
20. Gibellini D, Borderi M, Clo A, Morini S, Miserocchi A, Bon I, et al. HIV-related mechanisms in atherosclerosis and cardiovascular diseases. *J Cardiovasc Med.* (2013) 14:780–90. doi: 10.2459/JCM.0b013e3283619331
21. Dolan SE, Hadigan C, Killilea KM, Sullivan MP, Hemphill L, Lees RS, et al. Increased cardiovascular disease risk indices in HIV-infected women. *J Acquir Immune Defic Syndr.* (2005) 39:44–54. doi: 10.1097/01.qai.0000159323.59250.83
22. Saves M, Chene G, Ducimetiere P, Leport C, Le Moal G, Amouyel P, et al. Risk factors for coronary heart disease in patients treated for human immunodeficiency virus infection compared with the general population. *Clin Infect Dis.* (2003) 37:292–8. doi: 10.1086/375844
23. Group DADS, Friis-Moller N, Reiss P, Sabin CA, Weber R, Monforte A, et al. Class of antiretroviral drugs and the risk of myocardial infarction. *N Engl J Med.* (2007) 356:1723–35. doi: 10.1056/NEJMoa062744
24. Lo J, Abbara S, Shturman L, Soni A, Wei J, Rocha-Filho JA, et al. Increased prevalence of subclinical coronary atherosclerosis detected by coronary computed tomography angiography in HIV-infected men. *AIDS* (2010) 24:243–53. doi: 10.1097/QAD.0b013e328333ea9e
25. Oliviero U, Bonadies G, Apuzzi V, Foggia M, Bosso G, Nappa S, et al. Human immunodeficiency virus *per se* exerts atherogenic effects.

Atherosclerosis (2009) 204:586–9. doi: 10.1016/j.atherosclerosis.2008.10.012

26. Lundgren JD, Strategies for Management of Antiretroviral Therapy Study G, Babiker A, El-Sadr W, Emery S, Grund B, et al. Inferior clinical outcome of the CD4+ cell count-guided antiretroviral treatment interruption strategy in the SMART study: role of CD4+ Cell counts and HIV RNA levels during follow-up. *J Infect Dis.* (2008) 197:1145–55. doi: 10.1086/529523
27. Armah KA, McGinnis K, Baker J, Gibert C, Butt AA, Bryant KJ, et al. HIV status, burden of comorbid disease, and biomarkers of inflammation, altered coagulation, and monocyte activation. *Clin Infect Dis.* (2012) 55:126–36. doi: 10.1093/cid/cis406
28. Hsue PY, Hunt PW, Schnell A, Kalapus SC, Hoh R, Ganz P, et al. Role of viral replication, antiretroviral therapy, and immunodeficiency in HIV-associated atherosclerosis. *AIDS* (2009) 23:1059–67. doi: 10.1097/QAD.0b013e32832b514b
29. Funderburg NT, Mayne E, Sieg SF, Asaad R, Jiang W, Kalinowska M, et al. Increased tissue factor expression on circulating monocytes in chronic HIV infection: relationship to *in vivo* coagulation and immune activation. *Blood* (2010) 115:161–7. doi: 10.1182/blood-2009-03-210179
30. Hansen L, Parker I, Sutliff RL, Platt MO, Gleason RL, Jr. Endothelial dysfunction, arterial stiffening, and intima-media thickening in large arteries from HIV-1 transgenic mice. *Ann Biomed Eng.* (2013) 41:682–93. doi: 10.1007/s10439-012-0702-5
31. Solages A, Vita JA, Thornton DJ, Murray J, Heeren T, Craven DE, et al. Endothelial function in HIV-infected persons. *Clin Infect Dis.* (2006) 42:1325–32. doi: 10.1086/503261
32. Gokce N, Keaney JF Jr, Hunter LM, Watkins MT, Nedeljkovic ZS, Menzoian JO, et al. Predictive value of noninvasively determined endothelial dysfunction for long-term cardiovascular events in patients with peripheral vascular disease. *J Am College Cardiol.* (2003) 41:1769–75. doi: 10.1016/S0735-1097(03)00333-4
33. Suwaidi JA, Hamasaki S, Higano ST, Nishimura RA, Holmes DR, Jr., Lerman A. Long-term follow-up of patients with mild coronary artery disease and endothelial dysfunction. *Circulation* (2000) 101:948–54. doi: 10.1161/01.CIR.101.9.948
34. Loscalzo J. *Molecular Mechanisms of Atherosclerosis.* Boca Raton, FL: CRC Press (2004).
35. Ramji DP, Davies TS. Cytokines in atherosclerosis: key players in all stages of disease and promising therapeutic targets. *Cytokine Growth Factor Rev.* (2015) 26:673–85. doi: 10.1016/j.cytogfr.2015.04.003
36. Fiala M, Popik W, Qiao JH, Lossinsky AS, Alce T, Tran K, et al. HIV-1 induces cardiomyopathyby cardiomyocyte invasion and gp120, Tat, and cytokine apoptotic signaling. *Cardiovasc Toxicol.* (2004) 4:97–107. doi: 10.1385/CT:4:2:097
37. Huang MB, Khan M, Garcia-Barrio M, Powell M, Bond VC. Apoptotic effects in primary human umbilical vein endothelial cell cultures caused by exposure to virion-associated and cell membrane-associated HIV-1 gp120. *J Acquir Immune Defic Syndr.* (2001) 27:213–21. doi: 10.1097/00126334-200107010-00001
38. Ullrich CK, Groopman JE, Ganju RK. HIV-1 gp120- and gp160-induced apoptosis in cultured endothelial cells is mediated by caspases. *Blood* (2000) 96:1438–42.
39. Kanmogne GD, Kennedy RC, Grammas P. Analysis of human lung endothelial cells for susceptibility to HIV type 1 infection, coreceptor expression, and cytotoxicity of gp120 protein. *AIDS Res Hum Retroviruses* (2001) 17:45–53. doi: 10.1089/088922201750056771
40. Kanmogne GD, Kennedy RC, Grammas P. HIV-1 gp120 proteins and gp160 peptides are toxic to brain endothelial cells and neurons: possible pathway for HIV entry into the brain and HIV-associated dementia. *J Neuropathol Exp Neurol.* (2002) 61:992–1000. doi: 10.1093/jnen/61.11.992
41. Khan NA, Di Cello F, Stins M, Kim KS. Gp120-mediated cytotoxicity of human brain microvascular endothelial cells is dependent on p38 mitogen-activated protein kinase activation. *J Neurovirol.* (2007) 13:242–51. doi: 10.1080/13550280701286531
42. Acheampong EA, Parveen Z, Muthoga LW, Kalayeh M, Mukhtar M, Pomerantz RJ. Human Immunodeficiency virus type 1 Nef potently induces apoptosis in primary human brain microvascular endothelial cells via the activation of caspases. *J Virol.* (2005) 79:4257–69. doi: 10.1128/JVI.79.7.4257-4269.2005
43. Park IW, Ullrich CK, Schoenberger E, Ganju RK, Groopman JE. HIV-1 Tat induces microvascular endothelial apoptosis through caspase activation. *J Immunol.* (2001) 167:2766–71. doi: 10.4049/jimmunol.167.5.2766
44. Yang B, Akhter S, Chaudhuri A, Kanmogne GD. HIV-1 gp120 induces cytokine expression, leukocyte adhesion, and transmigration across the blood-brain barrier: modulatory effects of STAT1 signaling. *Microvasc Res.* (2009) 77:212–9. doi: 10.1016/j.mvr.2008.11.003
45. Park IW, Wang JF, Groopman JE. HIV-1 Tat promotes monocyte chemoattractant protein-1 secretion followed by transmigration of monocytes. *Blood* (2001) 97:352–8. doi: 10.1182/blood.V97.2.352
46. Westendorp MO, Shatrov VA, Schulze-Osthoff K, Frank R, Kraft M, Los M, et al. HIV-1 Tat potentiates TNF-induced NF-kappa B activation and cytotoxicity by altering the cellular redox state. *EMBO J.* (1995) 14:546–54. doi: 10.1002/j.1460-2075.1995.tb07030.x
47. Kanmogne GD, Schall K, Leibhart J, Knipe B, Gendelman HE, Persidsky Y. HIV-1 gp120 compromises blood-brain barrier integrity and enhances monocyte migration across blood-brain barrier: implication for viral neuropathogenesis. *J Cereb Blood Flow Metabol.* (2007) 27:123–34. doi: 10.1038/sj.jcbfm.9600330
48. Cota-Gomez A, Flores NC, Cruz C, Casullo A, Aw TY, Ichikawa H, et al. The human immunodeficiency virus-1 Tat protein activates human umbilical vein endothelial cell E-selectin expression via an NF-kappa B-dependent mechanism. *J Biol Chem.* (2002) 277:14390–9. doi: 10.1074/jbc.M108591200
49. Zidovetzki R, Wang JL, Chen P, Jeyaseelan R, Hofman F. Human immunodeficiency virus Tat protein induces interleukin 6 mRNA expression in human brain endothelial cells via protein kinase C- and cAMP-dependent protein kinase pathways. *AIDS Res Hum Retroviruses* (1998) 14:825–33. doi: 10.1089/aid.1998.14.825
50. Wang T, Green LA, Gupta SK, Kim C, Wang L, Almodovar S, et al. Transfer of intracellular HIV Nef to endothelium causes endothelial dysfunction. *PLoS ONE* (2014) 9:e91063. doi: 10.1371/journal.pone.0091063
51. Kanmogne GD, Primeaux C, Grammas P. HIV-1 gp120 proteins alter tight junction protein expression and brain endothelial cell permeability: implications for the pathogenesis of HIV-associated dementia. *J Neuropathol Exp Neurol.* (2005) 64:498–505. doi: 10.1093/jnen/64.6.498
52. Ren Z, Yao Q, Chen C. HIV-1 envelope glycoprotein 120 increases intercellular adhesion molecule-1 expression by human endothelial cells. *Lab Invest.* (2002) 82:245–55. doi: 10.1038/labinvest.3780418
53. Duan M, Yao H, Hu G, Chen X, Lund AK, Buch S. HIV Tat induces expression of ICAM-1 in HUVECs: implications for miR-221/-222 in HIV-associated cardiomyopathy. *PLoS ONE* (2013) 8:e60170. doi: 10.1371/journal.pone.0060170
54. Fan Y, Liu C, Qin X, Wang Y, Han Y, Zhou Y. The role of ERK1/2 signaling pathway in Nef protein upregulation of the expression of the intercellular adhesion molecule 1 in endothelial cells. *Angiology* (2010) 61:669–78. doi: 10.1177/0003319710364215
55. Liu K, Chi DS, Li C, Hall HK, Milhorn DM, Krishnaswamy G. HIV-1 Tat protein-induced VCAM-1 expression in human pulmonary artery endothelial cells and its signaling. *Am J Physiol Lung Cell Mol Physiol.* (2005) 289:L252–60. doi: 10.1152/ajplung.00200.2004
56. Shiu C, Barbier E, Di Cello F, Choi HJ, Stins M. HIV-1 gp120 as well as alcohol affect blood-brain barrier permeability and stress fiber formation: involvement of reactive oxygen species. *Alcohol Clin Exp Res.* (2007) 31:130–7. doi: 10.1111/j.1530-0277.2006.00271.x
57. Andras IE, Pu H, Deli MA, Nath A, Hennig B, Toborek M. HIV-1 Tat protein alters tight junction protein expression and distribution in cultured brain endothelial cells. *J Neurosci Res.* (2003) 74:255–65. doi: 10.1002/jnr.10762
58. Avraham HK, Jiang S, Lee TH, Prakash O, Avraham S. HIV-1 Tat-mediated effects on focal adhesion assembly and permeability in brain microvascular endothelial cells. *J Immunol.* (2004) 173:6228–33. doi: 10.4049/jimmunol.173.10.6228
59. Arese M, Ferrandi C, Primo L, Camussi G, Bussolino F. HIV-1 Tat protein stimulates *in vivo* vascular permeability and lymphomononuclear cell recruitment. *J Immunol.* (2001) 166:1380–8. doi: 10.4049/jimmunol.166.2.1380

60. Louboutin JP, Reyes BA, Agrawal L, Van Bockstaele EJ, Strayer DS. HIV-1 gp120 upregulates matrix metalloproteinases and their inhibitors in a rat model of HIV encephalopathy. *Euro J Neurosci.* (2011) 34:2015–23. doi: 10.1111/j.1460-9568.2011.07908.x
61. Chatterjee A, Black SM, Catravas JD. Endothelial nitric oxide (NO) and its pathophysiologic regulation. *Vasc Pharmacol.* (2008) 49:134–40. doi: 10.1016/j.vph.2008.06.008
62. Jiang J, Fu W, Wang X, Lin PH, Yao Q, Chen C. HIV gp120 induces endothelial dysfunction in tumour necrosis factor-alpha-activated porcine and human endothelial cells. *Cardiovasc Res.* (2010) 87:366–74. doi: 10.1093/cvr/cvq013
63. Price TO, Uras F, Banks WA, Ercal N. A novel antioxidant N-acetylcysteine amide prevents gp120- and Tat-induced oxidative stress in brain endothelial cells. *Exp Neurol.* (2006) 201:193–202. doi: 10.1016/j.expneurol.2006.03.030
64. Toborek M, Lee YW, Pu H, Malecki A, Flora G, Garrido R, et al. HIV-Tat protein induces oxidative and inflammatory pathways in brain endothelium. *J Neurochem.* (2003) 84:169–79. doi: 10.1046/j.1471-4159.85.s2.16_7.x
65. Turner BG, Summers MF. Structural biology of HIV. *J Mol Biol.* (1999) 285:1–32. doi: 10.1006/jmbi.1998.2354
66. Oh SK, Cruikshank WW, Raina J, Blanchard GC, Adler WH, Walker J, et al. Identification of HIV-1 envelope glycoprotein in the serum of AIDS and ARC patients. *J Acquir Immune Defic Syndr.* (1992) 5:251–6.
67. Schneider J, Kaaden O, Copeland TD, Oroszlan S, Hunsmann G. Shedding and interspecies type sero-reactivity of the envelope glycopolypeptide gp120 of the human immunodeficiency virus. *J General Virol.* (1986) 67(Pt 11):2533–8. doi: 10.1099/0022-1317-67-11-2533
68. Twu C, Liu NQ, Popik W, Bukrinsky M, Sayre J, Roberts J, et al. Cardiomyocytes undergo apoptosis in human immunodeficiency virus cardiomyopathy through mitochondrion- and death receptor-controlled pathways. *Proc Natl Acad Sci USA.* (2002) 99:14386–91. doi: 10.1073/pnas.212327899
69. Popovic M, Tenner-Racz K, Pelser C, Stellbrink HJ, van Lunzen J, Lewis G, et al. Persistence of HIV-1 structural proteins and glycoproteins in lymph nodes of patients under highly active antiretroviral therapy. *Proc Natl Acad Sci USA.* (2005) 102:14807–12. doi: 10.1073/pnas.0506857102
70. Anand AR, Ganju RK. HIV-1 gp120-mediated apoptosis of T cells is regulated by the membrane tyrosine phosphatase CD45. *J Biol Chem.* (2006) 281:12289–99. doi: 10.1074/jbc.M511786200
71. Anand AR, Prasad A, Bradley RR, Deol YS, Nagaraja T, Ren X, et al. HIV-1 gp120-induced migration of dendritic cells is regulated by a novel kinase cascade involving Pyk2, p38 MAP kinase, and LSP1. *Blood* (2009) 114:3588–600. doi: 10.1182/blood-2009-02-206342
72. Banda NK, Bernier J, Kurahara DK, Kurrle R, Haigwood N, Sekaly RP, et al. Crosslinking CD4 by human immunodeficiency virus gp120 primes T cells for activation-induced apoptosis. *J Exp Med.* (1992) 176:1099–106. doi: 10.1084/jem.176.4.1099
73. Freedman BD, Liu QH, Del Corno M, Collman RG. HIV-1 gp120 chemokine receptor-mediated signaling in human macrophages. *Immunol Res.* (2003) 27:261–76. doi: 10.1385/IR:27:2-3:261
74. Munshi N, Balasubramanian A, Koziel M, Ganju RK, Groopman JE. Hepatitis C and human immunodeficiency virus envelope proteins cooperatively induce hepatocytic apoptosis via an innocent bystander mechanism. *J Infect Dis.* (2003) 188:1192–204. doi: 10.1086/378643
75. Libby P, Ridker PM, Hansson GK. Progress and challenges in translating the biology of atherosclerosis. *Nature* (2011) 473:317–25. doi: 10.1038/nature10146
76. Otsuka F, Finn AV, Yazdani SK, Nakano M, Kolodgie FD, Virmani R. The importance of the endothelium in atherothrombosis and coronary stenting. *Nat Rev Cardiol.* (2012) 9:439–53. doi: 10.1038/nrcardio.2012.64
77. Huang MB, Bond VC. Involvement of protein kinase C in HIV-1 gp120-induced apoptosis in primary endothelium. *J Acquir Immune Defic Syndr.* (2000) 25:375–89. doi: 10.1097/00126334-200012150-00001
78. Yang X, Li Y, Li Y, Ren X, Zhang X, Hu D, et al. Oxidative stress-mediated atherosclerosis: mechanisms and therapies. *Front Physiol.* (2017) 8:600. doi: 10.3389/fphys.2017.00600
79. Green LA, Yi R, Petrusca D, Wang T, Elghouche A, Gupta SK, et al. HIV envelope protein gp120-induced apoptosis in lung microvascular endothelial cells by concerted upregulation of EMAP II and its receptor, CXCR3. *Am J Physiol Lung Cell Mol Physiol.* (2014) 306:L372–82. doi: 10.1152/ajplung.00193.2013
80. Sandoval YH, Atef ME, Levesque LO, Li Y, Anand-Srivastava MB. Endothelin-1 signaling in vascular physiology and pathophysiology. *Curr Vascu Pharmacol.* (2014) 12:202–14. doi: 10.2174/1570161112666140226122054
81. Matschurat S, Knies UE, Person V, Fink L, Stoelcker B, Ebenebe C, et al. Regulation of EMAP II by hypoxia. *Am J Pathol.* (2003) 162:93–103. doi: 10.1016/S0002-9440(10)63801-1
82. Hijmans JG, Stockleman K, Reiakvam W, Levy MV, Brewster LM, Bammert TD, et al. Effects of HIV-1 gp120 and tat on endothelial cell sensescence and senescence-associated microRNAs. *Physiol Rep.* (2018) 6:e13647. doi: 10.14814/phy2.13647
83. Katsuumi G, Shimizu I, Yoshida Y, Minamino T. Vascular senescence in cardiovascular and metabolic diseases. *Front Cardiovasc Med.* (2018) 5:18. doi: 10.3389/fcvm.2018.00018
84. Ferrante G, Condorelli G. Interleukin-6 trans-signaling and risk of future cardiovascular events: a new avenue for atheroprotection? *Cardiovasc Res.* (2018). doi: 10.1093/cvr/cvy233. [Epub ahead of print].
85. Takano Y, Shimokado K, Hata Y, Yoshida M. HIV envelope protein gp120-triggered CD4+ T-cell adhesion to vascular endothelium is regulated via CD4 and CXCR4 receptors. *Biochim Biophys Acta* (2007) 1772:549–55. doi: 10.1016/j.bbadis.2007.01.010
86. Granger DN, Senchenkova E. *Inflammation and the Microcirculation. Integrated Systems Physiology-From Cell to Function.* San Rafael, CA: Morgan and Claypool Life Sciences (2010).
87. Cioni C, Annunziata P. Circulating gp120 alters the blood-brain barrier permeability in HIV-1 gp120 transgenic mice. *Neurosci Lett.* (2002) 330:299–301. doi: 10.1016/S0304-3940(02)00814-5
88. Debaisieux S, Rayne F, Yezid H, Beaumelle B. The ins and outs of HIV-1 Tat. *Traffic* (2012) 13:355–63. doi: 10.1111/j.1600-0854.2011.01286.x
89. Poggi A, Carosio R, Fenoglio D, Brenci S, Murdaca G, Setti M, et al. Migration of V delta 1 and V delta 2 T cells in response to CXCR3 and CXCR4 ligands in healthy donors and HIV-1-infected patients: competition by HIV-1 Tat. *Blood* (2004) 103:2205–13. doi: 10.1182/blood-2003-08-2928
90. Mediouni S, Darque A, Baillat G, Ravaux I, Dhiver C, Tissot-Dupont H, et al. Antiretroviral therapy does not block the secretion of the human immunodeficiency virus tat protein. *Infect Disord Drug Targets* (2012) 12:81–6. doi: 10.2174/187152612798994939
91. Chang HC, Samaniego F, Nair BC, Buonaguro L, Ensoli B. HIV-1 Tat protein exits from cells via a leaderless secretory pathway and binds to extracellular matrix-associated heparan sulfate proteoglycans through its basic region. *AIDS* (1997) 11:1421–31. doi: 10.1097/00002030-199712000-00006
92. Barillari G, Gendelman R, Gallo RC, Ensoli B. The Tat protein of human immunodeficiency virus type 1, a growth factor for AIDS Kaposi sarcoma and cytokine-activated vascular cells, induces adhesion of the same cell types by using integrin receptors recognizing the RGD amino acid sequence. *Proc Natl Acad Sci USA.* (1993) 90:7941–5. doi: 10.1073/pnas.90.17.7941
93. Carey AN, Sypek EI, Singh HD, Kaufman MJ, McLaughlin JP. Expression of HIV-Tat protein is associated with learning and memory deficits in the mouse. *Behav Brain Res.* (2012) 229:48–56. doi: 10.1016/j.bbr.2011.12.019
94. Ensoli F, Fiorelli V, DeCristofaro M, Santini Muratori D, Novi A, Vannelli B, et al. Inflammatory cytokines and HIV-1-associated neurodegeneration: oncostatin-M produced by mononuclear cells from HIV-1-infected individuals induces apoptosis of primary neurons. *J Immunol.* (1999) 162:6268–77.
95. Wang T, Jiang Z, Hou W, Li Z, Cheng S, Green LA, et al. HIV Tat protein affects circadian rhythmicity by interfering with the circadian system. *HIV Med.* (2014) 15:565–70. doi: 10.1111/hiv.12154
96. Mitola S, Soldi R, Zanon I, Barra L, Gutierrez MI, Berkhout B, et al. Identification of specific molecular structures of human immunodeficiency virus type 1 Tat relevant for its biological effects on vascular endothelial cells. *J Virol.* (2000) 74:344–53. doi: 10.1128/JVI.74.1.344-353.2000
97. Vogel BE, Lee SJ, Hildebrand A, Craig W, Pierschbacher MD, Wong-Staal F, et al. A novel integrin specificity exemplified by binding of the alpha v beta 5 integrin to the basic domain of the HIV Tat protein and vitronectin. *J Cell Biol.* (1993) 121:461–8. doi: 10.1083/jcb.121.2.461

98. Albini A, Soldi R, Giunciuglio D, Giraudo E, Benelli R, Primo L, et al. The angiogenesis induced by HIV-1 tat protein is mediated by the Flk-1/KDR receptor on vascular endothelial cells. *Nat Med.* (1996) 2:1371–5. doi: 10.1038/nm1296-1371
99. Fiorelli V, Barillari G, Toschi E, Sgadari C, Monini P, Sturzl M, et al. IFN-gamma induces endothelial cells to proliferate and to invade the extracellular matrix in response to the HIV-1 Tat protein: implications for AIDS-Kaposi's sarcoma pathogenesis. *J Immunol.* (1999) 162:1165–70.
100. Margheri F, D'Alessio S, Serrati S, Pucci M, Del Rosso A, Benelli R, et al. The urokinase-type plasminogen activator, its receptor and u-PA inhibitor type-1 affect *in vitro* growth and invasion of Kaposi's sarcoma and capillary endothelial cells: role of HIV-Tat protein. *Int J Oncol.* (2005) 27:223–35. doi: 10.3892/ijo.27.1.223
101. Barillari G, Sgadari C, Palladino C, Gendelman R, Caputo A, Morris CB, et al. Inflammatory cytokines synergize with the HIV-1 Tat protein to promote angiogenesis and Kaposi's sarcoma via induction of basic fibroblast growth factor and the alpha v beta 3 integrin. *J Immunol.* (1999) 163:1929–35.
102. Urbinati C, Mitola S, Tanghetti E, Kumar C, Waltenberger J, Ribatti D, et al. Integrin alphavbeta3 as a target for blocking HIV-1 Tat-induced endothelial cell activation *in vitro* and angiogenesis *in vivo*. *Arterioscler Thromb Vasc Biol.* (2005) 25:2315–20. doi: 10.1161/01.ATV.0000186182.14908.7b
103. Rusnati M, Presta M. HIV-1 Tat protein and endothelium: from protein/cell interaction to AIDS-associated pathologies. *Angiogenesis* (2002) 5:141–51. doi: 10.1023/A:1023892223074
104. Sgadari C, Barillari G, Palladino C, Bellino S, Taddeo B, Toschi E, et al. Fibroblast growth factor-2 and the HIV-1 Tat protein synergize in promoting Bcl-2 expression and preventing endothelial cell apoptosis: implications for the pathogenesis of AIDS-associated Kaposi's sarcoma. *Int J Vasc Med.* (2011) 2011:452729. doi: 10.1155/2011/452729
105. Toschi E, Bacigalupo I, Strippoli R, Chiozzini C, Cereseto A, Falchi M, et al. HIV-1 Tat regulates endothelial cell cycle progression via activation of the Ras/ERK MAPK signaling pathway. *Mol Biol Cell* (2006) 17:1985–94. doi: 10.1091/mbc.e05-08-0717
106. Wu RF, Ma Z, Myers DP, Terada LS. HIV-1 Tat activates dual Nox pathways leading to independent activation of ERK and JNK MAP kinases. *J Biol Chem.* (2007) 282:37412–9. doi: 10.1074/jbc.M704481200
107. Dalvi P, Sharma H, Chinnappan M, Sanderson M, Allen J, Zeng R, et al. Enhanced autophagy in pulmonary endothelial cells on exposure to HIV-Tat and morphine: role in HIV-related pulmonary arterial hypertension. *Autophagy* (2016) 12:2420–38. doi: 10.1080/15548627.2016.1238551
108. Dhawan S, Puri RK, Kumar A, Duplan H, Masson JM, Aggarwal BB. Human immunodeficiency virus-1-tat protein induces the cell surface expression of endothelial leukocyte adhesion molecule-1, vascular cell adhesion molecule-1, and intercellular adhesion molecule-1 in human endothelial cells. *Blood* (1997) 90:1535–44.
109. Pieper GM, Olds CL, Bub JD, Lindholm PF. Transfection of human endothelial cells with HIV-1 tat gene activates NF-kappa B and enhances monocyte adhesion. *Ame J Physiol Heart Circ Physiol.* (2002) 283:H2315–21. doi: 10.1152/ajpheart.00469.2002
110. Andres V, Pello OM, Silvestre-Roig C. Macrophage proliferation and apoptosis in atherosclerosis. *Curr Opin Lipidol.* (2012) 23:429–38. doi: 10.1097/MOL.0b013e328357a379
111. Tousoulis D, Oikonomou E, Economou EK, Crea F, Kaski JC. Inflammatory cytokines in atherosclerosis: current therapeutic approaches. *Euro Heart J.* (2016) 37:1723–32. doi: 10.1093/eurheartj/ehv759
112. Pu H, Tian J, Flora G, Lee YW, Nath A, Hennig B, et al. HIV-1 Tat protein upregulates inflammatory mediators and induces monocyte invasion into the brain. *Mol Cell Neurosci.* (2003) 24:224–37. doi: 10.1016/S1044-7431(03)00171-4
113. Matzen K, Dirkx AE, oude Egbrink MG, Speth C, Gotte M, Ascherl G, et al. HIV-1 Tat increases the adhesion of monocytes and T-cells to the endothelium *in vitro* and *in vivo*: implications for AIDS-associated vasculopathy. *Virus Res.* (2004) 104:145–55. doi: 10.1016/j.virusres.2004.04.001
114. Flores SC, Marecki JC, Harper KP, Bose SK, Nelson SK, McCord JM. Tat protein of human immunodeficiency virus type 1 represses expression of manganese superoxide dismutase in HeLa cells. *Proc Natl Acad Sci USA.* (1993) 90:7632–6. doi: 10.1073/pnas.90.16.7632
115. Kestler HW III, Ringler DJ, Mori K, Panicali DL, Sehgal PK, Daniel MD, et al. Importance of the nef gene for maintenance of high virus loads and for development of AIDS. *Cell* (1991) 65:651–62. doi: 10.1016/0092-8674(91)90097-I
116. Kirchhoff F, Greenough TC, Brettler DB, Sullivan JL, Desrosiers RC. Brief report: absence of intact nef sequences in a long-term survivor with nonprogressive HIV-1 infection. *N Eng J Med.* (1995) 332:228–32. doi: 10.1056/NEJM199501263320405
117. Qiao X, He B, Chiu A, Knowles DM, Chadburn A, Cerutti A. Human immunodeficiency virus 1 Nef suppresses CD40-dependent immunoglobulin class switching in bystander B cells. *Nat Immunol.* (2006) 7:302–10. doi: 10.1038/ni1302
118. Qi M, Aiken C. Nef enhances HIV-1 infectivity via association with the virus assembly complex. *Virology* (2008) 373:287–97. doi: 10.1016/j.virol.2007.12.001
119. Sowinski S, Jolly C, Berninghausen O, Purbhoo MA, Chauveau A, Kohler K, et al. Membrane nanotubes physically connect T cells over long distances presenting a novel route for HIV-1 transmission. *Nat Cell Biol.* (2008) 10:211–9. doi: 10.1038/ncb1682
120. Duffy P, Wang X, Lin PH, Yao Q, Chen C. HIV Nef protein causes endothelial dysfunction in porcine pulmonary arteries and human pulmonary artery endothelial cells. *J Surg Res.* (2009) 156:257–64. doi: 10.1016/j.jss.2009.02.005
121. Lenassi M, Cagney G, Liao M, Vaupotic T, Bartholomeeusen K, Cheng Y, et al. HIV Nef is secreted in exosomes and triggers apoptosis in bystander CD4+ T cells. *Traffic* (2010) 11:110–22. doi: 10.1111/j.1600-0854.2009.01006.x
122. Kay DG, Yue P, Hanna Z, Jothy S, Tremblay E, Jolicoeur P. Cardiac disease in transgenic mice expressing human immunodeficiency virus-1 nef in cells of the immune system. *Am J Pathol.* (2002) 161:321–35. doi: 10.1016/S0002-9440(10)64184-3
123. Almodovar S, Hsue PY, Morelli J, Huang L, Flores SC, Lung HIVS. Pathogenesis of HIV-associated pulmonary hypertension: potential role of HIV-1 Nef. *Proc Am Thorac Soc.* (2011) 8:308–12. doi: 10.1513/pats.201006-046WR
124. Almodovar S, Knight R, Allshouse AA, Roemer S, Lozupone C, McDonald D, et al. Human Immunodeficiency Virus nef signature sequences are associated with pulmonary hypertension. *AIDS Res Hum Retroviruses* (2012) 28:607–18. doi: 10.1089/aid.2011.0021
125. Xue M, Yao S, Hu M, Li W, Hao T, Zhou F, et al. HIV-1 Nef and KSHV oncogene K1 synergistically promote angiogenesis by inducing cellular miR-718 to regulate the PTEN/AKT/mTOR signaling pathway. *Nucleic Acids Res.* (2014) 42:9862–79. doi: 10.1093/nar/gku583
126. Stolp B, Imle A, Coelho FM, Hons M, Gorina R, Lyck R, et al. HIV-1 Nef interferes with T-lymphocyte circulation through confined environments *in vivo*. *Proc Natl Acad Sci USA.* (2012) 109:18541–6. doi: 10.1073/pnas.1204322109
127. Lin S, Nadeau PE, Mergia A. HIV inhibits endothelial reverse cholesterol transport through impacting subcellular Caveolin-1 trafficking. *Retrovirology* (2015) 12:62. doi: 10.1186/s12977-015-0188-y
128. Bukrinsky M, Sviridov D. Human immunodeficiency virus infection and macrophage cholesterol metabolism. *J Leukocyte Biol.* (2006) 80:1044–51. doi: 10.1189/jlb.0206113
129. Mitka M. Exploring statins to decrease HIV-related heart disease risk. *JAMA* (2015) 314:657–9. doi: 10.1001/jama.2015.5498
130. Ryom L, Boesecke C, Bracchi M, Ambrosioni J, Pozniak A, Arribas J, et al. Highlights of the 2017 European AIDS Clinical Society (EACS) guidelines for the treatment of adult HIV-positive persons version 9.0. *HIV Med.* (2018) 19:309–15. doi: 10.1111/hiv.12600

15

Regulation of Type 2 Immunity in Myocardial Infarction

Jun-Yan Xu [1†], Yu-Yan Xiong [1†], Xiao-Tong Lu [2] and Yue-Jin Yang [1]*

[1] State Key Laboratory of Cardiovascular Disease, Department of Cardiology, Fuwai Hospital, National Center for Cardiovascular Diseases, Chinese Academy of Medical Science and Peking Union Medical College, Beijing, China, [2] National Cancer Center/National Clinical Research Center for Cancer/Cancer Hospital, Chinese Academy of Medical Sciences and Peking Union Medical College, Beijing, China

***Correspondence:**
Yue-Jin Yang
yangyjfw@126.com

[†] These authors have contributed equally to this work

Type 2 immunity participates in the pathogeneses of helminth infection and allergic diseases. Emerging evidence indicates that the components of type 2 immunity are also involved in maintaining metabolic hemostasis and facilitating the healing process after tissue injury. Numerous preclinical studies have suggested regulation of type 2 immunity-related cytokines, such as interleukin-4, -13, and -33, and cell types, such as M2 macrophages, mast cells, and eosinophils, affects cardiac functions after myocardial infarction (MI), providing new insights into the importance of immune modulation in the infarcted heart. This review provides an overview of the functions of these cytokines and cells in the setting of MI as well as their potential to predict the severity and prognosis of MI.

Keywords: myocardial infarction, type 2 immunity, interleukin, M2 macrophages, mast cells, eosinophils, immune modulation

INTRODUCTION

Type 2 immunity is characterized by the production of interleukin (IL)-4, IL-5, IL-9, IL-13, IL-25, IL-33, and thymic stromal lymphopoietin, as well as specific cell types including mast cells, eosinophils, basophils, alternatively activated M2 macrophages, type 2 innate lymphoid cells (ILC2), and T-helper (Th) 2 cells. It has mainly been considered to participate in the pathogeneses of helminth infection and allergic diseases. However, growing evidence suggests that these cell types and related cytokines are also involved in maintaining metabolic homeostasis and facilitating the healing process after tissue injury (1). Studies in experimental models and serum biomarker data from humans have proven the participation of type 2 immunity in the progression of myocardial infarction (MI). In this review, we will discuss several pivotal type 2 immunity-associated cytokines and cell types that modulate cardiac functions, following MI and their potential value as biomarkers of MI.

CYTOKINES

Activation of innate immunity and extensive inflammation are the typical pathological features of MI. Accumulating evidence suggests type 2 cytokines are critical participants in tissue repair and regeneration owing to their ability to regulate the functions of nearby cells and immunomodulation. Moreover, they may serve as ideal biomarkers to predict the severity and clinical outcomes of MI.

IL-4

IL-4 is an important Th2 cytokine with multiple biological functions, which mainly has an anti-inflammatory effect. Previous studies have demonstrated an association of elevated serum IL-4 with a reduced risk of cardiovascular diseases (2). Furthermore, the IL-4 level is lower in MI patients who later develop left ventricular dysfunction (3), indicating its cardioprotective properties.

One of the well-clarified mechanisms of IL-4 is in mediating myocardial repair via converting macrophages to the M2 phenotype. Administration of a long-acting IL-4 complex at 1 h after MI increases the proportion of cardiac M2 macrophages in both the infarct and border myocardium, along with increased tissue repair-related gene expression in M2 macrophages, and an improved cardiac structure (more connective tissue in the infarct zone) and functions. Further experiments suggested that IL-4 promotes fibrotic tissue formation via M2 macrophages rather than a direct interaction with cardiac fibroblasts. However, these effects are not observed when administrated at a late phase (7 or 28 days after MI), implying that IL-4 affects the early recruitment and polarization of M2 macrophages in the acute phase after MI (4). Similarly, injection of IL-4 plasmid DNA (carried by graphene oxide) around the border zone after coronary artery ligation largely reduces the number of inflammatory M1 macrophages, and polarizes macrophages to the reparative M2 phenotype in the mouse heart, leading to enhancement of cardiac functions (5).

IL-4 may also affect the functions of cardiac fibroblasts, thus participating in the profibrotic process directly. In the Ang II-induced hypertension model, wild-type (WT) mice exhibit higher cardiac fibrosis compared with $IL\text{-}4^{-/-}$ mice, as indicated by the increase in the interstitial collagen fraction and mRNA levels of procollagen type-I $\alpha1$ and procollagen type-III $\alpha1$. *In vitro* experiments have demonstrated that IL-4 promotes the expression of procollagen type-I $\alpha1$ and procollagen type-III $\alpha1$ in mouse cardiac fibroblasts via binding to IL-4Rα, and consequently increasing the production of collagen (6). Treatment of anti-IL-4 neutralizing antibodies reduces both the number and proliferation of fibroblasts as well as infiltration of $CD68^+$ macrophages (7). These findings suggest the sophisticated interaction between IL-4 and various cell types in the heart, which may lead to opposing outcomes under different pathological conditions.

IL-13

IL-13 also polarizes macrophages to the M2 phenotype through binding to IL-4Rα and activating the subsequent signal transducers and activators of transcription (STAT) 6 signaling pathway (8). In a mouse model of MI, IL-13 significantly increases in the myocardium with a peak on day 3. Further experiments in $IL\text{-}13^{-/-}$ mice suggested that IL-13 enhances cardiac functions by recruiting more monocytes/macrophages to the infarct and border area and inducing M2 macrophages. Interestingly, in contrast to the $IL\text{-}13^{-/-}$ female mice, $IL\text{-}13^{-/-}$ male mice exhibit a significant higher mortality and increased left ventricular dilation compared with WT mice after MI (9).

Recently, IL-13 was also found to induce mitosis of isolated cardiomyocytes when bound to IL-13R$\alpha1$. Through activation of the STAT3/periostin signaling pathway, IL-13 facilitates cardiac regeneration (10). Intraperitoneal administration of IL-13 significantly reduces the scar area and increases cardiomyocyte cell cycle activity/mitosis in a cardiomyocyte-specific *Gata4* knockout neonatal mouse after cryoinfarction (11). However, whether the salutary effects of IL-13 on the injured myocardium in the adult mouse model of MI are also partially related to its underlying regeneration property needs to be examined further.

IL-33

IL-33, a member of the IL-1 family, has an important role in adaptive and innate immunities (12). After tissue injury, IL-33 released by the damaged endothelial or epithelial cells promotes immune cell recruitment and tissue repair (13, 14). In the heart, IL-33 is mainly released by cardiac fibroblasts responding to biomechanical stress (15). The cognate receptors of IL-33 have two isoforms: transmembrane ST2 (ST2L) and soluble ST2 (sST2) (16). The long form ST2L is expressed on various kinds of immune cells such as macrophages, mast cells, basophils, Th2 cells, regulatory T cells, and ILC2 (17–22). Gene ablation of *IL-33* or *ST2* has demonstrated that the IL-33/ST2 signaling pathway is crucial for reducing cardiac hypertrophy, ventricular chamber dilation, and cardiac fibrosis under mechanical stress (15, 23). However, the soluble form sST2, which serves as a decoy receptor, may impede the cardioprotective effects by neutralizing IL-33 (24). Accumulating evidence suggests that the IL-33/ST2 system has a profound effect on cardiac functions and potential value to predict the severity and prognosis of acute coronary syndrome (ACS).

In rats, IL-33 is elevated significantly within the first 12 weeks after MI. However, the mRNA level of sST2 shows a similar pattern to inflammatory and fibrosis markers with a peak at 1 week, suggesting that sST2 impairs the cardioprotective effects at an early stage post-MI (25). Preclinical studies have demonstrated that early pharmacological treatment targeting the IL-33/ST2 system promotes cardiac functions in MI rats. Through downregulating and upregulating gene expression of sST2 and IL-33, respectively, mineralocorticoid receptor antagonists reduce cardiac fibrosis and mitigate inflammation responses in the infarcted myocardium (26). Furthermore, β-blocker significantly decreases the infarct size and promote cardiac functions by reducing the sST2 level (27).

Further experiments showed that IL-33 reduces hypoxia-induced apoptosis of cardiomyocytes *in vitro* through suppressing caspase-3 activity and increasing anti-apoptotic protein expression (cellular inhibitor of apoptosis protein 1, X-linked inhibitor of apoptosis protein, survivin, B-cell lymphoma 2, and B-cell lymphoma-extra large). In a rat model of myocardial ischemia-reperfusion (IR) injury, subcutaneous injection of IL-33 significantly reduces the infarct size and myocardial fibrosis. The benefits of IL-33 on cardiac functions were then abolished by *ST2* gene deletion, indicating that IL-33 exerts cardioprotective effects through combination with the ST2 receptor (28). In the diabetic myocardium, a low level of IL-33 is associated with chronic activation of protein kinase (PK) CβII that increases the vulnerability of the myocardium to IR injury. Exogenous IL-33 supplementation reduces the phosphorylation of PKCβII, cardiomyocyte apoptosis, and infarct size after cardiac IR injury. In addition, anoxia/reoxygenation-induced apoptosis of high glucose preconditioned cardiomyocytes and activation of PKCβII are alleviated by IL-33 *in vitro* (29). IL-33 treatment also significantly suppresses proinflammatory cytokine and chemokine expression, including IL-1β, IL-6, IL-17, tumor necrosis factor-α (TNF-α), monocyte chemoattractant protein (MCP)-1, and interferon-γ (IFN-γ)-induced protein 10, and reduces macrophage infiltration after MI. These effects are mediated by inhibition of p38 mitogen-activated protein kinase and nuclear factor kappa-light-chain-enhancer of activated B cells pathways (30).

Human studies have demonstrated that the circulating levels of IL-33 and sST2 are associated with the severity of ACS patients, and may thus serve as potential biomarkers. The serum level of IL-33 is significantly lower in patients with ACS compared with stable angina pectoris patients and control individuals (31, 32). Similarly, another study showed that the circulating level of IL-33 is significantly lower in ACS patients than in patients with coronary artery disease (33). In contrast, sST2 is negatively correlated with the outcomes of MI patients. For MI patients, serum sST2 immediately elevated on day 1 after MI and correlates positively with peak creatine kinase and negatively with the left ventricular ejection fraction (LVEF) (34). In addition, a higher sST2 level is observed in patients with a larger infarct size, lower LVEF, transmural infarction, and microvascular obstruction (35). These findings indicate that the sST2 level well-reflects the severity of myocardial injury. Moreover, sST2 can predict both short term (36–39) and long term (39–43) cardiac adverse events and mortality in ACS patients.

CELL TYPES

Apart from type 2 cytokines, the recruitment and activation of M2 macrophages, mast cells, and eosinophils, which are key type 2 immunity-related cell types, affect cardiac functions in the progression of MI via various mechanisms (**Figure 1**).

M2 Macrophages

So far, two subsets of macrophages have been identified in the heart, according to their different origins: (1) resident cardiac macrophages derived from the yolk sac and fetal liver during embryonic development and (2) macrophages differentiated from circulating monocytes when they migrate into hearts (44, 45). Although there are less macrophages in the myocardium compared with cardiomyocytes, endothelial cells, fibroblasts, and smooth muscle cells (46), they are indispensable for both cardiac homeostasis and myocardial repair. Based on surface markers and gene expression profiles, macrophages are generally divided into classically activated M1 and alternatively activated M2 macrophages, although their phenotypes and functions might be more complex *in vivo* (47, 48). After MI, the injured myocardium sequentially mobilizes Ly-6C^{high} monocytes and Ly-6C^{low} monocytes via C-C chemokine receptor type 2 and CX3C chemokine receptor 1, respectively (49). Ly-6C^{high} monocytes differentiate into M1 macrophages, which dominate in the heart before day 3 post-MI and are responsible for degradation of the extracellular matrix and clearance of cellular debris; whereas Ly-6C^{low} monocytes differentiate into M2 macrophages that are the prominent subset during day 4–7 post-MI and mainly involved in the healing process (50). Accumulating evidence suggests that M2 macrophages participate in the resolution of inflammation and cardiac repair, which benefits cardiac functions after MI. In the next sections, we will summarize their subpopulations, biological functions, modulation methods, and polarization mechanisms.

Subpopulations

In response to different stimuli or pathological stresses, M2 macrophages polarize into distinctive phenotypes, namely M2a, M2b, and M2c (51, 52). M2a macrophages can be elicited by IL-4 or IL-13 with increased levels of CD206 (53) and arginase 1 (54), which support cell growth, collagen formation, and tissue repair by promoting the biosynthesis of polyamine and proline (55). Chemokines, such as C-C motif chemokine ligand (CCL) 2 (56), CCL17 (57), CCL22 (58), and CCL24 (59), are overexpressed in M2a macrophages, contributing to the recruitment of eosinophils, basophils, and Th2 cells. In addition, fibronectin, β IG-H3, and factor VIII subunit A are overexpressed in M2a macrophages, which are associated with extracellular matrix deposition and tissue remodeling (60, 61). However, the production of proinflammatory cytokines, including IL-1, IL-6, and TNF-α, is low in M2a macrophages (62), whereas the level of anti-inflammatory cytokines, including IL-10 and transforming growth factor-β (TGF-β), is high (63). M2b macrophages (elicited by immune complexes or Toll-like receptor ligands) are characterized by a low level of IL-12 and high level of IL-10. In contrast to elevated anti-inflammatory cytokines in M2a and M2c macrophages, M2b macrophages exhibit increased proinflammatory cytokines including IL-1β, IL-6, and TNF-α (64, 65). Another obvious distinction between M2b and M2a is that M2b cells have higher expression of sphingosine kinase 1 enzyme (66). They similarly regulate the recruitment of immune cells (eosinophils, Th2 cells, and regulatory T cells) by selective production of CCL1 (67). In terms of M2c macrophages, they are induced by IL-10, TGF-β, or glucocorticoid stimulation and express a high level of the surface marker CD163 (68) with decreased proinflammatory cytokines (IL-6, IL-12, and TNF-α) and proinflammatory mediators (inducible nitric oxide synthase and cyclooxygenase) (69). Previous studies have shown high quantities of matrix metalloproteinases (MMP)-7, MMP-8, MMP-9, and tissue inhibitor of metalloproteinase-1 in M2c macrophages, suggesting their potential to regulate fibrosis after MI (68, 70, 71). M2c macrophages also express high levels of chemokines CCL16 and CCL18 that attract naïve T cells and eosinophils (51).

Biological Functions: Anti-inflammation, Angiogenesis, and Collagen Deposition

Macrophages are related to the processes of initiation, maintenance, and resolution of the inflammatory response

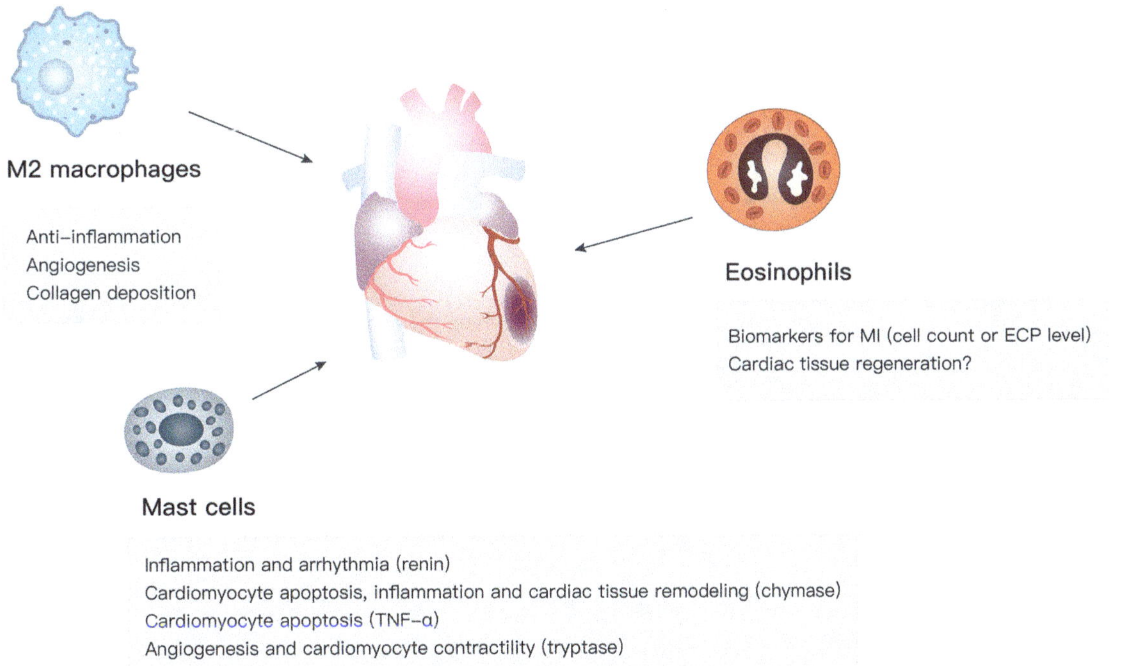

FIGURE 1 | Functions of M2 macrophages, mast cells, and eosinophils in MI.

and myocardial repair after MI (72, 73). Cardiac resident macrophages begin to apoptose by 2 h and almost vanish within 24 h after MI. In contrast, a considerable number of monocytes are recruited into the myocardium and then differentiate into macrophages, which peak at day 6 after MI (74). M2 macrophages, which dominate the infiltration during day 4–7 post-MI, facilitate the recovery of cardiac functions via secretion of anti-inflammatory cytokines, neovascularization, and collagen deposition (72) (**Figure 2**).

Anti-inflammation

Previous studies have demonstrated that an exaggerated inflammatory response increases ventricular dilatation and cardiac dysfunction after MI (75), whereas attenuated inflammation suppresses scar formation (76), and increases the risk of cardiac rupture (77). Hence, timely resolution of inflammation is crucial for myocardial repair.

Owing to the ability to secrete pro/anti-inflammatory cytokines, macrophages are essential modulators of the inflammatory process after MI. In *apoE*$^{-/-}$ atherosclerotic mice, prolonged presence of Ly-6C^{high} monocytes and higher proinflammatory gene expression in the infarcted myocardium hamper inflammation resolution and infarct healing (78), indicating the importance of timely infiltration by reparative M2 macrophages. Indeed, M2 macrophages restrict the expansion of inflammation through the release of anti-inflammatory cytokines including IL-10 and TGF-β. Further experiments demonstrated that IL-10 suppresses inflammation by restraining infiltration of inflammatory cells and the synthesis of inflammatory cytokines (IL-1β, IL-6, and TNF-α) *in vivo* (79). Early inhibition of TGF-β leads to increased infiltration of neutrophils and gene expression of IL-1β, TNF-α, and MCP-1, along with left ventricular dilation and decreased cardiac contractility, indicating that TGF-β protects the myocardium by regulating the inflammatory process (80).

Angiogenesis

Angiogenesis increases cardiac tissue perfusion, which makes it critical to salvage an infarcted myocardium. The beneficial effects of macrophages on cardiac functions are mediated partially by facilitating angiogenesis. Compared with WT mice, macrophage-deficient mice exhibit impaired angiogenesis and infarct healing (72). To further clarify the specific subtypes of macrophages that induce angiogenesis, circulating macrophages were depleted in the inflammatory phase (M1 macrophages) and healing phase (M2 macrophages), respectively. Consequently, there was a decline in quantity of microvascular α-actin$^+$ smooth muscle cells and CD31$^+$ endothelial cells in the infarcted myocardium when M2 macrophages were depleted (49). In addition, increased infiltration of M2 macrophages into myocardium after fibroblast growth factor (FGF)-2/hepatocyte growth factor administration is accompanied by enhanced angiogenesis (81). Simultaneously, M1, M2a, and M2c macrophages were injected subcutaneously into mice to determine their specific roles. In accordance with the above findings, compared with M1 macrophages, M2 macrophages had a higher angiogenic potential. When FGF-2 was neutralized in M2a or placental growth factor (PlGF) was blocked in M2c macrophages, angiogenesis and

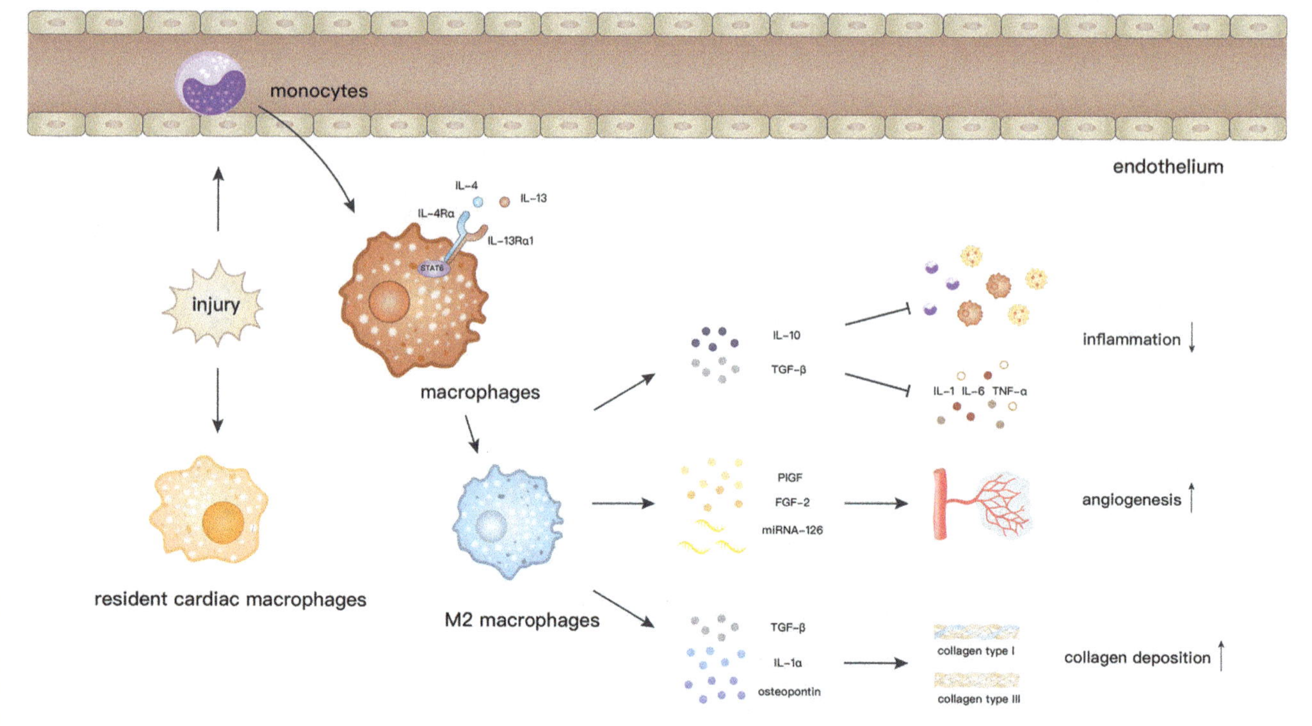

FIGURE 2 | After myocardial ischemic attack, resident cardiac macrophages begin to develop apoptose by 2 h and circulating monocytes infiltrate into the injury site and differentiate into macrophages. Elicited by IL-4 and IL-13, macrophages polarize toward the M2 phenotype through activation of STAT6. M2 macrophages facilitate the recovery of cardiac functions via secretion of anti-inflammatory cytokines, promoting angiogenesis and collagen deposition.

tube formation were reduced significantly, indicating that FGF signaling in M2a macrophages and PlGF signaling in M2c macrophages might be possible mechanisms of angiogenesis following MI (82). Apart from the release of angiogenic cytokines, M2 macrophages may regulate angiogenesis by transferring miRNAs. Angiogenic early outgrowth cells (EOCs), which are largely positive for M2 macrophage markers, were extracted from humans. Intramyocardial transplantation of EOCs from healthy donors into MI mice improved neovascularization in the infarct border zone and promoted cardiac repair. However, EOCs extracted from patients with chronic heart failure had loss of miRNA-126 and miRNA-130a and showed impaired cardiac neovascularization. Anti-miRNA-126 transfection decreased the angiogenic capacity of EOCs from healthy donors, whereas miRNA-126 mimic transfection increased the angiogenic capacity of EOCs from patients with chronic heart failure (83).

Collagen deposition

During the reparative phase after MI, collagen deposition in the infarcted myocardium stabilizes the damaged tissue and prevents infarct expansion and ventricular dysfunction. Depletion of macrophages decreases collagen deposition and wall thickness, increases left ventricular dilation, and leads to a high mortality after MI (72, 84). In contrast, injection of activated macrophages (73) or macrophage colony-stimulating factor (85) facilitates collagen deposition and myocardial repair.

M2 macrophage-depleted *Trib1*$^{-/-}$ mice were used to identify the contribution of M2 macrophages to cardiac repair. *Trib1*$^{-/-}$ mice exhibit decreased collagen fibril formation and more frequent cardiac rapture, whereas exogenous administration of IL-4, which promoted M2 macrophage polarization, increases the collagen volume in the infarct zone (86). Coculture with M2 macrophages isolated from the infarcted myocardium (86) or their secretome (87) enhances activation of cardiac fibroblasts *in vitro*. These effects might be ascribed to IL-1α and osteopontin, because gene expression of *Il1α* and *Spp1* is increased in M2 macrophages at 7 days after MI, and neutralization of IL-1α or osteopontin significantly reduces the fibroblast-myofibroblast transition when cocultured with M2 macrophages (86). Additionally, TGF-β released by M2 macrophages promotes synthesis of collagen type I and III (88, 89) through activation of Smad3 signaling in cardiac fibroblasts (90).

Modulation Methods and Polarization Mechanisms

Although numerous methods have been applied to promote the shift from M1 macrophages toward M2 macrophages after MI, the precise mechanisms of M1/M2 polarization have not been fully investigated in most studies (**Table 1**).

STAT proteins play an essential role in the immune response, inflammation, as well as cell growth and differentiation (127), and participate in various cardiovascular diseases (128, 129). It has been confirmed that IL-4 and IL-13 mediate macrophage polarization toward M2a macrophages depending

TABLE 1 | Modulation methods and mechanisms of macrophage polarization.

Modulation methods	Approaches	Animal strains	Pathological status	Polarization mechanisms	Biological effects	References
DRUG TREATMENT						
BIO	Intraperitoneal	SD rats	MI	Not investigated	Cardiac fibrosis↓ Cardiac function↑	(91)
N-propargyl caffeamide	Intraperitoneal	SD rats	MI	Not investigated	Infarct size↓	(92)
DAPT	Intravenous	SD rats	MI	Not investigated	Arrhythmia↓ Sympathetic hyperinnervation↓	(93)
Pyridostigmine	Contained in water	Wistar rats	MI	Not investigated	Anti-oxidant enzyme activity↓ Cytokine production↓	(94)
Pyridostigmine	Contained in water	Wistar rats	MI	Not investigated	LV diastolic function↑ Parasympathetic modulation↑ Sympathetic modulation↑	(95)
Eplerenone	Intracerebroventricular	Wistar rats	MI	Not investigated	Cardiomyocyte apoptosis↓ LVEF↑	(96)
Atorvastatin	Intragastric	Wistar rats	MI	Not investigated	Arrhythmia↓ Sympathetic hyperinnervation↓	(97)
Dapagliflozin	Intragastric	Wistar rats	MI	STAT3 signaling pathway	Cardiac contractility and relaxation↑ Cardiac fibrosis↓ Oxidative and nitrosative stress↓	(98)
Nicorandil	Intragastric	Wistar rats	MI	RhoA/Rho-kinase signaling↓	Cardiac contractility and relaxation↑ Cardiac fibrosis↓	(99)
HGF and FGF-2 contained microparticle	Intramyocardial	Wistar rats	MI	Not investigated	Angiogenesis↑	(81)
Telmisartan	Intragastric	Zucker diabetic fatty rats	IR injury	Ubiquitin-proteasome system↓	Cardiac function↑ Infarct size↓	(100)
Sitagliptin + G-CSF	Contained in food and intraperitoneal, respectively	C57/BL6 mice	MI	Not investigated	Cardiomyocyte hypertrophy↓ LV dilatation↓	(101)
Niacin	Intragastric	C57BL/6 mice	MI	PGD_2/DP1 axis↑	Cardiac function↑	(102)
Hydrogen sulfide	Intraperitoneal	C57BL/6 mice	MI	Lipolysis↑ fatty acid oxidation↑	Cardiac function↑ Survival↑	(103)
IL-2/Anti-IL-2 immune complex	Intraperitoneal	C57BL/6 mice	MI	Not investigated	Cardiomyocyte apoptosis↓ Infarct size↓ LV function↑	(104)
Long-acting IL-4 complex	Intraperitoneal	C57BL/6 mice	MI	Not investigated	Angiogenesis↑ Cardiomyocyte hypertrophy↓ Connective tissue formation↑ Infarct size↓	(4)
Topiramate	Intraperitoneal	C57BL/6 mice	MI	Not investigated	Cardiac rupture↓ Collagen density↑ Infarct size↓ Survival↑	(105)
BAY 60-6583	Intravenous	C57BL/6 mice	IR injury	PI3K/PKB pathway↑	Infarct size↓ Inflammation↓	(106)
Suppressing IRF5 by siRNA	Intravenous	C57BL/6 mice	MI	IRF5	Infarct healing↑	(107)
IL-10	Subcutaneous	C57BL/6J mice	MI	Not investigated	ECM deposition↓ Inflammation↓ LV function↑	(87)
Ω-Alkynyl arachidonic acid	Intraperitoneal	C57BL/6N mice	MI	Regulating cross-talk between PKM2, HIF-1α and iNOS	CK-MB↓ Infarct size↓	(108)

(Continued)

TABLE 1 | Continued

Modulation methods	Approaches	Animal strains	Pathological status	Polarization mechanisms	Biological effects	References
CRMP2 siRNA	Intravenous	*ApoE*$^{-/-}$ mice	MI	IRF5↓	Cardiac fibrosis↓ Inflammation↓ LVEF↑ Scar size↓ Survival↑	(109)
Graphene oxide-carried IL-4 plasmid DNA	Intramyocardial	Balb/C mice	MI	Not investigated	Angiogenesis↑ Cardiac fibrosis↓ Inflammatory cell infiltration↓ LV function↑ Survival↑	(5)
Hemin formulated in designed lipid-based particles	Intravenous	Balb/C mice	MI	Not investigated	Angiogenesis↑ Infarct-related regional function↑ Scar tissue↓	(110)
Histone deacetylase inhibitor	Intraperitoneal	CD1 mice	MI	Not investigated	Angiogenesis↑ LV dilation↓ LVEF↑	(111)
FGF-9	Intramyocardial	Db/db diabetic mice	MI	Not investigated	Cardiac function↑ Infarct size↓ Inflammation↓	(112)
Ac-SDKP	Intraperitoneal	Mice	MI	Not investigated	Cardiac function↑ Collagen deposition↓	(113)
HBSP	Subcutaneous injection	Rabbits	MI	Not investigated	Coronary atherosclerosis↓	(114)
GENE MODIFICATION						
Depletion of Caveolin-1	Gene modification	*Cav1*$^{-/-}$ mice	MI	TGF-β/Smad2↑	Cardiac fibrosis↑ Inflammatory cell infiltration↑ Survival↓	(115)
Depletion of Lp-PLA_2	Gene modification	*BmLp-PLA*$^{-/-}$ mice	MI	Not investigated	Angiogenesis↑ Collagen deposition↑ Infarct size↓ LVEF↑	(116)
Depletion of Wnt	Gene modification	*Cfms-icre;Wls*$^{fl/fl}$ mice	MI	Not investigated	Angiogenesis↑ Infarct-related regional function↑	(117)
Inhibition of PTP1B	Gene modification	*PTP1B*$^{-/-}$ mice	MI	Not investigated	Angiogenesis↑ LV Diastolic function↑ Myocardial perfusion↑	(118)
MIF deficiency	Gene modification	MIF deficient mice	MI	Not investigated	Cardiac remodeling↓ Cardiac rupture↓	(119)
Urokinase plasminogen activator overexpression	Gene modification	SR-uPA mice	MI	Not investigated	Cardiac fibrosis↑	(120)
CELL TRANSPLANTATION AND TISSUE ENGINEERING						
MSCs	Intramyocardial	SD rats	MI	Not investigated	Cardiac fibrosis↓ LVEF↑	(121)
MSCs	Intramyocardial	Macrophage depletion mice	MI	Not investigated	Infarct healing↑	(84)
BM-MSCs	Intravenous	NOD/SCID γ null mice	MI	IL-10 mediated	Cardiac function↑ Cardiac remodeling↓	(122)
FM-MSCs	Cell sheets	Lewis rats	MI	Not investigated	Angiogensis↑ Cardiac fibrosis↓ Cardiac function↑	(123)

(Continued)

TABLE 1 | Continued

Modulation methods	Approaches	Animal strains	Pathological status	Polarization mechanisms	Biological effects	References
Bone marrow transplantation	Intravenous	C57BL/6 mice	MI	Not investigated	Cardiac function↑ Cardiac remodeling↓ Survival↑ Wall thickness↑	(124)
Myocardial ECM patch	Sutured onto infarct area	Wistar rats	MI	Not investigated	Cardiac function↑	(125)
PHB patch	Patched on epicardial	Wistar rats	MI	Not investigated	Angiogenesis↑	(126)

BIO, (2'Z,3'E)-6-Bromoindirubin-3'-oxime; DAPT, N-N-(3,5-difluorophenacetylL-alanyl)-S-phenylglycine-t-butyl ester; LV, left ventricular; HGF, hepatocyte growth factor; G-CSF, granulocyte-colony stimulating factor; PI3K/PKB, phosphatidylinositol 3-kinase/ protein kinase B; ECM, extracellular matrix; PKM2, pyruvate kinase isozymes M2; HIF, hypoxia-inducible factor; Inos, inducible nitric oxide synthase; CRMP2, collapsin response mediator protein 2; Ac-SDKP, N-acetyl-seryl-aspartyl-lysyl-proline; HBSP, helix B surface peptide; Smad, mothers against decapentaplegic homolog 2; Lp-PLA2, lipoprotein-associated phospholipase A2; PTP1B, protein tyrosine phosphatase 1B; MIF, macrophage migration inhibitory factor; SR-uPA, overexpression of urokinase plasminogen activator; MSCs, mesenchymal stem cells; FM-MSCs, fetal membrane-derived mesenchymal stem cells; BM-MSCs, bone marrow-derived mesenchymal stem cells; PHB, poly(3-hydroxybutyrate).

on STAT6 signaling (130), whereas IFN-γ mediates macrophage polarization toward M1 macrophages depending on STAT1 signaling (131, 132). There is antagonism between STAT1 in M1 macrophages and STAT6 in M2 macrophages (133). Therefore, regulation of STAT1 and STAT6 axes is critical for the shift from M1 to M2 macrophages. Prostaglandin D_2 (PGD_2) participates in the resolution of inflammation (134) through binding to D prostanoid (DP1 and DP2) receptors (135). Macrophages express high levels of DP1 and DP2 (136), and activation of the DP1 receptor regulates macrophage infiltration and promotes inflammation resolution (137). In mice with macrophage-specific genetic deletion of DP1, macrophages are largely polarized to M1 phenotypes, leading to an extended inflammation period after MI with decreased myocardial repair. *In vitro* experiments showed that a DP1 receptor agonist inhibits Janus kinase 2/STAT1 phosphorylation by facilitating combination of the separated PKA regulatory IIα subunit and the transmembrane domain of IFN-γ receptor, which in turn induces STAT6 phosphorylation in macrophages (138). Similarly, another study confirmed that niacin activates the PGD_2/DP1 axis to polarize macrophages toward the M2 subtype and promotes cardiac healing post-MI (102). In addition, STAT3 is widely recognized as the primary transcription factor modulating IL-10 signaling in macrophages, and activation of the STAT3 pathway is a potential mechanism for polarization toward M2c macrophages (139, 140). Dapagliflozin, a selective sodium-dependent glucose transporter inhibitor, acts as an antioxidant and enhances STAT3 activity during myocardial ischemia. Simultaneously, dapagliflozin preferentially activates M2c macrophages by increasing IL-10 expression and attenuating myofibroblast infiltration during post-infarction remodeling (98).

Apart from STAT, interferon regulatory factor (IRF) 5 has been identified as another transcription factor modulating M1 macrophage polarization (141). In IRF5-silenced mice, expression of a M1 macrophage marker decreases, and the resolution of inflammation and infarct healing are augmented (107). By silencing upstream gene expression of collapsin response mediator protein-2, the level of IRF-5 decreases, which is accompanied by an increase of M2 macrophages. Such an M1/M2 switch is reversed by overexpression of IRF5 (109). These studies provide novel gene modification strategies to modulate M2 macrophage polarization.

Overall, targeting STAT and IRF signaling might be effective approaches to facilitate differentiation of macrophages toward the M2 phenotype, which is beneficial for cardiac repair after MI. More studies should be performed to investigate the precise mechanism of M2 polarization following MI (**Figure 3**).

Mast Cells

Mast cells arise from hematopoietic pluripotent precursors in bone marrow and then mature in response to proper stimuli such as stem cell factor (c-kit ligand) and IL-3 (142). In contrast to the various phenotypes of macrophages, mast cells appear to be simpler and their effects are largely mediated by degranulation. With regard to their perivascular location and abundant bioactive granules, such as chymases, tryptases, histamine, renin, and cathepsins (143), mast cells are assumed to actively participate in cardiovascular diseases. Cardiac mast cells exist in both the hearts of humans (144) and animals (145, 146), and are essential to maintain aminopeptidase activity in the normal heart (147). In addition, many mast cells accumulate in the subepicardial layer of the infarct zone after MI (148, 149), indicating their involvement in the pathological process. Although numerous studies have been conducted to elucidate the role of mast cells after MI, the effects of mast cells on the ischemic or infarcted myocardium are still controversial (**Figure 4**).

Ischemia-Reperfusion (IR) Injury and Ischemic Preconditioning (IPC)

Although timely and efficient reperfusion is the most critical therapy for MI, it may also induce continuing necrosis of cardiomyocytes and exacerbate inflammation because of IR injury. IPC is an effective approach to reduce myocardial IR injury and improve cardiac functions (150). It has been demonstrated that mast cells contribute to the protective effects of IPC against IR injury in the small intestines (151) and cerebrum (152). However, in the setting of myocardial IR injury,

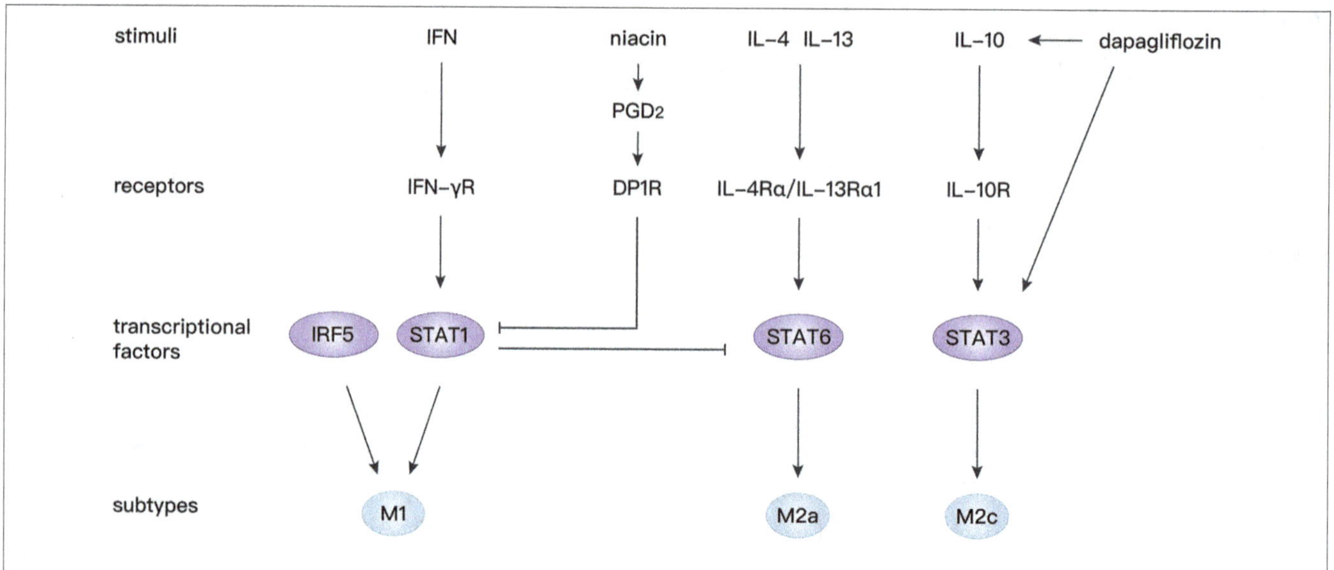

FIGURE 3 | Mechanisms of macrophage polarization after MI.

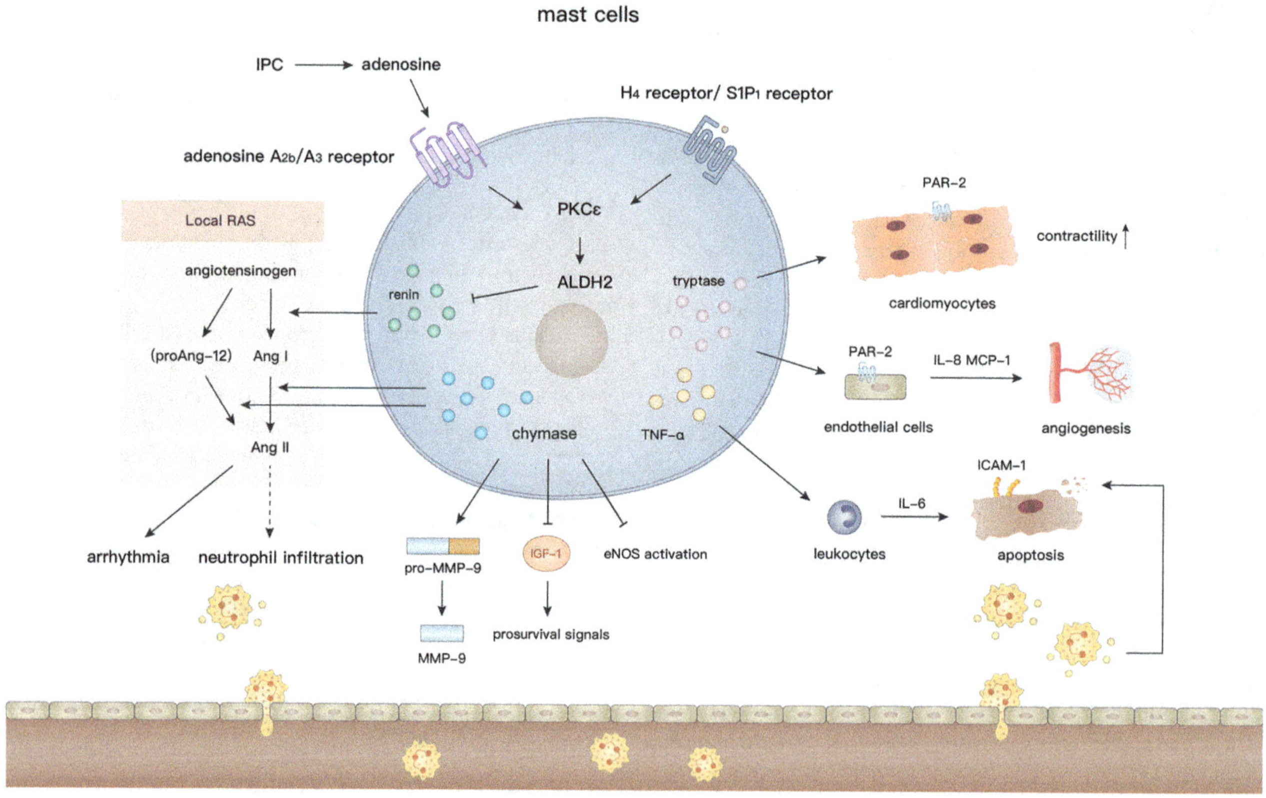

FIGURE 4 | In the setting of MI, the diverse biological effects of mast cells are largely mediated by their granules containing renin, chymase, tryptase, and TNF-α. Degranulation of mast cells induces activation of local RAS, inflammatory cell recruitment, angiogenesis, and regulation of cardiomyocyte contractility and apoptosis.

current evidence indicates that mast cell granules are generally deleterious and might augment myocardial injury.

Earlier studies did not find any association between mast cells and IR injury or IPC after MI, because their numbers and granular content are not affected after IPC (153), and neither a mast cell stabilizer nor mast cell degranulating compound 48/80 influence the antiarrhythmic effects of IPC (154, 155). Nevertheless, mast cell peroxidase, which is a marker of mast cell degranulation, exhibits a remarkable increase in the coronary perfusate after IPC or compound 48/80 pretreatment, indicating the potential involvement of mast cell degranulation in IPC (156). Further experiments demonstrated that norepinephrine preconditioning reduces myocardial injury by promoting degranulation (157, 158), whereas adrenoceptor blocker (158) or mast cell stabilizer (159) treatments during IPC largely decrease the degranulation of mast cells, and thus mitigate the salutary effects of IPC. These findings imply that IPC facilitates discharge of toxic substances via premature mast cell degranulation and consequently alleviate detrimental effects during the following prolonged ischemia. Additionally, inhibition of mast cell degranulation by an adenosine A_{2a} receptor agonist (160) or relaxin (161, 162) at the reperfusion phase reduces the oxidative injury, infarct size, and ventricular arrhythmia in an IR model.

More recently, mast cells have been reported to be a crucial source of renin in the myocardium (163) and thus elicit post-IR arrhythmia by activating the local renin angiotensin (Ang) system (RAS) (164, 165). After IPC, the level of adenosine elevates rapidly in the myocardium (166). *Ex vivo* experiments showed that adenosine further activates the PKCε/aldehyde dehydrogenase type 2 (ALDH2) pathway in cardiac mast cells via combination with adenosine A_{2b}/A_3 receptors, in turn, reduces the local secretion of renin and biosynthesis of Ang II, which induces arrhythmia by modulating sympathetic nerve endings (167). In accordance with the above findings, activation of G_i-coupled receptors, such as histamine-H_4 and sphingosine-1-phosphate-$S1P_1$ receptors on mast cells, also reduce the infarct size and the occurrence of arrhythmia through triggering the PKCε/ALDH2 pathway. In contrast, pharmacological inhibition of ALDH2 by glyceryl trinitrate treatment or gene modification (ALDH2*2 knock-in mice) abolishes the cardioprotective effects in IR models (168–170).

In addition to renin, IR injury can be caused by other granules in mast cells. Chymases effectively facilitate the conversion of Ang I (171, 172)/proAng-12 (173) (a proteolytic product of angiotensinogen) to Ang II, which may contribute to neutrophil infiltration via CXC chemokines (174) and cardiac tissue remodeling after IR injury. Interestingly, Ang II production is blocked by inhibition of chymases, but not Ang I-converting enzyme, suggesting that local chymase induced Ang II production is independent from classic RAS activation. In fact, inhibition of chymases protects cardiomyocytes from apoptosis after IR injury by reducing the level of pro-MMP-9, cleaved MMP-9, and neutrophil infiltration, and increasing activation of endothelial nitric oxide synthase (175). Moreover, mouse mast cell protease 4 (a homolog of human chymase) depletion significantly reduces the late, but not early, infarct area and improves left ventricular functions by ameliorating insulin-like growth factor-1 degradation and activating subsequent prosurvival signals (176). In addition, under oxidative stress, TNF-α, which is released during mast cell degranulation, is recognized as a crucial substance that induces cardiomyocyte apoptosis after IR. TNF-α upregulates transcription of *IL-6* in recruited leukocytes and subsequent induction of intracellular adhesion molecule-1 in cardiomyocytes, which mediates neutrophil adherence to cardiomyocytes and neutrophil-mediated cardiomyocyte injury (177, 178). Mast cell stabilizers (ketotifen and cromoglycate) inhibit TNF-α secretion (179) and may attenuate myocardial injury after IR. These findings indicate that inhibition of mast cell degranulation or the release of specific granules may be a promising strategy to alleviate IR injury.

Cardiac Fibrosis

Studies have demonstrated the profibrotic properties of mast cells under various pathological conditions, such as atrial fibrillation (180), valvular heart disease (181, 182), and heart failure (183, 184). However, in MI, credible evidence is lacking for the correlation between mast cells and cardiac fibrosis, except for some indirect observations. Mast cell precursors are recruited in the area of collagen deposition at 2–3 days after reperfusion, which is mediated by macrophage-derived stem cell factor (185). In the chronic phase of MI, *in situ* hybridization demonstrated that plasminogen activator inhibitor-1, which induces tissue fibrosis by inhibiting MMPs, mainly lies in cardiomyocytes and perivascular mast cells around the infarction border zone (186). In a rat model of MI, inhibition of chymases significantly reduces the fibrotic area and mRNA levels of collagen I, collagen III, and TGF β, which is important for the growth of fibroblasts (187). In addition, chymases facilitate the proliferation of fibroblasts in a dose-dependent manner *in vitro* (175). Additionally, bradykinin B_2 receptor antagonist (Hoe140) administration reduces the number of myofibroblasts and attenuates interstitial fibrosis post-MI, in accordance with the reduction in mast cell infiltration (188). More studies are needed to ascertain the functions of mast cells in cardiac fibrosis and their underlying mechanisms in MI.

Protective Properties

Despite the long-held view that mast cells and their degranulation are detrimental to myocardial repair, studies continue to uncover their favorable effects. Clinical studies have shown that a high level of baseline serum immunoglobulin E (>200 IU/ml) is associated with less cardiac arrest or cardiogenic shock events in MI patients. It was speculated that immunoglobulin E facilitates mast cell infiltration and degranulation in the ischemic myocardium and thus improves the prognosis (189). Indeed, in a canine model of myocardial IR injury, mast cells accumulate along the cardiac vasculature for 4 weeks or longer and exhibit a defect in granular content (tryptases and chymases). *In vitro* experiments demonstrated that mast cell tryptases upregulate the expression of angiogenic cytokines by endothelial cells, including IL-8 and MCP-1, which might be mediated by protease-activated receptor 2 (PAR2) activation (149). In addition, mast cell-deficient rats (c-kit deficiency) exhibit a decreased coronary microvessel density around the infarct zone, a larger infarct core, and poorer left ventricular functions compared with WT rats (190). Hence, the infiltration of mast cells might promote the angiogenic activity of cardiac endothelial cells and subsequent healing process in the infarcted myocardium via tryptase secretion. However, c-kit deficiency affects the functions of mast cells as well as other immune cells.

Models of specific depletion of tryptases, such as $Mcpt6^{-/-}$ mice (191), are necessary to verify the effects of tryptases *in vivo*. Recently, a more reliable c-kit-independent mast cell-deficient ($Cpa3^{cre/+}$) mouse was used to investigate the role of mast cells. Similarly, a large amount of mast cell progenitors, which mainly originated from white adipose tissue, were aggregated in the heart and differentiated into mature mast cells after MI. Although no differences were found in the capillary density, collagen deposition and the infarct size between $Cpa3^{cre/+}$ and WT mice, it demonstrated that mast cell-derived tryptases inhibit PKA activation and subsequent troponin I and myosin-binding protein C phosphorylation by promoting PAR-2 activation and, in turn, increase the Ca^{+} sensitivity and contractility of cardiomyocytes (192).

The underlying cardioprotective abilities of mast cells have also been illustrated by direct transplantation (mast cells or their granular components). Mast cell granules (MCGs) obtained by collecting a cell suspension after compound 48/80 stimulation has been proven to be therapeutic in MI. Early MCG injection at the infarct site augments myocardial angiogenesis and reduces cardiomyocyte apoptosis. Treatment with MCGs enhances endothelial cell migration, tube formation, and hypoxic resistance of cardiomyocytes *in vitro* (193). In addition, intracoronary functional mast cell implantation promotes cardiac fibroblast-to-myofibroblast conversion and angiogenesis compared with non-functional mast cells ($Kit^{W/W-V}$ mouse-derived mast cells), thereby preserving cardiac functions. However, these effects cannot be sustained long term (194). In addition, mast cells enhance cardiac functions by supporting the growth of stem cells. Mast cells or MCGs (extracted by freeze-thaw cycles and filtration) promote the migration and proliferation, but not myogenic differentiation, of mesenchymal stem cells (MSCs) via activation of the platelet-derived growth factor pathway in the early phase of MI. These effects may retain a sufficient number of MSCs for further myofibroblast differentiation in the healing phase (195).

Taken together, mast cell granules are very likely the main determinants in mediating beneficial effects after MI, including angiogenesis, cardiomyocyte contractility regulation, anti-apoptosis, hypoxia resistance, fibroblast-to-myofibroblast conversion, and the survival of stem cells. However, concerning the sophisticated composition of MCGs and different extraction methods, more studies are required to identify the key regulatory factors in their granules and to address the mechanisms using specific animal models.

Eosinophils

Eosinophils differentiate from multipotent progenitors in bone marrow and are then released into peripheral blood. They contain various kinds of specific granular contents including eosinophil cationic protein (ECP), eosinophil peroxidase, major basic protein, eosinophil-derived neurotoxin, cytokines, growth factors, chemokines, and enzymes (196). As an indispensable component of type 2 immunity, eosinophils comprehensively interact with other immune cells and participate in the process of helminth infection and allergic diseases through degranulation activity. Recent data suggest that eosinophils are also involved in the progression of MI owing to their proinflammatory and prothrombotic properties.

Biomarkers for ACS

In MI patients, serum ECP elevates significantly during the initial 2–3 days, whereas the number of eosinophils in peripheral blood decreases, indicating that eosinophils probably infiltrate into the infarcted myocardium and participate in the acute inflammatory process after MI (197). The activation and degranulation of eosinophils in the infarcted myocardium may affect the structure of heart and lead to cardiac rupture (198).

Many studies have investigated the relationship between eosinophils or ECP and clinical outcomes of MI patients. Patients with a higher eosinophil-to-leukocyte ratio at 24 h after admission have significantly higher occurrence of major adverse cardiovascular events (199). Similarly, baseline ECP levels before stent implantation are higher in patients who suffer major adverse cardiac events such as cardiac death, recurrent MI, and clinically driven target lesion revascularization (200, 201). However, it was also reported that a high level of eosinophils (blood samples collected within 72 h after admission) is associated with a lower 1-year risk of death after multivariate adjustment (202). In addition, severe ACS patients have lower blood eosinophils compared with less severe ACS patients (203, 204). The inconsistent results of the relationship between eosinophil numbers and clinical outcomes of MI patients may due to the timing of blood sample collection or different patient cohorts.

By analyzing thrombus aspiration samples during emergency coronary angiography, eosinophils were found to be largely contained in the coronary thrombus of ACS patients and associated with a larger thrombus area, indicated that eosinophils caused the occurrence of MI by facilitating thrombus growth in the coronary artery (204, 205). In accordance with the above results, eosinophil degranulation, ECP levels, and the thrombus score were higher in ST-segment elevation MI patients with major adverse cardiac events at the 1-year follow-up (206).

Potential Mediator of Tissue Repair

Growing evidence has demonstrated that eosinophils also induce tissue repair. In a mouse model of cardiotoxin-induced tibialis anterior muscle injury, eosinophils largely aggregate in the injured site and activate the IL-4/IL-13 signaling pathway in fibro/adipogenic progenitors via secretion of IL-4. Consequently, the proliferation of fibro/adipogenic progenitors facilitate myogenesis. The regeneration ability is impaired in ΔdblGATA mice (unique loss of eosinophil lineage) (207). Similarly, eosinophils are recruited into the liver after hepatic injury and release IL-4 that directly promotes hepatocyte proliferation via blinding to IL-4Rα on these cells (208). However, studies concerning the role of eosinophils in the injured myocardium are lacking. It will be intriguing to further clarify the role of eosinophils in MI with regard to their specific abilities.

CONCLUSION

Type 2 immunity-related cell types and cytokines participate in various physiological and pathological processes after MI. M2 macrophages inhibit the inflammatory response and promote angiogenesis and collagen deposition, thereby conferring benefits to the infarcted myocardium. Modulation of the macrophage polarization status is critical for myocardial repair. Although mast cells and their granules have been regarded as detrimental to myocardial healing, recent studies using more reliable mouse models have indicated that mast cell-derived tryptases actively regulate contractility of cardiomyocytes. Additionally, injection of MCGs preserves cardiac functions after MI by promoting angiogenesis, fibroblast-to-myofibroblast conversion, migration and proliferation of MSCs, and reducing cardiomyocyte apoptosis. In terms of eosinophils, the serum level of eosinophils and their granules, especially ECP, are closely related to the severity and clinical outcomes of ACS patients. Interestingly, two studies have revealed their underlying ability to activate intrinsic tissue repair of both muscular and hepatic injuries. However, these properties have not been tested in the setting of MI. Owing to the comprehensive interactions with immune and myocardial cells, type 2 cytokines have been proven to facilitate the recovery of cardiac functions after MI and serve as potential biomarkers to evaluate the severity and prognosis of MI. Nevertheless, the roles of basophils, ILC2, Th2 cells, and other type 2 cytokines in MI remain obscure. More studies are needed to further clarify the role of type 2 immunity in MI.

AUTHOR CONTRIBUTIONS

All authors made substantial contributions to the concept and interpretation of available evidence. J-YX, Y-YX, and X-TL drafted the manuscript and critically revised the manuscript for important intellectual content. All authors gave final approval of the manuscript for publication. All authors agree to be accountable for all aspects of the work and for ensuring that questions related to the accuracy or integrity of any part of the work are appropriately investigated and resolved.

FUNDING

This review was supported by grants from the CAMS Innovation Fund for Medical Sciences (2016-I2M-1-009) and the National Natural Science Foundation of China (81573957 and 81874461).

REFERENCES

1. Wynn TA. Type 2 cytokines: mechanisms and therapeutic strategies. *Nat Rev Immunol.* (2015) 15:271–82. doi: 10.1038/nri3831
2. Engelbertsen D, Andersson L, Ljungcrantz I, Wigren M, Hedblad B, Nilsson J, et al. T-helper 2 immunity is associated with reduced risk of myocardial infarction and stroke. *Arterioscler Thromb Vasc Biol.* (2013) 33:637–44. doi: 10.1161/ATVBAHA.112.300871
3. Szkodzinski J, Hudzik B, Osuch M, Romanowski W, Szygula-Jurkiewicz B, Polonski L, et al. Serum concentrations of interleukin-4 and interferon-gamma in relation to severe left ventricular dysfunction in patients with acute myocardial infarction undergoing percutaneous coronary intervention. *Heart Vessels* (2011) 26:399–407. doi: 10.1007/s00380-010-0076-2
4. Shintani Y, Ito T, Fields L, Shiraishi M, Ichihara Y, Sato N, et al. IL-4 as a Repurposed biological drug for myocardial infarction through augmentation of reparative cardiac macrophages: proof-of-concept data in mice. *Sci Rep.* (2017) 7:6877. doi: 10.1038/s41598-017-07328-z
5. Han J, Kim YS, Lim MY, Kim HY, Kong S, Kang M, et al. Dual roles of graphene oxide to attenuate inflammation and elicit timely polarization of macrophage phenotypes for cardiac repair. *ACS Nano* (2018) 12:1959–77. doi: 10.1021/acsnano.7b09107
6. Peng H, Sarwar Z, Yang XP, Peterson EL, Xu J, Janic B, et al. Profibrotic role for interleukin-4 in cardiac remodeling and dysfunction. *Hypertension* (2015) 66:582–9. doi: 10.1161/HYPERTENSIONAHA.115.05627
7. Kanellakis P, Ditiatkovski M, Kostolias G, Bobik A. A pro-fibrotic role for interleukin-4 in cardiac pressure overload. *Cardiovasc Res.* (2012) 95:77–85. doi: 10.1093/cvr/cvs142
8. Hershey GK. IL-13 receptors and signaling pathways: an evolving web. *J Allergy Clin Immunol.* (2003) 111:677–90; quiz: 91. doi: 10.1067/mai.2003.1333
9. Hofmann U, Knorr S, Vogel B, Weirather J, Frey A, Ertl G, et al. Interleukin-13 deficiency aggravates healing and remodeling in male mice after experimental myocardial infarction. *Circ Heart Fail.* (2014) 7:822–30. doi: 10.1161/CIRCHEARTFAILURE.113.001020
10. O'Meara CC, Wamstad JA, Gladstone RA, Fomovsky GM, Butty VL, Shrikumar A, et al. Transcriptional reversion of cardiac myocyte fate during mammalian cardiac regeneration. *Circ Res.* (2015) 116:804–15. doi: 10.1161/CIRCRESAHA.116.304269
11. Malek Mohammadi M, Kattih B, Grund A, Froese N, Korf-Klingebiel M, Gigina A, et al. The transcription factor GATA4 promotes myocardial regeneration in neonatal mice. *EMBO Mol Med.* (2017) 9:265–79. doi: 10.15252/emmm.201606602
12. Schmitz J, Owyang A, Oldham E, Song Y, Murphy E, McClanahan TK, et al. IL-33, an interleukin-1-like cytokine that signals via the IL-1 receptor-related protein ST2 and induces T helper type 2-associated cytokines. *Immunity* (2005) 23:479–90. doi: 10.1016/j.immuni.2005.09.015
13. Baekkevold ES, Roussigne M, Yamanaka T, Johansen FE, Jahnsen FL, Amalric F, et al. Molecular characterization of NF-HEV, a nuclear factor preferentially expressed in human high endothelial venules. *Am J Pathol.* (2003) 163:69–79. doi: 10.1016/S0002-9440(10)63631-0
14. Li J, Razumilava N, Gores GJ, Walters S, Mizuochi T, Mourya R, et al. Biliary repair and carcinogenesis are mediated by IL-33-dependent cholangiocyte proliferation. *J Clin Invest.* (2014) 124:3241–51. doi: 10.1172/JCI73742
15. Sanada S, Hakuno D, Higgins LJ, Schreiter ER, McKenzie AN, Lee RT. IL-33 and ST2 comprise a critical biomechanically induced and cardioprotective signaling system. *J Clin Invest.* (2007) 117:1538–49. doi: 10.1172/JCI30634
16. Bergers G, Reikerstorfer A, Braselmann S, Graninger P, Busslinger M. Alternative promoter usage of the Fos-responsive gene Fit-1 generates mRNA isoforms coding for either secreted or membrane-bound proteins related to the IL-1 receptor. *EMBO J.* (1994) 13:1176–88. doi: 10.1002/j.1460-2075.1994.tb06367.x
17. Wang M, Shen G, Xu L, Liu X, Brown JM, Feng D, et al. IL-1 receptor like 1 protects against alcoholic liver injury by limiting NF-κB activation in hepatic macrophages. *J Hepatol.* (2018) 68:109–17. doi: 10.1016/j.jhep.2017.08.023
18. Moritz DR, Rodewald HR, Gheyselinck J, Klemenz R. The IL-1 receptor-related T1 antigen is expressed on immature and mature mast cells and on fetal blood mast cell progenitors. *J Immunol.* (1998) 161:4866–74.
19. Tare N, Li H, Morschauser A, Cote-Sierra J, Ju G, Renzetti L, et al. KU812 cells provide a novel *in vitro* model of the human IL-33/ST2L axis: functional responses and identification of signaling pathways. *Exp Cell Res.* (2010) 316:2527–37. doi: 10.1016/j.yexcr.2010.04.007
20. Minutti CM, Drube S, Blair N, Schwartz C, McCrae JC, McKenzie AN, et al. Epidermal growth factor receptor expression licenses type-2 helper T cells to function in a T cell receptor-independent fashion. *Immunity* (2017) 47:710–22 e6. doi: 10.1016/j.immuni.2017.09.013
21. Biton J, Khaleghparast Athari S, Thiolat A, Santinon F, Lemeiter D, Herve R, et al. *In vivo* expansion of activated Foxp3+ regulatory T cells

and establishment of a type 2 immune response upon IL-33 treatment protect against experimental arthritis. *J Immunol.* (2016) 197:1708–19. doi: 10.4049/jimmunol.1502124
22. Monticelli LA, Sonnenberg GF, Abt MC, Alenghat T, Ziegler CG, Doering TA, et al. Innate lymphoid cells promote lung-tissue homeostasis after infection with influenza virus. *Nat Immunol.* (2011) 12:1045–54. doi: 10.1038/ni.2131
23. Veeraveedu PT, Sanada S, Okuda K, Fu HY, Matsuzaki T, Araki R, et al. Ablation of IL-33 gene exacerbate myocardial remodeling in mice with heart failure induced by mechanical stress. *Biochem Pharmacol.* (2017) 138:73–80. doi: 10.1016/j.bcp.2017.04.022
24. Kakkar R, Lee RT. The IL-33/ST2 pathway: therapeutic target and novel biomarker. *Nat Rev Drug Discov.* (2008) 7:827–40. doi: 10.1038/nrd2660
25. Sanchez-Mas J, Lax A, Asensio-Lopez Mdel C, Fernandez-Del Palacio MJ, Caballero L, Santarelli G, et al. Modulation of IL-33/ST2 system in postinfarction heart failure: correlation with cardiac remodelling markers. *Eur J Clin Invest.* (2014) 44:643–51. doi: 10.1111/eci.12282
26. Lax A, Sanchez-Mas J, Asensio-Lopez MC, Fernandez-Del Palacio MJ, Caballero L, Garrido IP, et al. Mineralocorticoid receptor antagonists modulate galectin-3 and interleukin-33/ST2 signaling in left ventricular systolic dysfunction after acute myocardial infarction. *JACC Heart Fail* (2015) 3:50–8. doi: 10.1016/j.jchf.2014.07.015
27. Xia J, Qu Y, Yin C, Xu D. Preliminary study of beta-blocker therapy on modulation of interleukin-33/ST2 signaling during ventricular remodeling after acute myocardial infarction. *Cardiol J.* (2017) 24:188–94. doi: 10.5603/CJ.a2016.0096
28. Seki K, Sanada S, Kudinova AY, Steinhauser ML, Handa V, Gannon J, et al. Interleukin-33 prevents apoptosis and improves survival after experimental myocardial infarction through ST2 signaling. *Circ Heart Fail* (2009) 2:684–91. doi: 10.1161/CIRCHEARTFAILURE.109.873240
29. Rui T, Zhang J, Xu X, Yao Y, Kao R, Martin CM. Reduction in IL-33 expression exaggerates ischaemia/reperfusion-induced myocardial injury in mice with diabetes mellitus. *Cardiovasc Res.* (2012) 94:370–8. doi: 10.1093/cvr/cvs015
30. Yin H, Li P, Hu F, Wang Y, Chai X, Zhang Y. IL-33 attenuates cardiac remodeling following myocardial infarction via inhibition of the p38 MAPK and NF-kappaB pathways. *Mol Med Rep.* (2014) 9:1834–8. doi: 10.3892/mmr.2014.2051
31. Liu CL, Shen DL, Zhu K, Tang JN, Wang XF, Zhang L, et al. Characterization of interleukin-33 and matrix metalloproteinase-28 in serum and their association with disease severity in patients with coronary heart disease. *Coron Artery Dis.* (2014) 25:498–504. doi: 10.1097/MCA.0000000000000117
32. Liu CL, Shen DL, Zhu K, Tang JN, Hai QM, Zhang JY. Levels of interleukin-33 and interleukin-6 in patients with acute coronary syndrome or stable angina. *Clin Invest Med.* (2013) 36:E234–41. doi: 10.25011/cim.v36i4.19957
33. Al Shahi H, Shimada K, Miyauchi K, Yoshihara T, Sai E, Shiozawa T, et al. Elevated circulating levels of inflammatory markers in patients with acute coronary syndrome. *Int J Vasc Med.* (2015) 2015:805375. doi: 10.1155/2015/805375
34. Weinberg EO, Shimpo M, De Keulenaer GW, MacGillivray C, Tominaga S, Solomon SD, et al. Expression and regulation of ST2, an interleukin-1 receptor family member, in cardiomyocytes and myocardial infarction. *Circulation* (2002) 106:2961–6. doi: 10.1161/01.CIR.0000038705.69871.D9
35. Weir RA, Miller AM, Murphy GE, Clements S, Steedman T, Connell JM, et al. Serum soluble ST2: a potential novel mediator in left ventricular and infarct remodeling after acute myocardial infarction. *J Am Coll Cardiol.* (2010) 55:243–50. doi: 10.1016/j.jacc.2009.08.047
36. Shimpo M, Morrow DA, Weinberg EO, Sabatine MS, Murphy SA, Antman EM, et al. Serum levels of the interleukin-1 receptor family member ST2 predict mortality and clinical outcome in acute myocardial infarction. *Circulation* (2004) 109:2186–90. doi: 10.1161/01.CIR.0000127958.21003.5A
37. O'Donoghue ML, Morrow DA, Cannon CP, Jarolim P, Desai NR, Sherwood MW, et al. Multimarker risk stratification in patients with acute myocardial infarction. *J Am Heart Assoc.* (2016) 5:e002586. doi: 10.1161/JAHA.115.002586
38. Marino R, Magrini L, Orsini F, Russo V, Cardelli P, Salerno G, et al. Comparison between soluble ST2 and high-sensitivity troponin I in predicting short-term mortality for patients presenting to the emergency department with chest pain. *Ann Lab Med.* (2017) 37:137–46. doi: 10.3343/alm.2017.37.2.137
39. Kohli P, Bonaca MP, Kakkar R, Kudinova AY, Scirica BM, Sabatine MS, et al. Role of ST2 in non-ST-elevation acute coronary syndrome in the MERLIN-TIMI 36 trial. *Clin Chem.* (2012) 58:257–66. doi: 10.1373/clinchem.2011.173369
40. Dhillon OS, Narayan HK, Khan SQ, Kelly D, Quinn PA, Squire IB, et al. Pre-discharge risk stratification in unselected STEMI: is there a role for ST2 or its natural ligand IL-33 when compared with contemporary risk markers? *Int J Cardiol.* (2013) 167:2182–8. doi: 10.1016/j.ijcard.2012.05.073
41. Dhillon OS, Narayan HK, Quinn PA, Squire IB, Davies JE, Ng LL. Interleukin 33 and ST2 in non-ST-elevation myocardial infarction: comparison with Global Registry of Acute Coronary Events Risk Scoring and NT-proBNP. *Am Heart J.* (2011) 161:1163–70. doi: 10.1016/j.ahj.2011.03.025
42. Jenkins WS, Roger VL, Jaffe AS, Weston SA, AbouEzzeddine OF, Jiang R, et al. Prognostic value of soluble ST2 after myocardial infarction: a community perspective. *Am J Med.* (2017) 130:1112 e9–e15. doi: 10.1016/j.amjmed.2017.02.034
43. Eggers KM, Armstrong PW, Califf RM, Simoons ML, Venge P, Wallentin L, et al. ST2 and mortality in non-ST-segment elevation acute coronary syndrome. *Am Heart J.* (2010) 159:788–94. doi: 10.1016/j.ahj.2010.02.022
44. Gomez Perdiguero E, Klapproth K, Schulz C, Busch K, Azzoni E, Crozet L, et al. Tissue-resident macrophages originate from yolk-sac-derived erythro-myeloid progenitors. *Nature* (2015) 518:547–51. doi: 10.1038/nature13989
45. Hoeffel G, Wang Y, Greter M, See P, Teo P, Malleret B, et al. Adult Langerhans cells derive predominantly from embryonic fetal liver monocytes with a minor contribution of yolk sac-derived macrophages. *J Exp Med.* (2012) 209:1167–81. doi: 10.1084/jem.20120340
46. Pinto AR, Ilinykh A, Ivey MJ, Kuwabara JT, D'Antoni ML, Debuque R, et al. Revisiting cardiac cellular composition. *Circ Res.* (2016) 118:400–9. doi: 10.1161/CIRCRESAHA.115.307778
47. Gleissner CA, Shaked I, Little KM, Ley K. CXC chemokine ligand 4 induces a unique transcriptome in monocyte-derived macrophages. *J Immunol.* (2010) 184:4810–8. doi: 10.4049/jimmunol.0901368
48. Mosser DM, Edwards JP. Exploring the full spectrum of macrophage activation. *Nat Rev Immunol.* (2008) 8:958–69. doi: 10.1038/nri2448
49. Nahrendorf M, Swirski FK, Aikawa E, Stangenberg L, Wurdinger T, Figueiredo JL, et al. The healing myocardium sequentially mobilizes two monocyte subsets with divergent and complementary functions. *J Exp Med.* (2007) 204:3037–47. doi: 10.1084/jem.20070885
50. Yan X, Anzai A, Katsumata Y, Matsuhashi T, Ito K, Endo J, et al. Temporal dynamics of cardiac immune cell accumulation following acute myocardial infarction. *J Mol Cell Cardiol.* (2013) 62:24–35. doi: 10.1016/j.yjmcc.2013.04.023
51. Mantovani A, Sica A, Sozzani S, Allavena P, Vecchi A, Locati M. The chemokine system in diverse forms of macrophage activation and polarization. *Trends Immunol.* (2004) 25:677–86. doi: 10.1016/j.it.2004.09.015
52. Colin S, Chinetti-Gbaguidi G, Staels B. Macrophage phenotypes in atherosclerosis. *Immunol Rev.* (2014) 262:153–66. doi: 10.1111/imr.12218
53. Stein M, Keshav S, Harris N, Gordon S. Interleukin 4 potently enhances murine macrophage mannose receptor activity: a marker of alternative immunologic macrophage activation. *J Exp Med.* (1992) 176:287–92. doi: 10.1084/jem.176.1.287
54. Modolell M, Corraliza IM, Link F, Soler G, Eichmann K. Reciprocal regulation of the nitric oxide synthase/arginase balance in mouse bone marrow-derived macrophages by TH1 and TH2 cytokines. *Eur J Immunol.* (1995) 25:1101–4. doi: 10.1002/eji.1830250436
55. Hesse M, Modolell M, La Flamme AC, Schito M, Fuentes JM, Cheever AW, et al. Differential regulation of nitric oxide synthase-2 and arginase-1 by type 1/type 2 cytokines *in vivo*: granulomatous pathology is shaped by the pattern of L-arginine metabolism. *J Immunol.* (2001) 167:6533–44. doi: 10.4049/jimmunol.167.11.6533
56. Gu L, Tseng S, Horner RM, Tam C, Loda M, Rollins BJ. Control of TH2 polarization by the chemokine monocyte chemoattractant protein-1. *Nature* (2000) 404:407–11. doi: 10.1038/35006097
57. Katakura T, Miyazaki M, Kobayashi M, Herndon DN, Suzuki F. CCL17 and IL-10 as effectors that enable alternatively activated macrophages to

inhibit the generation of classically activated macrophages. *J Immunol.* (2004) 172:1407–13. doi: 10.4049/jimmunol.172.3.1407

58. Andrew DP, Chang MS, McNinch J, Wathen ST, Rihanek M, Tseng J, et al. STCP-1 (MDC) CC chemokine acts specifically on chronically activated Th2 lymphocytes and is produced by monocytes on stimulation with Th2 cytokines IL-4 and IL-13. *J Immunol.* (1998) 161:5027–38.
59. Watanabe K, Jose PJ, Rankin SM. Eotaxin-2 generation is differentially regulated by lipopolysaccharide and IL-4 in monocytes and macrophages. *J Immunol.* (2002) 168:1911–8. doi: 10.4049/jimmunol.168.4.1911
60. Gratchev A, Guillot P, Hakiy N, Politz O, Orfanos CE, Schledzewski K, et al. Alternatively activated macrophages differentially express fibronectin and its splice variants and the extracellular matrix protein betaIG-H3. *Scand J Immunol.* (2001) 53:386–92. doi: 10.1046/j.1365-3083.2001.00885.x
61. Torocsik D, Bardos H, Nagy L, Adany R. Identification of factor XIII-A as a marker of alternative macrophage activation. *Cell Mol Life Sci.* (2005) 62:2132–9. doi: 10.1007/s00018-005-5242-9
62. Mantovani A, Locati M, Vecchi A, Sozzani S, Allavena P. Decoy receptors: a strategy to regulate inflammatory cytokines and chemokines. *Trends Immunol.* (2001) 22:328–36. doi: 10.1016/S1471-4906(01)01941-X
63. Gordon S. Alternative activation of macrophages. *Nat Rev Immunol.* (2003) 3:23–35. doi: 10.1038/nri978
64. Mantovani A, Sozzani S, Locati M, Allavena P, Sica A. Macrophage polarization: tumor-associated macrophages as a paradigm for polarized M2 mononuclear phagocytes. *Trends Immunol.* (2002) 23:549–55. doi: 10.1016/S1471-4906(02)02302-5
65. Anderson CF, Mosser DM. A novel phenotype for an activated macrophage: the type 2 activated macrophage. *J Leukoc Biol.* (2002) 72:101–6. doi: 10.1189/jlb.72.1.101
66. Edwards JP, Zhang X, Frauwirth KA, Mosser DM. Biochemical and functional characterization of three activated macrophage populations. *J Leukoc Biol.* (2006) 80:1298–307. doi: 10.1189/jlb.0406249
67. Sironi M, Martinez FO, D'Ambrosio D, Gattorno M, Polentarutti N, Locati M, et al. Differential regulation of chemokine production by Fcgamma receptor engagement in human monocytes: association of CCL1 with a distinct form of M2 monocyte activation (M2b, Type 2). *J Leukoc Biol.* (2006) 80:342–9. doi: 10.1189/jlb.1005586
68. Lurier EB, Dalton D, Dampier W, Raman P, Nassiri S, Ferraro NM, et al. Transcriptome analysis of IL-10-stimulated (M2c) macrophages by next-generation sequencing. *Immunobiology* (2017) 222:847–56. doi: 10.1016/j.imbio.2017.02.006
69. Valledor AF, Ricote M. Nuclear receptor signaling in macrophages. *Biochem Pharmacol.* (2004) 67:201–12. doi: 10.1016/j.bcp.2003.10.016
70. Spiller KL, Anfang RR, Spiller KJ, Ng J, Nakazawa KR, Daulton JW, et al. The role of macrophage phenotype in vascularization of tissue engineering scaffolds. *Biomaterials* (2014) 35:4477–88. doi: 10.1016/j.biomaterials.2014.02.012
71. Lolmede K, Campana L, Vezzoli M, Bosurgi L, Tonlorenzi R, Clementi E, et al. Inflammatory and alternatively activated human macrophages attract vessel-associated stem cells, relying on separate HMGB1- and MMP-9-dependent pathways. *J Leukoc Biol.* (2009) 85:779–87. doi: 10.1189/jlb.0908579
72. van Amerongen MJ, Harmsen MC, van Rooijen N, Petersen AH, van Luyn MJ. Macrophage depletion impairs wound healing and increases left ventricular remodeling after myocardial injury in mice. *Am J Pathol.* (2007) 170:818–29. doi: 10.2353/ajpath.2007.060547
73. Leor J, Rozen L, Zuloff-Shani A, Feinberg MS, Amsalem Y, Barbash IM, et al. *Ex vivo* activated human macrophages improve healing, remodeling, and function of the infarcted heart. *Circulation* (2006) 114(Suppl. 1):I94–100. doi: 10.1161/CIRCULATIONAHA.105.000331
74. Nahrendorf M, Sosnovik DE, Waterman P, Swirski FK, Pande AN, Aikawa E, et al. Dual channel optical tomographic imaging of leukocyte recruitment and protease activity in the healing myocardial infarct. *Circ Res.* (2007) 100:1218–25. doi: 10.1161/01.RES.0000265064.46075.31
75. Soehnlein O, Lindbom L. Phagocyte partnership during the onset and resolution of inflammation. *Nat Rev Immunol.* (2010) 10:427–39. doi: 10.1038/nri2779
76. Heymans S, Luttun A, Nuyens D, Theilmeier G, Creemers E, Moons L, et al. Inhibition of plasminogen activators or matrix metalloproteinases prevents cardiac rupture but impairs therapeutic angiogenesis and causes cardiac failure. *Nat Med.* (1999) 5:1135–42. doi: 10.1038/13459
77. Matsui Y, Ikesue M, Danzaki K, Morimoto J, Sato M, Tanaka S, et al. Syndecan-4 prevents cardiac rupture and dysfunction after myocardial infarction. *Circ Res.* (2011) 108:1328–39. doi: 10.1161/CIRCRESAHA.110.235689
78. Panizzi P, Swirski FK, Figueiredo JL, Waterman P, Sosnovik DE, Aikawa E, et al. Impaired infarct healing in atherosclerotic mice with Ly-6C(hi) monocytosis. *J Am Coll Cardiol.* (2010) 55:1629–38. doi: 10.1016/j.jacc.2009.08.089
79. Krishnamurthy P, Rajasingh J, Lambers E, Qin G, Losordo DW, Kishore R. IL-10 inhibits inflammation and attenuates left ventricular remodeling after myocardial infarction via activation of STAT3 and suppression of HuR. *Circ Res.* (2009) 104:e9–18. doi: 10.1161/CIRCRESAHA.108.188243
80. Ikeuchi M, Tsutsui H, Shiomi T, Matsusaka H, Matsushima S, Wen J, et al. Inhibition of TGF-beta signaling exacerbates early cardiac dysfunction but prevents late remodeling after infarction. *Cardiovasc Res.* (2004) 64:526–35. doi: 10.1016/j.cardiores.2004.07.017
81. Barbay V, Houssari M, Mekki M, Banquet S, Edwards-Levy F, Henry JP, et al. Role of M2-like macrophage recruitment during angiogenic growth factor therapy. *Angiogenesis* (2015) 18:191–200. doi: 10.1007/s10456-014-9456-z
82. Jetten N, Verbruggen S, Gijbels MJ, Post MJ, De Winther MP, Donners MM. Anti-inflammatory M2, but not pro-inflammatory M1 macrophages promote angiogenesis *in vivo*. *Angiogenesis* (2014) 17:109–18. doi: 10.1007/s10456-013-9381-6
83. Jakob P, Doerries C, Briand S, Mocharla P, Krankel N, Besler C, et al. Loss of angiomiR-126 and 130a in angiogenic early outgrowth cells from patients with chronic heart failure: role for impaired *in vivo* neovascularization and cardiac repair capacity. *Circulation* (2012) 126:2962–75. doi: 10.1161/CIRCULATIONAHA.112.093906
84. Ben-Mordechai T, Holbova R, Landa-Rouben N, Harel-Adar T, Feinberg MS, Abd Elrahman I, et al. Macrophage subpopulations are essential for infarct repair with and without stem cell therapy. *J Am Coll Cardiol.* (2013) 62:1890–901. doi: 10.1016/j.jacc.2013.07.057
85. Yano T, Miura T, Whittaker P, Miki T, Sakamoto J, Nakamura Y, et al. Macrophage colony-stimulating factor treatment after myocardial infarction attenuates left ventricular dysfunction by accelerating infarct repair. *J Am Coll Cardiol.* (2006) 47:626–34. doi: 10.1016/j.jacc.2005.09.037
86. Shiraishi M, Shintani Y, Shintani Y, Ishida H, Saba R, Yamaguchi A, et al. Alternatively activated macrophages determine repair of the infarcted adult murine heart. *J Clin Invest.* (2016) 126:2151–66. doi: 10.1172/JCI85782
87. Jung M, Ma Y, Iyer RP, DeLeon-Pennell KY, Yabluchanskiy A, Garrett MR, et al. IL-10 improves cardiac remodeling after myocardial infarction by stimulating M2 macrophage polarization and fibroblast activation. *Basic Res Cardiol.* (2017) 112:33. doi: 10.1007/s00395-017-0622-5
88. Eghbali M, Tomek R, Sukhatme VP, Woods C, Bhambi B. Differential effects of transforming growth factor-beta 1 and phorbol myristate acetate on cardiac fibroblasts. Regulation of fibrillar collagen mRNAs and expression of early transcription factors. *Circ Res.* (1991) 69:483–90. doi: 10.1161/01.RES.69.2.483
89. Chua CC, Chua BH, Zhao ZY, Krebs C, Diglio C, Perrin E. Effect of growth factors on collagen metabolism in cultured human heart fibroblasts. *Connect Tissue Res.* (1991) 26:271–81. doi: 10.3109/03008209109152444
90. Bujak M, Ren G, Kweon HJ, Dobaczewski M, Reddy A, Taffet G, et al. Essential role of Smad3 in infarct healing and in the pathogenesis of cardiac remodeling. *Circulation* (2007) 116:2127–38. doi: 10.1161/CIRCULATIONAHA.107.704197
91. Kim YS, Jeong H-Y, Kim AR, Kim W-H, Cho H, Um J, et al. Natural product derivative BIO promotes recovery after myocardial infarction via unique modulation of the cardiac microenvironment. *Sci Rep.* (2016) 6:30726. doi: 10.1038/srep30726
92. Cheng Y, Yang C, Luo D, Li X, Le XC, Rong J. N-Propargyl caffeamide skews macrophages towards a resolving M2-like phenotype against myocardial ischemic injury via activating Nrf2/HO-1 pathway and inhibiting NF-kB pathway. *Cell Physiol Biochem.* (2018) 47(6):2544–57. doi: 10.1159/000491651
93. Yin J, Hu H, Li X, Xue M, Cheng W, Wang Y, et al. Inhibition of Notch signaling pathway attenuates sympathetic hyperinnervation together with

the augmentation of M2 macrophages in rats post-myocardial infarction. *Am J Physiol Cell Physiol.* (2016) 310:C41–53. doi: 10.1152/ajpcell.00163.2015

94. Bezerra OC, França CM, Rocha JA, Neves GA, Souza PRM, Teixeira Gomes M, et al. Cholinergic stimulation improves oxidative stress and inflammation in experimental myocardial infarction. *Sci Rep.* (2017) 7:13687. doi: 10.1038/s41598-017-14021-8
95. Rocha JA, Ribeiro SP, França CM, Coelho O, Alves G, Lacchini S, et al. Increase in cholinergic modulation with pyridostigmine induces anti-inflammatory cell recruitment soon after acute myocardial infarction in rats. *Am J Physiol Regul Integr Comp Physiol.* (2016) 310:R697–706. doi: 10.1152/ajpregu.00328.2015
96. Rafatian N, Westcott KV, White RA, Leenen FHH. Cardiac macrophages and apoptosis after myocardial infarction: effects of central MR blockade. *Am J Physiol Regul Integr Comp Physiol.* (2014) 307:R879–87. doi: 10.1152/ajpregu.00075.2014
97. Yang N, Cheng W, Hu H, Xue M, Li X, Wang Y, et al. Atorvastatin attenuates sympathetic hyperinnervation together with the augmentation of M2 macrophages in rats postmyocardial infarction. *Cardiovasc Ther.* (2016) 34:234–44. doi: 10.1111/1755-5922.12193
98. Lee TM, Chang NC, Lin SZ. Dapagliflozin, a selective SGLT2 Inhibitor, attenuated cardiac fibrosis by regulating the macrophage polarization via STAT3 signaling in infarcted rat hearts. *Free Radic Biol Med.* (2017) 104:298–310. doi: 10.1016/j.freeradbiomed.2017.01.035
99. Lee T-M, Lin S-Z, Chang N-C. Nicorandil regulates the macrophage skewing and ameliorates myofibroblasts by inhibition of RhoA/Rho-kinase signalling in infarcted rats. *J Cell Mol Med.* (2018) 22:1056–69. doi: 10.1111/jcmm.13130
100. Di Filippo C, Rossi C, Ferraro B, Maisto R, De Angelis A, Ferraraccio F, et al. Involvement of proteasome and macrophages M2 in the protection afforded by telmisartan against the acute myocardial infarction in Zucker diabetic fatty rats with metabolic syndrome. *Mediators Inflamm.* (2014) 2014:972761. doi: 10.1155/2014/972761
101. Gross L, Paintmayer L, Lehner S, Brandl L, Brenner C, Grabmaier U, et al. FDG-PET reveals improved cardiac regeneration and attenuated adverse remodelling following Sitagliptin + G-CSF therapy after acute myocardial infarction. *Eur Heart J Cardiovasc Imaging* (2016) 17:136–45. doi: 10.1093/ehjci/jev237
102. Kong D, Li J, Shen Y, Liu G, Zuo S, Tao B, et al. Niacin promotes cardiac healing after myocardial infarction through activation of the myeloid prostaglandin D2 receptor subtype 1. *J Pharmacol Exp Ther.* (2017) 360:435–44. doi: 10.1124/jpet.116.238261
103. Miao L, Shen X, Whiteman M, Xin H, Shen Y, Xin X, et al. Hydrogen sulfide mitigates myocardial infarction via promotion of mitochondrial biogenesis-dependent M2 polarization of macrophages. *Antioxid Redox Signal* (2016) 25:268–81. doi: 10.1089/ars.2015.6577
104. Zeng Z, Yu K, Chen L, Li W, Xiao H, Huang Z. Interleukin-2/Anti-Interleukin-2 immune complex attenuates cardiac remodeling after myocardial infarction through expansion of regulatory T cells. *J Immunol Res.* (2016) 2016:8493767. doi: 10.1155/2016/8493767
105. Wang Z, Huang S, Sheng Y, Peng X, Liu H, Jin N, et al. Topiramate modulates post-infarction inflammation primarily by targeting monocytes or macrophages. *Cardiovasc Res.* (2017) 113:475–87. doi: 10.1093/cvr/cvx027
106. Tian Y, Piras BA, Kron IL, French BA, Yang Z. Adenosine 2B receptor activation reduces myocardial reperfusion injury by promoting anti-inflammatory macrophages differentiation via PI3K/Akt pathway. *Oxid Med Cell Longev.* (2015) 2015:585297. doi: 10.1155/2015/585297
107. Courties G, Heidt T, Sebas M, Iwamoto Y, Jeon D, Truelove J, et al. *In vivo* silencing of the transcription factor IRF5 reprograms the macrophage phenotype and improves infarct healing. *J Am Coll Cardiol.* (2014) 63:1556–66. doi: 10.1016/j.jacc.2013.11.023
108. Cheng Y, Feng Y, Xia Z, Li X, Rong J. ω-Alkynyl arachidonic acid promotes anti-inflammatory macrophage M2 polarization against acute myocardial infarction via regulating the cross-talk between PKM2, HIF-1α and iNOS. *Biochim Biophys Acta Mol Cell Biol Lipids* (2017) 1862:1595–605. doi: 10.1016/j.bbalip.2017.09.009
109. Zhou L-S, Zhao G-L, Liu Q, Jiang S-C, Wang Y, Zhang D-M. Silencing collapsin response mediator protein-2 reprograms macrophage phenotype and improves infarct healing in experimental myocardial infarction model. *J Inflamm (Lond)* (2015) 12:11. doi: 10.1186/s12950-015-0053-8
110. Ben-Mordechai T, Kain D, Holbova R, Landa N, Levin L-P, Elron-Gross I, et al. Targeting and modulating infarct macrophages with hemin formulated in designed lipid-based particles improves cardiac remodeling and function. *J Control Release* (2017) 257:21–31. doi: 10.1016/j.jconrel.2017.01.001
111. Kimbrough D, Wang SH, Wright LH, Mani SK, Kasiganesan H, LaRue AC, et al. HDAC inhibition helps post-MI healing by modulating macrophage polarization. *J Mol Cell Cardiol.* (2018) 119:51–63. doi: 10.1016/j.yjmcc.2018.04.011
112. Singla DK, Singla RD, Abdelli LS, Glass C. Fibroblast growth factor-9 enhances M2 macrophage differentiation and attenuates adverse cardiac remodeling in the infarcted diabetic heart. *PLoS ONE* (2015) 10:e0120739. doi: 10.1371/journal.pone.0120739
113. Ma X, Yuan Y, Zhang Z, Zhang Y, Li M. An analog of Ac-SDKP improves heart functions after myocardial infarction by suppressing alternative activation (M2) of macrophages. *Int J Cardiol.* (2014) 175:376–8. doi: 10.1016/j.ijcard.2014.05.016
114. Ueba H, Shiomi M, Brines M, Yamin M, Kobayashi T, Ako J, et al. Suppression of coronary atherosclerosis by helix B surface Peptide, a nonerythropoietic, tissue-protective compound derived from erythropoietin. *Mol Med.* (2013) 19:195–202. doi: 10.2119/molmed.2013.00037
115. Shivshankar P, Halade GV, Calhoun C, Escobar GP, Mehr AJ, Jimenez F, et al. Caveolin-1 deletion exacerbates cardiac interstitial fibrosis by promoting M2 macrophage activation in mice after myocardial infarction. *J Mol Cell Cardiol.* (2014) 76:84–93. doi: 10.1016/j.yjmcc.2014.07.020
116. He S, Chousterman BG, Fenn A, Anzai A, Nairz M, Brandt M, et al. Lp-PLA2 antagonizes left ventricular healing after myocardial infarction by impairing the appearance of reparative macrophages. *Circ Heart Fail* (2015) 8:980–7. doi: 10.1161/CIRCHEARTFAILURE.115.002334
117. Palevski D, Levin-Kotler L-P, Kain D, Naftali-Shani N, Landa N, Ben-Mordechai T, et al. Loss of macrophage wnt secretion improves remodeling and function after myocardial infarction in mice. *J Am Heart Assoc.* (2017) 6:e004387. doi: 10.1161/JAHA.116.004387
118. Besnier M, Galaup A, Nicol L, Henry J-P, Coquerel D, Gueret A, et al. Enhanced angiogenesis and increased cardiac perfusion after myocardial infarction in protein tyrosine phosphatase 1B-deficient mice. *FASEB J.* (2014) 28:3351–61. doi: 10.1096/fj.13-245753
119. White DA, Su Y, Kanellakis P, Kiriazis H, Morand EF, Bucala R, et al. Differential roles of cardiac and leukocyte derived macrophage migration inhibitory factor in inflammatory responses and cardiac remodelling post myocardial infarction. *J Mol Cell Cardiol.* (2014) 69:32–42. doi: 10.1016/j.yjmcc.2014.01.015
120. Carlson S, Helterline D, Asbe L, Dupras S, Minami E, Farris S, et al. Cardiac macrophages adopt profibrotic/M2 phenotype in infarcted hearts: Role of urokinase plasminogen activator. *J Mol Cell Cardiol.* (2017) 108:42–49. doi: 10.1016/j.yjmcc.2016.05.016
121. Cho D-I, Kim MR, Jeong H-y, Jeong HC, Jeong MH, Yoon SH, et al. Mesenchymal stem cells reciprocally regulate the M1/M2 balance in mouse bone marrow-derived macrophages. *Exp Mol Med.* (2014) 46:e70. doi: 10.1038/emm.2013.135
122. Dayan V, Yannarelli G, Billia F, Filomeno P, Wang X-H, Davies JE, et al. Mesenchymal stromal cells mediate a switch to alternatively activated monocytes/macrophages after acute myocardial infarction. *Basic Res Cardiol.* (2011) 106:1299–310. doi: 10.1007/s00395-011-0221-9
123. Ishikane S, Hosoda H, Yamahara K, Akitake Y, Kyoungsook J, Mishima K, et al. Allogeneic transplantation of fetal membrane-derived mesenchymal stem cell sheets increases neovascularization and improves cardiac function after myocardial infarction in rats. *Transplantation* (2013) 96:697–706. doi: 10.1097/TP.0b013e31829f753d
124. Protti A, Mongue-Din H, Mylonas KJ, Sirker A, Sag CM, Swim MM, et al. Bone marrow transplantation modulates tissue macrophage phenotype and enhances cardiac recovery after subsequent acute myocardial infarction. *J Mol Cell Cardiol.* (2016) 90:120–8. doi: 10.1016/j.yjmcc.2015.12.007
125. Sarig U, Sarig H, de-Berardinis E, Chaw S-Y, Nguyen EBV, Ramanujam VS, et al. Natural myocardial ECM patch drives cardiac progenitor based restoration even after scarring. *Acta Biomater.* (2016) 44:209–20. doi: 10.1016/j.actbio.2016.08.031

126. Castellano D, Blanes M, Marco B, Cerrada I, Ruiz-Saurí A, Pelacho B, et al. A comparison of electrospun polymers reveals poly(3-hydroxybutyrate) fiber as a superior scaffold for cardiac repair. *Stem Cells Dev.* (2014) 23:1479–90. doi: 10.1089/scd.2013.0578
127. Levy DE, Darnell JE Jr. Stats: transcriptional control and biological impact. *Nat Rev Mol Cell Biol.* (2002) 3:651–62. doi: 10.1038/nrm909
128. Grote K, Luchtefeld M, Schieffer B. JANUS under stress–role of JAK/STAT signaling pathway in vascular diseases. *Vascul Pharmacol.* (2005) 43:357–63. doi: 10.1016/j.vph.2005.08.021
129. Sun H, Wang Y. Interferon regulatory factors in heart: stress response beyond inflammation. *Hypertension* (2014) 63:663–4. doi: 10.1161/HYPERTENSIONAHA.113.02795
130. Martinez FO, Helming L, Gordon S. Alternative activation of macrophages: an immunologic functional perspective. *Annu Rev Immunol.* (2009) 27:451–83. doi: 10.1146/annurev.immunol.021908.132532
131. Meraz MA, White JM, Sheehan KC, Bach EA, Rodig SJ, Dighe AS, et al. Targeted disruption of the Stat1 gene in mice reveals unexpected physiologic specificity in the JAK-STAT signaling pathway. *Cell* (1996) 84:431–42. doi: 10.1016/S0092-8674(00)81288-X
132. Darnell JE, Jr., Kerr IM, Stark GR. Jak-STAT pathways and transcriptional activation in response to IFNs and other extracellular signaling proteins. *Science* (1994) 264:1415–21. doi: 10.1126/science.8197455
133. Ohmori Y, Hamilton TA. IL-4-induced STAT6 suppresses IFN-gamma-stimulated STAT1-dependent transcription in mouse macrophages. *J Immunol.* (1997) 159:5474–82.
134. Buckley CD, Gilroy DW, Serhan CN. Proresolving lipid mediators and mechanisms in the resolution of acute inflammation. *Immunity* (2014) 40:315–27. doi: 10.1016/j.immuni.2014.02.009
135. Joo M, Sadikot RT. PGD synthase and PGD2 in immune resposne. *Mediators Inflamm.* (2012) 2012:503128. doi: 10.1155/2012/503128
136. Sandig H, Pease JE, Sabroe I. Contrary prostaglandins: the opposing roles of PGD2 and its metabolites in leukocyte function. *J Leukoc Biol.* (2007) 81:372–82. doi: 10.1189/jlb.0706424
137. Rajakariar R, Hilliard M, Lawrence T, Trivedi S, Colville-Nash P, Bellingan G, et al. Hematopoietic prostaglandin D2 synthase controls the onset and resolution of acute inflammation through PGD2 and 15-deoxyDelta12 14 PGJ2. *Proc Natl Acad Sci USA.* (2007) 104:20979–84. doi: 10.1073/pnas.0707394104
138. Kong D, Shen Y, Liu G, Zuo S, Ji Y, Lu A, et al. PKA regulatory IIalpha subunit is essential for PGD2-mediated resolution of inflammation. *J Exp Med.* (2016) 213:2209–26. doi: 10.1084/jem.20160459
139. Murray PJ. Understanding and exploiting the endogenous interleukin-10/STAT3-mediated anti-inflammatory response. *Curr Opin Pharmacol.* (2006) 6:379–86. doi: 10.1016/j.coph.2006.01.010
140. Williams L, Bradley L, Smith A, Foxwell B. Signal transducer and activator of transcription 3 is the dominant mediator of the anti-inflammatory effects of IL-10 in human macrophages. *J Immunol.* (2004) 172:567–76. doi: 10.4049/jimmunol.172.1.567
141. Krausgruber T, Blazek K, Smallie T, Alzabin S, Lockstone H, Sahgal N, et al. IRF5 promotes inflammatory macrophage polarization and TH1-TH17 responses. *Nat Immunol.* (2011) 12:231–8. doi: 10.1038/ni.1990
142. Gurish MF, Austen KF. Developmental origin and functional specialization of mast cell subsets. *Immunity* (2012) 37:25–33. doi: 10.1016/j.immuni.2012.07.003
143. Wernersson S, Pejler G. Mast cell secretory granules: armed for battle. *Nat Rev Immunol.* (2014) 14:478–94. doi: 10.1038/nri3690
144. Sperr WR, Bankl HC, Mundigler G, Klappacher G, Grossschmidt K, Agis H, et al. The human cardiac mast cell: localization, isolation, phenotype, and functional characterization. *Blood* (1994) 84:3876–84.
145. Frangogiannis NG, Burns AR, Michael LH, Entman ML. Histochemical and morphological characteristics of canine cardiac mast cells. *Histochem J.* (1999) 31:221–9. doi: 10.1023/A:1003541332070
146. Dewald O, Ren G, Duerr GD, Zoerlein M, Klemm C, Gersch C, et al. Of mice and dogs: species-specific differences in the inflammatory response following myocardial infarction. *Am J Pathol.* (2004) 164:665–77. doi: 10.1016/S0002-9440(10)63154-9
147. Monis B, Weinberg T. Aminopeptidase activity in myocardial infarction of man. A histochemical study. *Am J Pathol.* (1964) 44:867–76.
148. Engels W, Reiters PH, Daemen MJ, Smits JF, van der Vusse GJ. Transmural changes in mast cell density in rat heart after infarct induction *in vivo*. *J Pathol.* (1995) 177:423–9. doi: 10.1002/path.1711770414
149. Somasundaram P, Ren G, Nagar H, Kraemer D, Mendoza L, Michael LH, et al. Mast cell tryptase may modulate endothelial cell phenotype in healing myocardial infarcts. *J Pathol.* (2005) 205:102–11. doi: 10.1002/path.1690
150. Hausenloy DJ, Yellon DM. Ischaemic conditioning and reperfusion injury. *Nat Rev Cardiol.* (2016) 13:193–209. doi: 10.1038/nrcardio.2016.5
151. Xing D, Zhang R, Li S, Huang P, Luo C, Hei Z, et al. Pivotal role of mast cell carboxypeptidase A in mediating protection against small intestinal ischemia-reperfusion injury in rats after ischemic preconditioning. *J Surg Res.* (2014) 192:177–86. doi: 10.1016/j.jss.2014.05.050
152. Rehni AK, Bhateja P, Singh N, Jaggi AS. Implication of mast cell degranulation in ischemic preconditioning-induced prevention of cerebral injury. *Fundam Clin Pharmacol.* (2008) 22:179–88. doi: 10.1111/j.1472-8206.2008.00567.x
153. Wang P, Downey JM, Cohen MV. Mast cell degranulation does not contribute to ischemic preconditioning in isolated rabbit hearts. *Basic Res Cardiol.* (1996) 91:458–67. doi: 10.1007/BF00788727
154. Humphreys RA, Kane KA, Parratt JR. Lack of involvement of mast cell degranulation in the antiarrhythmic effect of preconditioning in rats. *J Cardiovasc Pharmacol.* (1998) 31:418–23. doi: 10.1097/00005344-199803000-00013
155. Davani S, Muret P, Royer B, Kantelip B, Frances C, Millart H, et al. Ischaemic preconditioning and mast cell histamine release: microdialysis of isolated rat hearts. *Pharmacol Res.* (2002) 45:383–90. doi: 10.1006/phrs.2001.0960
156. Parikh V, Singh M. Resident cardiac mast cells and the cardioprotective effect of ischemic preconditioning in isolated rat heart. *J Cardiovasc Pharmacol.* (1997) 30:149–56. doi: 10.1097/00005344-199708000-00001
157. Parikh V, Singh M. Possible role of cardiac mast cells in norepinephrine induced myocardial preconditioning. *Methods Find Exp Clin Pharmacol.* (1999) 21:269–74. doi: 10.1358/mf.1999.21.4.538177
158. Parikh V, Singh M. Possible role of adrenergic component and cardiac mast cell degranulation in preconditioning-induced cardioprotection. *Pharmacol Res.* (1999) 40:129–37. doi: 10.1006/phrs.1999.0501
159. Parikh V, Singh M. Cardiac mast cell stabilization and cardioprotective effect of ischemic preconditioning in isolated rat heart. *J Cardiovasc Pharmacol.* (1998) 31:779–85. doi: 10.1097/00005344-199805000-00018
160. Rork TH, Wallace KL, Kennedy DP, Marshall MA, Lankford AR, Linden J. Adenosine A2A receptor activation reduces infarct size in the isolated, perfused mouse heart by inhibiting resident cardiac mast cell degranulation. *Am J Physiol Heart Circ Physiol.* (2008) 295:H1825–33. doi: 10.1152/ajpheart.495.2008
161. Nistri S, Cinci L, Perna AM, Masini E, Mastroianni R, Bani D. Relaxin induces mast cell inhibition and reduces ventricular arrhythmias in a swine model of acute myocardial infarction. *Pharmacol Res.* (2008) 57:43–8. doi: 10.1016/j.phrs.2007.11.001
162. Nistri S, Cinci L, Perna AM, Masini E, Bani D. Mast cell inhibition and reduced ventricular arrhythmias in a swine model of acute myocardial infarction upon therapeutic administration of relaxin. *Inflamm Res.* (2008) 57(Suppl. 1):S7–8. doi: 10.1007/s00011-007-0602-6
163. Silver RB, Reid AC, Mackins CJ, Askwith T, Schaefer U, Herzlinger D, et al. Mast cells: a unique source of renin. *Proc Natl Acad Sci USA.* (2004) 101:13607–12. doi: 10.1073/pnas.0403208101
164. Mackins CJ, Kano S, Seyedi N, Schafer U, Reid AC, Machida T, et al. Cardiac mast cell-derived renin promotes local angiotensin formation, norepinephrine release, and arrhythmias in ischemia/reperfusion. *J Clin Invest.* (2006) 116:1063–70. doi: 10.1172/JCI25713
165. Aldi S, Marino A, Tomita K, Corti F, Anand R, Olson KE, et al. E-NTPDase1/CD39 modulates renin release from heart mast cells during ischemia/reperfusion: a novel cardioprotective role. *FASEB J.* (2015) 29:61–9. doi: 10.1096/fj.14-261867
166. Headrick JP. Ischemic preconditioning: bioenergetic and metabolic changes and the role of endogenous adenosine. *J Mol Cell Cardiol.* (1996) 28:1227–40. doi: 10.1006/jmcc.1996.0113
167. Koda K, Salazar-Rodriguez M, Corti F, Chan NY, Estephan R, Silver RB, et al. Aldehyde dehydrogenase activation prevents reperfusion arrhythmias

by inhibiting local renin release from cardiac mast cells. *Circulation* (2010) 122:771–81. doi: 10.1161/CIRCULATIONAHA.110.952481
168. Marino A, Sakamoto T, Robador PA, Tomita K, Levi R. S1P receptor 1-mediated anti-renin-angiotensin system cardioprotection: pivotal role of mast cell aldehyde dehydrogenase type 2. *J Pharmacol Exp Ther.* (2017) 362:230–42. doi: 10.1124/jpet.117.241976
169. Marino A, Levi R. Salvaging the ischemic heart: Gi-coupled receptors in mast cells activate a PKC/ALDH2 pathway providing anti-RAS cardioprotection. *Curr Med Chem.* (2018) 25:4416–31. doi: 10.2174/0929867325666180214115127
170. Aldi S, Takano K, Tomita K, Koda K, Chan NY, Marino A, et al. Histamine H4-receptors inhibit mast cell renin release in ischemia/reperfusion via protein kinase C epsilon-dependent aldehyde dehydrogenase type-2 activation. *J Pharmacol Exp Ther.* (2014) 349:508–17. doi: 10.1124/jpet.114.214122
171. Urata H, Kinoshita A, Misono KS, Bumpus FM, Husain A. Identification of a highly specific chymase as the major angiotensin II-forming enzyme in the human heart. *J Biol Chem.* (1990) 265:22348–57.
172. Wei CC, Hase N, Inoue Y, Bradley EW, Yahiro E, Li M, et al. Mast cell chymase limits the cardiac efficacy of Ang I-converting enzyme inhibitor therapy in rodents. *J Clin Invest.* (2010) 120:1229–39. doi: 10.1172/JCI39345
173. Prosser HC, Forster ME, Richards AM, Pemberton CJ. Cardiac chymase converts rat proAngiotensin-12 (PA12) to angiotensin II: effects of PA12 upon cardiac haemodynamics. *Cardiovasc Res.* (2009) 82:40–50. doi: 10.1093/cvr/cvp003
174. Nabah YN, Mateo T, Estelles R, Mata M, Zagorski J, Sarau H, et al. Angiotensin II induces neutrophil accumulation *in vivo* through generation and release of CXC chemokines. *Circulation* (2004) 110:3581–6. doi: 10.1161/01.CIR.0000148824.93600.F3
175. Oyamada S, Bianchi C, Takai S, Chu LM, Sellke FW. Chymase inhibition reduces infarction and matrix metalloproteinase-9 activation and attenuates inflammation and fibrosis after acute myocardial ischemia/reperfusion. *J Pharmacol Exp Ther.* (2011) 339:143–51. doi: 10.1124/jpet.111.179697
176. Tejada T, Tan L, Torres RA, Calvert JW, Lambert JP, Zaidi M, et al. IGF-1 degradation by mouse mast cell protease 4 promotes cell death and adverse cardiac remodeling days after a myocardial infarction. *Proc Natl Acad Sci USA.* (2016) 113:6949–54. doi: 10.1073/pnas.1603127113
177. Youker KA, Hawkins HK, Kukielka GL, Perrard JL, Michael LH, Ballantyne CM, et al. Molecular evidence for induction of intracellular adhesion molecule-1 in the viable border zone associated with ischemia-reperfusion injury of the dog heart. *Circulation* (1994) 89:2736–46. doi: 10.1161/01.CIR.89.6.2736
178. Frangogiannis NG, Lindsey ML, Michael LH, Youker KA, Bressler RB, Mendoza LH, et al. Resident cardiac mast cells degranulate and release preformed TNF-alpha, initiating the cytokine cascade in experimental canine myocardial ischemia/reperfusion. *Circulation* (1998) 98:699–710. doi: 10.1161/01.CIR.98.7.699
179. Gilles S, Zahler S, Welsch U, Sommerhoff CP, Becker BF. Release of TNF-alpha during myocardial reperfusion depends on oxidative stress and is prevented by mast cell stabilizers. *Cardiovasc Res.* (2003) 60:608–16. doi: 10.1016/j.cardiores.2003.08.016
180. Liao CH, Akazawa H, Tamagawa M, Ito K, Yasuda N, Kudo Y, et al. Cardiac mast cells cause atrial fibrillation through PDGF-A-mediated fibrosis in pressure-overloaded mouse hearts. *J Clin Invest.* (2010) 120:242–53. doi: 10.1172/JCI39942
181. Helske S, Lindstedt KA, Laine M, Mayranpaa M, Werkkala K, Lommi J, et al. Induction of local angiotensin II-producing systems in stenotic aortic valves. *J Am Coll Cardiol.* (2004) 44:1859–66. doi: 10.1016/j.jacc.2004.07.054
182. Helske S, Syvaranta S, Kupari M, Lappalainen J, Laine M, Lommi J, et al. Possible role for mast cell-derived cathepsin G in the adverse remodelling of stenotic aortic valves. *Eur Heart J.* (2006) 27:1495–504. doi: 10.1093/eurheartj/ehi706
183. Hara M, Ono K, Hwang MW, Iwasaki A, Okada M, Nakatani K, et al. Evidence for a role of mast cells in the evolution to congestive heart failure. *J Exp Med.* (2002) 195:375–81. doi: 10.1084/jem.20002036
184. Matsumoto T, Wada A, Tsutamoto T, Ohnishi M, Isono T, Kinoshita M. Chymase inhibition prevents cardiac fibrosis and improves diastolic dysfunction in the progression of heart failure. *Circulation* (2003) 107:2555–8. doi: 10.1161/01.CIR.0000074041.81728.79
185. Frangogiannis NG, Perrard JL, Mendoza LH, Burns AR, Lindsey ML, Ballantyne CM, et al. Stem cell factor induction is associated with mast cell accumulation after canine myocardial ischemia and reperfusion. *Circulation* (1998) 98:687–98. doi: 10.1161/01.CIR.98.7.687
186. Takeshita K, Hayashi M, Iino S, Kondo T, Inden Y, Iwase M, et al. Increased expression of plasminogen activator inhibitor-1 in cardiomyocytes contributes to cardiac fibrosis after myocardial infarction. *Am J Pathol.* (2004) 164:449–56. doi: 10.1016/S0002-9440(10)63135-5
187. Kanemitsu H, Takai S, Tsuneyoshi H, Nishina T, Yoshikawa K, Miyazaki M, et al. Chymase inhibition prevents cardiac fibrosis and dysfunction after myocardial infarction in rats. *Hypertens Res.* (2006) 29:57–64. doi: 10.1291/hypres.29.57
188. Koike MK, de Carvalho Frimm C, de Lourdes Higuchi M. Bradykinin B2 receptor antagonism attenuates inflammation, mast cell infiltration and fibrosis in remote myocardium after infarction in rats. *Clin Exp Pharmacol Physiol.* (2005) 32:1131–6. doi: 10.1111/j.1440-1681.2005.04309.x
189. Szczeklik A, Sladek K, Szczerba A, Dropinski J. Serum immunoglobulin E response to myocardial infarction. *Circulation* (1988) 77:1245–9. doi: 10.1161/01.CIR.77.6.1245
190. Yamaki T, Iwai-Takano M, Yaoita H, Ogawa K, Tajima H, Takeishi Y, et al. Participation of mast cells in angiogenesis in the border zone of myocardial infarction in rats. *J Med Ultrason (2001)* (2009) 36:119–27. doi: 10.1007/s10396-009-0229-z
191. Shin K, Watts GF, Oettgen HC, Friend DS, Pemberton AD, Gurish MF, et al. Mouse mast cell tryptase mMCP-6 is a critical link between adaptive and innate immunity in the chronic phase of *Trichinella spiralis* infection. *J Immunol.* (2008) 180:4885–91. doi: 10.4049/jimmunol.180.7.4885
192. Ngkelo A, Richart A, Kirk JA, Bonnin P, Vilar J, Lemitre M, et al. Mast cells regulate myofilament calcium sensitization and heart function after myocardial infarction. *J Exp Med.* (2016) 213:1353–74. doi: 10.1084/jem.20160081
193. Kwon JS, Kim YS, Cho AS, Cho HH, Kim JS, Hong MH, et al. The novel role of mast cells in the microenvironment of acute myocardial infarction. *J Mol Cell Cardiol.* (2011) 50:814–25. doi: 10.1016/j.yjmcc.2011.01.019
194. Shao Z, Nazari M, Guo L, Li SH, Sun J, Liu SM, et al. The cardiac repair benefits of inflammation do not persist: evidence from mast cell implantation. *J Cell Mol Med.* (2015) 19:2751–62. doi: 10.1111/jcmm.12703
195. Nazari M, Ni NC, Ludke A, Li SH, Guo J, Weisel RD, et al. Mast cells promote proliferation and migration and inhibit differentiation of mesenchymal stem cells through PDGF. *J Mol Cell Cardiol.* (2016) 94:32–42. doi: 10.1016/j.yjmcc.2016.03.007
196. Rosenberg HF, Dyer KD, Foster PS. Eosinophils: changing perspectives in health and disease. *Nat Rev Immunol.* (2013) 13:9–22. doi: 10.1038/nri3341
197. Hallgren R, Venge P, Cullhed I, Olsson I. Blood eosinophils and eosinophil cationic protein after acute myocardial infarction or corticosteroid administration. *Br J Haematol.* (1979) 42:147–54. doi: 10.1111/j.1365-2141.1979.tb03707.x
198. Atkinson JB, Robinowitz M, McAllister HA, Virmani R. Association of eosinophils with cardiac rupture. *Hum Pathol.* (1985) 16:562–8. doi: 10.1016/S0046-8177(85)80105-2
199. Konishi T, Funayama N, Yamamoto T, Morita T, Hotta D, Nishihara H, et al. Prognostic value of eosinophil to leukocyte ratio in patients with ST-elevation myocardial infarction undergoing primary percutaneous coronary intervention. *J Atheroscler Thromb.* (2017) 24:827–40. doi: 10.5551/jat.37937
200. Niccoli G, Schiavino D, Belloni F, Ferrante G, La Torre G, Conte M, et al. Pre-intervention eosinophil cationic protein serum levels predict clinical outcomes following implantation of drug-eluting stents. *Eur Heart J.* (2009) 30:1340–7. doi: 10.1093/eurheartj/ehp120
201. Niccoli G, Sgueglia GA, Conte M, Cosentino N, Minelli S, Belloni F, et al. Eosinophil cationic protein and clinical outcome after bare metal stent implantation. *Atherosclerosis* (2011) 215:166–9. doi: 10.1016/j.atherosclerosis.2010.11.044
202. Shiyovich A, Gilutz H, Plakht Y. White blood cell subtypes are associated with a greater long-term risk of death after acute myocardial infarction. *Tex Heart Inst J.* (2017) 44:176–88. doi: 10.14503/THIJ-16-5768

203. Odeberg J, Freitag M, Forssell H, Vaara I, Persson ML, Odeberg H, et al. Influence of pre-existing inflammation on the outcome of acute coronary syndrome: a cross-sectional study. *BMJ Open* (2016) 6:e009968. doi: 10.1136/bmjopen-2015-009968
204. Jiang P, Wang DZ, Ren YL, Cai JP, Chen BX. Significance of eosinophil accumulation in the thrombus and decrease in peripheral blood in patients with acute coronary syndrome. *Coron Artery Dis.* (2015) 26:101–6. doi: 10.1097/MCA.0000000000000186
205. Sakai T, Inoue S, Matsuyama TA, Takei M, Ota H, Katagiri T, et al. Eosinophils may be involved in thrombus growth in acute coronary syndrome. *Int Heart J.* (2009) 50:267–77. doi: 10.1536/ihj.50.267
206. Niccoli G, Calvieri C, Flego D, Scalone G, Imaeva A, Sabato V, et al. Allergic inflammation is associated with coronary instability and a worse clinical outcome after acute myocardial infarction. *Circ Cardiovasc Interv.* (2015) 8:e002554. doi: 10.1161/CIRCINTERVENTIONS.115.002554
207. Heredia JE, Mukundan L, Chen FM, Mueller AA, Deo RC, Locksley RM, et al. Type 2 innate signals stimulate fibro/adipogenic progenitors to facilitate muscle regeneration. *Cell* (2013) 153:376–88. doi: 10.1016/j.cell.2013.02.053
208. Goh YP, Henderson NC, Heredia JE, Red Eagle A, Odegaard JI, Lehwald N, et al. Eosinophils secrete IL-4 to facilitate liver regeneration. *Proc Natl Acad Sci USA.* (2013) 110:9914–9. doi: 10.1073/pnas.1304046110

16

The Antidiabetic and Antinephritic Activities of *Auricularia cornea* (An Albino Mutant Strain) via Modulation of Oxidative Stress in the db/db Mice

Di Wang[1,2†], *Xue Jiang*[2†], *Shanshan Teng*[2], *Yaqin Zhang*[2], *Yang Liu*[1], *Xiao Li*[1*] *and Yu Li*[1*]

[1] *Engineering Research Center of Chinese Ministry of Education for Edible and Medicinal Fungi, Jilin Agricultural University, Changchun, China,* [2] *School of Life Sciences, Jilin University, Changchun, China*

***Correspondence:**
Xiao Li
lxmogu@163.com
Yu Li
fungi966@163.com

† *These authors have contributed equally to this work*

This study first systematically analyzed the constituents of an albino mutant strain of *Auricularia cornea* (AU). After 8 weeks of continuous treatment with metformin (Met) (0.1 g/kg) and AU (0.1 and 0.4 g/kg), db/db mice showed hypoglycemic functioning, indicated by reduced bodyweight, food intake, plasma glucose, serum levels of glycated hemoglobin A1c and glucagon, hepatic levels of phosphoenolpyruvate carboxykinase and lucose-6-phosphatasem, and increased serum levels of insulin. The effect of hypolipidemic functions were indicated by suppressed levels of total cholesterol and triglyceride, and enhanced levels of hepatic glycogen and high-density lipoprotein cholesterol. The renal protective effect of AU was confirmed by the protection in renal structures and the regulation of potential indicators of nephropathy. The anti-oxidative and anti-inflammatory effects of AU were verified by a cytokine array combined with an enzyme-linked immunosorbent assay. AU decreased the expression of protein kinase C α and $\beta 2$ and phosphor-nuclear factor-κB, and enhanced the expression of catalase, nuclear respiratory factor 2 (Nrf2), manganese superoxide dismutase 2, heme oxygenase-1 and−2, heat shock protein 27 (HSP27), HSP60, and HSP70 in the kidneys of db/db mice. The results confirmed that AU's anti-diabetic and anti-nephritic effects are related to its modulation on oxidative stress.

Keywords: ***Auricularia cornea*, diabetes, diabetic nephropathy, oxidative stress, inflammation**

INTRODUCTION

Diabetes mellitus (DM) is a progressive metabolic disease characterized by an imbalance in glucose homeostasis, impaired insulin secretion, and abnormal lipid and carbohydrate metabolism (1). The prevalence of DM has increased four-fold in the past three decades, and the global diabetic population is ~382 million (2).

Long-term hyperglycemia can induce secondary complications such as renal damage (3). Diabetic nephropathy (DN), a major cause of end-stage renal disease and cardiovascular disease (4), is characterized by an elevated lipid profile and increased oxidative stress (5). DN affects around 30% of patients with type 1 and 25% of patients with type 2 diabetes, which indicates excessive morbidity and mortality (4). Hyperglycemia induces the excessive production of mitochondrial superoxide and leads directly to the overproduction of reactive oxygen species (ROS), which can cause tubulointerstitial fibrosis and inflammatory cell infiltration (6). The accumulation of inflammatory cells in the glomerulus of DN patients stimulates the secretion of cytokines and chemokines, which transfer inflammatory cells to damaged areas (7).

ROS can be eliminated by nuclear respiratory factor 2 (Nrf2), a type of leucine zipper transcription factor that regulates the expression of phase 2 detoxification genes such as heme oxygenase 1 (HO-1) (8). Severe kidney damage has been observed in Nrf2 knockout diabetic mice (9). Nuclear factor-κB (NF-κB), an important inflammatory transcription factor, can be activated by extremely high levels of proinflammatory cytokines and consequently helps to generate more pro-inflammatory mediators under pathological conditions, including diabetes (10). NF-κB participates in the cellular response to stimulations, including ROS (11).

The conventional therapeutic agents for diabetes cannot effectively restore β-cell function, and the long-term nature of the treatment causes multiple side effects, including peripheral hyperinsulinemia, and hypoglycemia and increased cardiovascular risks (12, 13). These therapeutic strategies suppress blood glucose levels and reduce hypertension by blocking the renin-angiotensin system, which has a negative therapeutic effect on diabetic complications such as DN (5). Therefore, alternative agents with fewer side effects and greater activities against complications are needed. Edible fungi, which contain plenty of bioactive components with few adverse effects, are reported to show various pharmacological activities (14). Our previous studies confirmed that the antidiabetic activities of *Cordyceps militaris*, *Paecilomyces hepialid,* and *Inonotus obliquus* are related to the regulation of oxidative stress in diet-streptozotocin-induced diabetic Sprague-Dawley rats models (15–17). An albino mutant strain of *Auricularia cornea* entitled Yu Muer (AU) was first reported and cultured by the research team led by Prof. Li (the Chinese Academy of Engineering) at Jilin Agricultural University, Jilin, China. AU exhibits antineoplastic activity and antioxidant effects in H22 bearing mice (18). However, the antidiabetic and antinephritic activities of AU and their underlying mechanisms have not been reported.

The db/db mouse model exhibits insulin resistance at around 2 weeks of age and eventually develops hyperglycemia induced by β cell failure at 4–8 weeks, which accurately reflects the pathophysiology of diabetes (19). In the present study, the antidiabetic and antinephritic activities of AU and its possible oxidative stress related mechanisms were analyzed on db/db mice.

MATERIALS AND METHODS

Detection of AU Components

The cultured fruitbodies of AU (provided by Prof. Li's group at Jilin Agricultural University, Jilin, China) were shattered by a crusher and dry stored for the follow-up experiment. **Figure S1** presents a picture of AU.

Main Components Analysis

The main components of AU, including total protein, total sugar, reducing sugar, crude fat, total ash, crude fiber, and total flavones, were assessed by the Kjeldahl method (20), phenol-sulfuric acid method (21), direct titration (22), Soxhlet extraction (23), combustion method (24), double differences method (25), and UV spectrophotometry (26), respectively. Total triterpenoids and mannitol were assessed by high performance liquid chromatography (HPLC) (27, 28).

Fatty Acids Analysis

AU was extracted with a 1:1 ratio of ether: petroleum ether (V:V) via evaporation at 80°C, then 0.5 M of NaOH in a methanol solution and 25% Boron trifluoride (BF3) were added stepwise and incubated at 60°C for 30 and 20 min, respectively. Finally, a saturated solution of NaCl and hexane was mixed with the samples, and the levels of fatty acids were analyzed using a gas chromatography-mass spectrometer (QP2010, Shimadzu, Japan) (29).

Amino Acids Analysis

AU was hydrolyzed by HCl (6 mol/L) at 110°C for 24 h, and the amino acid composition of AU was analyzed by HPLC using an Agilent 1260 (Agilent, California, America) equipped Agilent C18 column (4.6 × 250 mm × 5 μm) at 1.0 mL/min with mobile phase A (25 mM acetate buffer, pH 5.8) and mobile phase B (acetonitrile) (30).

Minerals Analysis

AU (0.5 g) was placed in a digestion tank and mixed with nitric acid (5 mL) to digest for 27 min (at 100, 140, 160, and 180°C, 3 min of each, and at 190°C for 15 min). The levels of minerals including zinc (Zn), kalium (K), ferrum (Fe), manganese (Mn), natrium (Na), cuprum (Cu), and calcium (Ca) were detected using inductively coupled plasma optical emission spectrometry (ICP-OES, optima 8,000) (31), and lead (Pb), selenium (Se), mercury (Hg), chromium (Cr), cadmium (Cd), and arsenic (As) were analyzed using inductively coupled plasma mass spectrometry (Thermo Fisher Scientific ICAPQ) (32).

Animal Care and Experimental Design

The experimental animal protocol was approved by the Animal Ethics Committee of Jilin University (20170301). All procedures were carried out on the basis of the Laboratory Animal Care and Use recommendations, which are intended to reduce the use of animals and minimize animal distress. The male db/db mice and wild db/+ littermates in a C57BLKs/J background [8 weeks, SCXK (Su) 2015-0001] were purchased from the Nanjing Biomedical Research Institute of Nanjing University (Nanjing, China). Mice were housed at a temperature of 23 ± 1°C and humidity of 60% with a 12-h light-dark cycle (lights on 07:00–19:00) and free access to food and water. After 1 week of adaptation, the db/db mice with non-random blood glucose levels >11.1 mmol/L were considered to be diabetes. The mice were randomly divided into four groups (n = 12/group) and treated with 4.0 mL/kg of physiological saline (model group), Met at 0.1 g/kg (positive control group) and AU at doses of 0.1 and 0.4 g/kg (AU-treated groups) by gavage once per day, respectively, for eight consecutive weeks. The db/+ mice (n = 12) were orally treated with 4.0 mL/kg of physiological saline (control group) for eight consecutive weeks. AU fruiting body was pulverized using the ultrafine grinder (XDW-6A, Ji'nan Tatsu Micro Machinery Co.. Ltd., Ji'nan, China) and mixed with physiological saline. Before administration, the mixture was shaken up. Throughout the experimental period, the body weights and blood glucose concentrations of the mice were measured once a week. Due to the limited amount of sera and tissues, we randomly stagger samples to guarantee a sample size of 10 for each of the following assays.

Sample Collection and Parameter Determination

The mice were fasted for 2 h before sacrifice. Blood samples were collected and then centrifuged at 3,000 rpm for 10 min twice, and the collected sera were stored at −80°C. Tissues (kidney and liver) were harvested and washed in ice-cold physiological saline solution. Half of each tissue was homogenized in double distilled water and/or a radioimmunoprecipitation assay (RIPA) buffer (Sigma-Aldrich, USA) containing 1% protease inhibitor cocktail and 2% phenylmethanesulfonyl fluoride (Sigma-Aldrich, USA) and stored at −80°C for the subsequent experiment, while the other half was embedded with 10% neutral phosphate-buffered formalin for histopathological examination. Enzyme-linked immunosorbent assay (ELISA) commercial kits (Shanghai Yuanye Bio-Technology Co. Ltd., Shanghai, China) were used to determine the levels of granulocyte colony-stimulating factor (G-CSF, CK-E20002), glycated hemoglobin A1c (GhbA1c; CK-E20512), insulin (INS, CK-E20353), total cholesterol (TC; CK-E91839), triglyceride (TG; CK-E91733), high-density lipoprotein cholesterol (HDL-C; CK-E93031), alanine aminotransferase (ALT; CK-E90314), aspartate aminotransferase (AST; CK-E91386), and glucagon (GC; CK-E92275) in serum; the levels of interleukin (IL)-2 (CK-E20010), IL-1β (CK-E20533), IL-10 (CK-E20005), ROS (CK-E91516), microalbuminuria (MAU/ALB, CK-E95121), 6-keto-prostaglandin F1α (6-K-PGF1α; CK-E30144), and matrix metalloproteinase-9 (MMP-9; CK-E90157) in kidney; the level of N-acetyl-β-D-glucosidase (NAG; CK-E20276) in urine; the levels of phosphoenolpyruvate carboxykinase (PEPCK; CK-E93964) and glucose-6-phosphatase (G-6-Pase; CK-E94770) in liver; and the levels of glutathione peroxidase (GSH-Px; CK-E92669), superoxide dismutase (SOD; CK-E20348). and catalase (CAT; CK-E92636) in serum and kidney. Glycogen assay kits (A043) (Nanjing Jiancheng Bioengineering Institute, Nanjing, China) were used to detect the level of hepatic glycogen.

Proteome Profiling of Kidney

Twenty-six cytokines from the kidney samples of db/db mice were quantified using a Cytokine Array Kit (ARY018, R&D Systems, Minneapolis, MN). Briefly, the kidney was excised and homogenized in RIPA buffer with 1% protease inhibitor cocktail (Sigma-Aldrich, USA). After centrifugation at 10,000 rpm for 10 min, the protein concentration of the supernatant was quantitated using a bicinchoninic acid (BCA) protein assay kit (Merck Millipore, USA). Membranes containing 26 different cytokine antibodies were blocked with BSA for 1 h at room temperature and then incubated with 100 μg of protein supernatant mixed with a cocktail of biotinylated detection antibodies. Streptavidin-HRP and chemiluminescence were used to detect the antibodies bound to the membrane antibodies. The membranes were then exposed and quantified using Image J software (National Institutes of Health, Bethesda, MD).

Western Blot

One part of the kidney tissues obtained from the db/db mice was homogenized in RIPA buffer with a 1% protease inhibitor cocktail on ice for 30 min. After centrifugation (10,000 rpm for 10 min) and elimination of the precipitate, total protein concentrations were determined by BCA protein assay kit (Merck Millipore, USA). Denatured protein samples (40 μg) were subjected to 12% sodium dodecyl sulfate-polyacrylamide gel electrophoresis (SDS-PAGE) (Bio-Rad, USA) and then electro blotted onto 0.45 μm PVDF membranes (Bio Basic, Inc., USA). After blocking with 5% bovine serum albumin (BSA) for 4 h, the transferred membranes were incubated overnight at 4°C in the corresponding primary antibodies (at a dilution of 1:2,000) containing total-NF-κB (t-NF-κB, ab32536), phosphor-NF-κB (p-NF-κB, ab86299), Nrf2 (ab137550), catalase (CAT, ab16731), HO-1 (ab68477), HO-2 (ab90492), manganese superoxide dismutase 2 (SOD2, ab13533), protein kinase C alpha (PKC-α, ab23513), PKC β2 (ab32026), heat shock protein 27 (HSP27, ab12351), HSP 60 (ab45134), and HSP70 (ab181606) (Abcam, Cambridge, USA), and the reference protein glyceraldehyde-3-phosphate dehydrogenase (GAPDH; ABS16) (Merck Millipore, Darmstadt, Germany). The transferred membranes were washed five times with TBS buffer and then incubated with horseradish peroxidase-conjugated goat anti-rabbit secondary antibody (sc-3836) (Santa Cruz Biotechnology, Santa Cruz, USA) for 4 h at 4°C. The protein bands were established and fixed by Immobilon Western HRP substrate (Millipore Corporation, Billerica, USA). The relative intensity of protein expression was quantified using Image J software (National Institutes of Health, Bethesda, MD).

Histopathological Observation

Ten percent formalin-fixed kidney tissues were dehydrated in ethyl alcohol (from 70 to 100%) and dealcoholized in xylene. Subsequently, the tissues were embedded in paraffin and cut into 5-mm thick sections. Sections were then deparaffinized in xylene and rehydrated in ethyl alcohol (from 100 to 70%) in reverse order. All specimens were stained with hematoxylin and eosin (H&E) and periodic acid Schiff (PAS) and assessed for kidney damage and inflammation under an inverted microscope CKX41 (Olympus, Japan).

Statistical Analysis

All data were expressed as the mean ± S.E.M. Differences were determined by one-way analysis of variance followed by *post-hoc* multiple comparisons (Dunn's test) using SPSS 16.0 software (IBM Corporation, Armonk, USA). Statistical significance was declared for *p*-values under 0.05.

RESULTS

Composition of AU

The AU consisted of 56.9% total sugar, 2.8% reducing sugar, 8.1% protein, 4.2% total ash, 2.4% crude fat, 8.0% crude fiber and 3.1 $\times$ 10^{-4}% total triterpenoids (**Table 1**). Among 17 types of amino acid detected, the concentrations of glutamic acid, aspartic acid, leucine and arginine were higher than others (**Table 1**). Seven minerals, Zn, Fe, Mn, Ca, Cu, Na, and K were detected in AU (**Table 1**).

The concentrations of Pb, Cr, As, and Se in the AU were below the limit of detection, and the AU didn't contain Hg or Cd (**Table 1**). Among 35 types of fatty acid tested, only 16 types of fatty acid were existed in the AU (**Table 2**).

The Hypoglycemic Effect of AU on db/db Mice

Compared with db/+ mice, the db/db mice showed increased bodyweight and changes in the organ indices of the kidney, spleen and liver (P < 0.001, **Table 3**). After 8 weeks of administration of AU at doses of 0.1 and 0.4 g/kg, bodyweight was reduced by 9.1 and 13.6%, respectively (P < 0.05, **Table 3**). AU at 0.4 g/kg strongly enhanced the kidney and spleen indices and reduced the liver indices (P < 0.05, **Table 3**). The high levels of food intake observed in the db/db mice were also suppressed by Met and AU after 8 weeks of administration (P < 0.05; **Table S1**).

Increased blood glucose levels were observed in the db/db mice compared with the db/+ mice. Similar to Meet, AU remitted

TABLE 1 | Main components of AU.

	Compounds	Contents (%)	Compounds	Contents (%)	Compounds	Contents (%)
Main components	Total protein	8.1	Total sugar	56.9	Reducing sugar	2.8
	Crude fat	2.4	Total ash	4.2	Crude fiber	8.0
	Total triterpenoids ($\times 10^{-4}$)	3.1	Total flavones	ND[I]	Mannitol	ND[II]
Amino acid	Aspartic acid (Asp)	0.6	Glutamic acid (Glu)	0.7	Cystine (Cys)	0.3
	Serine (Ser)	0.4	Glycine (Gly)	0.3	Histidine (His)	0.2
	Arginine (Arg)	0.5	L-Threonine (Thr)	0.3	Alanine (Ala)	0.4
	Proline (Pro)	0.3	Tyrosine (Tyr)	0.2	Valine (Val)	0.3
	DL-Methionine (Met) ($\times 10^{-2}$)	6.0	Isoleucine (Ile)	0.2	Leucine (Leu)	0.5
	Phenylalanine (Phe)	0.4	Lysine (Lys)	0.3		
Minerals	Zinc (Zn) ($\times 10^{-3}$)	3.6	Ferrum (Fe) ($\times 10^{-3}$)	4.3	Manganese (Mn) ($\times 10^{-3}$)	0.5
	Calcium (Ca)	0.1	Cuprum (Cu) ($\times 10^{-3}$)	0.6	Natrium (Na) ($\times 10^{-2}$)	1.7
	Kalium (K)	1.1	Lead (Pb) ($\times 10^{-5}$)	1.2	Mercury (Hg)	ND[III]
	Chromium (Cr) ($\times 10^{-4}$)	5.0	Arsenic (As) ($\times 10^{-6}$)	4.0	Cadmium (Cd)	ND[III]
	Selenium (Se) ($\times 10^{-6}$)	2.6				

AU, Auricularianigricans; ND, not detected; ND[I], the detection limit was 1 g/kg; ND[II], the detection limit was 0.056 g/kg; ND[III], the detection limit was 20 µg/kg.

TABLE 2 | The composition and percentage content of fatty acids.

Compounds	Contents (%)	Compounds	Contents (%)	Compounds	Contents (%)
Octoic acid (C8:0)	ND[I]	Heptadecenoic acid (C17:1) ($\times 10^{-3}$)	4.0	Docosanoic acid (C22:0) ($\times 10^{-2}$)	2.2
Capric acid (C10:0)	ND[II]	Stearic acid (C18:0)	0.2	Eicosatrienoic acid (C20:3n6)	ND[XI]
Undecanoic acid (C11:0)	ND[III]	Trans-oleic acid (C18:1n9t) ($\times 10^{-3}$)	2.0	Erucic acid (C22:1n9)	ND[XII]
Lauric acid (C12:0)	ND[IV]	Oleic acid (C18:1n9c)	0.6	Eicosatrienoic acid (C20:3n3)	ND[XIII]
Tridecanoic acid (C13:0)	ND[V]	Trans-linoleic acid (C18:2n6t)	ND[VII]	Arachidonic acid (C20:4n6)	ND[XIV]
Myristic acid (C14:0) ($\times 10^{-3}$)	4.0	Linoleic acid (C18:2n6c)	0.8	Tricosanoic acid (C23:0) ($\times 10^{-3}$)	4.0
Myristoleic acid (C14:1)	ND[VI]	Arachidic acid (C20:0) ($\times 10^{-2}$)	1.3	Docosadienoic acid (C22:2n6)	ND[XV]
Pentadecanoic acid (C15:0) ($\times 10^{-2}$)	3.4	γ-linolenic acid (C18:3n6)	ND[VIII]	Eicosapentaenoic acid (C20:5n3)	ND[XVI]
Pentadecenoic acid (C15:1)	ND[VII]	Eicosenoic acid (C20:1n9) ($\times 10^{-2}$)	2.8	Tetracosanoic acid (C24:0) ($\times 10^{-2}$)	3.8
Hexadecanoic acid (C16:0)	0.3	α-linolenic acid (C18:3n3)	ND[IX]	Nervonic acid (C24:1n9)	ND[XVII]
Palmitoleic acid (C16:1) ($\times 10^{-3}$)	4.0	Heneicosanoic acid (C21:0)	ND[X]	Docosahexaenoic acid (C22:6n3)	ND[XVIII]
Heptadecanoic acid (C17:0) ($\times 10^{-3}$)	8.0	Eicosadienoic acid (C20:2) ($\times 10^{-3}$)	3.0		

ND, not detected; ND[I], the detection limit was 4.20 mg/kg; ND[II], the detection limit was 3.83 mg/kg; ND[III], the detection limit was 3.54 mg/kg; ND[IV], the detection limit was 2.99 mg/kg; ND[V], the detection limit was 2.91 mg/kg; ND[VI], the detection limit was 2.82 mg/kg; ND[VII], the detection limit was 2.64 mg/kg; ND[VIII], the detection limit was 2.51 mg/kg; ND[IX], the detection limit was 2.36 mg/kg; ND[X], the detection limit was 2.05 mg/kg; ND[XI], the detection limit was 2.68 mg/kg; ND[XII], the detection limit was 2.42 mg/kg; ND[XIII], the detection limit was 3.21 mg/kg; ND[XIV], the detection limit was 4.66 mg/kg; ND[XV], the detection limit was 2.88 mg/kg; ND[XVI], the detection limit was 3.31 mg/kg; ND[XVII], the detection limit was 4.83 mg/kg; ND[XVIII], the detection limit was 4.33 mg/kg.

TABLE 3 | The effects of AU on body weights and organ indices.

	Week	db/+	db/db	0.1 g/kg Met	0.1 g/kg AU	0.4 g/kg AU
Body weights (g)	1	20.0 ± 0.3	43.0 ± 0.5###	43.1 ± 0.8	43.9 ± 0.4	44.3 ± 0.8
	2	21.1 ± 0.3	45.1 ± 0.7###	44.9 ± 0.7	44.7 ± 0.5	44.8 ± 1.0
	3	21.0 ± 0.3	45.3 ± 0.7###	44.6 ± 1.0	43.8 ± 0.9	44.7 ± 1.2
	4	20.9 ± 0.4	45.5 ± 1.0###	44.1 ± 0.8	45.4 ± 0.9	45.4 ± 1.1
	5	21.0 ± 0.3	47.7 ± 0.9###	44.0 ± 0.8*	46.1 ± 0.9	45.9 ± 1.1
	6	21.8 ± 0.3	52.4 ± 0.9###	46.6 ± 0.9**	50.6 ± 0.7	47.1 ± 1.4*
	7	21.6 ± 0.3	53.6 ± 0.6###	48.9 ± 1.2*	49.0 ± 1.0*	48.4 ± 1.5*
	8	22.0 ± 0.3	54.7 ± 0.6###	50.1 ± 1.1**	49.5 ± 1.2*	49.0 ± 1.7*
	9	21.9 ± 0.6	55.9 ± 0.5###	52.6 ± 0.3**	50.8 ± 1.4*	48.3 ± 2.1*
Organ indices (%)	Kidney	1.28 ± 0.03	0.69 ± 0.02###	0.78 ± 0.03*	0.80 ± 0.07	0.85 ± 0.05*
	Spleen	0.34 ± 0.06	0.14 ± 0.03###	0.14 ± 0.01	0.21 ± 0.06**	0.20 ± 0.08*
	Liver	4.04 ± 0.12	6.78 ± 0.14###	6.66 ± 0.13	6.52 ± 0.19	6.11 ± 0.11*

*The data were analyzed using a one-way ANOVA and they are expressed as means ± S.E.M. (n = 10). ###$P < 0.001$ vs. db/+ mice; *$P < 0.05$, and **$P < 0.01$ vs. non-treated db/db mice.*

the increased levels of blood glucose ($P < 0.05$, **Figure 1A**). The db/db mice showed significantly elevated levels of GHbA1c and GC and diminished levels of INS in serum, all of which were reversed after administration with Met and AU ($P < 0.05$, **Figures 1B–D**).

The Hypolipidemic and Liver Protective Effects of AU on db/db Mice

Hyperlipoproteinemia is a common complication of DM (33). Compared with vehicle-treated db/db mice, serum TG and TC levels were significantly decreased ($P < 0.05$, **Figures 2A,B**); while the serum HDL-C concentration was increased ($P < 0.05$, **Figure 2C**) after 8 weeks of AU treatment.

The liver plays a significant role in blood glucose homeostasis, lipid metabolism, and glucose storage (34). ALT and AST, which remain at high levels in diabetes patients, reflect the impaired liver function (35). Similar to Meet, the 8-week AU treatment resulted in 11.2 and 14.0% reductions in the serum levels of ALT and AST, respectively ($P < 0.05$, **Figures 2D,E**).

Gluconeogenesis is one of the major pathways for the production of endogenous glucose. PEPCK and G-6-Pase are two rate-limiting enzymes that regulate hepatic gluconeogenesis (36). Compared with the db/+ mice, enhanced levels of PEPCK, and G-6-Pase ($P < 0.001$, **Figures 2F,G**) were observed in the db/db mice, which were suppressed by Met and AU ($P < 0.05$, **Figures 2F,G**). AU enhanced hepatic glycogen levels by >94.1% in db/db mice ($P < 0.01$, **Figure 2H**). AU and Met improved vacuolar degeneration of hepatocytes in the db/db mice in pathological examinations, further confirming their hepatoprotective effects (**Figure 2I**).

The Renal Protection of AU on db/db Mice

As a specific and sensitive index of renal tubular damage (37), the high levels of NAG in urine were significantly reduced by AU in the db/db mice ($P < 0.01$; **Figure 3A**). Furthermore, 8 weeks of AU administration resulted in an 11.5% increment in serum levels of G-CSF ($P < 0.05$, **Figure 3B**), a 36.6% reduction in renal levels of MAU/ALB ($P < 0.01$, **Figure 3C**), and a 21.2% reduction in renal levels of 6-keto-PGF1α ($P < 0.05$, **Figure 3D**). Meanwhile, AU at 0.1 g/kg enhanced the renal levels of MMP-9 by 38.5% ($P < 0.05$, **Figure 3E**) in the db/db mice.

The tubulointerstitial and glomerular damage caused by DN is closely related to inflammatory cytokines (12). Among the detected inflammatory cytokines, 8 weeks of AU administration resulted in a reduction of >28.9% in IL-2 levels and an increment of >24.2% in IL-10 levels in the kidney of the db/db mice ($P < 0.05$, **Figures 3F,G**).

The renal protective effect of AU was further confirmed by the H&E and PAS staining. The neutrophil infiltrations in renal papillae, inflammatory cell infiltrations, and thickened basement membrane of renal tubular epithelial cells in the db/db mice were all improved by 8 weeks of AU and Met administration (**Figures 3H,I**). Encouragingly, AU had no effect on the organ structures of the spleen, indicating its safe use in animals (**Figure S2**).

Antioxidative Effects of AU on db/db Mice

The cytokines-related to inflammation and oxidative stress in the kidneys of db/db mice treated with AU were systematically screened using high-throughput renal antibody chip analysis. Among the 26 detected cytokines, AU influenced the levels of HSP27, HSP60, HSP70, and SOD2 oxidative stress-related cytokines in the kidney (**Figure S3** and **Table S2**). The overproduction of superoxide induced by hyperglycemia leads to cellular damage, which can be equilibrated by the activities of antioxidant and redox factors (38). Based on the results of the cytokine array assay and ELISA detection, the underproduction of CAT, GSH-Px, and SOD were noted in the kidneys of the db/db mice ($P < 0.05$, **Table 4**), all of which were significantly enhanced by Met and AU administration ($P < 0.05$, **Table 4**). Eight weeks of AU administration resulted in a >26.6% reduction in ROS levels in the kidneys of the db/db mice ($P < 0.05$, **Table 4**). AU also enhanced the serum levels of CAT, GSH-Px, and SOD in the db/db mice ($P < 0.05$, **Figure S4**).

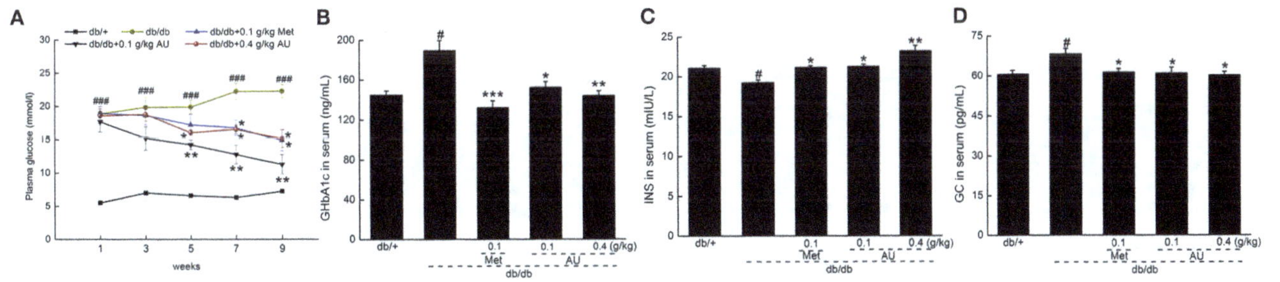

FIGURE 1 | The hypoglycemic effect of AU on db/db mice. **(A)** AU reduced the fasting plasma glucose in db/db mice. AU regulated the serum levels of **(B)** GHbA1c, **(C)** INS, and **(D)** GC in db/db mice after 8 week administration. The data were expressed as means ± S.E.M. ($n = 10$) and analyzed using a one-way ANOVA. # $P < 0.05$ vs. db/+ mice, ### $P < 0.001$ vs. db/+ mice, *$P < 0.05$, **$P < 0.01$ and ***$P < 0.001$ vs. non-treated db/db mice. GHbA1c, glycated hemoglobin A1c; INS, insulin; GC, glucagon.

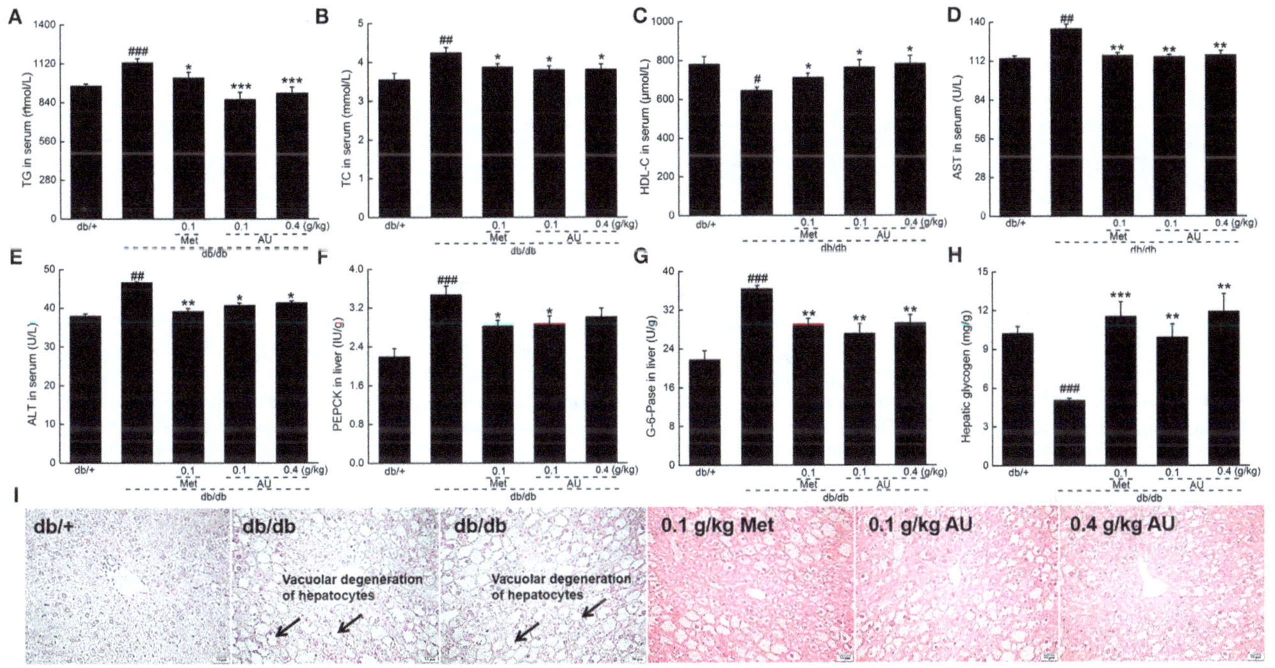

FIGURE 2 | The hypolipidemic and liver protective effects of AU on db/db mice. AU regulated the serum levels of **(A)** TG, **(B)** TC, **(C)** HDL-C, **(D)** AST, and **(E)** ALT in db/db mice. AU reduced the levels of **(F)** PEPCK and **(G)** G-6-Pase in liver and enhanced the levels of **(H)** hepatic glycogen in db/db mice. The data were expressed as means ± S.E.M. ($n = 10$) and analyzed using a one way ANOVA. #$P < 0.05$, ##$P < 0.01$, and ###$P < 0.001$ vs. db/+ mice, *$P < 0.05$, **$P < 0.01$, and *** $P < 0.001$ vs. non-treated db/db mice. **(I)** Histopathological analysis in liver via H&E staining (scale bar: 50 μm; magnification: 200×). TG, triglyceride; TC, total cholesterol; HDL-C, high-density lipoprotein cholesterol; AST, aspartate aminotransferase; ALT, alanine aminotransferase; PEPCK, phosphoenolpyruvate carboxykinase; G-6-Pase, glucose-6-phosphatase; H&E, hematoxylin eosin.

Based on the results of the high-throughput renal antibody chip analysis, we further studied the effects of AU on oxidative stress. Compared with the model mice, the expressions levels of PKC-α, PKC-β2, and p-NF-κB in kidney tissues were significantly downregulated by AU ($P < 0.05$, **Figure 4A**). Met and AU administration increased the expression levels of HSP27, HSP60, and HSP70 by western blot, as a validation of the high-throughput renal antibody chip analysis ($P < 0.05$, **Figure 4B**). The expressions levels of Nrf2, HO-1, HO-2, SOD2, and CAT were significantly upregulated in the kidneys of the db/db mice after 8 weeks of AU administration, indicating its antioxidant activities ($P < 0.05$, **Figure 4C**).

DISCUSSION

AU contains multifarious nutritive materials (7 varieties of mineral, 17 varieties of amino acid, and 16 varieties of fatty acid). Polysaccharides extracted from fungi show various pharmacological activities, including antidiabetic properties (17). Selenium, an essential trace element, helps to prevent diabetes

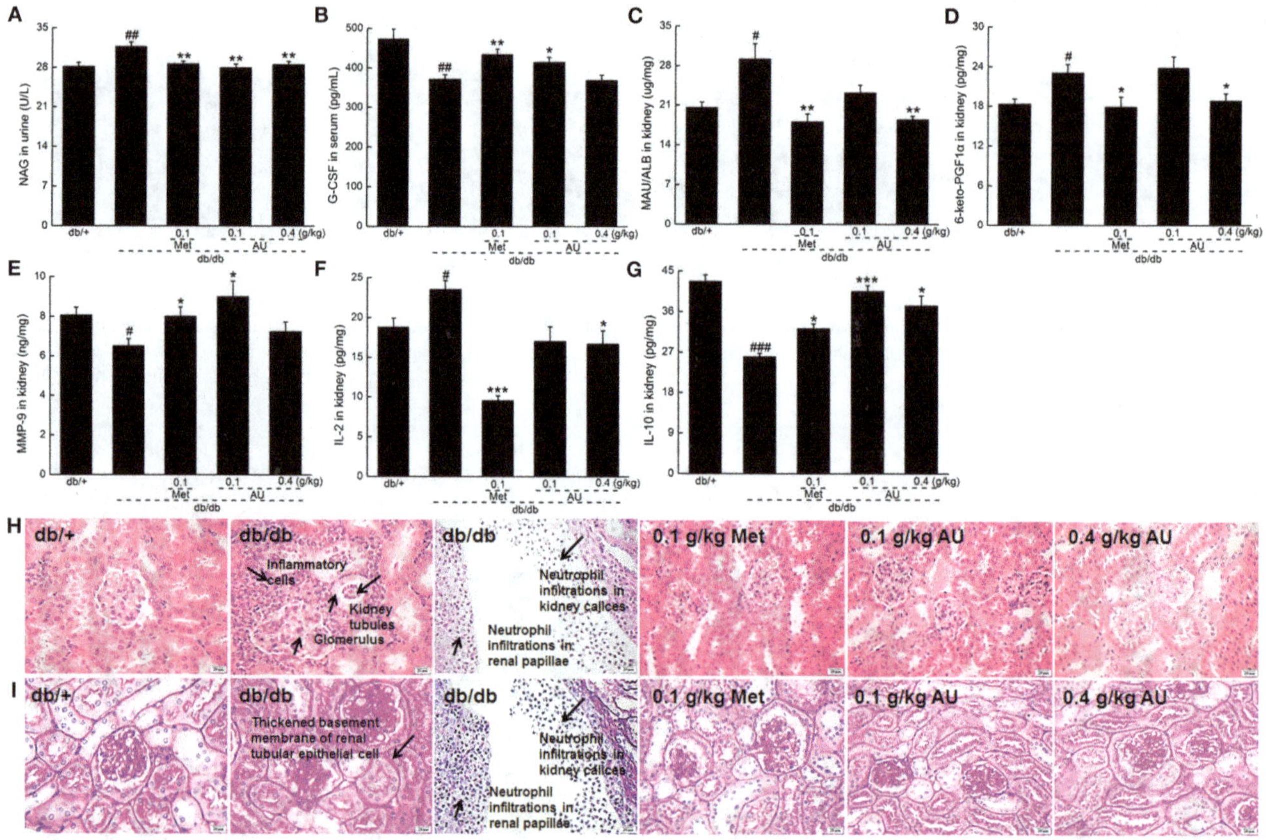

FIGURE 3 | The renal protection of AU via anti-inflammation on db/db mice. **(A)** AU reduced the NAG levels in urine of db/db mice. **(B)** AU enhanced the serum levels of G-CSF in db/db mice. AU reduced the levels of **(C)** MAU/ALB and **(D)** 6-keto-PGF1α and enhanced the levels of **(E)** MMP-9 in kidney of db/db mice. AU reduced the levels of **(F)** IL-2 and enhanced the levels of **(G)** IL-10 in kidney of db/db mice. The data were analyzed using a one-way ANOVA and they are expressed as means ± S.E.M. ($n = 10$). #$P < 0.05$, and ##$P < 0.01$ vs. db/+ mice, ### $P < 0.001$ vs. db/+ mice, *$P < 0.05$, **$P < 0.01$, and ***$P < 0.001$ vs. non-treated db/db mice. Histopathological analysis in kidney via **(H)** H&E staining (scale bar: 20 μm; magnification: 400×) and **(I)** PAS staining (scale bar: 20 μm; magnification: 400×). NAG, N-acetyl-β-D-glucosidase; G-CSF, granulocyte colony-stimulating factor; MAU/ALB, microalbuminuria; 6-keto-PGF1α, 6-keto-prostaglandin F1α; MMP-9, matrix metalloproteinase-9; IL, interleukin; H&E, hematoxylin eosin; PAS, periodic acid Schiff.

TABLE 4 | The effects of AU on oxidative stress related factors in kidney of mice.

	db/+	db/db	0.1 g/kg Met	0.1 g/kg AU	0.4 g/kg AU
CAT (U/mg)	9.0 ± 0.5	7.2 ± 0.3#	8.7 ± 0.6*	10.0 ± 1.1*	8.3 ± 0.4*
GSH-Px (U/mg)	74.3 ± 6.6	44.1 ± 2.1###	53.1 ± 3.9*	65.1 ± 6.3**	58.5 ± 5.3*
SOD (U/mg)	37.0 ± 2.6	25.3 ± 2.1##	32.9 ± 2.7*	35.5 ± 3.3*	34.2 ± 3.4*
ROS (U/mg)	48.6 ± 0.3	66.1 ± 4.9#	41.0 ± 1.8***	48.5 ± 4.8*	44.8 ± 2.3**

*The data were analyzed using a one-way ANOVA and they are expressed as means ± S.E.M. ($n = 10$). #$P < 0.05$, ##$P < 0.01$, and ###$P < 0.001$ vs. db/+ mice; *$P < 0.05$, **$P < 0.01$, and ***$P < 0.001$ vs. non-treated db/db mice. CAT, catalase; GSH-Px, glutathione peroxidase; SOD, superoxide dismutase; ROS, reactive oxygen species.*

effectively via antioxidation (14). Based on the contents of AU and our experimental data, we successfully confirmed that AU exhibited a hypoglycemic effect by reducing blood glucose levels, modulating glucose tolerance, and recovering the serum levels of GHbA1c, GC, and INS. The high level of food intake observed in the db/db mice was strongly reversed by Met and AU. AU appeared to affect glucose metabolism mainly by reducing body weight and altering appetite. Among patients with diabetes, 55–80% have glycogen deposition abnormalities and steatohepatitis in their livers. Patients also showed a decreased entry rate of glucose into peripheral tissues, elevated hepatic glucose production, and gluconeogenesis (39). The glucose disposal and glycogen accumulation stimulated by insulin is an important way of regulating glucose concentration (34). Glycogen, a primary intracellular storable form of glucose, can be produced by gluconeogenesis. PEPCK and G-6-Pase are two rate-limiting enzymes that regulate hepatic gluconeogenesis and accelerate the transformation of glycogen, fat, and protein into glucose. The

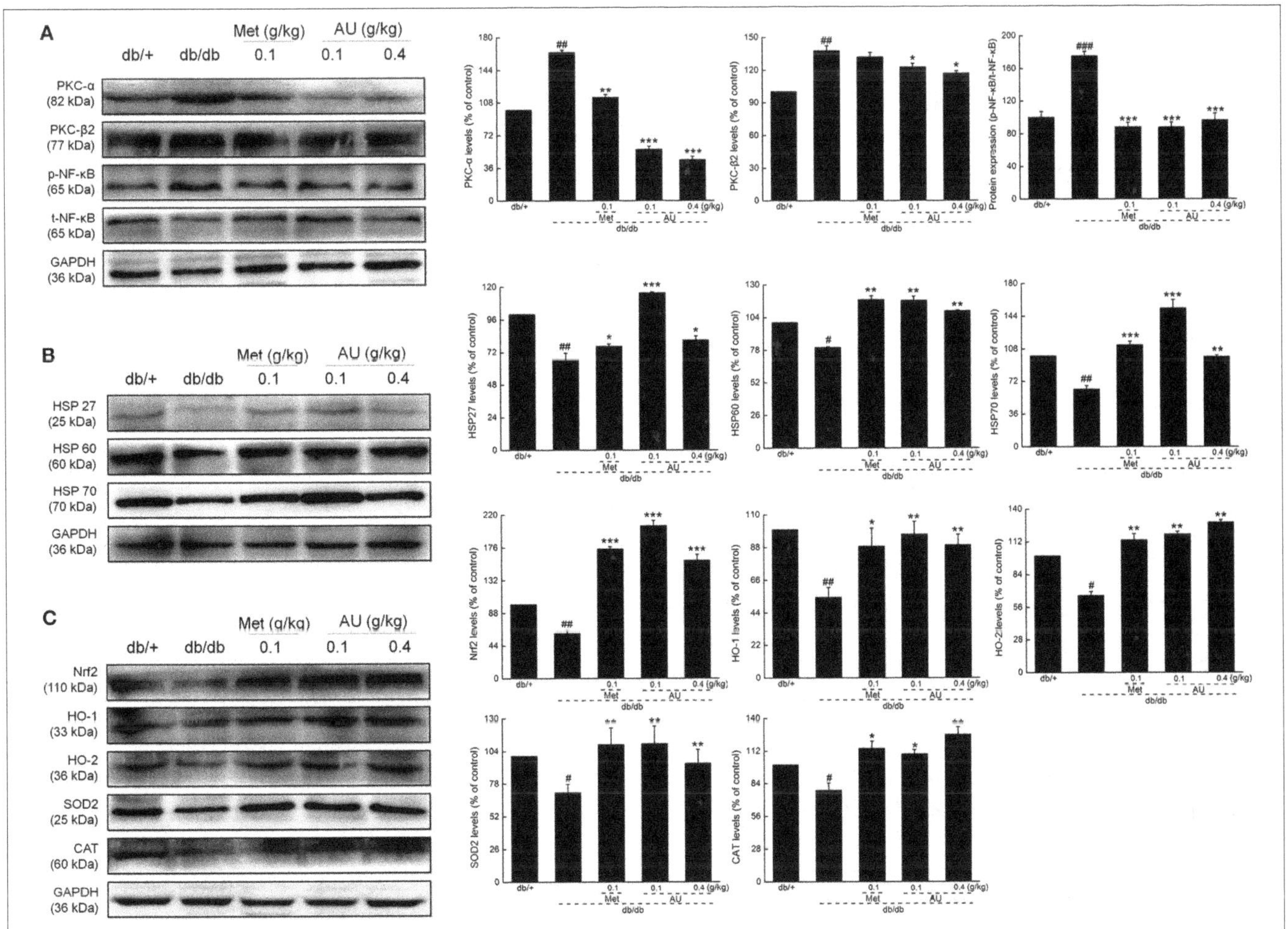

FIGURE 4 | The anti-oxidation and anti-inflammation of AU may be related to Nrf2 signaling. **(A)** AU reduced the expression levels of PKC-α, PKC β2, and p-NF-κB in the kidney of db/db mice. **(B)** AU enhanced the expression levels of HSP26, HSP60, and HSP70 in the kidney of db/db mice. **(C)** AU enhanced the expression levels of Nrf2, HO-1, HO-2, SOD2, and CAT in the kidney of db/db mice. The data on quantified protein expression were normalized to the levels of GAPDH, except for p-NF-κB, which was normalized to the expression levels of t-NF-κB. The data were analyzed using a one-way ANOVA and they are expressed as means ± S.E.M. ($n = 10$). #$P < 0.05$, ##$P < 0.01$, and ###$P < 0.001$ vs. db/+ mice, *$P < 0.05$, **$P < 0.01$, and ***$P < 0.001$ vs. non-treated db/db mice. PKC, protein kinase C; NF-κB, nuclear factor-κB; HSP, heat shock protein; Nrf2, nuclear respiratory factor 2; HO-1, heme oxygenase 1; HO-2, heme oxygenase 2; SOD2, manganese superoxide dismutase 2; CAT, catalase; GAPDH, glyceraldehyde-3-phosphate dehydrogenase.

inhibition of PEPCK and G-6-Pase expression can effectively regulate the increased blood glucose (36, 40), which is consistent with the results of our present study. Lipid peroxidation caused by hyperglycemia induces liver damage in diabetes (41). Insufficient insulin leads to the accumulation of lipids, specifically TG and TC, in hyperglycemic patients, and thus causes diabetes-related complications (42). The accumulation of excessive adipose cells in the liver leads to hepatic steatosis and further fatty liver damage (43). The beneficial effects of AU on lipid metabolism indices and liver structures strongly confirmed its protective effect on the liver in the db/db mice. Combined with hyperglycemia and insulin resistance during the development of DN, oxidative stress, and inflammation are reported to be involved in inducing tubular fibrosis and mesangial expansion (44). The renal protective effect of AU was demonstrated by the down-regulation of the levels of NAG in urine and MAU/ALB in the kidney, and up-regulation of the levels of G-CSF and MMP-9 in the kidney of the db/db mice. Microalbuminuria is an early predictive risk factor for nephropathy, which can lead to abnormalities in the kidney tissues such as nodules and expansions of the mesangium (45). The fibrinolytic activity of MMP-9 plays a beneficial role in preventing crescentic proliferative glomerulonephritis in mice (46). G-CSF reduces pro-inflammatory cytokine expression and prevents the endothelialization of damaged vascular tissue (47), which helps to stop the progression of DN in rats (48).

Intense inflammatory reaction is accompanied by the progression of DN, which can develop into nephritides in the late stage (49). AU increased the levels of IL-2 and IL-10 in the kidneys of db/db mice, further demonstrating its renoprotective effect. Proinflammatory CD4+ cells are activated by the overproduction of IL-2, leading to the deterioration of glomerular damage by recruiting neutrophils (50). As an efficient anti-inflammatory cytokine, IL-10 can improve hyperglycemia, and insulin resistance (51). NF-κB signaling is exacerbated in the glomeruli and renal tubes in patients with DN, and regulates the expression of inflammatory mediators and proinflammatory cytokines (10, 52). Hyperglycemia in diabetes leads to the activation of PKC, which further enhances the activation of NF-κB (53). The renal protection of AU in db/db mice may be partially related to its anti-inflammatory effects via the regulation of NF-κB signaling.

Hyperglycemia and lipotoxicity, a state induced by dyslipidemia, lead to renal injury due to oxidative stress through the production of excess ROS (54). Oxidative stress triggers inflammatory reactions, such as basement membrane thickening and inflammatory cell infiltration, by activating NF-κB signaling, and finally exacerbates kidney damage in DN (49, 55). On the one hand, heat shock proteins (HSPs) contribute to protein homeostasis, accelerate regeneration, and minimize injury, thus protecting cells against various stressors such as oxidative stress as part of the defense system (56). Alternatively, oxidative damage can be prevented by enhancing the activities of antioxidant enzymes including CAT, GSH-Px, and SOD, which strengthen the response of the antioxidant defense system (57). SOD catalyzes the translation of superoxide radicals into hydrogen peroxide, which is then decomposed into oxygen and water by CAT, thus preventing the accumulation of ROS (58). AU successfully regulated Nrf2 and its downstream targets. Nrf2 can neutralize ROS by activating and regulating intracellular antioxidant effects (59). Preventing the degradation of Nrf2 resulted in the transcription of downstream antioxidant enzymes such as HO-1 and SOD (60). Evidence suggests that Nrf2-dependent ARE activation influences the upregulation of HSPs such as HSP70 (61). The antidiabetic and antinephritic activities of AU in db/db mice may be partially related to its anti-oxidative and anti-inflammatory activities via Nrf2 signaling. However, more experiments need to be performed to prove Nrf2 is a downstream effector of AU to perform antioxidative effects.

There were some limitations to our present study. High-throughput renal antibody chip analysis shows that AU influences the levels of apoptosis-related cytokines in kidneys, which we failed to detect in the present study. We will further investigate the anti-apoptotic effects of AU as part of its renal protection effect in db/db mice. Although we detected the main components of the albino mutant strain of *A. cornea*, based on the present results, we are still hard to conclude which compounds cause the antidiabetic and antinephritic activities. In our ongoing experiments, we have already separated the polysaccharides from the albino mutant strain of *A. cornea*, which showed hyperglycemic effects in db/db mice. We will further study whether the polysaccharides are responsible for these effects in AU. Furthermore, we only proved that AU attenuated diabetes and its following kidney oxidative pressure and inflammation. However, AU's pharmacological effect at macroalbuminuria stage still needs further investigation.

In conclusion, the anti-diabetic and anti- nephritic effects of AU and its possible anti-oxidation and anti-inflammation mechanisms-possible related to Nrf2 signaling- were explored in db/db diabetic models.

ETHICS STATEMENT

The experimental animal protocol was approved by the Animal Ethics Committee of Jilin University (20170301). All efforts were carried out on the basis of the recommendations of Laboratory Animal Care and Use, which were made to reduce the use of animals and minimize animal distress. The male db/db mice and wild db/+ littermates in a C57BLKs/J background [8 weeks, SCXK (Su) 2015-0001] were purchased from the Nanjing Biomedical Research Institute of Nanjing University (Nanjing, China). Animals were housed at the temperature of 23 ± 1°C and humidity of 60% with a 12-h light-dark cycle (lights on 07:00–19:00) and free access to food and water.

AUTHOR CONTRIBUTIONS

XL and YuL: conceptualization. XJ, ST, YZ, and YaL: experiment and result. DW and XJ: article writing. All authors listed have made a substantial, direct and intellectual contribution to the work, and approved it for publication.

FUNDING

This work was supported by the Special Fund for Agro-scientific Research in the Public Interest (No. 201503137), the Science and Technology Bureau of Changchun (No.15SS11), the Key Scientific and Technological Project of Jilin Province in China (Grant No. YYZX201609), and the Special Projects of the Cooperation between Jilin University and Jilin Province of China (Grant No. SXGJSF2017-1).

REFERENCES

1. Saha MR, Dey P, Sarkar I, De Sarker D, Haldar B, Chaudhuri TK, et al. Acacia nilotica leaf improves insulin resistance and hyperglycemia associated acute hepatic injury and nephrotoxicity by improving systemic antioxidant status in diabetic mice. *J Ethnopharmacol.* (2018) 210:275–86. doi: 10.1016/j.jep.2017.08.036
2. Borgohain MP, Chowdhury L, Ahmed S, Bolshette N, Devasani K, Das TJ, et al. Renoprotective and antioxidative effects of methanolic *Paederia foetida* leaf extract on experimental diabetic nephropathy in rats. *J Ethnopharmacol.* (2017) 198:451–9. doi: 10.1016/j.jep.2017.01.035
3. Foster SR, Dilworth LL, Omoruyi FO, Thompson R, Alexander-Lindo RL. Pancreatic and renal function in streptozotocin-induced type 2 diabetic rats administered combined inositol hexakisphosphate and inositol supplement.

Biomed Pharmacother. (2017) 96:72–7. doi: 10.1016/j.biopha.2017.09.126

4. Yuan D, Liu XM, Fang Z, Du LL, Chang J, Lin SH. Protective effect of resveratrol on kidney in rats with diabetic nephropathy and its effect on endoplasmic reticulum stress. *Eur Rev Med Pharmaco.* (2018) 22:1485–93. doi: 10.26355/eurrev_201803_14497
5. Cui Y, Shi Y, Bao Y, Wang S, Hua Q, Liu Y. Zingerone attenuates diabetic nephropathy through inhibition of nicotinamide adenine dinucleotide phosphate oxidase 4. *Biomed Pharmacother.* (2018) 99:422–30. doi: 10.1016/j.biopha.2018.01.051
6. Krishan P, Singh G, Bedi O. Carbohydrate restriction ameliorates nephropathy by reducing oxidative stress and upregulating HIF-1alpha levels in type-1 diabetic rats. *J Diabetes Metab Disord.* (2017) 16:47. doi: 10.1186/s40200-017-0331-5
7. Hu X, Zhang X, Jin G, Shi Z, Sun W, Chen F. Geniposide reduces development of streptozotocin-induced diabetic nephropathy via regulating nuclear factor-kappa B signaling pathways. *Fundamen Clini Pharmacol.* (2017) 31:54–63. doi: 10.1111/fcp.12231
8. Ha Kim K, Sadikot RT, Yeon Lee J, Jeong HS, Oh YK, Blackwell TS, et al. Suppressed ubiquitination of Nrf2 by p47(phox) contributes to Nrf2 activation. *Free Rad Biol Med.* (2017) 113:48–58. doi: 10.1016/j.freeradbiomed.2017.09.011
9. Guo W, Tian D, Jia Y, Huang W, Jiang M, Wang J, et al. MDM2 controls NRF2 antioxidant activity in prevention of diabetic kidney disease. *Biochim Biophys Acta.* (2018) 1865:1034–45. doi: 10.1016/j.bbamcr.2018.04.011
10. Lee H, Lim Y. Tocotrienol-rich fraction supplementation reduces hyperglycemia-induced skeletal muscle damage through regulation of insulin signaling and oxidative stress in type 2 diabetic mice. *J Nutr Biochem.* (2018) 57:77–85. doi: 10.1016/j.jnutbio.2018.03.016
11. Moniruzzaman M, Ghosal I, Das D, Chakraborty SB. Melatonin ameliorates H2O2-induced oxidative stress through modulation of Erk/Akt/NFkB pathway. *Biol Res.* (2018) 51:17. doi: 10.1186/s40659-018-0168-5
12. Ding L, Lu S, Wang Y, Chen H, Long W, Ma C, et al. BPI-3016, a novel long-acting hGLP-1 analogue for the treatment of Type 2 diabetes mellitus. *Pharmacol Res.* (2017) 122:130–9. doi: 10.1016/j.phrs.2017.05.007
13. Liu C-W, WangY-C, Hsieha C-C, Lu H-C, Chiang D-C. Guava (*Psidium guajava* Linn.) leaf extract promotes glucose uptake and glycogen accumulation by modulating the insulin signaling pathway in high-glucose-induced insulin-resistant mouse FL83B cells. *Process Biochem.* (2015) 50:1128–35. doi: 10.1016/j.procbio.2015.03.022
14. Liu Y, You Y, Li Y, Zhang L, Yin L, Shen Y, et al. The characterization, selenylation, and antidiabetic activity of mycelial polysaccharides from Catathelasma ventricosum. *Carbohydr Polym.* (2017) 174:72–81. doi: 10.1016/j.carbpol.2017.06.050
15. Dong Y, Jing T, Meng Q, Liu C, Hu S, Ma Y, et al. Studies on the antidiabetic activities of *Cordyceps militaris* extract in diet-streptozotocin-induced diabetic Sprague-Dawley rats. *BioMed Res Int.* (2014) 2014:160980. doi: 10.1155/2014/160980
16. Wang J, Teng L, Liu Y, Hu W, Chen W, Hu X, et al. Studies on the antidiabetic and antinephritic activities of paecilomyces hepiali water extract in diet-streptozotocin-induced diabetic sprague dawley rats. *J Diabetes Res.* (2016) 2016:4368380. doi: 10.1155/2016/4368380
17. Wang J, Hu W, Li L, Huang X, Liu Y, Wang D, et al. Antidiabetic activities of polysaccharides separated from Inonotus obliquus via the modulation of oxidative stress in mice with streptozotocin-induced diabetes. *PLoS ONE.* (2017) 12:e0180476. doi: 10.1371/journal.pone.0180476
18. Cao Yuchun BH, Li Xiao, Bau T, Li Yu. Anti-tumor activities of *Auricularia cornea* fruiting body extract in H22 bearing mice. *Mycosystema.* (2017) 36:10. doi: 10.13346/j.mycosystema.160243
19. Senturk B, Demircan BM, Ozkan AD, Tohumeken S, Delibasi T, Guler MO, et al. Diabetic wound regeneration using heparin-mimetic peptide amphiphile gel in db/db mice. *Biomater Sci.* (2017) 5:1293–303. doi: 10.1039/C7BM00251C
20. Sáez-Plaza P, Michałowski T, Navas MJ, Asuero AG, Wybraniec S. An overview of the kjeldahl method of nitrogen determination. part early history I, chemistry of the procedure, and titrimetric finish. *Criti Rev Anal Chem.* (2013) 43:178–223. doi: 10.1080/10408347.2012.751786
21. Chow PS, Landhausser SM. A method for routine measurements of total sugar and starch content in woody plant tissues. *Tree Physiol.* (2004) 24:1129–36. doi: 10.1093/treephys/24.10.1129
22. Xue P, Zhao Y, Wen C, Cheng S, Lin S. Effects of electron beam irradiation on physicochemical properties of corn flour and improvement of the gelatinization inhibition. *Food Chem.* (2017) 233:467–75. doi: 10.1016/j.foodchem.2017.04.152
23. De Santiago E, Dominguez-Fernandez M, Cid C, De Pena MP. Impact of cooking process on nutritional composition and antioxidants of cactus cladodes (*Opuntia ficus-indica*). *Food Chem.* (2018) 240:1055–62. doi: 10.1016/j.foodchem.2017.08.039
24. Jurak E, Punt AM, Arts W, Kabel MA, Gruppen H. Fate of carbohydrates and lignin during composting and mycelium growth of *Agaricus bisporus* on wheat straw based compost. *PLoS ONE.* (2015) 10:e0138909. doi: 10.1371/journal.pone.0138909
25. Tesfaye T, Sithole B, Ramjugernath D, Chunilall V. Valorisation of chicken feathers: characterisation of chemical properties. *Waste Manage.* (2017) 68:626–35. doi: 10.1016/j.wasman.2017.06.050
26. Zhao C, Zhao X, Zhang J, Zou W, Zhang Y, Li L. Screening of bacillus strains from sun vinegar for efficient production of flavonoid and phenol. *Indian J Microbiol.* (2016) 56:498–503. doi: 10.1007/s12088-016-0602-8
27. Chen B, Ke B, Ye L, Jin S, Jie F, Zhao L, et al. Isolation and varietal characterization of *Ganoderma* resinaceum from areas of *Ganoderma lucidum* production in China. *Sci Hortic.* (2017) 224:109–14. doi: 10.1016/j.scienta.2017.06.002
28. Wang X, Wang X, Guo Y. Rapidly simultaneous determination of six effective components in cistanche tubulosa by near infrared spectroscopy. *Molecules.* (2017) 22:843. doi: 10.3390/molecules22050843
29. Massouras T, Triantaphyllopoulos KA, Theodossiou I. Chemical composition, protein fraction and fatty acid profile of donkey milk during lactation. *Int Dairy J.* (2017) 75:83–90. doi: 10.1016/j.idairyj.2017.06.007
30. Wang YQ, Ye DQ, Zhu BQ, Wu GF, Duan CQ. Rapid HPLC analysis of amino acids and biogenic amines in wines during fermentation and evaluation of matrix effect. *Food Chem.* (2014) 163:6–15. doi: 10.1016/j.foodchem.2014.04.064
31. Peyton DP, Healy MG, Fleming GTA, Grant J, Wall D, Morrison L, et al. Nutrient, metal and microbial loss in surface runoff following treated sludge and dairy cattle slurry application to an Irish grassland soil. *Sci Total Environ.* (2016) 541:218–229. doi: 10.1016/j.scitotenv.2015.09.053
32. Santos WPC, Ribeiro NM, Santos D, Korn GAM, Lopes MV. Bioaccessibility assessment of toxic and essential elements in produced pulses, Bahia, Brazil. *Food Chem.* (2018) 240:112–22. doi: 10.1016/j.foodchem.2017.07.051
33. Yu J, Cui P-J, Zeng W-L, Xie X-L, Liang W-J, Lin G-B, et al. Protective effect of selenium-polysaccharides from the mycelia of *Coprinus comatus* on alloxan-induced oxidative stress in mice. *Food Chem.* (2009) 117:42–7. doi: 10.1016/j.foodchem.2009.03.073
34. Shen SC, Cheng FC, Wu NJ. Effect of guava (*Psidium guajava* Linn.) leaf soluble solids on glucose metabolism in type 2 diabetic rats. *Phytother Res.* (2008) 22:1458–64. doi: 10.1002/ptr.2476
35. Karim N, Jeenduang N, Tangpong J. Anti-glycemic and anti-hepatotoxic effects of mangosteen vinegar rind from garcinia mangostana against HFD/STZ-induced type II diabetes in mice. *Pol J Food Nutr Sci.* (2018) 68:163–9. doi: 10.1515/pjfns-2017-0018
36. Cui X, Qian DW, Jiang S, Shang EX, Zhu ZH, Duan JA. Scutellariae radix and coptidis rhizoma improve glucose and lipid metabolism in T2DM rats via regulation of the metabolic profiling and MAPK/PI3K/Akt signaling pathway. *Int J Mol Sci.* (2018) 19:3634. doi: 10.3390/ijms19113634
37. El-Ashmawy NE, Khedr EG, El-Bahrawy HA, El-Berashy SA. Effect of human umbilical cord blood-derived mononuclear cells on diabetic nephropathy in rats. *Biomed Pharmacother.* (2017) 97:1040–5. doi: 10.1016/j.biopha.2017.10.151
38. Noratto GD, Chew BP, Atienza LM. Red raspberry (*Rubus idaeus* L.) intake decreases oxidative stress in obese diabetic (db/db) mice. *Food Chem.* (2017) 227:305–14. doi: 10.1016/j.foodchem.2017.01.097
39. Abdel-Moneim A, El-Twab SMA, Yousef AI, Reheim ESA, Ashour MB. Modulation of hyperglycemia and dyslipidemia in experimental type 2 diabetes by gallic acid and p-coumaric acid: the role of

adipocytokines and PPARgamma. *Biomed Pharmacother.* (2018) 105:1091–7. doi: 10.1016/j.biopha.2018.06.096

40. Guo Y, Dai R, Deng Y, Sun L, Meng S, Xin N. Hypoglycemic activity of the extracts of Belamcanda chinensis leaves (BCLE) on KK-A(y) mice. *Biomed Pharmacother.* (2018) 110:449–55. doi: 10.1016/j.biopha.2018.11.094
41. Taghizadeh M, Rashidi AA, Taherian AA, Vakili Z, Mehran M. The protective effect of hydroalcoholic extract of rosa canina (Dog Rose) fruit on liver function and structure in streptozotocin-induced diabetes in rats. *J Dietary Suppl.* (2018) 15:624–35. doi: 10.1080/19390211.2017.1369205
42. Palazhy S, Viswanathan V. Lipid abnormalities in type 2 diabetes mellitus patients with overt nephropathy. *Diabetes Metab J.* (2017) 41:128–34. doi: 10.4093/dmj.2017.41.2.128
43. Elaidy SM, Hussain MA, El-Kherbetawy MK. Time-dependent therapeutic roles of nitazoxanide on high-fat diet/streptozotocin-induced diabetes in rats: effects on hepatic peroxisome proliferator-activated receptor-gamma receptors. *Can J Physiol Pharmacol.* (2018) 96:485–97. doi: 10.1139/cjpp-2017-0533
44. Mima A. Renal protection by sodium-glucose cotransporter 2 inhibitors and its underlying mechanisms in diabetic kidney disease. *J Diabetes Compl.* (2018) 32:720–5. doi: 10.1016/j.jdiacomp.2018.04.011
45. Hieshima K, Suzuki T, Sugiyama S, Kurinami N, Yoshida A, Miyamoto F, et al. Smoking cessation ameliorates microalbuminuria with reduction of blood pressure and pulse rate in patients with already diagnosed diabetes mellitus. *J Clini Med Res.* (2018) 10:478–85. doi: 10.14740/jocmr3400w
46. Lelongt B, Bengatta S, Delauche M, Lund LR, Werb Z, Ronco PM. Matrix metalloproteinase 9 protects mice from anti–glomerular basement membrane nephritis through its fibrinolytic activity. *J Exp Med.* (2001) 193:793–802. doi: 10.1084/jem.193.7.793
47. Gong J-H, Dong J-Y, Xie T, Lu S-L. Influence of high glucose and AGE environment on the proliferation, apoptosis, paracrine effects, and cytokine expression of human adipose stem cells *in vitro*. *Int J Diabetes Dev Countr.* (2017) 38:228–37. doi: 10.1007/s13410-017-0574-1
48. So BI, Song YS, Fang CH, Park JY, Lee Y, Shin JH, et al. G-CSF prevents progression of diabetic nephropathy in rat. *PLoS ONE.* (2013) 8:e38493. doi: 10.1371/journal.pone.0077048
49. Xu HL, Wang XT, Cheng Y, Zhao JG, Zhou YJ, Yang JJ, et al. Ursolic acid improves diabetic nephropathy via suppression of oxidative stress and inflammation in streptozotocin-induced rats. *Biomed Pharmacother.* (2018) 105:915–21. doi: 10.1016/j.biopha.2018.06.055
50. Bertelli R, Di Donato A, Cioni M, Grassi F, Ikehata M, Bonanni A, et al. LPS nephropathy in mice is ameliorated by IL-2 independently of regulatory T cells activity. *PLoS ONE.* (2014) 9:e111285. doi: 10.1371/journal.pone.0111285
51. Denys A, Udalova IA, Smith C, Williams LM, Ciesielski CJ, Campbell J, et al. Evidence for a dual mechanism for IL-10 suppression of TNF- production that does not involve inhibition of p38 mitogen-activated protein kinase or NF- B in primary human macrophages. *J Immunol.* (2002) 168:4837–45. doi: 10.4049/jimmunol.168.10.4837
52. Mousum SA, Ahmed S, Gawali B, Kwatra M, Ahmed A, Lahkar M. Nyctanthes arbor-tristis leaf extract ameliorates hyperlipidemia- and hyperglycemia-associated nephrotoxicity by improving anti-oxidant and anti-inflammatory status in high-fat diet-streptozotocin-induced diabetic rats. *Inflammopharmacology.* (2018) 26:1415–28. doi: 10.1007/s10787-018-0497-6
53. Hamzawy M, Gouda SAA, Rashid L, Attia Morcos M, Shoukry H, Sharawy N. The cellular selection between apoptosis and autophagy: roles of vitamin D, glucose and immune response in diabetic nephropathy. *Endocrine.* (2017) 58:66–80. doi: 10.1007/s12020-017-1402-6
54. Shao M, Lu X, Cong W, Xing X, Tan Y, Li Y, et al. Multiple low-dose radiation prevents type 2 diabetes-induced renal damage through attenuation of dyslipidemia and insulin resistance and subsequent renal inflammation and oxidative stress. *PLoS ONE.* (2014) 9:e92574. doi: 10.1371/journal.pone.0092574
55. Gargouri B, Bhatia HS, Bouchard M, Fiebich BL, Fetoui H. Inflammatory and oxidative mechanisms potentiate bifenthrin-induced neurological alterations and anxiety-like behavior in adult rats. *Toxicol Lett.* (2018) 294:73–86. doi: 10.1016/j.toxlet.2018.05.020
56. Lappalainen J, Oksala NKJ, Laaksonen DE, Khanna S, Kokkola T, Kaarniranta K, et al. Suppressed heat shock protein response in the kidney of exercise-trained diabetic rats. *Scand J Med Sci Sports.* (2018) 28:1808–17. doi: 10.1111/sms.13079
57. Singh P, Prasad SM. Antioxidant enzyme responses to the oxidative stress due to chlorpyrifos, dimethoate and dieldrin stress in palak (*Spinacia oleracea* L.) and their toxicity alleviation by soil amendments in tropical croplands. *Sci Total Environ.* (2018) 630:839–48. doi: 10.1016/j.scitotenv.2018.02.203
58. Zhang C, Zhang L, Liu H, Zhang J, Hu C, Jia L. Antioxidation, anti-hyperglycaemia and renoprotective effects of extracellular polysaccharides from *Pleurotus eryngii* SI-04. *Int J Biol Macromol.* (2018) 111:219–28. doi: 10.1016/j.ijbiomac.2018.01.009
59. Lin YC, Chang YH, Yang SY, Wu KD, Chu TS. Update of pathophysiology and management of diabetic kidney disease. *J Formosan Med Assoc.* (2018) 117:662–75. doi: 10.1016/j.jfma.2018.02.007
60. Giribabu N, Karim K, Kilari EK, Salleh N. *Phyllanthus niruri* leaves aqueous extract improves kidney functions, ameliorates kidney oxidative stress, inflammation, fibrosis, and apoptosis and enhances kidney cell proliferation in adult male rats with diabetes mellitus. *J Ethnopharmacol.* (2017) 205:123–37. doi: 10.1016/j.jep.2017.05.002
61. Alani B, Salehi R, Sadeghi P, Khodagholi F, Digaleh H, Jabbarzadeh-Tabrizi S, et al. Silencing of Hsp70 intensifies 6-OHDA-induced apoptosis and Hsp90 upregulation in PC12 cells. *J Mol Neurosci.* (2015) 55:174–83. doi: 10.1007/s12031-014-0298-3

17

Macrophage Lysophosphatidylcholine Acyltransferase 3 Deficiency-Mediated Inflammation is not Sufficient to Induce Atherosclerosis in a Mouse Model

Hui Jiang [1,2], *Zhiqiang Li* [1,2], *Chongmin Huan* [1,2,3] *and Xian-Cheng Jiang* [1,2*]

[1] Department of Cell Biology, State University of New York Downstate Medical Center, Brooklyn, NY, United States,
[2] Molecular and Cellular Cardiology Program, VA New York Harbor Healthcare System, Brooklyn, NY, United States,
[3] Department of Surgery, State University of New York Downstate Medical Center, Brooklyn, NY, United States

***Correspondence:**
Xian-Cheng Jiang
XJiang@downstate.edu

Mammalian cell membrane phosphatidylcholines (PCs), the major phospholipids, exhibit diversity which is controlled by Lands' cycle or PC remodeling pathway. Lysophosphatidylcholine acyltransferase (LPCAT) is one of the major players in the pathway and plays an important role in maintaining cell membrane structure and function. LPCAT3 is highly expressed in macrophages, however, its role in mediating inflammation is still not understood, since contradictory results were reported previously. The order of LPCAT mRNA levels in mouse macrophages is as follows: LPCAT3 > LPCAT1 > LPCAT2 >> LPCAT4. In order to investigate the role of *LPCAT3* in macrophages, we prepared myeloid cell-specific *Lpcat3* knockout (KO) mice and found that the deficiency significantly reduced certain polyunsaturated phosphatidylcholines, such as 16:0/20:4, 18:1/18:2, 18:0/20:4, and 18:1/20:4 in macrophage plasma membrane. *Lpcat3* deficiency significantly increased toll like receptor 4 protein and phosphorylated c-Src in membrane lipid rafts, and increased LPS-induced IL-6 and TNFα releasing through activation of MAP kinases and NFκB. Moreover, the ablation of LPCAT3 in macrophages significantly increase of M1 macrophages. However, macrophage deletion of *Lpcat3* in (LDL receptor) *Ldlr* KO mice, both male and female, on a Western type diet, did not have a significant impact on atherogenesis. In conclusion, LPCAT3 is one of LPCATs in macrophages, involved in PC remodeling. LPCAT3 deficiency has no effect on cholesterol efflux. However, the deficiency promotes macrophage inflammatory response, but such an effect has a marginal influence on the development of atherosclerosis.

Keywords: lysophosphatidylcholine acyltransferase 3 (LPCAT3), phosphatidylcholine remodeling, macrophage Lpcat3 gene knockout mice, inflammation, atherosclerosis

INTRODUCTION

Phosphatidylcholines (PCs), the major phospholipids, on mammalian cell membrane exhibit structural diversity (1, 2). Polyunsaturated PCs ensure the fluidity of cell membrane. In macrophages, the plasma membrane provides a platform that mediates inflammation. lipopolysaccharide (LPS) or peptidoglycan treatment promotes the assembly of the toll like receptor (TLR) complex in lipid rafts (3–5). We found that a decrease in macrophage plasma membrane sphingomyelin level can effectively prevent inflammatory responses by reducing TLR4 expression (6–8), thus decreasing atherosclerosis (6, 7, 9). It is also reported that cellular lipids are important regulators of c-Scr activation by altering the recruitment of C-Scr to the plasma membrane (10) and many studies also have shown a critical role for c-Src in macrophage-mediated inflammatory responses (11). It is known that the composition of polyunsaturated PCs in membranes is regulated by LPCATs (12–14).

There are four isoforms for LPCAT (13, 15–18). The major isoform in the liver and macrophage is LPCAT3 (14, 18–20). LPCAT3 exhibits an acyl donor preference toward polyunsaturated fatty acid-CoA molecules like arachidonoyl-CoA (18, 21). Modifications of polyunsaturated PC composition on cell membrane have an impact on many biological processes (22–27). We found that *Lpcat3* deficiency significantly reduces polyunsaturated PCs on the hepatocytes and enterocytes and impacts plasma lipid metabolism (28).

The development of atherosclerosis is closely related with inflammation. Macrophage-derived foam cells in the vessel wall can produce many pro-inflammatory chemokines and cytokines (29) which promote atherogenesis. Previously, one study showed that *Lpcat3* silencing significantly increased LPS-mediated inflammatory response in macrophages and this could be due to the decrease of macrophage membrane polyunsaturated PCs (14). On the contrary, another study indicated that *Lpcat3* silencing did not influence macrophage LPS-induced inflammatory response, although PC composition changes were also observed (19). We still do not understand the discrepancy of both studies and still do not know whether PC remodeling in macrophage has an impact on inflammation. Very recently, it has been reported that *Lpcat3* deficiency in hematopoietic cells influence cholesterol and phospholipid metabolism and promotes atherosclerosis in a mouse model (30). However, macrophage specific *Lpcat3* deficiency on atherosclerosis is still not precisely evaluated. In this study, we utilized myeloid cell-specific *Lpcat3* deficient mice to study the effect of *Lpcat3* deficiency on cholesterol efflux, inflammation, and atherosclerosis. We hypothesized that alterations in the levels of macrophage membrane polyunsaturated PCs affect membrane fluidity, cholesterol efflux and inflammatory responses.

MATERIALS AND METHODS

Generation of Myeloid Cell-Specific *Lpcat3*-Deficient Mice

Lpcat3-Flox mice (28) were crossed with LysM-Cre transgenic mice (Jackson Laboratory) to establish *Lpcat3*-Flox/LysM-Cre mice according to the strategy (**Figure 1A**). We used both male and female mice, with C57BL/6 background and at age of 12-week-old. Our studies were approved by the Institutional Animal Care and Use Committee of State University of New York Downstate Medical Center.

Abbreviations: LPCAT3, lysophosphatidylcholine acyltransferase 3; PC, phosphatidylcholine; KO, knockout; cre, cre recombinase; LPS, lipopolysaccharide; TLR4, toll like 4 receptor; WT, wild type.

Bone Marrow-Derived Macrophage Isolation

Mice were sacrificed by CO_2. Bone marrow cells were isolated and macrophages were cultured as we did before (7). To eliminated the effect of FBS on macrophage surface PC composition, medium was changed to serum-free medium (0.2% BSA DMEM) for 24 h before all *in vitro* experiments.

mRNA Measurement

Total RNA was extracted from the cells using Trizol method (Invitrogen). The Superscript^{TM} III First-strand Synthesis kit (Invitrogen) was used for cDNA synthesis. SYBR Select Master Mix kit (Applied Biosystems) was used for PCR with following program: activation at 95°C for 10 min followed by 40 amplification cycles of 95°C for 15 s and 60°C for 60 s. The gene encoding Gapdh was used as internal controls. Relative gene expression is expressed as the mean ± SD. Mouse *Lpcat3* primers: forward, TTTCTGGTTCCGCTGCATGT, reverse, CCGACAGAATGCACACTCCTTC; *Gapdh* primers: forward, TGTAGACCATGTAGTTGAGGTCA; reverse, AGGTC GGTGTGAACGGATTTG. *Lpcat1* primers: forward, CGTGA ATATGTGGTCGCCTTG, reverse, ATGCTGCCATCCTCA GGAGAT. Lpcat2 primers: forward, GTCCAGCAGACTACG ATCAGTG, reverse, CTTATTGGATGGGTCAGCTTTTC. Lpcat4 primers: forward, TTCGGTTTCAGAGGATACGACAA, reverse, AATGTCTGGATTGTCGGACTGAA.

Measurement of Total LPCAT3 Activity and PC Subspecies

LPCAT3 activity was measured according to a published protocol, using NBD-lysoPC and arachidonoyl-CoA as subtracts (20). Liquid chromatography-coupled tandem mass spectrometry (LC-MS/MS) was used for the measurement of PC subspecies as described (20).

M1/M2 Measurement

Control and *Lpcat3* KO mice were euthanized by CO_2, and peritoneal macrophages were harvested by washing abdominal cavity with cold PBS. Harvested peritoneal resident macrophages were made to single-cell suspensions. Cells were then blocked with 0.5% BSA (w/v) and 2% FBS (v/v) in PBS and then stained with antibodies F4/80 (1:600 dilutions; BD Bioscience), CD11b (1:600 dilutions; BD Bioscience), and CD80 (1:600 dilutions; BD Bioscience) or CD206 (1: 400; Thermo Fisher). After being washed 3 times, cells were suspended in PBS and analyzed by Flow-cytometery.

Western Blot for Macrophage Lipid Rafts Lyn, TLR4, Total c-Scr, and Phosphorylated c-Scr

Macrophages (50×10^6), derived from Bone marrow, were homogenized. A previously reported method was used for lipid rafts isolation (8). Equal amount of protein from all fragments were used for Western blots with specific antibodies to Lyn

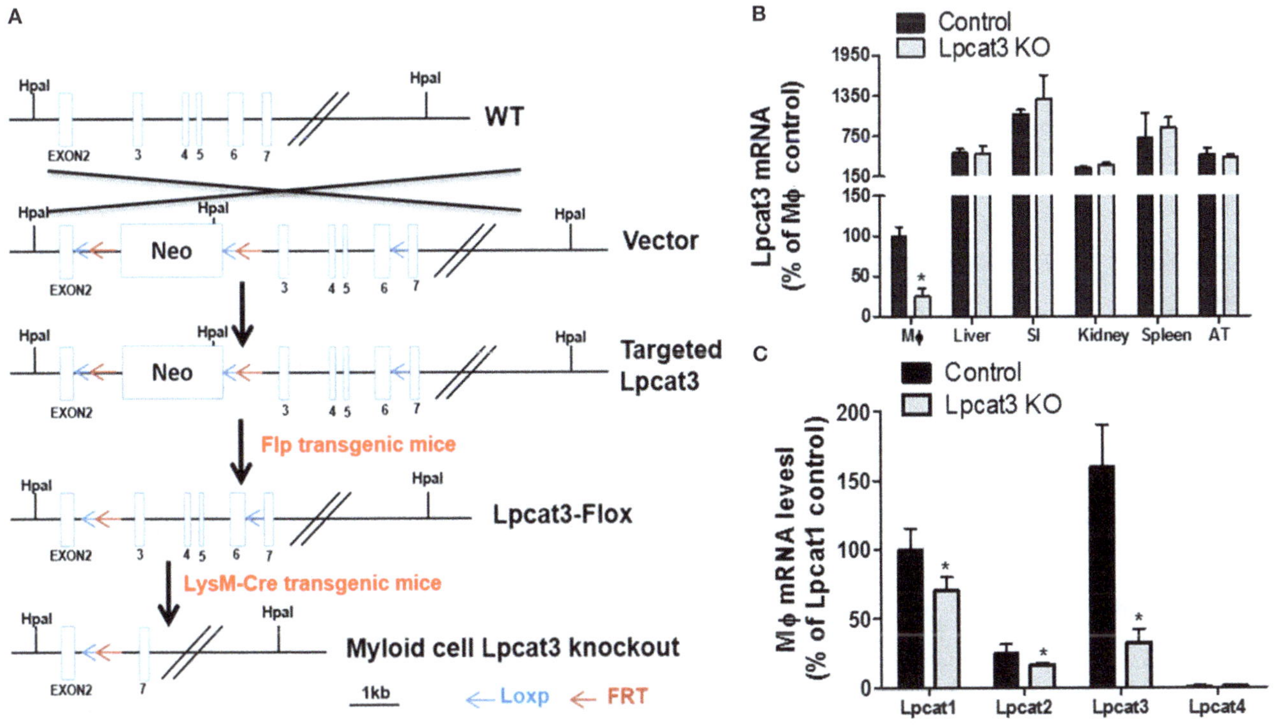

FIGURE 1 | Myeloid cell-specific *Lpcat3* KO mouse preparation. **(A)** Strategy for myeloid cell-specific *Lpcat3*-deficient mice preparation. **(B)** LPCAT3 mRNA tissue distribution. (SI, small intestine; AT, adipose tissue) **(C)** Macrophage LPCAT1, LPCAT2, and LPCAT3 mRNA tissue distribution. mRNAs were measured by Real-time PCR. Values are mean ± SD, $n = 4$, $^*P < 0.01$.

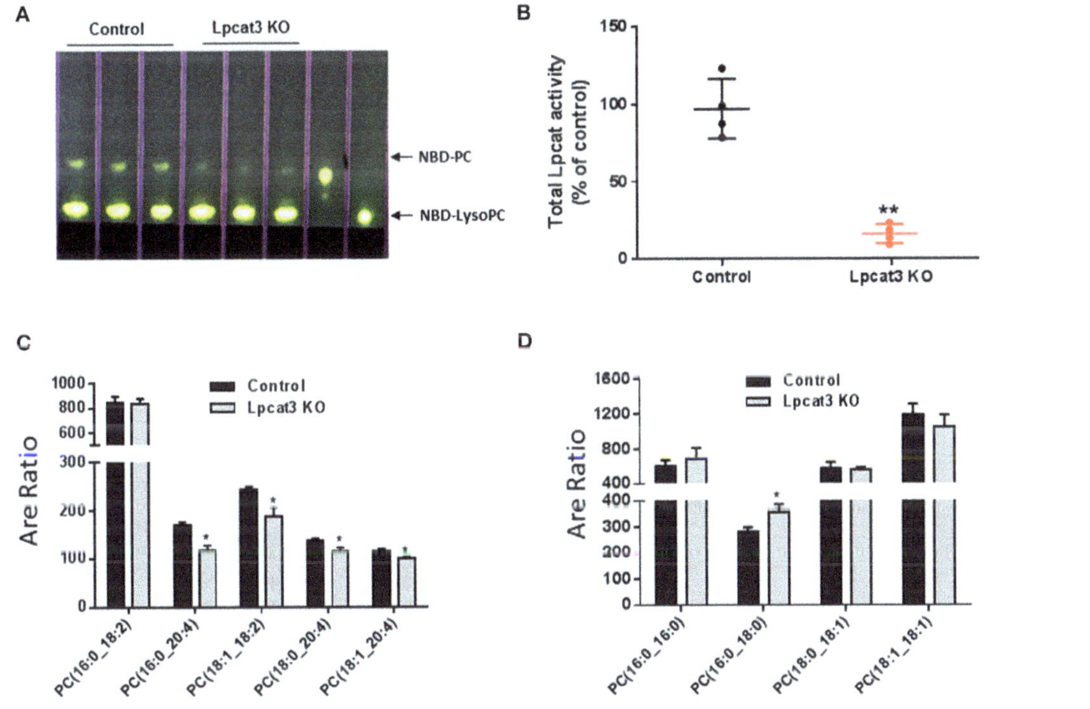

FIGURE 2 | LPCAT3 activity and PC composition measurements. **(A,B)** LPCAT3 activity measurement and quantification. The detail procedure was stated in "Materials and Methods." **(C,D)** PC subspecies measured by LC/MS/MS. Values are mean ± SD, $n = 3\text{–}4$, $^*P < 0.05$, $^{**}P < 0.01$.

(Santa Cruz), TLR4 (Santa Cruz), total c-Scr (Cell Signaling), and phospho-Src-Tyr416 (Cell Signaling).

TNF-α and IL-6 Measurements

Bone marrow–derived macrophages were treated with 10 ng/ml LPS for 16 h and TNF- α and IL-6 released to the medium were analyzed with ELISA kits (eBiosciences).

Western Blot for Macrophage p38 and p42/44

To eliminate lipoprotein effect from FBS to cell surface PC composition, Bone marrow-derived macrophage from Control and *Lpcat3* KO mice were changed to serum-free medium 24 h before experiment. Macrophages were then treated with 1 μg/ml LPS in 0.2% BSA DMEM for 0, 10, and 20 min. Cells were washed with cold PBS and harvested. Cells were homogenized in TSE buffer (50 mM Tris, 200 mM NaCl, 1 mM EDTA, pH 7.5). Cell lysates were used for Western blots with antibodies against p38 and p42/44 (Cell Signaling). The maximum intensity of each band was measured by Image-Pro Plus version 4.5 software (Media Cybernetics Inc.).

Nuclear Preparation and Western Blot for P65

We isolated macrophage nucleus using a Kit (Thermo Scientific). The nuclear preperation was utilized for Western blot with specific antibodies to p65 (Santa Cruz) and anti-histone 3 (H3).

Isolation of Lipid Rafts

Bone marrow-derived macrophages (50×10^6) were homogenized and lipid rafts were isolated by a previously reported method (8).

Cholesterol Efflux (*ex vivo*) Measurement

Bone marrow-derived macrophages were labeled with [^{3}H]cholesterol carried by acetylated-LDL. The cholesterol efflux was measured by an established method (7).

Bone Marrow Transplantation and Atherosclerosis Study Model

Ldlr KO female or male mice (age 8 weeks, Jackson Laboratory) were utilized. Bone marrow transplantation was performed as previously described (7). After 8 weeks transplantation, all mice were on a high fat high cholesterol diet for 3 months.

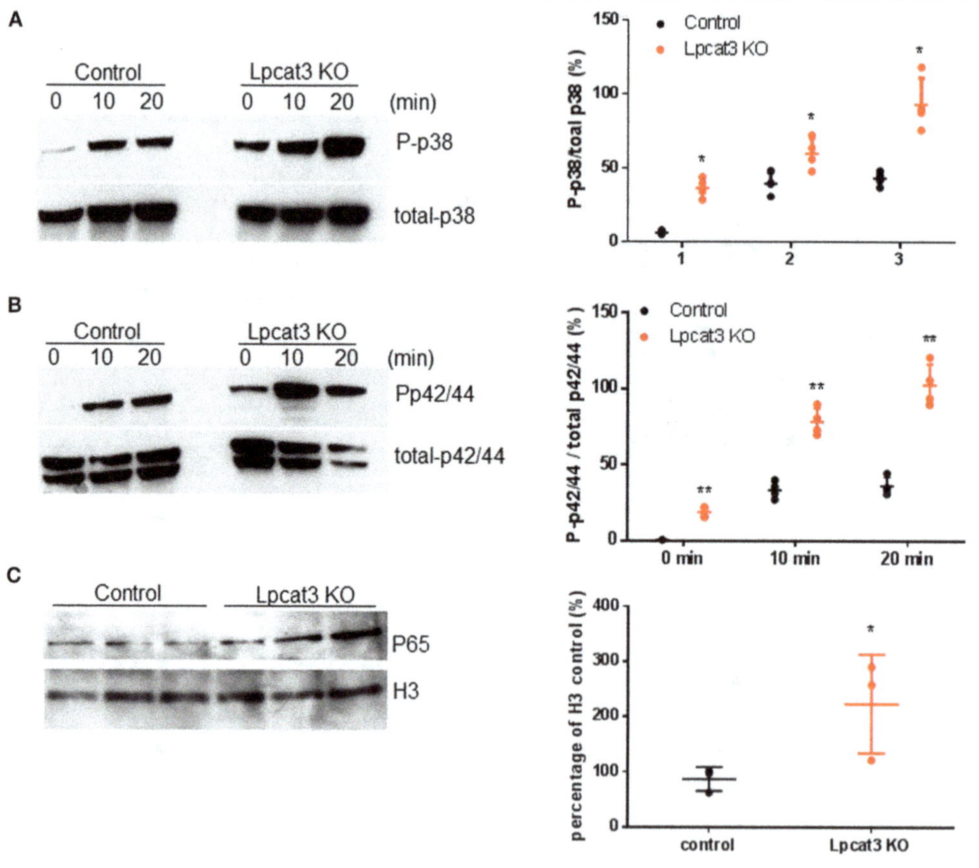

FIGURE 3 | *Lpcat3* KO macrophages promotes p38, p42/44, and NFκB activation. WT and *Lpcat3* KO macrophages were treated with 1 μg/ml LPS. **(A)** Western blot and quantitative display of total p38 and phosphorylated p38. **(B)** Western blot and quantitative display of total p42/44 and phosphorylated p42/44. Macrophage nucleus were isolated and p65 was measured by Western blot. **(C)** Western blot and quantitative display of p65. Values are mean ± SD, $n = 3$–4, *$P < 0.01$; **$P < 0.01$.

Mouse Atherosclerotic Lesion Measurement

We used the method which we reported before for atherosclerotic lesion measurement (7).

Statistical Analysis

Mean ± SD is expressed for each results. Data between two groups were analyzed by the unpaired, two-tailed Student's *t*-test, and among multiple groups by ANOVA followed by the Student-Newman-Keuls (SNK) test.

RESULTS

Production of Myeloid Cell-Specific *Lpcat3*-Deficient Mice

To produce myeloid cell-specific *Lpcat3* KO mice, we crossed *Lpcat3*-Flox mice with LysM-Cre transgenic mice. We collected bone marrow derived macrophage, liver, small intestine, adipose tissue, kidney, spleen from the homozygous KO male mice. Compared with controls, *Lpcat3* mRNA level was decreased by 80% in the macrophage but no other tissues (**Figure 1B**). We also noticed that among the tested tissues, macrophage is the lowest one for LPCAT3 expression (**Figure 1B**). Moreover, we found that, besides LPCAT3, LPCAT1, and LPCAT2 are also LPCAT isoforms expressed in macrophages and both may also play important roles in PC remodeling in the cell. This is different from the liver and small intestine, where LPCAT1, LPCAT2, and LPCAT4 are negligible (28). Compared with controls, the mRNA levels of LPCAT1 and LPCAT2 were significantly reduced by 30 and 35%, respectively, in *Lpcat3* KO macrophages (**Figure 1C**). We then measured total LPCAT3 activity using NBD-lysoPC and arachidonoyl-CoA (14) in the macrophage homogenate and found it was decreased by 80% compared with controls (**Figures 2A,B**). Similar results were obtained with female mice (data not shown).

Effect of *Lpcat3* Deficiency on Macrophage Inflammation, Cholesterol Efflux, and ER Stress

PC subspecies populations in macrophage homogenates were analyzed by LC/MS/MS. We found that *Lpcat3* deficiency decreased the amount of polyunsaturated PCs (16:0/20:4, 18:1/18:2, 18:0/20:4, and 18:1/20:4) in the membrane (**Figure 2C**), while other PCs have no significant changes except 16:0/18:0 which was increased (**Figure 2D**). These changes could affect macrophage mediated inflammatory response.

We investigated to consequence of *Lpcat3* deficiency in macrophage inflammatory responses. After LPS (1 μg/ml) treatment, *Lpcat3* KO macrophages significantly increased levels of phosphorylated p38 and p42/44 (**Figures 3A,B**). We also measured nucleus NFκB subunit p65 and found it was increased in *Lpcat3* KO macrophages (**Figure 3C**).

We then sought to investigate TLR4 levels in the KO macrophages and controls, since TLR4 is upstream of NFκB and MAP kinase. Lipid rafts play essential role in TLR4-mediated signaling (4, 31), thus, we examined whether *Lpcat3* deficiency affects TLR4 levels in the lipid rafts. We isolated lipid rafts which are enriched with Lyn kinase (marker of lipid rafts) (**Figure 4A**) and different subspecies of sphingomyelin (**Figure 4B**), as reported before (7). As seen on **Figure 4A**, lipid raft regions contain much more TLR4 protein compared with controls.

A recent report indicated that c-Src phosphorylation (activation)-mediated NFκB activation and then TNFα elevation could participate in macrophage activation and inflammation

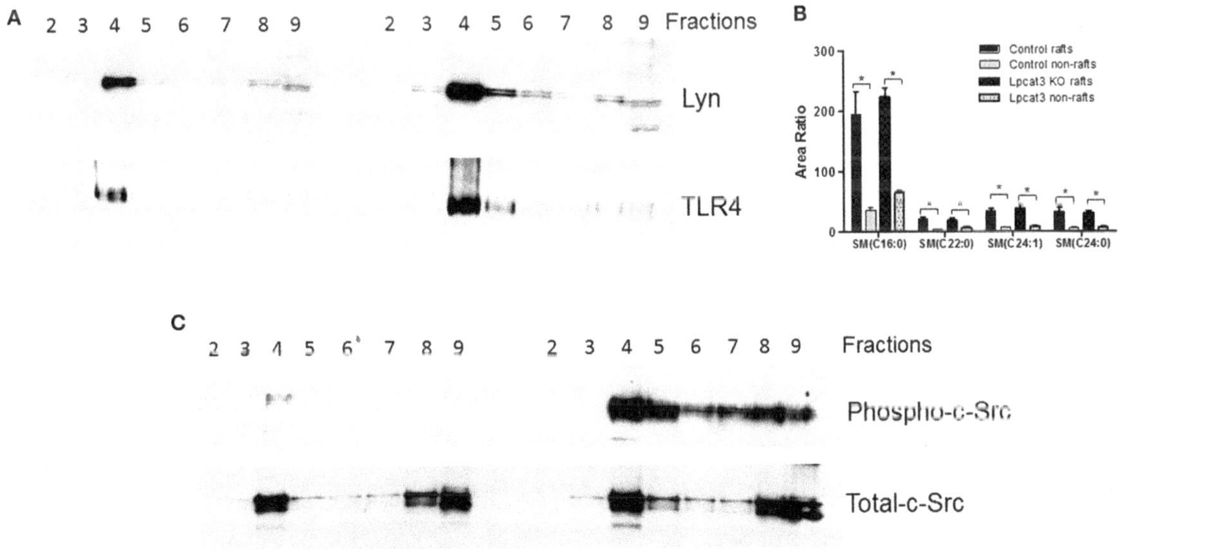

FIGURE 4 | Lipid rafts TLR4 and phosphorylated c-Src measurement. Macrophage lipid rafts isolated according a method in "Materials and Methods." **(A)** Western blot of Lyn Kinase (a lipid rafts marker) and TLR4 in each fractions from lipid rafts isolation. **(B)** LC/MS/MS measurement for sphingomyelin levels in rafts and non-rafts regions. **(C)** Western blot of phosphorylated c-Src and total c-Src in each fractions from lipid rafts isolation. The picture is the representative of three experiments. $^*p <$ 0.05.

(32). We found that *Lpcat3* deficiency dramatically increased phosphorylated c-Src in macrophage lipid rafts (**Figure 4C**) as assessed by Western blot using phospho-Src-Tyr416 antibody.

To further confirm the impact of macrophage *Lpcat3* deficiency mediated inflammation, we utilized F4/80, CD11b, and CD80 antibodies to label M1 and F4/80, CD11b, and CD206 antibody to label M2 macrophages, respectively, then measured abundancy of both macrophages using Flow cytometry. We found that *Lpcat3* deficiency significantly increased M1 (**Figure 5A**) but not M2 macrophages (**Figure 5B**). We further treated macrophages with LPS and IL-4, respectively. We found that LPS treatment significantly increased IL-1β mRNA levels in the deficient macrophages (**Figure 5C**), while IL-4 treatment had no effect on arginase1 (**Figure 5D**) but increased CD206 mRNA levels (**Figure 5E**).

We also determined the impact of the deficiency-related proinflammatory cytokine production. We stimulated the macrophage with LPS and found that *Lpcat3* deficiency significantly promotes IL-6 and TNFα secretion from macrophages, compared with controls (**Figures 5F,G**).

A previous study indicated that fetal liver derived *Lpcat3* deficient macrophage reduced cholesterol efflux (30). We first utilized Ac-LDL to load bone marrow derived macrophages with cholesterol and we did not find a difference in cholesterol accumulation between control and *Lpcat3* deficiency (**Figure 6A**). We then utilized Ac-LDL and [^{3}H]-cholesterol to load the cells with [^{3}H]-cholesterol and then evaluated cholesterol efflux using apoA-I. We also did not find significant difference between control and *Lpcat3* deficiency (**Figure 6B**). We further measured mRNA levels of ABCA1 and ABCG1, both transporters are involved in cholesterol efflux, and we did not find any significant changes (**Figure 6C**).

It has been reported that *Lpcat3* knockdown in macrophages exacerbated mRNAs of genes which are involved in ER stress (14). We measured mRNA levels of BIP, IRE1α, and PERK in control and *Lpcat3* KO microphages and found that BIP mRNA was significantly reduced while mRNA levels of IRE1α and PERK had no significant difference (**Figure 6D**).

Bone Marrow Transplantation and Atherosclerosis Evaluation

To evaluate the impact of the *Lpcat3* deficiency on atherosclerosis, we transplanted *Lpcat3* KO or wide type (WT) bone marrow into lethally irradiated *Ldlr* KO mice to produce *Lpcat3* KO→*Ldlr* KO (experimental) and WT→*Ldlr*

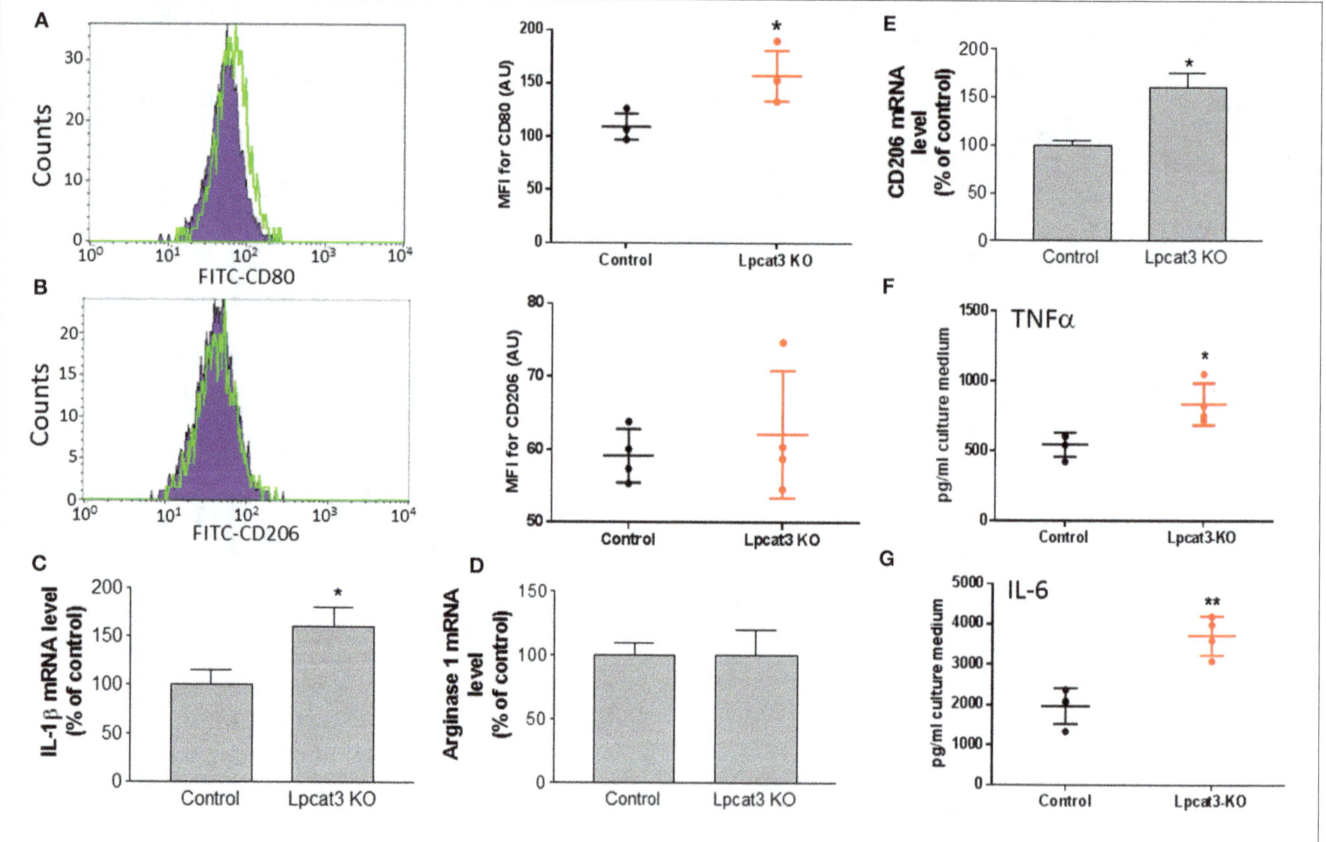

FIGURE 5 | Evaluation of inflammation in *Lpcat3* KO macrophages. **(A,B)** M1/M2 macrophage measurement. Harvested peritoneal macrophages were made to single-cell suspensions. Cells were stained with antibodies F4/80, CD11b, and CD80 or CD206. Cell suspension was analyzed by Flow cytometry. **(C)** Macrophages were treated 10 ng/ml LPS for 16 h, IL-1β mRNA was measured. **(D,E)** Macrophages were treated 20 ng/ml IL-4 for 24 h, arginase-1, and CD206 mRNAs were measured, respectively. **(F,G)** Macrophages were treated with 10 ng/ml LPS for 16 h and TNF-α and IL-6 released to the medium were analyzed with ELISA kits (eBiosciences). Values are mean ± SD, n = 3–4, *P < 0.01; **P < 0.01.

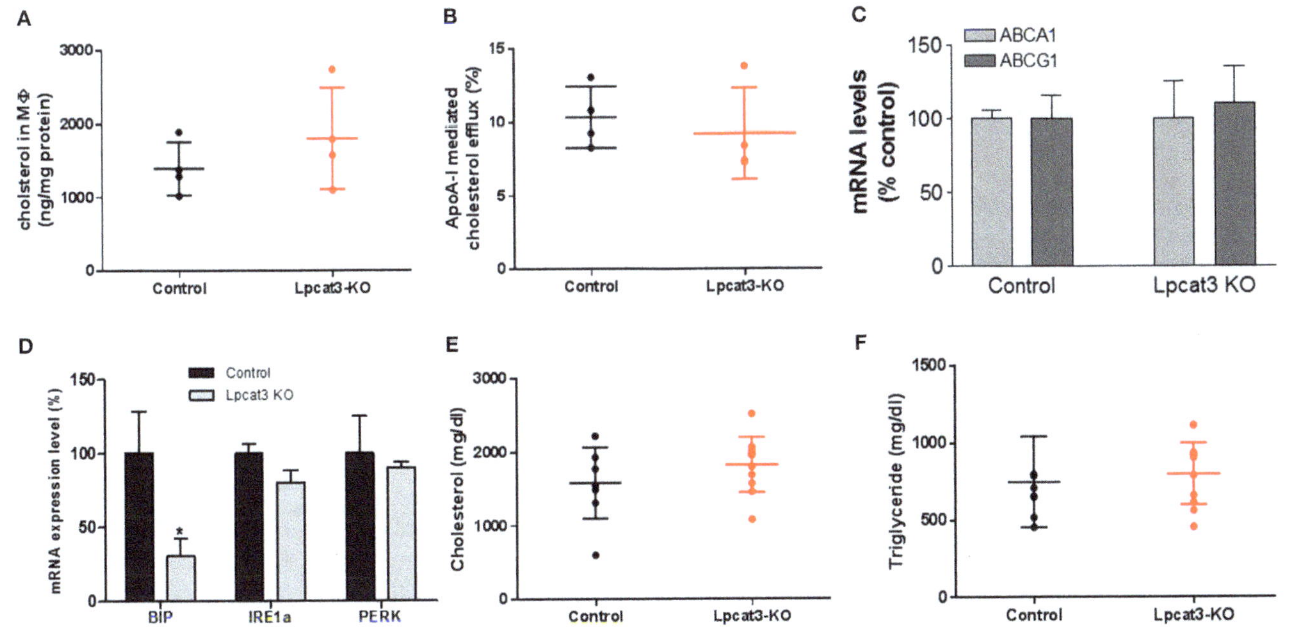

FIGURE 6 | Measurements of cholesterol loading and efflux, ER stress markers, and plasma lipids. WT and *Lpcat3* KO bone marrow derived macrophages were labeled with [^{3}H]cholesterol carried by acetylated-LDL. **(A)** Cellular cholesterol measurement after acetylated-LDL loading. **(B)** ApoA-I mediated cholesterol efflux. **(C)** mRNA levels of ABCA1 and ABCG1. **(D)** mRNA levels of ER stress markers (BIP, IRE1α, and PERK) were measured by real time PCR. **(E,F)** Plasma cholesterol and triglyceride levels in WT→*Ldlr* KO and *Lpcat3* KO→*Ldlr* KO mice. Values are mean ± SD, $n = 4$–8, *$P < 0.01$.

KO (control) mice. We then fed the animal with a high fat high cholesterol diet (0.15% cholesterol, 20% saturated fat) for 3 months. We found no significant changes in plasma lipid cholesterol and triglyceride levels (**Figures 6E,F**). We also found that there was no difference in body weight gain in these animals (data not shown).

Finally, we evaluated atherosclerosis in these mice. We found that, after 3 months on a high fat high cholesterol diet, all mice had lesions in the aortic arch. However, *Lpcat3* KO→*Ldlr* KO mice did not show significant bigger lesions than that of the WT→*Ldlr* KO mice (**Figures 7A–E**). The male mice also showed same results (**Figures 8A–E**).

DISCUSSION

In this study, we have demonstrated that depletion of the *Lpcat3* in macrophages induced a significant 1) reduction of polyunsaturated PCs on cell membrane; 2) induction of M1 macrophages in peritoneal region; and 3) induction of macrophage inflammation through TLR4 and c-Src pathways. However, myeloid cell-specific *Lpcat3* deficiency did not significantly increase atherosclerosis in *Ldlr* KO female and male mice fed a high fat high cholesterol diet for 3 months.

One of the key findings of this study is that LPCAT3 is one of the LPCATs in macrophages (**Figure 1C**). LPCAT1, LPCAT2, and LPCAT3 can make contribution to PC remodeling in macrophages. LyM-Cre-mediated *Lpcat3* ablation significantly reduced macrophage LPCAT3 activity (80%) (**Figure 2B**) and reduced polyunsaturated PC levels on the plasma membrane of macrophages (**Figure 2C**), but not saturated and monounsaturated PCs (**Figure 2D**).

Another key finding of this study is that LyM-Cre-mediated macrophage *Lpcat3* deficiency has pro-inflammation properties. A previous study indicated that LPCAT3 siRNA significantly increased LPS-mediated inflammatory response in macrophages (14). We found that *Lpcat3* deficiency-mediated macrophage plasma membrane polyunsaturated PC levels reduction can induce TLR4 expression in the lipid rafts (**Figure 4A**), thereby inducing both MAP kinase and NFκB (**Figure 3**) activation and promoting inflammatory cytokine productions (**Figures 5C,D**). Cellular lipids function are important regulators of c-Src activation by altering the recruitment of C-Src to lipid rafts in the plasma membrane (10). Studies have shown a critical role for c-Src in macrophage-mediated inflammatory responses (11). c-Src activates MAP kinases (33–35) and NFκB (36–38). A recent report indicated that c-Src phosphorylation (activation) could participate in macrophage inflammation through NFκB activation and TNFα elevation (32). We found that *Lpcat3* deficiency dramatically increased phosphorylated-c-Src in macrophage lipid rafts (**Figure 4C**), indicating, besides TLR4 pathway, c-Src pathway might also play an important role in *Lpcat3*-dificiency-mediated effect in macrophages.

It has been reported that acute *Lpcat3* knockdown in hepatocytes and macrophage exacerbated ER stress (14). However, the same group of researchers reported that genetic deletion of *Lpcat3* from the liver did not influence the expression of ER stress markers (39). Previously, we also found that *Lpcat3* deficiency in small intestine had no effect on ER stress markers (40). We found in this study that besides a significant reduction of BIP, IRE1, and PERK had no significant changes (**Figure 6C**).

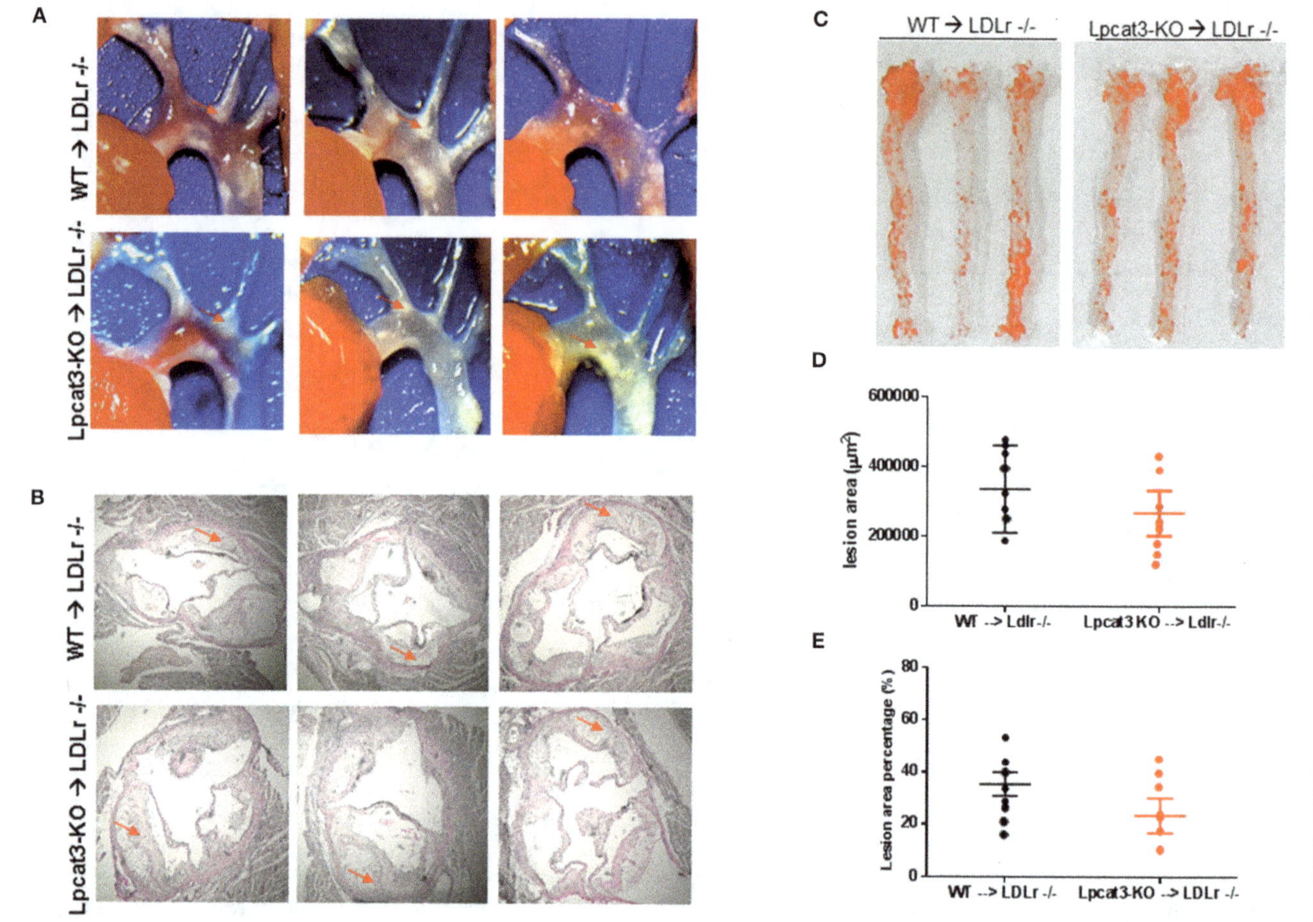

FIGURE 7 | Atherosclerosis measurement in male WT→*Ldlr* KO and *Lpcat3* KO→*Ldlr* KO mice. **(A)** Aortic arches with atherosclerotic plaques (white areas). **(B)** Aortic root assay for lesion areas after H&E staining. Six alternate sections (10 μm thick) sliced from paraffin-fixed aortic root tissues of each transplanted mouse were used for the analysis. **(C)** *En face* aortic plaque analysis after Oil Red O staining. **(D)** Quantitative display of root assay. **(E)** Quantitative display of *en face* assay. Red arrows indicate lesion area. Values are mean ± SD. *N* = 8–9.

We compared our results in this study with a very recent similar study (30). We noticed the following similarity and differences. First of all, we utilized bone marrow derived macrophages from myeloid cell-specific *Lpcat3*-deficient mice, while Thomas et al. utilized fetal liver cells derived macrophages from whole body *Lpcat3* deficient mice. LyM-Cre could only mediate 80% LPCAT3 deficiency (**Figures 2A,B**) instead of 100% (30). Secondly, both macrophages displayed major reductions in the arachidonate content of phosphatidylcholines (**Figure 2C**). Thirdly, we found macrophage *Lpcat3* deficiency have no effect on Ac-LDL-mediated cholesterol accumulation as well as cholesterol efflux (**Figures 6A,B**), while Thomas et al. found that *Lpcat3* deficiency cause an increase in the ratio of free to esterified cholesterol and a reduction in cholesterol efflux in macrophages. Fourthly, we found that macrophage *Lpcat3* deficiency promote inflammation, while the other study did not find changes in macrophage inflammatory response. Finally, we found that myeloid cell-specific *Lpcat3*-deficiency had no significant changes in atherogenesis (**Figures 7**, **8**), while, hematopoietic-specific *Lpcat3*-deficiency promotes atherosclerosis (30).

Although we cannot explain why there was a different outcome of myeloid cell-specific *Lpcat3* deficiency and hematopoietic cell-specific *Lpcat3* deficiency, in terms of mouse atherosclerosis, we speculate that, owning to their hematopoietic origin, *Lpcat3* KO fetal liver also harbored *Lpcat3* KO B-cells, T-cells, mast cells, and granulocytes in the *Lpcat3* KO chimeric mice (*Lpcat3* KO fetal liver cells →*Ldlr* KO) (30). Thus, it is impossible to rule out the possible contributions of these cells in the development of atherogenesis. We prepared myeloid cell-specific *Lpcat3*-deficient mice and transplanted their bone marrow into *Ldlr* KO mice, and then evaluate atherosclerosis in these mice (**Figures 7**, **8**). Nevertheless, we still cannot rule out the contribution of cells besides macrophages in myeloid cell lineage (41).

We also speculate that *Lpcat3* deficiency-mediated changes in macrophage might not be sufficient enough to have an impact on atherogenesity. In PC remodeling system, besides LPCAT3, there are LPCAT1, LPCAT2, and LPCAT4 (13, 15–17). In this study, we indicated that LPCAT1 and LPCAT2 are expressed in macrophages, whereas LPCAT4 expression level is negligible

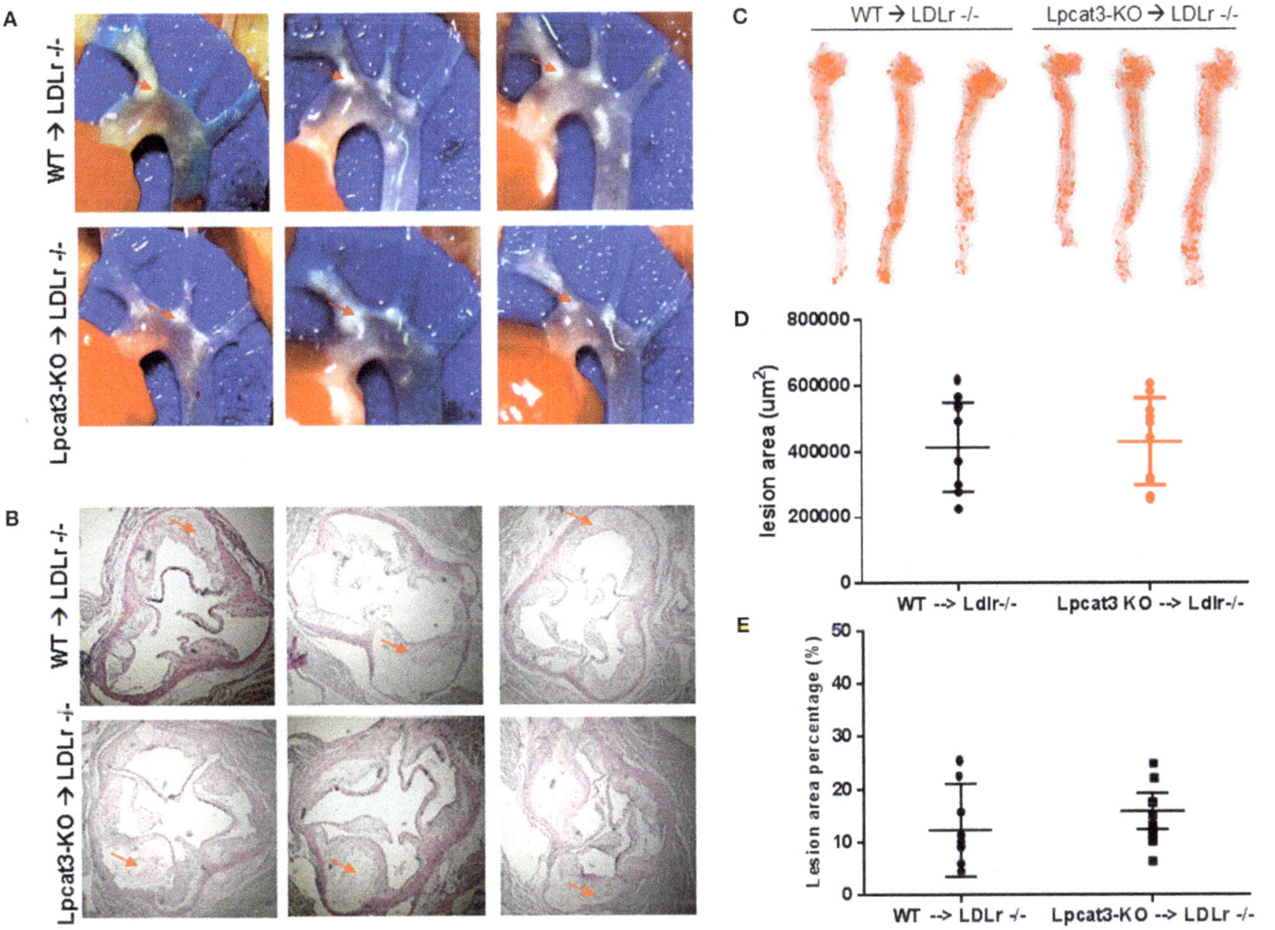

FIGURE 8 | Atherosclerosis measurement in female WT→*Ldlr* KO and *Lpcat3* KO→*Ldlr* KO mice. **(A)** Aortic arches with atherosclerotic plaques (white areas). **(B)** Aortic root assay for lesion areas after H&E staining. Six alternate sections (10 μm thick) sliced from paraffin-fixed aortic root tissues of each transplanted mouse were used for the analysis. **(C)** *En face* aortic plaque analysis after Oil Red O staining. **(D)** Quantitative display of root assay. **(E)** Quantitative display of *en face* assay. Red arrows indicate lesion area. Values are mean ± SD. $N = 8$–9.

(**Figure 1D**). Thus, LPCAT1, LPCAT2, and LPCAT3 can all play role in PC remodeling in macrophages. This is different from hepatocytes and enterocyte where LPCAT3 is the major LPCAT (28). LPCAT1 and LPCAT2 are not only involved in PC remodeling activity but also involved in production of platelet activating factor (PAF) (17, 42), a potent proinflammatory phospholipid (43, 44). We found that LPCAT3 deficiency has an impact on downregulation of LPCAT1 and LPCAT2 (**Figure 1D**) and this could result in reduction of PAF or could be due to regulating lysoPC and/or arachidonic acid (14, 19) availability in macrophages. Further studies are needed to evaluate this LPCAT3 deficiency-mediated effect.

There is limitation of bone marrow transplantation approach of this study. The transplanted macrophage containing LDL receptor. However, LDL receptor contained macrophages have negligible effect on high fat high cholesterol diet induced atherosclerosis in *Ldlr* KO mice (45). Thus, many researchers including us, in the last 20 years, did similar bone marrow transplantation and evaluate atherosclerosis relevance of the genes, which we are interested in, in *Ldlr* KO mice under atherogenic diet.

In conclusion, LPCAT3 contributes to PC remodeling in mouse macrophages and PC composition in macrophage plasma membranes. *Lpcat3* deficiency promotes inflammation. However, such an effect has no significant effect on the development of atherosclerosis.

AUTHOR CONTRIBUTIONS

HJ, ZL, and CH did the experiments. X-CJ composed and finalized the manuscript.

FUNDING

This work was supported by NIH Grants RO1HL-139582 and VA Merit award 000900-01.

REFERENCES

1. Holub BJ, Kuksis A. Metabolism of molecular species of diacylglycerophospholipids. *Adv Lipid Res.* (1978) 16:1–125. doi: 10.1016/B978-0-12-024916-9.50007-X
2. MacDonald JI, Sprecher H. Phospholipid fatty acid remodeling in mammalian cells. *Biochim Biophys Acta* (1991) 1084:105–21. doi: 10.1016/0005-2760(91)90209-Z
3. Triantafilou M, Triantafilou K. Lipopolysaccharide recognition: CD14, TLRs and the LPS-activation cluster. *Trends Immunol.* (2002) 23:301–4. doi: 10.1016/S1471-4906(02)02233-0
4. Triantafilou M, Miyake K, Golenbock DT, Triantafilou K. Mediators of innate immune recognition of bacteria concentrate in lipid rafts and facilitate lipopolysaccharide-induced cell activation. *J Cell Sci.* (2002) 115 (Pt 12):2603–11.
5. Soong G, Reddy B, Sokol S, Adamo R, Prince A. TLR2 is mobilized into an apical lipid raft receptor complex to signal infection in airway epithelial cells. *J Clin Invest.* (2004) 113:1482–9. doi: 10.1172/JCI200420773
6. Liu J, Huan C, Chakraborty M, Zhang H, Lu D, Kuo MS, et al. Macrophage sphingomyelin synthase 2 deficiency decreases atherosclerosis in mice. *Circ Res.* (2009) 105:295–303. doi: 10.1161/CIRCRESAHA.109.194613
7. Chakraborty M, Lou C, Huan C, Kuo MS, Park TS, Cao G, et al. Myeloid cell-specific serine palmitoyltransferase subunit 2 haploinsufficiency reduces murine atherosclerosis. *J Clin Investig.* (2013) 123:1784–97. doi: 10.1172/JCI60415
8. Hailemariam TK, Huan C, Liu J, Li Z, Roman C, Kalbfeisch M, et al. Sphingomyelin synthase 2 deficiency attenuates NFkappaB activation. *Arterioscler Thromb Vasc Biol.* (2008) 28:1519–26. doi: 10.1161/ATVBAHA.108.168682
9. Li Z, Fan Y, Liu J, Li Y, Huan C, Bui HH, et al. Impact of sphingomyelin synthase 1 deficiency on sphingolipid metabolism and atherosclerosis in mice. *Arterioscler Thromb Vasc Biol.* (2012) 32:1577–84. doi: 10.1161/ATVBAHA.112.251538
10. Holzer RG, Park EJ, Li N, Tran H, Chen M, Choi C, et al. Saturated fatty acids induce c-Src clustering within membrane subdomains, leading to JNK activation. *Cell* (2011) 147:173–84. doi: 10.1016/j.cell.2011.08.034
11. Byeon SE, Yi YS, Oh J, Yoo BC, Hong S, Cho JY. The role of Src kinase in macrophage-mediated inflammatory responses. *Mediators Inflamm.* (2012) 2012:512926. doi: 10.1155/2012/512926
12. Lee HC, Inoue T, Imae R, Kono N, Shirae S, Matsuda S, et al. Caenorhabditis elegans mboa-7, a member of the MBOAT family, is required for selective incorporation of polyunsaturated fatty acids into phosphatidylinositol. *Mol Biol Cell* (2008) 19:1174–84. doi: 10.1091/mbc.e07-09-0893
13. Hishikawa D, Shindou H, Kobayashi S, Nakanishi H, Taguchi R, Shimizu T. Discovery of a lysophospholipid acyltransferase family essential for membrane asymmetry and diversity. *Proc Nat Acad Sci USA.* (2008) 105:2830–5. doi: 10.1073/pnas.0712245105
14. Rong X, Albert CJ, Hong C, Duerr MA, Chamberlain BT, Tarling EJ, et al. LXRs regulate ER stress and inflammation through dynamic modulation of membrane phospholipid composition. *Cell Metabol.* (2013) 18:685–97. doi: 10.1016/j.cmet.2013.10.002
15. Chen X, Hyatt BA, Mucenski ML, Mason RJ, Shannon JM. Identification and characterization of a lysophosphatidylcholine acyltransferase in alveolar type II cells. *Proc Nat Acad Sci USA.* (2006) 103:11724–9. doi: 10.1073/pnas.0604946103
16. Nakanishi H, Shindou H, Hishikawa D, Harayama T, Ogasawara R, Suwabe A, et al. Cloning and characterization of mouse lung-type acyl-CoA:lysophosphatidylcholine acyltransferase 1 (LPCAT1). Expression in alveolar type II cells and possible involvement in surfactant production. *J Biol Chem.* (2006) 281:20140–7. doi: 10.1074/jbc.M600225200
17. Shindou H, Hishikawa D, Nakanishi H, Harayama T, Ishii S, Taguchi R, et al. A single enzyme catalyzes both platelet-activating factor production and membrane biogenesis of inflammatory cells. Cloning and characterization of acetyl-CoA:LYSO-PAF acetyltransferase. *J Biol Chem.* (2007) 282:6532–9. doi: 10.1074/jbc.M609641200
18. Zhao Y, Chen YQ, Bonacci TM, Bredt DS, Li S, Bensch WR, et al. Identification and characterization of a major liver lysophosphatidylcholine acyltransferase. *J Biol Chem.* (2008) 283:8258–65. doi: 10.1074/jbc.M710422200
19. Ishibashi M, Varin A, Filomenko R, Lopez T, Athias A, Gambert P, et al. Liver x receptor regulates arachidonic acid distribution and eicosanoid release in human macrophages: a key role for lysophosphatidylcholine acyltransferase 3. *Arterioscler Thromb Vasc Biol.* (2013) 33:1171–9. doi: 10.1161/ATVBAHA.112.300812
20. Li Z, Ding T, Pan X, Li Y, Li R, Sanders PE, et al. Lysophosphatidylcholine acyltransferase 3 knockdown-mediated liver lysophosphatidylcholine accumulation promotes very low density lipoprotein production by enhancing microsomal triglyceride transfer protein expression. *J Biol Chem.* (2012) 287:20122–31. doi: 10.1074/jbc.M111.334664
21. Kazachkov M, Chen Q, Wang L, Zou J. Substrate preferences of a lysophosphatidylcholine acyltransferase highlight its role in phospholipid remodeling. *Lipids* (2008) 43:895–902. doi: 10.1007/s11745-008-3233-y
22. Ariyama H, Kono N, Matsuda S, Inoue T, Arai H. Decrease in membrane phospholipid unsaturation induces unfolded protein response. *J Biol Chem.* (2010) 285:22027–35. doi: 10.1074/jbc.M110.126870
23. Bergo MO, Gavino BJ, Steenbergen R, Sturbois B, Parlow AF, Sanan DA, et al. Defining the importance of phosphatidylserine synthase 2 in mice. *J Biol Chem.* (2002) 277:47701–8. doi: 10.1074/jbc.M207734200
24. Chen M, Mason RP, Tulenko TN. Atherosclerosis alters the composition, structure and function of arterial smooth muscle cell plasma membranes. *Biochim Biophys Acta* (1995) 1272:101–12. doi: 10.1016/0925-4439(95)00073-D
25. Li Y, Ge M, Ciani L, Kuriakose G, Westover EJ, Dura M, et al. Enrichment of endoplasmic reticulum with cholesterol inhibits sarcoplasmic-endoplasmic reticulum calcium ATPase-2b activity in parallel with increased order of membrane lipids: implications for depletion of endoplasmic reticulum calcium stores and apoptosis in cholesterol-loaded macrophages. *J Biol Chem.* (2004) 279:37030–9. doi: 10.1074/jbc.M405195200
26. Steenbergen R, Nanowski TS, Nelson R, Young SG, Vance JE. Phospholipid homeostasis in phosphatidylserine synthase-2-deficient mice. *Biochim Biophys Acta* (2006) 1761:313–23. doi: 10.1016/j.bbalip.2006.03.005
27. Wiedmer T, Zhao J, Li L, Zhou Q, Hevener A, Olefsky JM, et al. Adiposity, dyslipidemia, and insulin resistance in mice with targeted deletion of phospholipid scramblase 3 (PLSCR3). *Proc Natl Acad Sci USA.* (2004) 101:13296–301. doi: 10.1073/pnas.0405354101
28. Kabir I, Li Z, Bui HH, Kuo MS, Gao G, Jiang XC. Small intestine but not liver lysophosphatidylcholine acyltransferase 3 (Lpcat3) deficiency has a dominant effect on plasma lipid metabolism. *J Biol Chem.* (2016) 291:7651–60. doi: 10.1074/jbc.M115.697011
29. Libby P. Inflammation in atherosclerosis. *Nature* (2002) 420:868–74. doi: 10.1038/nature01323
30. Thomas C, Jalil A, Magnani C, Ishibashi M, Quere R, Bourgeois T, et al. LPCAT3 deficiency in hematopoietic cells alters cholesterol and phospholipid homeostasis and promotes atherosclerosis. *Atherosclerosis* (2018) 275:409–18. doi: 10.1016/j.atherosclerosis.2018.05.023
31. Plociennikowska A, Hromada-Judycka A, Borzecka K, Kwiatkowska K. Co-operation of TLR4 and raft proteins in LPS-induced pro-inflammatory signaling. *Cell Mol Life Sci.* (2015) 72:557–81. doi: 10.1007/s00018-014-1762-5
32. Cheng XL, Ding F, Li H, Tan XQ, Liu X, Cao JM, et al. Activation of AMPA receptor promotes TNF-alpha release via the ROS-cSrc-NFkappaB signaling cascade in RAW264.7 macrophages. *Biochem Biophys Res Commun.* (2015) 461:275–80. doi: 10.1016/j.bbrc.2015.04.015
33. Luttrell LM, Hawes BE, van Biesen T, Luttrell DK, Lansing TJ, Lefkowitz RJ. Role of c-Src tyrosine kinase in G protein-coupled receptor- and Gbetagamma subunit-mediated activation of mitogen-activated protein kinases. *J Biol Chem.* (1996) 271:19443–50. doi: 10.1074/jbc.271.32.19443
34. Bondzi C, Litz J, Dent P, Krystal GW. Src family kinase activity is required for Kit-mediated mitogen-activated protein (MAP) kinase activation, however loss of functional retinoblastoma protein makes MAP kinase activation unnecessary for growth of small cell lung cancer cells. *Cell Growth Differ.* (2000) 11:305–14.
35. Kim MJ, Byun JY, Yun CH, Park IC, Lee KH, Lee SJ. c-Src-p38 mitogen-activated protein kinase signaling is required for Akt activation in response to ionizing radiation. *Mol Cancer Res.* (2008) 6:1872–80. doi: 10.1158/1541-7786.MCR-08-0084
36. Lluis JM, Buricchi F, Chiarugi P, Morales A, Fernandez-Checa JC. Dual role of mitochondrial reactive oxygen species in hypoxia signaling: activation of

nuclear factor-{kappa}B via c-SRC and oxidant-dependent cell death. *Cancer Res.* (2007) 67:7368–77. doi: 10.1158/0008-5472.CAN-07-0515

37. Jalal DI, Kone BC. Src activation of NF-kappaB augments IL-1beta-induced nitric oxide production in mesangial cells. *J Am Soc Nephrol.* (2006) 17:99–106. doi: 10.1681/ASN.2005070693
38. Brady RR, Loveridge CJ, Dunlop MG, Stark LA. c-Src dependency of NSAID-induced effects on NF-kappaB-mediated apoptosis in colorectal cancer cells. *Carcinogenesis* (2011) 32:1069–77. doi: 10.1093/carcin/bgr077
39. Rong X, Wang B, Dunham MM, Hedde PN, Wong JS, Gratton E, et al. Lpcat3-dependent production of arachidonoyl phospholipids is a key determinant of triglyceride secretion. *eLife* (2015) 4:e06557. doi: 10.7554/eLife.06557
40. Li Z, Jiang H, Ding T, Lou C, Bui HH, Kuo MS, et al. Deficiency in lysophosphatidylcholine acyltransferase 3 reduces plasma levels of lipids by reducing lipid absorption in mice. *Gastroenterology* (2015) 149:1519–29. doi: 10.1053/j.gastro.2015.07.012
41. Clausen BE, Burkhardt C, Reith W, Renkawitz R, Forster I. Conditional gene targeting in macrophages and granulocytes using LysMcre mice. *Transgen Res.* (1999) 8:265–77. doi: 10.1023/A:1008942828960
42. Harayama T, Shindou H, Ogasawara R, Suwabe A, Shimizu T. Identification of a novel noninflammatory biosynthetic pathway of platelet-activating factor. *J Biol Chem.* (2008) 283:11097–106. doi: 10.1074/jbc.M708909200
43. Shimizu T. Lipid mediators in health and disease: enzymes and receptors as therapeutic targets for the regulation of immunity and inflammation. *Ann Rev Pharmacol Toxicol.* (2009) 49:123–50. doi: 10.1146/annurev.pharmtox.011008.145616
44. Prescott SM, Zimmerman GA, McIntyre TM. Platelet-activating factor. *J Biol Chem.* (1990) 265:17381–4.
45. Linton MF, Babaev VR, Gleaves LA, Fazio S. A direct role for the macrophage low density lipoprotein receptor in atherosclerotic lesion formation. *J Biol Chem.* (1999) 274:19204–10. doi: 10.1074/jbc.274.27.19204

18

BLTR1 in Monocytes Emerges as a Therapeutic Target For Vascular Inflammation with a Subsequent Intimal Hyperplasia in a Murine Wire-Injured Femoral Artery

Seung E. Baek [1,2], *So Y. Park* [1,2], *Sun S. Bae* [1,2], *Koanhoi Kim* [1], *Won S. Lee* [1] and *Chi D. Kim* [1,2*]

[1] *Department of Pharmacology, School of Medicine, Pusan National University, Yangsan, South Korea,* [2] *Gene and Cell Therapy Research Center for Vessel-Associated Diseases, Pusan National University, Yangsan, South Korea*

***Correspondence:**
Chi D. Kim
chidkim@pusan.ac.kr

Given the importance of high-mobility group box 1 (HMGB1) and 5-lipoxygenase (5-LO) signaling in vascular inflammation, we investigated the role of leukotriene signaling in monocytes on monocyte-to-macrophage differentiation (MMD) induced by HMGB1, and on vascular inflammation and subsequent intimal hyperplasia in a mouse model of wire-injured femoral artery. In cultured primary bone marrow-derived cells (BMDCs) stimulated with HMGB1, the number of cells with macrophage-like morphology was markedly increased in association with an increased expression of CD11b/Mac-1, which were attenuated in cells pre-treated with Zileuton, a 5-LO inhibitor as well as in 5-LO-deficient BMDCs. Of various leukotriene receptor inhibitors examined, which included leukotriene B4 receptors (BLTRs) and cysteinyl leukotriene receptors (cysLTRs), the BLTR1 inhibitor (U75302) exclusively suppressed MMD induction by HMGB1. The importance of BLTR1 in HMGB1-induced MMD was also observed in BMDCs isolated from BLTR1-deficient mice and BMDCs transfected with BLTR1 siRNA. Although leukotriene B4 (LTB4) had minimal direct effects on MMD in control and 5-LO-deficient BMDCs, MMD attenuation by HMGB1 in 5-LO-deficient BMDCs was significantly reversed by exogenous LTB4, but not in BLTR1-deficient BMDCs, suggesting that LTB4/BLTR1-mediated priming of monocytes is a prerequisite of HMGB1-induced MMD. *In vivo*, both macrophage infiltration and intimal hyperplasia in our wire-injured femoral artery were markedly attenuated in BLTR1-deficient mice as compared with wild-type controls, but these effects were reversed in BLTR1-deficient mice transplanted with monocytes from control mice. These results suggest that BLTR1 in monocytes is a pivotal player in MMD with subsequent macrophage infiltration into neointima, leading to vascular remodeling after vascular injury.

Keywords: high mobility group box 1, 5-lipoxygenase, leukotriene B4 receptor, monocyte-to-macrophage differentiation, vascular restenosis, intimal hyperplasia

INTRODUCTION

Vascular endoluminal interventional procedures injure vascular walls, and result in the release endogenous damage-associated molecular patterns (DAMPs) (1, 2). Of the various DAMP proteins, high mobility group box 1 protein (HMGB1) has emerged as an important regulator of inflammatory responses resulting from tissue injury (3–5), and been implicated as an active player in vascular inflammation with resultant intimal hyperplasia after arterial injury (6). In a previous study, we found HMGB1 enhanced monocyte-to-macrophage differentiation (MMD) and resultant vascular inflammation in injured vasculature (7), and thus, we suggested coordinated relationships exist between local vascular injury and pattern recognition receptor-related signals in the process of vascular inflammation.

Monocyte recruitment to injured tissues, their subsequent transformation into macrophages, and the overproduction of inflammatory cytokines are major steps in the process of vascular inflammation (8, 9). These sequential events stimulate vascular smooth muscle cell (VSMC) proliferation and extracellular matrix deposition in neointima, which result in intimal hyperplasia and vascular occlusion (10). Furthermore, several key proteins involved in the leukotriene cascades, such as, 5-lipoxygenase (5-LO) and arachidonate 5-lipoxygenase activating protein (FLAP), and leukotriene (LT) receptors are highly expressed in human atherosclerotic plaque (11–13), which suggests their potential involvements in vascular inflammation.

Previous studies have reported genetic targeting of 5-LO reduced lesion size in atherosclerosis prone mouse strains (14–16). Likewise, in a previous study, we found 5-LO importantly contributed to the development of atherosclerosis by increasing the expressions of adhesion molecules on monocytes, and thus, increasing monocyte adhesion to vascular endothelium (17). In FLAP-deficient mice, neointima hyperplasia in injured arteries was significantly attenuated by reducing inflammatory cytokine release from FLAP-deficient macrophages (18), which suggested 5-LO in macrophages plays a pivotal role in vascular inflammation. However, although 5-LO in inflammatory cells has been proposed to be an important player in the development of vascular inflammation (12, 19), the importance of 5-LO signaling pathways in monocytes in vascular inflammation with subsequent vascular remodeling in injured vasculatures remains unclear.

Leukotrienes (LTs) are considered to mediate inflammatory responses in various cardiovascular diseases characterized by vascular inflammation (20). LTs exert their actions via four subclasses of receptors, such as, BLT1 and BLT2 (receptors for LTB4), and CysLT1 and CysLT2 (receptors for cysteinyl-leukotrienes) (21). Previous studies have implicated LT receptor activation in atherogenesis and vascular remodeling after angioplasty (21, 22), and studies on the genetic and pharmacological targeting of BLTR1 in atherosclerotic mouse strains further supported the involvement of leukotriene-signaling in vascular inflammation (23–25). However, the precise role of BLTR1 signaling in monocytes in the process of vascular inflammation remains unclear.

In a previous study, we described the importance of 5-LO in monocytes during vascular inflammation (7). However, our incomplete understanding of how 5-LO signaling pathways in monocytes contribute to vascular inflammation explains the incapability of current treatments to prevent vascular remodeling in the injured vasculatures. Given the importance of HMGB1 and 5-LO signaling in monocytes during vascular inflammation, we investigated the role of leukotriene signaling in monocytes on MMD induced by HMGB1. To further determine the contribution of 5-LO signaling in monocytes in macrophage infiltration into neointima lesions, we also investigated the importance of BLTR1 signaling in monocytes in vascular inflammation and subsequent intimal hyperplasia using BLTR1-deficient mice and BLTR1-deficient mice transplanted with monocytes from WT mice.

Abbreviations: HMGB1, High mobility group box 1 protein; 5-LO, 5-Lipoxygenase; MMD, monocyte to macrophage differentiation; BMDC, Bone marrow derived cell; BLTR, receptor for leukotriene B4; CysLTR, receptor for cysteinyl-leukotrienes; DAMP, Damage-associated molecular patterns; VSMC, Vascular smooth muscle cell; FLAP, 5-Lipoxygenase activating protein; LT, Leukotriene; LTB4, Leukotriene B4; BMDM, Bone marrow derived monocyte; PBMC, Peripheral blood mononuclear cell; LDPI, Laser Doppler perfusion imaging; H&E, Hematoxylin and Eosin; α-SMA, alpha-smooth muscle actin; DAPI, 4′6-Diamidino-2-phenylindole; WT, Wild-type.

MATERIALS AND METHODS

Ethics Statement and Animals

All experiments involving animals conformed with the Guide for the Care and Use of Laboratory Animals published by the US National Institute of Health (NIH Publication No. 85-23, 2011 revision), and all animal-related experimental protocols were approved by the Pusan National University Institutional Animal Care and Use Committee of the College of Medicine (PNU-2016-1310). Genotyping, including that of 5-LO-deficient mice and BLTR1-deficient mice, was performed by PCR using a protocol provided by the Jackson Laboratory (Harlan Nossan, ITA). Wild-type (WT) control mice (C57BL/6J) were purchased from the Jackson Laboratory. Animals were housed in an air-conditioned room at 22–25°C and kept under a 12-h light/dark cycle. Food and water were provided *ad libitum*.

Vascular Injury Models and Blood Flow Measurement

C57BL/6J (WT), 5-LO-deficient and BLTR1-deficient male mice (7 wk-old) were subjected to right femoral artery injury using a 0.25 mm diameter angioplasty guidewire under chloral hydrate (450 mg/kg, intraperitoneal injection) anesthesia and aseptic conditions, as previously described (26). The adequacy of anesthesia was confirmed by response to toe pinch. Wire-injured femoral arteries were harvested from mice euthanized by carbon dioxide insufflations and cervical dislocation, and then cross sectioned (4 μm). Tissue sections were stained with hematoxylin and eosin (H&E) and immunohistological marker antibodies. Femoral arterial blood flow was measured using a laser Doppler perfusion imaging (LDPI) analyzer (Moor Instruments, Devon, UK) at 0, 1, 2, 3, and 4 wks after femoral artery injury. The changes in blood flow were calculated using the colors of histogram pixels.

Chemicals and Antibodies

Zileuton and alpha-smooth muscle actin (α-SMA) antibody were purchased from Sigma-Aldrich (St. Louis, MO, USA). LTB4, U75302 and REV5901 were from Cayman Chemical Inc (Ann Arbor, MI, USA). MK 886 was purchased from EMD Serono (Rockland, MA, USA), HMGB1 from R&D systems (Minneapolis, MN, USA), CD11b antibody from Abcam (Cambridge, MA, USA), and BLTR1 antibody from Biorbyt (Cambridge, UK). CD36, CD14, β-actin, and 5-LO antibodies were purchased from Santa Cruz Biotechnology (Santa Cruz, CA, USA), R-phycoerythrin PE-conjugated mouse anti-human CD11b/Mac-1 antibody and PE-conjugated mouse IgG isotype control antibody from BD (San Diego, CA, USA). Horseradish peroxidase (HRP)-conjugated IgG antibody was used as the secondary antibody from Santa Cruz Biotechnology. Restriction enzymes were purchased from Promega (Madison, WI, USA). 5-LO and BLTR1 siRNA oligonucleotides were synthesized by Bioneer (Daejeon, ROK). siRNA molecules were transfected into cells using Lipofectamine 2000 siRNA transfection reagent (Invitrogen, Carlsbad, CA, USA). PCR primers were from Bioneer.

Isolation of Bone Marrow-Derived Cells and Culture

Bone marrow derived cells (BMDCs) were isolated from mice (7 wks, male) euthanized by carbon dioxide insufflation and cervical dislocation. Briefly, after bone marrow cells were harvested from femurs and tibiae, red blood cells were lysed using lysing buffer (Sigma-Aldrich) and incubated in RPMI1640 containing 10% heat-inactivated fetal bovine serum (FBS) for 24 h. Non-adherent cells were harvested and centrifuged at 1300 rpm for 10 min, and the cell pellets so obtained were washed twice with PBS and resuspended in RPMI 1640 containing 10% FBS. BMDCs were maintained in RPMI 1640 containing 10% FBS and antibiotic-antimycotic (Life technologies, Carlsbad, CA, USA) at 37°C. Cells (5×10^5/mL) were seeded and cultured for 24 h in complete medium for further experiments.

Flow Cytometric Analysis

BMDCs were resuspended in fluorescence activated cell sorter (FACS) buffer (PBS containing 1% FCS and 0.05% NaN_3), to assess the surface expression of CD11b/Mac-1 protein. Cells were incubated with a FcR blocker to block non-specific antibody binding, and then incubated with PE-conjugated anti-mouse CD11b antibody (1:500). Analysis was performed using a FACS Calibur and CELLQUESTPRO software BD, and 1×10^4 cells were recorded per sample. Live cells were gated based on size (FSC) and granularity (SSC), and then CD11b/Mac-1 expression was analyzed. Fluorescence was analyzed by FACS as described above.

Reverse Transcription-PCR Analysis

Total RNA was isolated from cells using QIAzol (Qiagen, Hilden, Germany) and reverse transcribed into cDNA using the Improm-II Reverse Transcription System (Promega). cDNA amplification was performed using primers specific for 5-LO (forward, 5′-ATTGCCATCCAGCTCAACCAAACC-3′; reverse, 5′-TGGCGATACCAAACACCTCAGACA-3′). 5-LO mRNA levels in BMDCs were quantified by RT-PCR using GAPDH mRNA as the internal standard. Relative intensities were expressed as fold changes vs. GAPDH.

Western Blot Analysis

BMDC lysates were prepared in ice-cold lysis buffer, and equal amounts of proteins were separated on 8~10% polyacrylamide gel under reducing conditions, and then transferred to nitrocellulose membranes (Amersham-Pharmacia Biotech, Piscataway, NJ, USA). Membranes were blocked with 5% skim milk in TBST and incubated overnight with primary antibody (1:1000) in 5% skim milk. Blots were washed with TBST, incubated with HRP-conjugated secondary antibody for 2 h, and developed using ECL Western blot detection reagents (Amersham-Pharmacia Biotech). Membranes were re-blotted with anti-β-actin antibody (Santa Cruz Biotechnology) as an internal control. Signals from bands were quantified using US-SCAN-IT gel 5.1 software (Silk Scientific, Orem, Utah, USA). Results were expressed as relative densities.

Quantitative Real-Time Reverse Transcription Analysis

Total RNA was isolated from cells using QIAzol (Qiagen) and reverse transcribed into cDNA using the Improm-II Reverse Transcription System (Promega). BLTR1 gene expression was determined by real-time PCR using 1 ng of reverse-transcribed cDNA and a LightCycler 96 system equipped with LightCycler DNA Master SYBR Green I (Roche Molecular Biochemicals, Mannheim, Germany). PCR was performed under the following conditions: 95°C for 10 min followed by 50 amplification cycles of 95°C for 10 s, 45°C for 10 s, and 72°C for 10 s. Amplification efficiencies were calculated and normalized with respect to mouse GAPDH. The PCR primers used were as follows: forward, 5'-TTACCACCTGGTGAACCTGGTGGAA-3'; reverse, 5'-TTCGAAGACTCAGGAATGGTGGAG-3'. Quantities were calculated using standard curves.

Measurement of LTB4 Production

LTB4 production was measured in extracellular medium using an LTB4 assay kit (Cayman Chemical Inc., Ann Arbor, MI, USA) according to the manufacturer's instructions. Briefly, BMDCs were stimulated with HMGB1 (100 ng/ml), and LTB4 levels in concentrated media were quantified by ELISA (Bio-Tek Instrument Inc., Winooski, VT, USA).

Preparation of BLTR1 siRNA and *in vitro* Transfection

Small interfering RNA (siRNA) for BLTR1 and scrambled siRNA (negative control) were designed and synthesized using a Silencer™ siRNA construction kit purchased from Bioneer. The sequences of BLTR1 siRNA and scrambled siRNA were 5′-GAUCUGCGCUCCGAACUAUdTdT-3′ and 5′-AUAGUUCGGAGCGCAGAUCdTdT-3′, respectively. For siRNA transfection, cells were seeded and transfected with BLTR1 siRNA using Lipofectamine 2000 (Invitrogen, NY, USA) according to the manufacturer's protocol. Transfection efficiencies were monitored using a fluorescent oligonucleotide (BLOCK-iT Fluorescent Oligo; Invitrogen) and estimated to be between 80 and 90%.

Immunofluorescence Analysis

Wire-injured femoral arteries were harvested and serial paraffin sections (4 μm) of femoral arteries were incubated with mouse-anti α-SMA (1:400) and rabbit-anti CD36 (1:200) antibodies. Alexa488-conjugated IgG and Alexa594-conjugated IgG (Abcam) were used to detect immunofluorescence signals for α-SMA and CD36, respectively. After nuclei were visualized by staining with 0.1 μg/ml diamidino-2-phenylindole (DAPI), slides were mounted in Vectashield. Fluorescence images were visualized by scanning confocal microscopy (LSM 510, Carl Zeiss, Oberkochen, Germany), and analyzed by National Institutes of Health (NIH) image software (Image J, NIH, USA).

Transplantation of Bone Marrow-Derived Monocytes

BMDCs were harvested from the femurs and tibiae of mice (7 wks, male), which had been euthanized by carbon dioxide insufflation and cervical dislocation, and bone marrow-derived monocytes (BMDMs, CD11b-positive cells) were then separated using MACS technology (Miltenyi, Bergisch Gladbach, GER) using a standard procedure. BMDCs were then stained with fluorochrome-labeled monoclonal anti-CD11b, sorted using a BD ARIAIII cell sorter (Becton Dickinson, San Jose, CA, USA), washed, and resuspended at 1×10^7 cells/ml. Recipient BLTR1-deficient mice were administered 1×10^7 BMDMs per mouse by tail vein injection. The expressions of BLTR1 mRNA and protein in peripheral blood monocytes (PBMCs) isolated from three groups of BMDMs-transplanted mice (WTWT mice, WT monocytes into WT mice; KOKO mice, BLTR1-deficient monocytes into BLTR1-deficient mice; and WTKO mice, WT monocytes into BLTR1-deficient mice) were determined by Real Time PCR and immunocytochemistry, respectively.

Statistical Analysis

Results were expressed as means ± SEMs. One way analysis of variance (ANOVA) followed by Turkey's multiple comparison test was used to determine the significance of differences. Statistical significance was accepted for P values < 0.05.

RESULTS

A Role for 5-LO in MMD Induced by HMGB1

The effects of HMGB1 on the expression of 5-LO mRNA and protein in BMDCs were determined using semi-quantitative RT-PCR and Western blot analysis. In previous studies, HMGB1 were secreted to 10–100 ng/ml physiologically or pathologically (27, 28). Thus, BMDCs were treated with HMGB1 at concentrations of 100 ng/ml in our study. As shown in **Figure 1A**, HMGB1 at concentration of 100 ng/ml increased the mRNA and protein expression of 5-LO in a time-dependent manner in BMDCs and THP-1 cells (**Supplementary Figure 1**), which were attenuated by inhibition of various receptors for HMGB1 (**Supplementary Figure 2**). To determine the functional role of 5-LO increased in HMGB1-stimulated cells, LTB4 production in HMGB1-treated cells was measured using ELISA. As shown in **Figure 1B**, LTB4 production in HMGB1-stimulated cells was gradually increased up to 24 h (approximately 10 ng/10^7 cells), suggesting the potential involvement of 5-LO-derived LTs in MMD induction by HMGB1.

To evaluate the potential role for 5-LO on MMD induction by HMGB1, we determined the effects of Zileuton (10 or 30 μM), a 5-LO inhibitor, on MMD induced by HMGB1. When the cellular morphology of HMGB1-stimulated BMDCs were photographed under a phase contrast microscope, the majority of cells had a macrophage-like morphology, were larger than non-stimulated cells, and strongly adherent and irregular or spindle shaped. Immunocytochemistry of HMGB1-stimulated BMDCs also revealed that the surface expression of CD11b/Mac-1 (red) was markedly increased, which was significantly attenuated by pre-treatment with Zileuton, suggesting a potential role for 5-LO in MMD induced by HMGB1 (**Figure 1C**).

Participation of BLTR1 Signaling in Monocytes During HMGB1-Induced MMD

To evaluate the role of leukotriene (LT) receptor signaling in monocytes during HMGB1-induced MMD, BMDCs were stimulated with HMGB1 (100 ng/ml) for 10 days in the presence of various leukotriene receptor inhibitors, including U75302 (a BLTR1 inhibitor), LY255283 (a BLTR2 inhibitor), REV5901 (a cysLTR1 inhibitor), and HAMI3379 (a cysLTR2 inhibitor). As shown in **Figure 2**, flow cytometric analysis showed an increase in the surface expression of CD11b/Mac-1 on BMDCs stimulated with HMGB1, which were attenuated dose-dependently by pretreatment with a BLTR1 inhibitor (U75302), but not by BLTR2 and cysLTR inhibitors. To further identify the role of BLTR1 in monocytes, we determined HMGB1-induced CD11b/Mac-1 expression in BLTR1-deficient BMDCs. As shown in **Figure 3**, HMGB1-induced expression of CD11b/Mac-1 on BMDCs was markedly attenuated in BLTR1-depleted cells using siRNA as well as in BLTR1-deficient cells isolated from BLTR1-deficient mice, suggesting a pivotal involvement of BLTR1 in HMGB1-induced MMD.

Exogenous LTB4 Augmented HMGB1-Induced MMD in 5-LO-Deficient BMDCs, but Not in BLTR1-Deficient BMDCs

On the basis of the hypothesis that 5-LO-derived LTB4 in HMGB1-stimulated cells might play an important role in the process of MMD, the effects of exogenous LTB4 on MMD were investigated in 5-LO-deficient cells. Although LTB4 (1–10 ng/ml) had minimal direct effects on MMD in control and 5-LO-deficient BMDCs (**Supplementary Figure 3**), the attenuated MMD in 5-LO-deficient cells stimulated with HMGB1 was

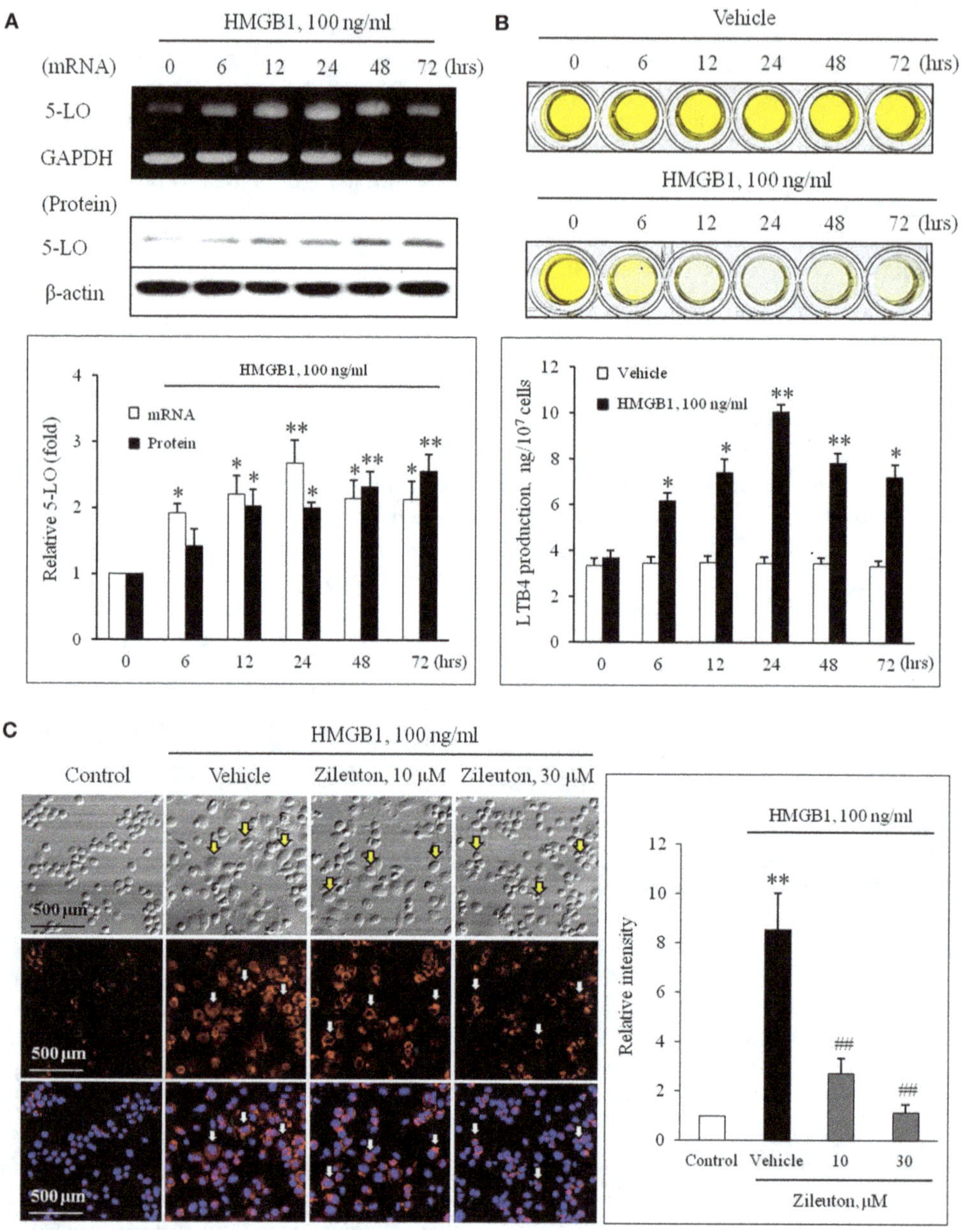

FIGURE 1 | Role of 5-LO in monocytes on monocyte-to-macrophage differentiation (MMD) induced by HMGB1. **(A)** Time-courses of the expressions of 5-LO mRNA and protein in BMDCs stimulated with HMGB1 (100 ng/ml) were determined using RT-PCR and Western blot, respectively. Bottom: Blot densities were quantified and presented as the means ± SEMs of 6–7 independent experiments. $^*P < 0.05$; $^{**}P < 0.01$ vs. corresponding value at 0 h. **(B)** Time-course of LTB4 production in vehicle- or HMGB1 (100 ng/ml)-stimulated BMDCs as determined by ELISA. Bottom: Color signals were quantified, and data were presented as the means ± SEMs of 6–7 independent experiments. $^*P < 0.05$; $^{**}P < 0.01$ vs. value at 0 h. **(C)** Representative immunocytochemical images of BMDCs stimulated with HMGB1. BMDCs were pre-treated with Zileuton at 10 or 30 μM for 1 h, and then stimulated with HMGB1 (100 ng/ml) for 10 days. Cells were stained with anti-CD11b/Mac-1 (red) and DAPI (blue), and then morphological changes and CD11b/Mac-1 expressions were photographed under a phase contrast microscope. Arrows indicate cells with a macrophage-like morphology. Right: Images were analyzed using Image J, and data were presented as the means ± SEMs of 3–4 independent experiments. $^{**}P < 0.01$ vs. control, $^{\#\#}P < 0.01$ vs. vehicle.

significantly reversed to the control level when cells were pre-treated with LTB4 at 10 ng/ml, a concentration comparable to that produced in HMGB1 (100 ng/ml)-stimulated control cells (**Figure 4**), which indicated the importance of the role played by LTB4 in HMGB1-induced MMD. Interestingly, the attenuated MMD by HMGB1 in BLTR1-deficient cells was not reversed by pre-treating cells with exogenous LTB4 (**Figure 4**). Collectively, these findings indicate the important role of LTB4-BLTR1 signaling in HMGB1-induced MMD in monocytes.

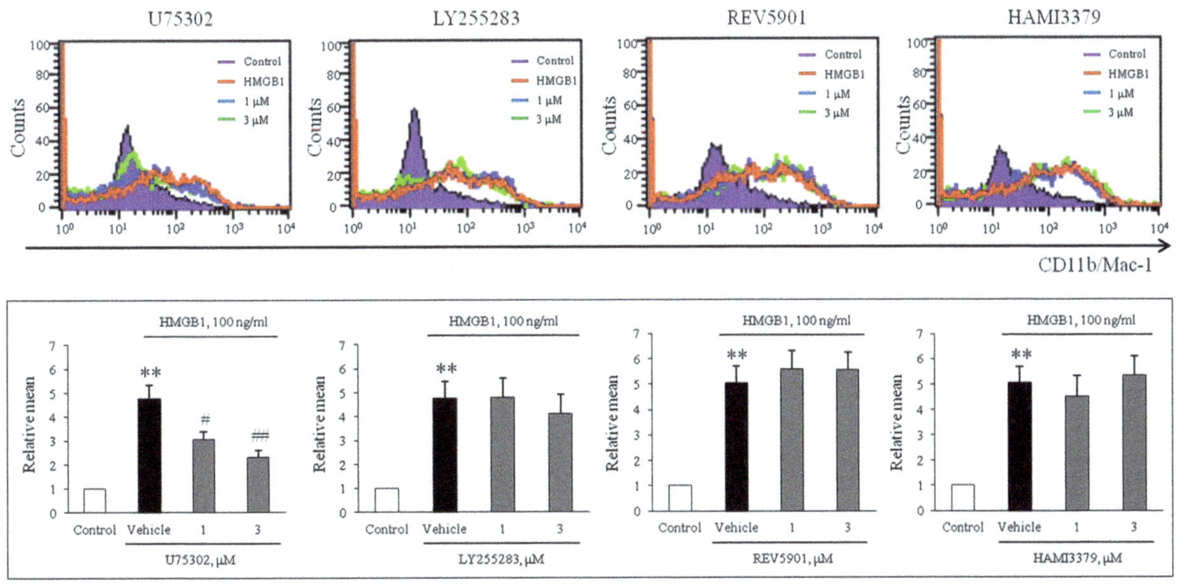

FIGURE 2 | A potential role of BLTR1 signaling in monocytes on HMGB1-induced MMD. Representative flow cytometric images of CD11b/Mac-1 expression in BMDCs treated with HMGB1 (100 ng/ml) in the presence or absence of inhibitors for BLTR1 (U75302), BLTR2 (LY255283), cysLTR1 (REV5901), and cysLTR2 (HAMI3379). Bottom: Surface expressions of CD11b/Mac-1 on macrophages were expressed as mean fluorescent intensities. Quantified data were presented as the means ± SEMs of 7–8 independent experiments. $^{**}P < 0.01$ vs. control, $^{\#}P < 0.05$; $^{\#\#}P < 0.01$ vs. vehicle.

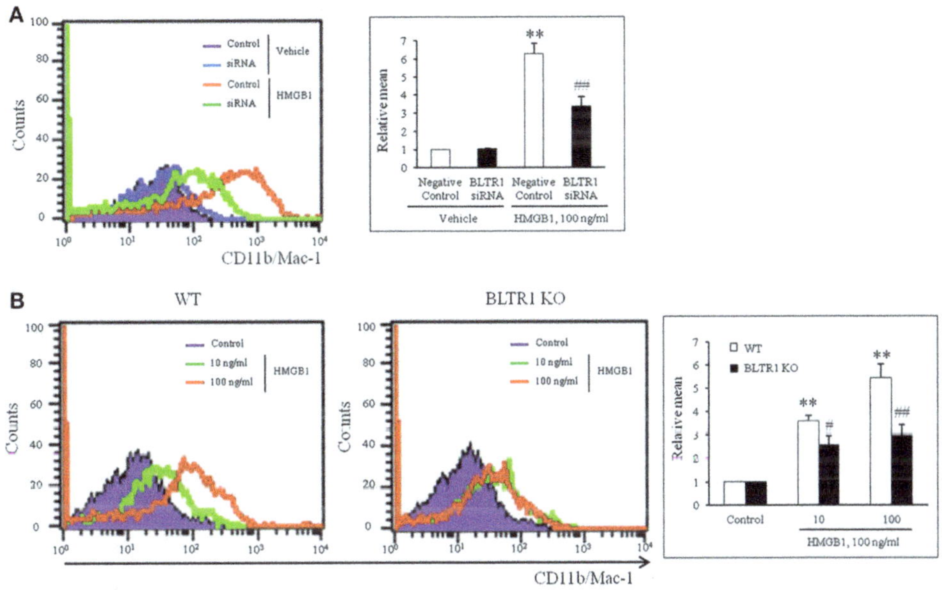

FIGURE 3 | Identification of the role played by BLTR1 in monocytes during HMGB1-induced MMD. **(A)** Representative flow cytometric images of CD11b/Mac-1 expression in BLTR1-depleted BMDCs. BMDCs were transfected with negative control or BLTR1 siRNA for 48 h, and then stimulated with HMGB1 (100 ng/ml) for 10 days. Right: Mean fluorescent intensities were quantified, and data were presented as the means ± SEMs of 5–6 independent experiments. $^{**}P < 0.01$ vs. corresponding negative control in vehicle, $^{\#\#}P < 0.01$ vs. negative control in HMGB1. **(B)** Representative flow cytometric images of CD11b/Mac-1 expression in BLTR1-deficient BMDCs. BMDCs isolated from wild-type (WT) or BLTR1-deficient (KO) mice were stimulated with HMGB1 for 10 days, and then cellular expressions of CD11b/Mac-1 were determined by flow cytometry. Right: Differential interface flow cytometric images of CD11b/Mac-1 expression were quantified, and data were presented as the means ± SEMs of 4–5 independent experiments. $^{**}P < 0.01$ vs. corresponding control, $^{\#}P < 0.05$; $^{\#\#}P < 0.01$ vs. corresponding value in WT mice.

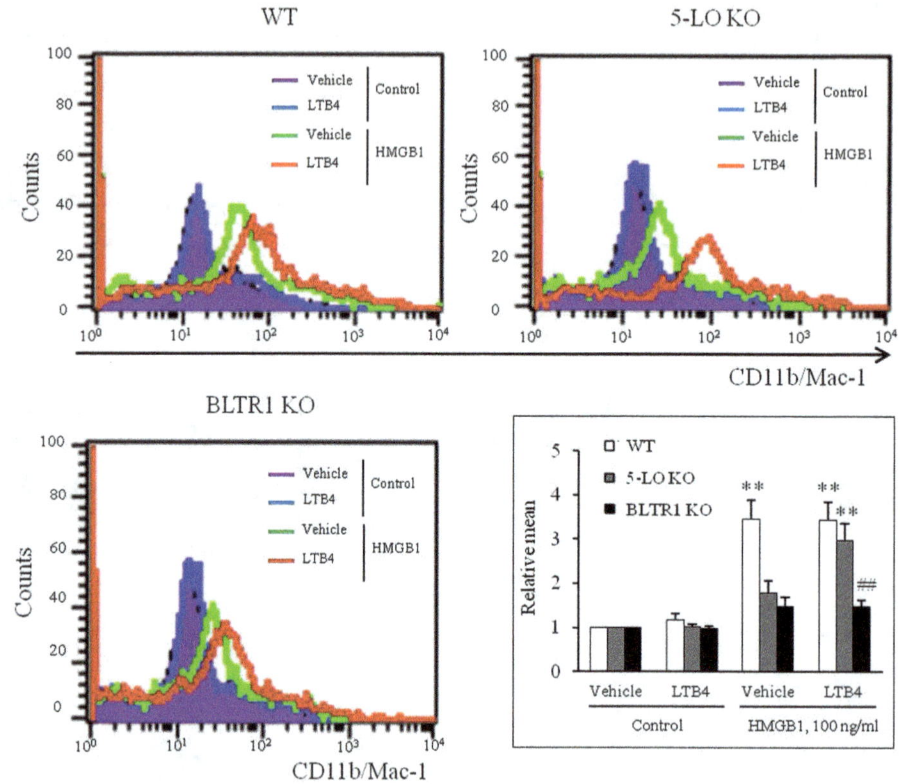

FIGURE 4 | Role of LTB4-BLTR1 signaling in monocytes on HMGB1-induced MMD. Representative flow cytometric images of CD11b/Mac-1 expression in HMGB1-stimulated BMDCs in the presence or absence of exogenous LTB4. BMDCs isolated from wild-type (WT), 5-LO-deficient (KO), and BLTR1-KO mice, were incubated with LTB4 (10 ng/ml) for 1 h, and then treated with HMGB1 (100 ng/ml) to induce MMD. The cellular expressions of CD11b/Mac-1 were determined by flow cytometry. Bottom right: Differential CD11b/Mac-1 expressions in interface flow cytometric images were quantified, and data were presented as the means ± SEMs of 8–9 independent experiments. $^{**}P < 0.01$ vs. corresponding value in control, $^{\#\#}P < 0.01$ vs. corresponding value in WT mice.

Role of BLTR1 in Vascular Inflammation and Neointima Formation in Wire-Injured Vasculature

To investigate the potential involvement of HMGB1 in the progression of vascular inflammation and neointima formation, we determined the levels of HMGB1 in the injured vasculatures. At 4 wks after wire injury, HMGB1 levels were markedly increased in neointima lesions of the injured vasculatures from both control and BLTR1-deficient mice. However, blood flow changes and neointima formation in the injured vasculatures were attenuated in BLTR1-deficient mice compared to those of control mice. Likewise, macrophage infiltration into neointima was also markedly attenuated in BLTR1-deficient mice (**Figure 5**), suggesting BLTR1 contributed to vascular inflammation and subsequent neointima formation induced by damage-associated mediators secreted in the injured vasculatures.

To investigate the contribution of BLTR1 in monocytes to macrophage infiltration of neointima lesions, BMDMs of WT mice were adoptively transferred into BLTR1-deficient mice. When BLTR1 mRNA levels in PBMCs isolated from the three groups of BMDM-transplanted mice (WTWT, WT monocytes into WT mice; WTKO, WT monocytes into BLTR1-deficient mice; and KOKO, BLTR1-deficient monocytes into BLTR1-deficient mice) were determined by Real Time PCR, an increase in BLTR1 mRNA levels in the monocytes of recipient mice was detected at 1 and 5 wks after adoptive transplantation (**Figure 6A**). Likewise, an increase in BLTR1 protein levels observed in monocytes of recipient mice was also detected at 5 wks after adoptive transplantation (**Figure 6B**). As shown in **Figure 6C**, intimal hyperplasia and macrophage infiltration were significantly increased in WT monocyte-recipient mice (WTKO) comparing with that in BLTR1-deficient mice transferred with BLTR1-deficient BMDMs (KOKO). These observations suggested that BLTR1 in monocytes played a critical role in the infiltration of macrophage into neointima lesions, and that they influenced neointima formation in our murine model of femoral artery injury.

DISCUSSION

In this study, we investigated the importance of leukotriene signaling in monocytes on monocyte-to-macrophage differentiation and vascular inflammation and resultant intimal hyperplasia in a mouse model of wire-injured femoral artery. In cultured primary BMDCs, genetic or pharmacological

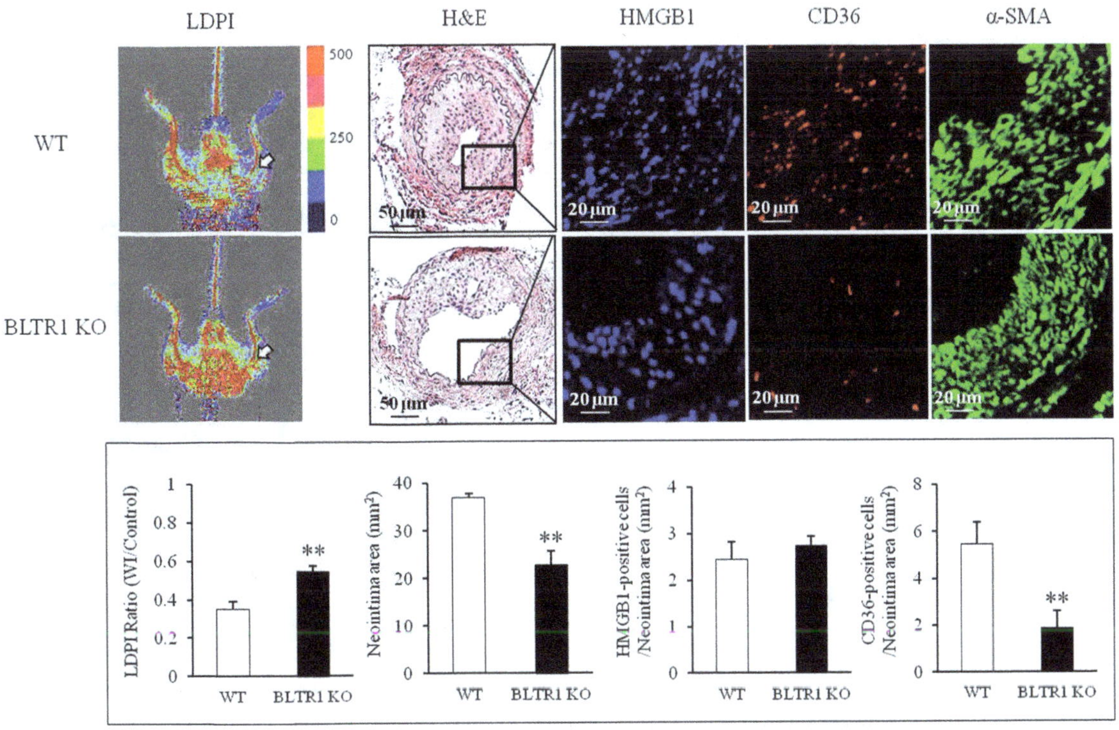

FIGURE 5 | Involvement of BLTR1 in macrophage infiltration and neointima formation in wire-injured femoral arteries. Doppler images: Blood flow in the femoral arteries of WT and BLTR1-deficient (KO) mice at 4 wks after wire injury (WI) was assessed using a LDPI analyzer. In these color-coded images, red hue indicates regions of maximum perfusion, medium perfusion values are shown in yellow, and lowest perfusion values are represented as blue. Arrows indicate blood flow in an injured femoral artery. Photographs are representative of 5-6 independent experiments. H&E: Cross sections of mouse femoral arteries were prepared at 4 wks after WI, and stained with H&E. HMGB1 and CD36: HMGB1 and macrophage infiltration in the indicated neointima were stained with anti-HMGB1 antibody and anti-CD36 antibody, respectively. α-SMA: VSMCs were stained with anti-α-SMA antibody. Images are representative of 5–6 independent experiments. Bottom: LDPI ratio was quantified as the ratio of the blue-to-red pixels in the injured artery (WI) vs. non-injured arteries (Control). Neointima volumes in the cross sections of injured femoral artery were determined using an image analyzer. Numbers of HMGB1-positive and CD36-positive cells in neointima area were quantified, and data were presented as the means ± SEMs of 3-4 independent experiments. $^{**}P < 0.01$ vs. WT mice.

inhibition of the 5-lipoxygenase pathway in monocytes attenuated MMD induced by HMGB1, an endogenous damage-associated molecular patterns. Among various inhibitors for leukotriene receptors, U75302, a BLTR1 inhibitor, exclusively attenuated MMD induced by HMGB1. The importance of BLTR1 signaling during HMGB1-induced MMD was also demonstrated using BLTR1-deficient BMDCs. Thus, BLTR1 signaling in monocytes was suggested as a pivotal player in MMD induced by HMGB1, leading to vascular inflammation after vascular injury.

MMD is a key event in the process of vascular inflammation, which results in the remodeling of the injured vasculatures (29). Thus, an understanding of the fundamental molecular mechanisms that underlie this differentiation is an important aspect of identifying new therapeutic strategies. In our previous study, the importance of 5-LO in monocytes was identified using genetic and pharmacological inhibition of the 5-LO pathway in monocytes (7). In addition, in accordance with previous report by Yu et al. (18) in which disruption of the LT synthesis/response pathway in myeloid cells restrained several components of response to injury, we showed in a previous *in vivo* study 5-LO in monocytes played a pivotal role in vascular inflammation and resultant restenosis (7). However, although the importance of 5-LO in monocytes during MMD with subsequent vascular inflammation was identified, the 5-LO-linked signaling in monocytes mediating MMD need to be identified to develop specific target-based therapeutics, because 5-LO in monocytes exert its action via production of various leukotrienes (LT) including LTB4 and cysteinyl LTs.

Leukotrienes exert their actions via four subclasses of 7-transmembrane G-protein-coupled cell surface receptors. BLTR1 and BLTR2 are high and low affinity receptors of LTB4, respectively, whereas CysLT1 and CysLT2 are activated by cysteinyl-LTs (30–32). Thus, we stimulated BMDCs in the presence of various inhibitors for LT receptors including LTB4 receptors (BLTR1 or BLTR2) or cysteinyl LT receptors (cysLTR1 or cysLTR2). In our present study, U75302 (a BLTR1 inhibitor) exclusively attenuated MMD induced by HMGB1 among various inhibitors. The importance of BLTR1 in monocytes on HMGB1-induced MMD was also demonstrated using BLTR1-deficient cells. Moreover, HMGB1 increased 5-LO expression in monocytes with subsequent production of LTB4 in the

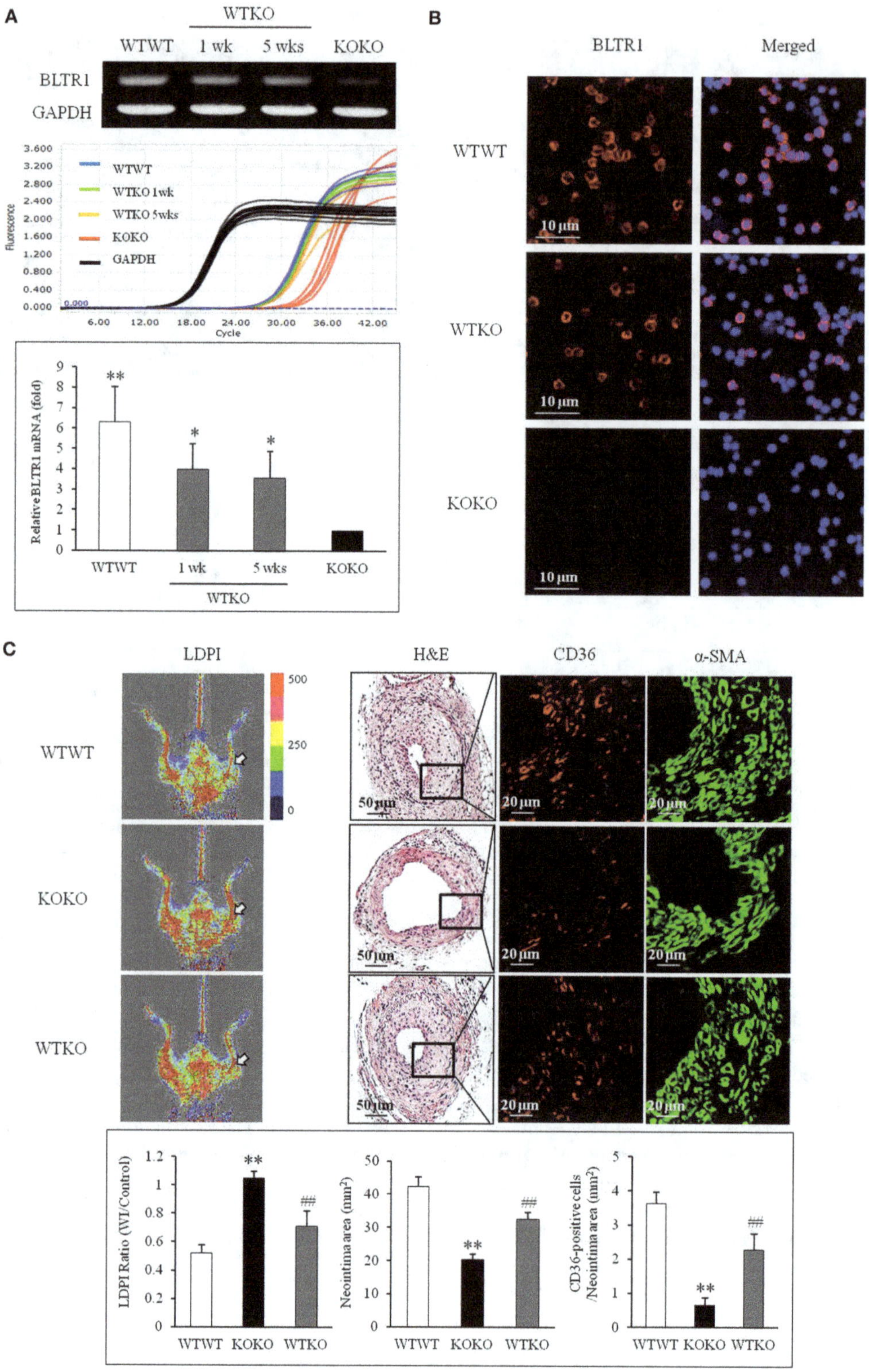

FIGURE 6 | Identification of a pivotal role for BLTR1 in monocytes on vascular inflammation and neointima formation in the wire-injured femoral artery. **(A)** Expressions of BLTR1 mRNA in PBMCs isolated from three groups of mice transplanted with BMDMs (WTWT, WT cells into WT mice; KOKO, BLTR1-deficient cells into BLTR1-deficient mice; and WTKO, WT cells into BLTR1-deficient mice) were determined by Real Time PCR. PCR signals were quantified, and data were presented as the means ± SEMs of 4–5 independent experiments. $^*P < 0.05$; $^{**}P < 0.01$ vs. KOKO mice. **(B)** Expressions of BLTR1 protein in PBMCs isolated from these three groups of mice at 5 wks post-transplantation were determined by immunocytochemistry. Photographs are representative of 3–4 independent experiments.

(Continued)

FIGURE 6 | (C) Doppler imaging: Blood flow in the femoral arteries of WTWT, WTKO, and KOKO mice at 4 wks after wire injury were monitored using a LDPI analyzer. Arrows indicate blood flow in the injured femoral artery. Photographs are representative of 4–5 independent experiments. H&E: Cross sections of the femoral arteries of WTWT, WTKO, and KOKO mice at 4 wks after wire injury were stained with H&E. CD36 & α-SMA: Infiltrating macrophages in indicated neointima was stained with anti-CD36 antibody, and VSMCs were stained with anti-α-SMA antibody. Photographs are representative of 4–5 independent experiments. Bottom: LDPI ratio was quantified as the ratio of the blue-to-red pixels in the injured artery (WI) vs. non-injured arteries (Control). Neointima volumes were determined using an image analyzer. Numbers of CD36-positive cells within neointima area in the injured artery of WT and BLTR1-deficient mice were quantified, and data were expressed as the means ± SEMs of 4–5 independent experiments. $^{**}P < 0.01$ vs. WTWT mice, $^{\#\#}P < 0.01$ vs. KOKO mice.

present study, suggesting that HMGB1 might induce MMD via production of 5-LO-mediated production of LTB4.

To determine the direct functional role of exogenous LTB4 on MMD, BMDCs were stimulated with various concentrations of LTB4 in the absence or presence of HMGB1. We found that LTB4 had minimal effects on MMD in cells from control, 5-LO-deficient and BLTR1-deficient mice. However, MMD suppression by HMGB1 was significantly reversed by exogenous LTB4 in 5-LO-deficient cells, but not in BLTR1-deficient cells, suggesting LTB4/BLTR1 signaling as a pivotal player for HMGB1-induced MMD. Thus, LTB4/BLTR1-mediated priming of monocytes is considered as an essential prerequisite for HMGB1-induced MMD based on the previous report that exogenous LTB4 potentiated the priming effect of cytokines on human monocytes (33). However, further studies are remained to determine the precise roles of these signals in cell priming.

The molecular processes that initiate inflammation in arterial walls after mechanical injury are not fully understood. Recently, endogenous molecules released during cell death and stress, termed DAMPs, could activate pattern recognition receptors and lead to inflammation, because endoluminal vascular interventional procedures cause stretching of vessel walls and subsequent cell necrosis (34). Thus, coordinated relationships exist between local vascular injury and pattern recognition receptor-related signals in the process of vascular inflammation (20). Of the various DAMPs, HMGB1 has emerged as an important regulator of inflammatory responses resulting from tissue injury (3, 4), and has been implicated as an active player in vascular inflammation leading to intimal hyperplasia after arterial injury (6). Reportedly, HMGB1 is known to have pro-inflammatory cytokine-like activity, promote chemotaxis, and stimulate cellular migration and growth (35). Interestingly, in a previous study we found HMGB1 enhanced MMD and caused vascular inflammation (7). Collectively, these observations suggest that HMGB1-related signals in monocytes might be considered therapeutic targets for the treatment of vascular inflammation.

In our *in vivo* study, both macrophage infiltration and intimal hyperplasia in the wire-injured femoral artery were markedly attenuated in BLTR1-deficient mice compared to that in wild-type control mice. Although the importance of BLTR1 in vascular smooth muscle cells in the intimal hyperplasia has been reported previously (16), we expected the potential role for BLTR1 in monocytes in vascular inflammation on the basis of our *in vitro* data in which the BLTR1 signaling in monocytes played a pivotal role in MMD induced by HMGB1. To confirm the contribution of BLTR1 in monocytes in macrophage infiltration into neointimal lesion, BMDMs isolated from WT mice were adoptively transferred into BLTR1-deficient mice as previously described (7, 18). In our present study, intimal hyperplasia and macrophage infiltration were significantly greater in BLTR1-deficient mice administered WT BMDMs than those in BLTR1 deficient mice administered BLTR1-deficient BMDMs. Based on these results, it was suggested that BLTR1 in monocytes played a pivotal role in MMD induced by HMGB1, and subsequent macrophage infiltration in the injured vasculatures with neointima formation in our murine wire-injured femoral artery model.

AUTHOR CONTRIBUTIONS

SEB and CDK designed and performed experiments, analyzed the experimental data, and wrote the manuscript, and SSB, KK, and WSL contributed to data analysis. SYP performed experiments. All authors approved the final manuscript.

FUNDING

This research was supported by the Basic Science Research Program (NRF-2016R1A2B2011509) and by the Medical Research Center (MRC) Program (NRF-2015R1A5A2009656) through the National Research Foundation of Korea (NRF) grant funded by the Korean government (MSIP).

REFERENCES

1. Land WG. Chronic allograft dysfunction: a model disorder of innate immunity. *Biomed J.* (2013) 36:209–28. doi: 10.4103/2319-4170.117622
2. Cai JJ, Wen J, Bauer E, Zhong H, Yuan H, Chen AF. The role of HMGB1 in cardiovascular biology: danger signals. *Antioxid Redox Signal* (2015) 23:1351–69. doi: 10.1089/ars.2015.6408
3. Venereau E, Schiraldi M, Uguccioni M, Bianchi ME. HMGB1 and leukocyte migration during trauma and sterile inflammation. *Mol Immunol.* (2013) 55:76–82. doi: 10.1016/j.molimm.2012.10.037
4. Izuishi K, Tsung A, Jeyabalan G, Critchlow ND, Li J, Tracey KJ, et al. Cutting edge: high-mobility group box 1 preconditioning protects against liver ischemia-reperfusion injury. *J Immunol.* (2006) 176:7154–8. doi: 10.4049/jimmunol.176.12.7154

5. Liaw PC, Ito T, Iba T, Thachil J, Zeerleder S. DAMP and DIC: the role of extracellular DNA and DNA-binding proteins in the pathogenesis of DIC. *Blood Rev.* (2016) 30:257–61. doi: 10.1016/j.blre.2015.12.004
6. Cai J, Yuan H, Wang Q, Yang H, Al-Abed Y, Hua Z, et al. HMGB1-driven inflammation and intimal hyperplasia after arterial injury involves cell-specific actions mediated by TLR4. *Arterioscler Thromb Vasc Biol.* (2015) 35:2579–93. doi: 10.1161/ATVBAHA.115.305789
7. Baek SE, Jang MA, Lee SJ, Park SY, Bae SS, Kim CD. 5-Lipoxygenase in monocytes emerges as a therapeutic target for intimal hyperplasia in a murine wire-injured femoral artery. *Biochim Biophys Acta.* (2017) 1863:2210–19. doi: 10.1016/j.bbadis.2017.06.012
8. La Gruta NL, Kedzierska K, Stambas J, Doherty PC. A question of self-preservation: immunopathology in influenza virus infection. *Immunol Cell Biol.* (2007) 85:85–92. doi: 10.1038/sj.icb.7100026
9. Shi C, Pamer EG. Monocyte recruitment during infection and inflammation. *Nat Rev Immunol.* (2011) 11:762–74. doi: 10.1038/nri3070
10. Welt FG, Rogers C. Inflammation and restenosis in the stent era. *Arterioscler Thromb Vasc Biol.* (2002) 22:1769–76. doi: 10.1161/01.ATV.0000037100.44766.5B
11. Spanbroek R, Grabner R, Lotzer K, Hildner M, Urbach A, Ruhling K, et al. Expanding expression of the 5-lipoxygenase pathway within the arterial wall during human atherogenesis. *Proc Natl Acad Sci USA.* (2003) 100:1238–43. doi: 10.1073/pnas.242716099
12. Lotzer K, Funk CD, Habenicht AJ. The 5-lipoxygenase pathway in arterial wall biology and atherosclerosis. *Biochim Biophys Acta.* (2005) 1736:30–7. doi: 10.1016/j.bbalip.2005.07.001
13. Poeckel D, Funk CD. The 5-lipoxygenase/leukotriene pathway in preclinical models of cardiovascular disease. *Cardiovasc Res.* (2010) 86:243–53. doi: 10.1093/cvr/cvq016
14. Mehrabian M, Allayee H, Wong J, Shi W, Wang XP, Shaposhnik Z, et al. Identification of 5-lipoxygenase as a major gene contributing to atherosclerosis susceptibility in mice. *Circ Res.* (2002) 91:120–6. doi: 10.1161/01.RES.0000028008.99774.7F
15. Ghazalpour A, Wang X, Lusis AJ, Mehrabian M. Complex inheritance of the 5-lipoxygenase locus influencing atherosclerosis in mice. *Genetics* (2006) 173:943–51. doi: 10.1534/genetics.106.057455
16. Back M, Bu DX, Branstrom R, Sheikine Y, Yan ZQ, Hansson GK. Leukotriene B4 signaling through NF-kappaB-dependent BLT1 receptors on vascular smooth muscle cells in atherosclerosis and intimal hyperplasia. *Proc Natl Acad Sci USA.* (2005) 102:17501–6. doi: 10.1073/pnas.0505845102
17. Lee SJ, Choi EK, Seo KW, Bae JU, Kim YH, Park SY, et al. 5-Lipoxygenase plays a pivotal role in endothelial adhesion of monocytes via an increased expression of Mac-1. *Cardiovasc Res.* (2013) 99:724–33. doi: 10.1093/cvr/cvt135
18. Yu Z, Ricciotti E, Miwa T, Liu S, Ihida-Stansbury K, Landersberg G, et al. Myeloid cell 5-lipoxygenase activating protein modulates the response to vascular injury. *Circ Res.* (2013) 112:432–40. doi: 10.1161/CIRCRESAHA.112.300755
19. Khan R, Spagnoli V, Tardif JC, LAllier PL. Novel anti-inflammatory therapies for the treatment of atherosclerosis. *Atherosclerosis* (2015) 240:497–509. doi: 10.1016/j.atherosclerosis.2015.04.783
20. Back M, Weber C, Lutgens E. Regulation of atherosclerotic plaque inflammation. *J Intern Med.* (2015) 278:462–82. doi: 10.1111/joim.12367
21. Back M, Hansson GK. Leukotriene receptors in atherosclerosis. *Ann Med.* (2006) 38:493–502. doi: 10.1080/07853890600982737
22. Li RC, Haribabu B, Mathis SP, Kim J, Gozal D. Leukotriene B4 receptor-1 mediates intermittent hypoxia-induced atherogenesis. *Am J Respir Crit Care Med.* (2011) 184:124–31. doi: 10.1164/rccm.201012-2039OC
23. Aiello RJ, Bourassa PA, Lindsey S, Weng W, Freeman A, Showell HJ. Leukotriene B4 receptor antagonism reduces monocytic foam cells in mice. *Arterioscler Thromb Vasc Biol.* (2002) 22:443–9. doi: 10.1161/hq0302.105593
24. Subbarao K, Jala VR, Mathis S, Suttles J, Zacharias W, Ahamed J, et al. Role of leukotriene B4 receptors in the development of atherosclerosis: potential mechanisms. *Arterioscler Thromb Vasc Biol.* (2004) 24:369–75. doi: 10.1161/01.ATV.0000110503.16605.15
25. Heller EA, Liu E, Tager AM, Sinha S, Roberts JD, Koehn SL, et al. Inhibition of atherogenesis in BLT1-deficient mice reveals a role for LTB4 and BLT1 in smooth muscle cell recruitment. *Circulation* (2005) 112:578–86. doi: 10.1161/CIRCULATIONAHA.105.545616
26. Roque M, Fallon JT, Badimon JJ, Zhang WX, Taubman MB, Reis ED. Mouse model of femoral artery denudation injury associated with the rapid accumulation of adhesion molecules on the luminal surface and recruitment of neutrophils. *Arterioscler Thromb Vasc Biol.* (2000) 20:335–42. doi: 10.1161/01.ATV.20.2.335
27. Hirata Y, Kurobe H, Higashida M, Fukuda D, Shimabukuro M, Tanaka K, et al. HMGB1 plays a critical role in vascular inflammation and lesion formation via toll-like receptor 9. *Atherosclerosis* (2013) 231:227–33. doi: 10.1016/j.atherosclerosis.2013.09.010
28. Alleva LM, Budd AC, Clark IA. Systemic release of high mobility group box 1 protein during severe murine influenza. *J Immunol.* (2008) 181:1454–9. doi: 10.4049/jimmunol.181.2.1454
29. Ogle ME, Segar CE, Sridhar S, Botchwey EA. Monocytes and macrophages in tissue repair: implications for immunoregenerative biomaterial design. *Exp Biol Med.* (2016) 241:1084–97. doi: 10.1177/1535370216650293
30. Brink C, Dahlen SE, Drazen J, Evans JF, Hay DW, Nicosia S, et al. International union of pharmacology XXXVII. Nomenclature for leukotriene and lipoxin receptor. *Pharmacol Rev.* (2003) 55:195–227. doi: 10.1124/pr.55.1.8
31. Back M. Functional characteristics of cysteinyl-leukotriene receptor subtypes. *Life Sci.* (2002) 71:611–22. doi: 10.1016/S0024-3205(02)01733-2
32. Riccioni G, Zanasi A, Vitulano N, Mancini B, DOrazio N. Leukotrienes in atherosclerosis: new target insights and future therapy perspectives. *Mediators Inflamm.* (2009) 2009:737282. doi: 10.1155/2009/737282
33. Dugas N, Dugas B, Kolb JP, Yamaoka K, Delfraiss JF, Damais C. Role of leukotriene B4 in the interleukin-4-induced human mononuclear phagocyte activation. *Immunology* (1996) 88:384–8. doi: 10.1046/j.1365-2567.1996.d01-658.x
34. Zheng Y, Gardner SE, Clarke MC. Cell death, damage-associated molecular patterns, and sterile inflammation in cardiovascular disease. *Arterioscler Thromb Vasc Biol.* (2011) 31:2781–6. doi: 10.1161/ATVBAHA.111.224907
35. Andersson U, Tracey KJ. HMGB1 is a therapeutic target for sterile inflammation and infection. *Annu Rev Immunol.* (2011) 29:139–62. doi: 10.1146/annurev-immunol-030409-101323

19

CD8$^+$-T Cells with Specificity for a Model Antigen in Cardiomyocytes can Become Activated After Transverse Aortic Constriction but do not Accelerate Progression to Heart Failure

Carina Gröschel[1,2†], André Sasse[1†], Sebastian Monecke[1,2], Charlotte Röhrborn[1], Leslie Elsner[1], Michael Didié[2,3,4], Verena Reupke[5], Gertrude Bunt[6], Andrew H. Lichtman[7], Karl Toischer[2,4], Wolfram-Hubertus Zimmermann[2,3], Gerd Hasenfuß[2,4] and Ralf Dressel[1,2]*

[1] Institute of Cellular and Molecular Immunology, University Medical Center Göttingen, Göttingen, Germany, [2] DZHK (German Center for Cardiovascular Research), Partner Site Göttingen, Göttingen, Germany, [3] Institute of Pharmacology and Toxicology, University Medical Center Göttingen, Göttingen, Germany, [4] Department of Cardiology and Pneumology, University Medical Center Göttingen, Göttingen, Germany, [5] Central Animal Facility, University Medical Center Göttingen, Göttingen, Germany, [6] Clinical Optical Microscopy, Department of Neuropathology, University Medical Center Göttingen, Göttingen, Germany, [7] Department of Pathology, Brigham and Women's Hospital, Harvard Medical School, Boston, MA, United States

***Correspondence:**
Ralf Dressel
rdresse@gwdg.de

† These authors have contributed equally to this work

Heart failure due to pressure overload is frequently associated with inflammation. In addition to inflammatory responses of the innate immune system, autoimmune reactions of the adaptive immune system appear to be triggered in subgroups of patients with heart failure as demonstrated by the presence of autoantibodies against myocardial antigens. Moreover, T cell-deficient and T cell-depleted mice have been reported to be protected from heart failure induced by transverse aortic constriction (TAC) and we have shown recently that CD4$^+$-helper T cells with specificity for an antigen in cardiomyocytes accelerate TAC-induced heart failure. In this study, we set out to investigate the potential contribution of CD8$^+$-cytotoxic T cells with specificity to a model antigen (ovalbumin, OVA) in cardiomyocytes to pressure overload-induced heart failure. In 78% of cMy-mOVA mice with cardiomyocyte-specific OVA expression, a low-grade OVA-specific cellular cytotoxicity was detected after TAC. Adoptive transfer of OVA-specific CD8$^+$-T cells from T cell receptor transgenic OT-I mice before TAC did not increase the risk of OVA-specific autoimmunity in cMy-mOVA mice. After TAC, again 78% of the mice displayed an OVA-specific cytotoxicity with on average only a three-fold higher killing of OVA-expressing target cells. More CD8$^+$ cells were present after TAC in the myocardium of cMy-mOVA mice with OT-I T cells (on average 17.5/mm^2) than in mice that did not receive OVA-specific CD8$^+$-T cells (3.6/mm^2). However, the extent of fibrosis was similar in both groups. Functionally, as determined by echocardiography, the adoptive transfer of

OVA-specific CD8+-T cells did not significantly accelerate the progression from hypertrophy to heart failure in cMy-mOVA mice. These findings argue therefore against a major impact of cytotoxic T cells with specificity for autoantigens of cardiomyocytes in pressure overload-induced heart failure.

Keywords: autoimmunity, autoantigen, pressure overload, cytotoxic T cells, adoptive transfer, transgenic T cell receptor, heart failure

INTRODUCTION

In many clinical studies signs of inflammation have been observed during the progression of chronic heart failure (1). Inflammation is thereby not restricted to heart failure occurring in the cause of classic inflammatory cardiomyopathies. It can occur also in response to hemodynamic overload (2). Increased levels of pro-inflammatory cytokines including interleukin (IL)-6 and tumor necrosis factor (TNF)-α were observed in the circulation of patients with pressure overload (3, 4). However, clinical studies targeting TNF-α by anti-inflammatory drugs have been largely unsuccessful in the therapy of heart failure (5, 6). Therefore, the pathophysiological basis of the inflammatory response to hemodynamic load needs to be further investigated to identify better therapeutic targets.

In addition to the unspecific immune response to tissue damage or cellular stress that is mediated by cells of the innate immune system, autoimmune responses of the adaptive immune system to myocardial antigens can contribute to the progression of heart failure. This is most obvious from studies of autoantibodies against myocardial antigens. Antibodies, e.g., against β1-adreno-receptors and M2-acetylcholine-receptors were found after transverse aortic constriction (TAC) in animal models (7). In patients, such autoantibodies of the IgG isotype can directly impair cardiac function (8, 9) and are therefore promising therapeutic targets (10, 11). Autoreactive T helper cells must also exist in these patients, since their help is required for immunoglobulin class switching to IgG in the autoreactive B cells.

We have recently demonstrated that T helper cells with specificity for an antigen in cardiomyocytes can contribute to the progression of heart failure after TAC also independently of autoantibodies (12). For this purpose, cMy-mOVA mice expressing the model antigen ovalbumin (OVA) on cardiomyocytes (13) were crossed with OT-II mice (14) expressing a transgenic T cell receptor (TCR) on CD4+-T cells with specificity for OVA. In the resulting double-transgenic cMy-mOVA-OT-II mice, progression from hypertrophy to heart failure after TAC was accelerated compared to cMy-mOVA mice. No OVA-specific antibodies were found after TAC but more T cells infiltrated the myocardium of cMy-mOVA-OT-II than cMy-mOVA mice where they could directly contribute to maladaptive cardiac remodeling (12).

It has not been investigated so far, whether CD8+-cytotoxic T lymphocytes (CTL) with specificity for an antigen in cardiomyocytes become also activated in response to pressure overload and contribute to the progression of heart failure. To address these questions, we analyzed whether CD8+-T cells with specificity against OVA become activated in cMy-mOVA mice after TAC. Moreover, we adoptively transferred CD8+-T cells with specificity for OVA from OT-I mice, carrying a transgenic TCR with specificity for OVA on CD8+-T cells (15), into cMy-mOVA mice before TAC to investigate whether they would contribute to the progression of heart failure. We show here that CTL with specificity for an antigen in cardiomyocytes indeed can become activated after TAC but fail to accelerate progression into heart failure.

MATERIALS AND METHODS

Animal Experiments

All animal experiments were approved by the responsible agency (Niedersächsisches Landesamt für Lebensmittelsicherheit und Verbraucherschutz) and were carried out in compliance with German and European legislation (Directive 2010/63/EU). OVA-transgenic cMy-mOVA (13), TCR-transgenic OT-I (15), and double-transgenic cMy-mOVA-OT-I mice were bred in the central animal facility at the University Medical Center Göttingen under specific pathogen-free conditions in individually ventilated cages and in a 12 h light-dark cycle. Both, OT-I and cMy-mOVA mice have a C57BL/6 background. Mice aged between 8 and 12 weeks were used for experiments. Male and female mice were equally distributed but otherwise randomly assigned to the experimental groups. The cMy-mOVA mice that received OVA-specific CD8+-T cells purified by magnetic activated cell sorting (MACS) from lymph nodes of OT-I mice are designated cMy-mOVA+OT-I mice. The adoptive transfer of 10^7 CD8+-T cells was performed by intravenous injection into the tail vein 1 day before surgery.

TAC and sham surgery was performed as described previously (12, 16). Briefly, the mice received intraperitoneal injections of medetomidin (0.5 mg/kg), midazolam (5 mg/kg), and fentanyl (0.05 mg/kg) for anesthesia. The transversal aorta was displayed after horizontal incision at the jugulum and a 26-gauge needle was tied against the aorta. The surgical thread was not tied in sham-operated mice. The skin was closed after removal of the needle and the anesthesia was reversed by subcutaneous injection of atipamezol (2.5 mg/kg) and flumazenil (0.5 mg/kg). The mice received buprenorphine (60 μg/kg) subcutaneously 1 h after surgery for further analgesia. Metamizole (1.33 mg/ml) had to be added to the drinking water for 1 week to achieve long-term analgesia.

The pressure gradient over the aortic ligature was measured using pulsed wave Doppler 3 days after surgery. At this time point, approximately 50 μl blood were taken from the orbital sinus of the mice to determine the presence of adoptively transferred $CD8^+$-T cells in the blood of cMy-mOVA+OT-I mice. For echocardiography, the mice were anesthetized with 3-% isoflurane, and temperature, respiration, and ECG-controlled anesthesia was maintained with 1.5-% isoflurane.

At the end of the experiments, 10 weeks after the operation, the mice were sacrificed in isoflurane anesthesia by cervical dislocation. The hearts were excised, perfused via the aorta with 0.9% NaCl and after weighting of the ventricles, one-third of the heart from the middle part was fixed in 3.7% formaldehyde solution overnight and the other two thirds oriented toward the basis and the apex of the heart were snap frozen in liquid nitrogen. Finally, spleens were harvested and placed in Dulbecco's modified Eagle medium (DMEM) on ice for further analysis.

Echocardiography

A Vevo2100 (VisualSonics, Toronto, Canada) system with a 30 MHz center frequency transducer was used for transthoracic echocardiography. B-mode recordings (16, 17) were used to determine the long axis in systole (Ls) and diastole (Ld), the end-diastolic (LVIDd) and end-systolic (LVIDs) left ventricular (LV) chamber diameter and the anterior and posterior wall thickness in systole (AWThs and PWThs) and diastole (AWThd and PWThd), the area of the endocardium in systole (Area s) and diastole (Area d) and the area of the epicardium in systole (Epi s). The recordings and analyses were done blinded to the treatment of the mice. Fractional area shortening (FAS) was calculated as (Area d–Area s)/Area d × 100. The ejection fraction (EF) was calculated as (5/6 × Area d × Ld−5/6 × Area s × Ls)/(5/6 × Area d × Ld) × 100. Echocardiographic LV weight (LVW) was estimated using the formula: 1.05 × 5/6 x (Epi s × (Ls + (AWThs + PWThs)/2)–Area s × Ls).

Histology and Immunohistochemistry

Formaldehyde-fixed heart samples were embedded in paraffin before 5 μm sections were cut. Collagen was visualized by Sirius Red staining to measure the extent of fibrosis as described previously (12, 17). Presence of immune cells in the myocardium was determined by immunohistochemistry (12, 18) using anti-CD3 (1:200, MCA1477, rat IgG_1, ABD Serotec, Oxford, UK), anti-CD4 (1:200, clone 4SM95, rat IgG_1, eBiosciences, Frankfurt, Germany), anti-CD8 (1:200, clone 4SM15, rat IgG_{2a}, eBiosciences), anti-CD45R(B220) (1:200, clone RA3-6B2, rat IgG_{2a}, Biolegend, Fell, Germany), and anti-F4/80 monoclonal antibodies (1:200, clone A3-1, rat IgG_{2b}, Biolegend), respectively. For all antibodies except anti-F4/80, antigen retrieval was performed by boiling the slides 5 times for 5 min in sodium citrate buffer (10 mmol/L sodium citrate, pH 6, 0.05% Tween 20). Polyclonal biotinylated goat anti-rat IgG secondary antibodies (1:200, 112-065-062, Jackson laboratories) and HRP-conjugated streptavidin (405210, Biolegend) served as secondary and tertiary reagents.

The slides were scanned with a 20x objective (UPlanApo, NA 0.75) using the dotSlide SL slide scanner (Olympus, Hamburg, Germany) equipped with a peltier-cooled XC10 camera. The extent of fibrosis and the numbers of stained cells in two complete heart sections were quantified using cellSens Dimensions software (Olympus) by a scientist blinded to the treatment of the mice. Fibrotic areas were determined as the proportion of the area of collagen relative to the sum of the area of collagen and the area of cardiomyocytes.

Lymphocyte Preparation

Lymphocytes were obtained from lymph nodes of OT-I mice for adoptive transfers and from spleens of the cMy-mOVA and cMy-mOVA+OT-I mice in the experiments for analysis using a Tenbroeck homogenizer. Untouched $CD3^+CD8^+$ cells from OT-I mice were obtained by MACS (130-104-075, Miltenyi Biotec GmbH, Bergisch Gladbach, Germany) according to the manufacturer's protocol. The $CD8^+$-T cells were incubated for 5 min with 5 μM of the dye carboxyfluorescein succinimidyl ester (CFSE; C-1157, Invitrogen) in phosphate buffered saline (PBS)/0.1% bovine serum albumin at 37°C and washed 3 times with DMEM containing 10% fetal calf serum (FCS) before adoptive transfer. The splenocytes of experimental animals were subjected to a removal of erythrocytes by incubation for 5 min in lysis buffer (155 mM NH_4Cl, 10 mM $KHCO_3$, 0.1 mM EDTA, pH 7.4-7.8).

Flow Cytometry

Flow cytometry was performed as described previously (19) on a FACS Calibur flow cytometer (BD Biosciences, Heidelberg, Germany) using CellQuestPro data acquisition and analysis software. Antibodies used for flow cytometry (anti-CD3, clone 17A2, rat IgG_{2b}, PE-labeled; anti-CD8, clone 53-6.7, rat IgG_{2a} PE/Cy5-labeled; anti-TCRVβ5.1/5.2, clone MR9-4, mouse IgG_1, FITC-labeled) and the respective isotype controls were purchased from Biolegend. The anti-$H2K^b$/SIINFEKL antibody (clone 25-D1.16, mouse IgG_1, APC-labeled) was obtained from BD Biosciences. For staining of cell surface antigens, 5×10^5 cells were incubated in 100 μl PBS with 1 μg of the respective primary monoclonal antibody for 30 min at 4°C before washing with PBS. Blood samples were directly stained and processed with BD FACS Lysing Solution (#349202, Becton Dickinson) according to the manufacturer's instructions.

Target Cells to Determine OVA-Specific Cytotoxicity

To monitor OVA-specific cytotoxicity, an enhanced green fluorescent protein (eGFP) or OVA-eGFP fusion protein expression cassette under control of an ubiquitously active hEF1α/CAG composite promoter in the pEGFP-1 vector (Clontech, Heidelberg, Germany) was introduced into the mouse leukemia cell line RMA (20), which carries the major histocompatibility complex (MHC) haplotype ($H2^b$). For transfection, 10^7 cells were mixed with 40 μg of the linearized vector before electroporation (250 mV and 960 μF). Successfully transfected cells were selected with 1,000 ng/ml G418 for 2 weeks before single cell clones were picked. Expression of eGFP was determined by flow cytometry to select stably transfected clones. The characterization of the selected clones expressing eGFP (RMA-con) or the OVA-eGFP fusion protein (RMA-OVA) is shown in **Supplementary Figure 1**.

Cytotoxicity Assay

The cytotoxic effector cells were used either directly at the day of preparation (day 0) or after restimulation with OVA for 4 days in ^{51}Cr-release assays. For restimulation, the splenocytes were cultured in round-bottomed microtiter plates (5 × 10^5 cells per well) in DMEM with 1 µM OVA and 10 ng/ml mouse IL-2 (#12340026, Immunotools, Friesoythe, Germany). Target cells were labeled by incubating 1 x 10^6 cells in 200 µl DMEM containing 100 µl FCS and 50 µCi $Na_2^{51}CrO_4$ (Hartmann Analytic, Braunschweig, Germany) for 1 h at 37°C and washed three times with DMEM. Effector cells were added to 5 x 10^3 ^{51}Cr-labeled target cells in triplicates at various effector to target (E:T) ratios in 200 µl DMEM with 10% FCS per well of round-bottomed microtiter plates. The E:T ratios always indicate the ratio of $CD3^+CD8^+$ effector cells to target cells. Spontaneous release was determined by incubation of target cells in the absence of effector cells. The microtiter plates were centrifuged for 5 min at 40x g, incubated at 37°C for 4 h, and then centrifuged again. Supernatant and sediment were separately taken to determine radioactivity in each well using a MicroBeta^2 counter (PerkinElmer Life Sciences, Köln, Germany). Percentage of specific lysis was calculated by subtracting percent spontaneous ^{51}Cr-release (20). The resistance of parental RMA cells and the transfected clones to killing by MACS-separated IL-2-activated natural killer (NK) cells was determined by ^{51}Cr-release assays in comparison to YAC-1 target cells as described previously (21).

Statistics

Results are shown as means with standard error of the mean (SEM). The data were evaluated with the SPSS software (IBM, Armonk, NY, USA). Analyses of variance (ANOVA) was used to compare data sets with more than two experimental groups and the Bonferroni *post hoc* test was employed for subsequent comparisons between the groups. Cytotoxicity data were analyzed by 2-way ANOVA adjusted for E:T ratios. Mixed linear models with the specification auto-regressive process AR (1) were employed to analyze alterations over time in the echocardiography data sets. Data of two groups such as sham and TAC were compared by t-test. If the Levene test indicated inequality of variances, an unequal variance t-test has been used instead of Student's t-test. The Kolmogorov-Smirnov test was used to assess normal distribution. More than two groups of not normally distributed data were analyzed by the Kruskal-Wallis test. The Mann-Whitney U-test was used to compare two groups of not normally distributed data. The Kruskal-Wallis test and the U-test were also used frequently when only some data within a related set of data were not normally distributed in order to allow for uniform reporting of the analyses. The Bonferroni-Holm correction was used to adjust for multiple testing in *post hoc* comparisons of two groups. Categorical data were analyzed by Fisher's exact test. The survival curves of mice were compared by Log Rank (Cox-Mantel) tests. P-values of < 0.05 in two-sided tests were considered to be significant and three levels of significance are usually indicated in the figures ($^*P < 0.05$, $^{**}P < 0.01$, $^{***}P < 0.001$).

RESULTS

OVA-Specific CTL Can Become Activated in cMy-mOVA Mice After TAC

The investigation of the potential role of CTL in cardiac autoimmunity elicited by pressure overload is hampered by the lack of known relevant autoantigens. Therefore, we used cMy-mOVA mice that express OVA on the plasma membrane of cardiomyocytes (13) to determine whether a CTL response to this model antigen occurs after TAC. Splenocytes were harvested 10 weeks after TAC or sham surgery and re-stimulated *in vitro* for 4 days with 1 µM OVA. Afterwards, the cells were used as effector cells in ^{51}Cr release assays against mouse leukemia RMA cells, which express either an OVA-EGFP fusion protein (RMA-OVA), and are therefore targets for OVA-specific CTL, or EGFP only as control (RMA-con). The characteristics of these target cell lines that were generated to measure OVA-specific CTL responses are shown in **Supplementary Figure 1**. Both, RMA-con and RMA-OVA cells were hardly killed by splenocytes from sham-operated mice (**Figure 1A**). Splenocytes from TAC-operated mice, in contrast, killed RMA-OVA cells significantly better than RMA-con cells (**Figure 1B**). The presence of an OVA-specific cellular cytotoxic activity against RMA target cells, which are resistant against NK cells, demonstrates that indeed OVA-specific CTL became activated in response to cardiac pressure overload although the specific lysis of OVA-expressing target cells was on average still low. In accord with these data, a significantly higher proportion of mice that underwent TAC (77.8%) than sham surgery (23.1%) exerted a higher cytotoxic activity against RMA-OVA than RMA-con cells ($P = 0.0274$, Fisher's exact test; **Figure 1C**). Notably, in some mice, the OVA-specific cytotoxicity after TAC was considerably higher than on average (**Figure 1D**), whereas in others no OVA-specific CTL activity was detected (**Figure 1E**).

OVA-Specific $CD8^+$-T Cells Do Not Accelerate Progression of cMy-mOVA Mice Into Heart Failure

The observation of a cytotoxic activity against a myocardial antigen after TAC justified further investigation. To increase the likelihood and potentially also the strength of an OVA-specific CTL response after TAC, we crossed cMy-mOVA mice with OT-I mice to obtain animals that express OVA on cardiomyocytes and have $CD8^+$-T cells mostly with specificity for this antigen. Previously, we have used this strategy successfully to generate cMy-mOVA-OT-II mice that have $CD4^+$-T cells with specificity for OVA (12). Unexpectedly, all of these double-transgenic cMy-mOVA-OT-I mice died before reaching an age of 10 days (**Supplementary Figure 2A**). Their myocardium did not display an infiltration of $CD3^+$-T cells (**Supplementary Figure 2B**) making it unlikely that a vigorous autoimmune response of OVA-specific CTL to OVA-expressing cardiomyocytes was the underlying reason of death. However, we could not continue to bread these mice to determine the actual reason of death and decided to circumvent this problem by adoptively transferring

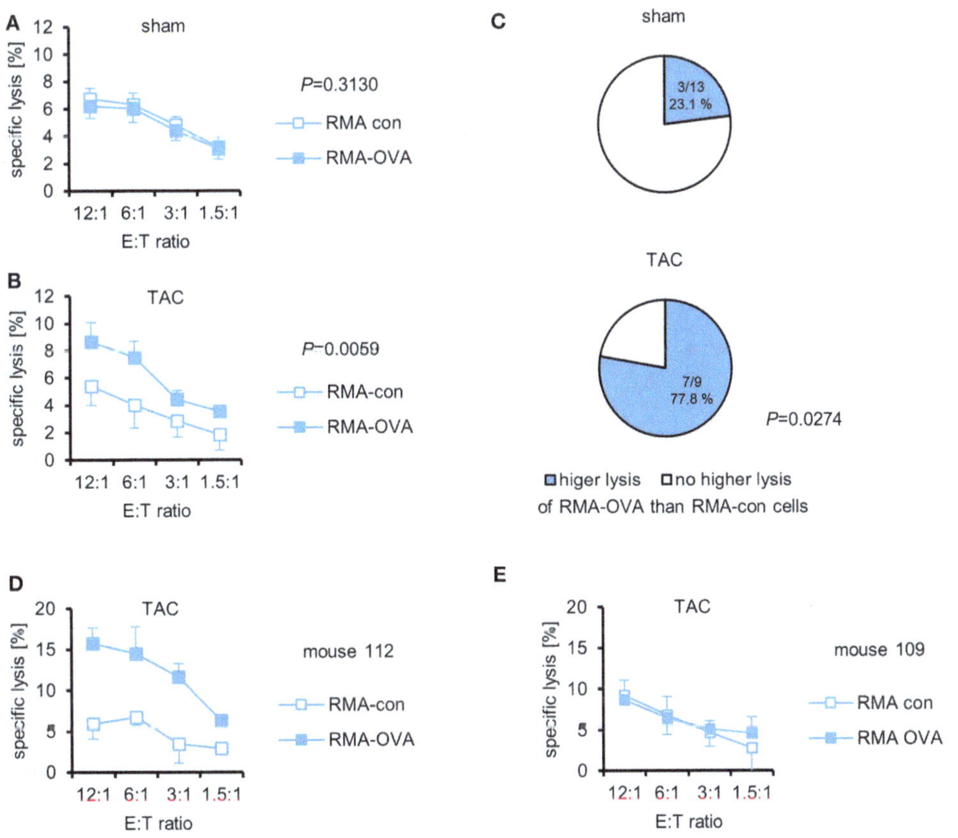

FIGURE 1 | OVA-specific CTL become activated in cMy-mOVA mice after TAC. The cytotoxic activity of splenocytes against RMA-OVA and RMA-con target cells was determined by ^{51}Cr-release assays at several CD3^{+}CD8^{+} effector cell to target cell (E:T) ratios 10 weeks after **(A)** sham (n = 13) or **(B)** TAC (n = 9) surgery. Means and standard errors of the mean (SEM) are displayed. Differences between sham and TAC-operated mice were analyzed by 2-way ANOVA adjusted for the E:T ratios and the respective P-values are indicated. **(C)** The proportion of mice exerting a higher cytotoxic activity against RMA-OVA than RMA-con cells is displayed. The difference between sham and TAC-operated mice has been analyzed by Fisher's exact test and the P-value is displayed. **(D)** The OVA-specific cellular cytotoxicity was higher in some mice after TAC. Means and SEM of triplets are shown for mouse 112. **(E)** The lack of an OVA-specific cytotoxicity in mouse 109 that also underwent TAC is shown for comparison.

OVA-specific CD8^{+}-T cells from OT-I mice into cMy-mOVA mice before surgery.

Thus, cMy-mOVA mice received at day 1 before TAC or sham surgery 10^7 MACS-separated CFSE-labeled CD3^{+}CD8^{+} cells from OT-I mice (cMy-mOVA+OT-I) or PBS (cMy-mOVA) by intravenous injection (n = 14 per group). The transgenic TCR of OT-I mice was detected by a TCRVβ5.1/5.2-specific antibody. The purity of the transferred CD8^{+}-T cells carrying the transgenic Vβ5.1/5.2^{+} TCR was >90% (**Supplementary Figure 3**). Three days after surgery, the pressure gradient over the aortic ligature was determined using pulsed wave Doppler. In all mice that underwent TAC an aortic stenosis was obtained. The pressure gradients in mice that had received CD8^{+}-T cells from OT-I mice before TAC was not significantly different from control mice after TAC (**Supplementary Figure 4A**). At day 3 after surgery, also blood was taken to verify by flow cytometry the successful transfer of OT-I-derived cells. On average about 2% of the lymphocytes in the blood were CD3^{+}CFSE^{+} OT-I-derived T cells (**Supplementary Figure 4B**) suggesting that most transferred cells were at this time point in other compartments than the peripheral blood. Signs of a dilution of CFSE due to cell proliferation were not observed in the non-lymphocyte-depleted recipients. Six mice (3 after sham and 3 after TAC intervention) were at this point excluded from further analysis since <0.5% of the lymphocytes in the blood of the recipients were CD3^{+}CFSE^{+} T cells. A few additional mice (sham: n = 3, TAC: n = 4) were operated and already sacrificed at the end of the first week in order to exclude an early loss of the transferred T cells. Similar proportions (on average 2.3%) of CFSE-labeled T cells were found among the splenocytes of sham and TAC-operated mice (**Supplementary Figure 4C**). Furthermore, the proportion of TCRVβ5.1/5.2^{+}-T cells was increased in these mice compared to cMy-mOVA mice (n = 7) that did not receive OT-I-derived T cells (**Supplementary Figure 4D**), indicating that OVA-specific T cells were still present in both sham and TAC-operated mice 1 week after the intervention.

Echocardiography was performed to determine heart function 3 days before and 1, 4, and 8 weeks after the intervention. Cardiac hypertrophy developed within 1 week after TAC as indicated

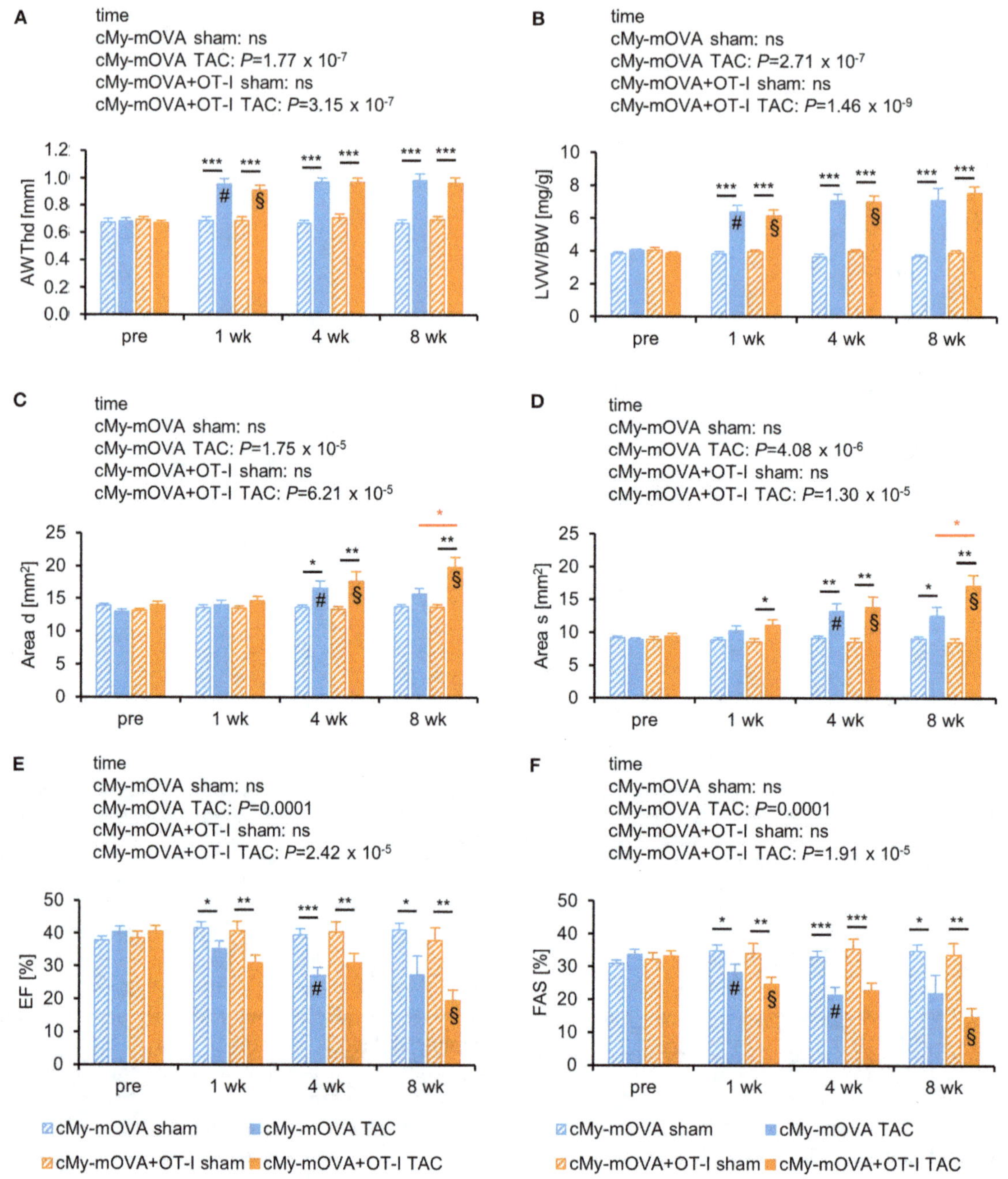

FIGURE 2 | OVA-specific CD8^{+}-T cells promote cardiac dilatation but do not accelerate the progression from hypertrophy to heart failure after TAC in cMy-mOVA mice. Echocardiography was performed in cMy-mOVA and in cMy-mOVA+OT-I mice before (pre; $n = 14$ per group for cMy-mOVA and $n = 11$ per group for cMy-mOVA+OT-I mice) as well as 1 week ($n = 14$ for cMy-mOVA and $n = 11$ for cMy-mOVA+OT-I mice), 4 weeks ($n = 14$ cMy-mOVA and $n = 11$ (sham) or 10 (TAC) for cMy-mOVA+OT-I mice), and 8 weeks ($n = 14$ (sham) or 10 (TAC) for cMy-mOVA and $n = 11$ (sham) or 9 (TAC) for cMy-mOVA+OT-I mice) after sham or TAC surgery. **(A)** Anterior wall thickness in diastole (AWThd), **(B)** left ventricular weight/body weight (LVW/BW) ratio, **(C)** area of the endocardium in diastole (Area d), **(D)** area of the endocardium in systole (Area s), **(E)**, ejection fraction (EF), and **(F)** fractional area shortening (FAS) were determined and means plus SEM are displayed. Differences between the time points within each experimental group were analyzed by a mixed linear model (time) and the *P*-values are given in the panels. Significant differences in the Bonferroni *post hoc* test ($P < 0.05$) compared to the previous time point are indicated for cMy-mOVA (#) and cMy-mOVA+OT-I mice (§). Differences between sham and TAC groups at a given time point were analyzed by *t*-tests and significant differences are indicated by black bars (*$P < 0.05$, **$P < 0.01$, ***$P < 0.001$). Similarly, differences between cMy-mOVA and cMy-mOVA+OT-I mice after TAC were analyzed and red bars and stars indicate significant *P*-values.

by the anterior wall thickness in diastole (AWTHd; **Figure 2A**) and the left ventricular weight/body weight (LVW/BW) ratio (**Figure 2B**). A dilation of the left ventricle occurred in both experimental groups between the first and the fourth week as indicated by an increase of the area of the endocardium in diastole (Area d; **Figure 2C**) and the area of the endocardium in systole (Area s; **Figure 2D**). Notably, the dimensions of Area d and Area s further progressed from week 4 to week 8 only in cMy-mOVA+OT-I mice and both parameters were greater in the mice with OVA-specific CTL than in cMy-mOVA mice 8 weeks after TAC. However, heart function after TAC measured as ejection fraction (EF; **Figure 2E**) or fractional area shortening (FAS; **Figure 2F**) was not significantly different between cMy-mOVA+OT-I and cMy-mOVA mice at any time point. On average EF and FAS were, however, more reduced 10 weeks after TAC in cMy-mOVA+OT-I than cMy-mOVA mice. When the development of heart failure over time was analyzed for the individual groups, a significant reduction of the EF was observed in cMy-mOVA mice between week 1 and week 4 and in cMy-mOVA+OT-I mice between week 4 and week 8 (**Figure 2E**). The FAS was reduced in both cMy-mOVA+OT-I and cMy-mOVA mice already 1 week after TAC and declined further until week 4 in cMy-mOVA mice and from week 4 to week 8 in cMy-mOVA+OT-I mice. In summary, the presence of $CD8^+$-T cells with specificity for an antigen in cardiomyocytes appeared to promote left ventricular dilation but failed to significantly accelerate the progression from hypertrophy to heart failure at least during the time period analyzed here.

All sham-operated mice survived until the end of the experiment and did not show any clinical signs of sickness during the course of the experiment. Four of the 14 cMy-mOVA mice died or had to be sacrificed before the end of the experiment due to illness (**Supplementary Figure 5A**). Of the 11 cMy-mOVA+OT-I mice, 9 remained in the experiment until the end of the observation time (**Supplementary Figure 5B**). The survival of the mice that had received OT-I-derived $CD8^+$-T cells before TAC was not different from controls [$P = 0.5608$; Log Rank (Cox-Mantel) test], suggesting that the ventricular dilation observed in echocardiography does not translate into an enhanced heart failure related mortality.

More T Cells Infiltrate the Myocardium of cMy-mOVA+OT-I Than cMy-mOVA Mice, but Fibrosis and Cardiac Hypertrophy Are Similar

The mice were sacrificed 10 weeks after surgery. The infiltration of the myocardium with cells of the immune system was assessed by immunohistochemistry (**Figure 3A**). More $CD3^+$-T cells were present in the myocardium of TAC than sham-operated mice (**Figure 3B**). Notably, more $CD3^+$-T cells infiltrated the myocardium of cMy-mOVA+OT-I than cMy-mOVA mice after TAC but also after sham surgery. The same pattern was observed when the numbers of $CD8^+$ cells were determined (**Figure 3C**), suggesting that adoptively transferred OT-I-derived $CD8^+$-T cells were enriched in the myocardium of the cMy-mOVA+OT-I mice. $CD4^+$ T cells (**Figure 3D**) and $CD45R(B220)^+$ B cells (**Figure 3E**) as well as $F4/80^+$ myeloid cells (**Figure 3F**), which include monocytes and macrophages, increased in numbers after TAC but were not more abundant in cMy-mOVA+OT-I than cMy-mOVA mice, arguing for a specific enrichment of the OVA-specific $CD8^+$-T cells in the OVA-expressing myocardium.

The cardiac hypertrophy after TAC at autopsy measured as ventricular weight/body weight ratio was similar in cMy-mOVA and cMy-mOVA+OT-I mice (**Figure 4A**). Myocardial fibrosis was analyzed on Sirius Red stained complete cross-sections (**Figures 4A,B**) and found to be similarly increased in cMy-mOVA and cMy-mOVA+OT-I mice after TAC (**Figures 4A,C**).

OVA-Specific CTL Can Become Activated in cMy-mOVA+OT Mice After TAC and Have a Higher Cytotoxic Activity Than OVA-Specific CTL in cMy-mOVA Mice

At autopsy, splenocytes were harvested. The proportion of $CD3^+CD8^+$ cells was analyzed by flow cytometry and found to be similar in mice that had received $CD8^+$-T cells from OT-I mice and controls (**Supplementary Figure 4E**). The proportion of $CD3^+TCRV\beta5.1/5.2^+$-T cells was not increased among the splenocytes of cMy-mOVA+OT-I mice (**Supplementary Figure 4F**), suggesting that the transferred $CD8^+$-T cells were either in other compartments or mostly lost at this time point. When the splenocytes were then directly used as effector cells in ^{51}Cr-release assays against RMA-con and RMA-OVA target cells, they did not exert any OVA-specific cytotoxicity. However, following a restimulation with 1 μM OVA for 4 days, an OVA-specific cellular cytotoxicity was detected in both sham and TAC-operated mice (**Figure 5A**). It was much higher in TAC than sham-operated cMy-mOVA+OT-I mice because the RMA-OVA cells were killed significantly better by splenocytes from TAC than sham-operated mice ($P = 0.009$, 2-way ANOVA adjusted for E:T ratios), in contrast to RMA-con cells ($P = 0.5905$, 2-way ANOVA adjusted for E:T ratios). OVA-restimulated splenocytes from a significantly higher proportion of cMy-mOVA+OT-I mice that underwent TAC (77.8%) than sham surgery (20.0%) exerted an OVA-specific cytotoxic activity ($P = 0.0230$, Fisher's exact test; **Figure 5B**). These frequencies were very similar to those observed in cMy-mOVA mice (**Figure 1C**). Therefore, we compared the OVA-specific CTL activity in cMy-mOVA and cMy-mOVA+OT-I mice. It was not different in sham-operated cMy-mOVA and cMy-mOVA+OT-I mice but after TAC splenocytes from cMy-mOVA+OT-I mice killed RMA-OVA cells significantly better than splenocytes from cMy-mOVA mice (**Figure 5C**). In conclusion, this suggests that the risk to elicit OVA-specific CTL activity is not increased after adoptive transfer of OT-I-derived $CD8^+$-T cells. However, if (presumably very few) OVA-specific CTL become activated in response to TAC in an animal, they can exert a higher cytotoxic activity upon antigen-specific restimulation, if the high affinity OT-I-derived $CD8^+$-T cells had been transferred.

DISCUSSION

In recent years clear evidence has been accumulated that autoimmune responses can contribute to the progression of heart failure. This is best documented by the presence of autoantibodies with direct cardio-depressive effects in subgroups of patients with dilative cardiomyopathy, in which the therapeutic removal of those antibodies by immunoadsorption

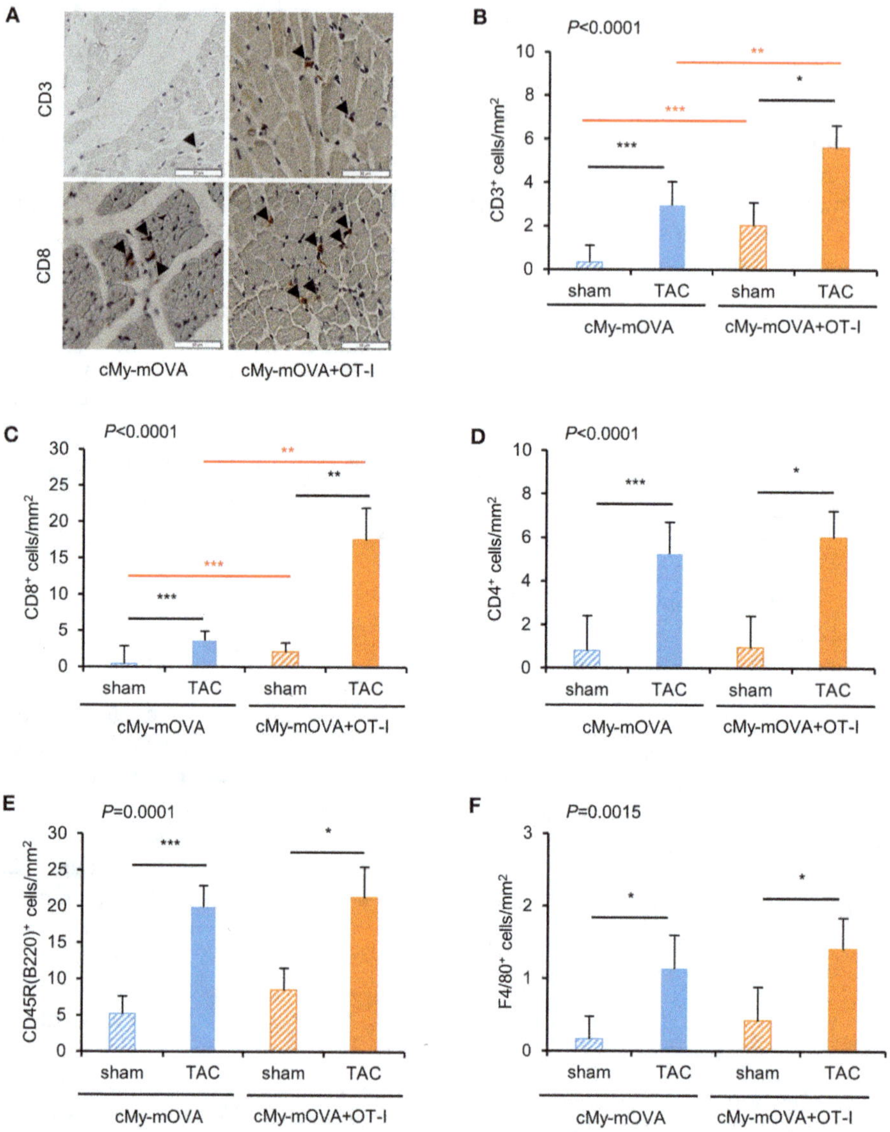

FIGURE 3 | More infiltration of $CD3^+$ and $CD8^+$ cells in the myocardium of cMy-mOVA+OT-I than cMy-mOVA mice. **(A)** The infiltration of $CD3^+$ and $CD8^+$ cells was analyzed by immunohistochemistry in the myocardium of sham and TAC-operated cMy-mOVA and cMy-mOVA+OT-I as illustrated here. The bars indicate 50 μm. The arrow heads point to $CD3^+$ or $CD8^+$ cells, respectively. The numbers of infiltrating $CD3^+$-T cells **(B)**, $CD8^+$ cells **(C)** $CD4^+$ cells **(D)**, $CD45R(B220)^+$ B cells **(E)** and $F4/80^+$ monocytes/macrophages **(F)** were determined in the myocardium after 10 weeks in sham and TAC-operated cMy-mOVA (sham $n = 14$, TAC $n = 10$) and cMy-mOVA+OT-I mice (sham $n = 11$, TAC $n = 9$) and means plus SEM are shown. The *P*-value of a Kruskal-Wallis test comparing all groups is indicated. Differences between two groups were analyzed by *U*-tests and significant *P*-values are given in the panels ($^*P < 0.05$, $^{**}P < 0.01$, $^{***}P < 0.001$). The Bonferroni-Holm correction was used to adjust for multiple testing in the two group comparisons.

is beneficial (11). Notably, similar autoantibodies were also found in animal models of pressure overload (7). More recently, the investigation of the role of T cells in the pathophysiology of pressure overload has been initiated. Our interest in this topic has been stimulated by the finding that pressure overload after TAC, but not volume overload after aorto-caval shunt, was associated with myocardial inflammation and induced a gene expression profile indicating an activation of T cell receptor signaling pathways in the myocardium (16).

The impact of T cells in the pathophysiology of pressure overload has been investigated initially in T cell-deficient and T cell-depleted mice. Mice lacking a functional recombination activation gene 2 (*Rag2*), which do not have B and T cells, were reported to be protected from the transition from hypertrophy to heart failure after TAC (22). Similarly, TCRα-deficient mice or mice in which T cells were depleted by administration of anti-CD3 antibodies, had a preserved cardiac function after TAC (23). Recently, it has been demonstrated that blocking of T cell activation by abatacept, a cytotoxic T-lymphocyte-associated

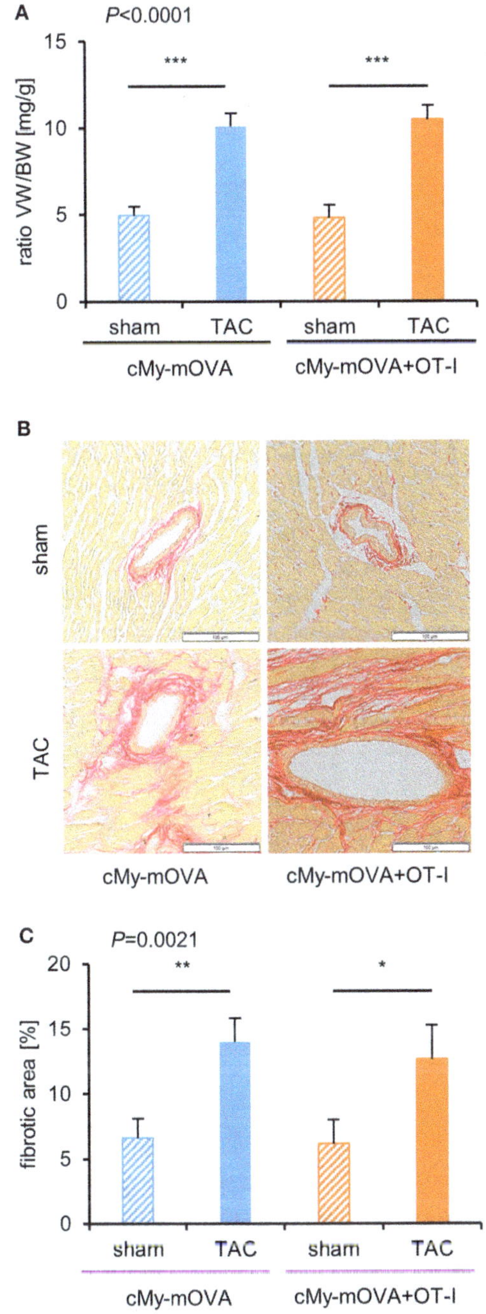

FIGURE 4 | Similar cardiac hypertrophy and fibrosis in cMy-mOVA and cMy-mOVA+OT-I mice after TAC. **(A)** The ventricular weight/body weight (VW/DW) ratio was determined at autopsy after 10 weeks in sham and TAC-operated cMy-mOVA and cMy-mOVA+OT-I mice. **(B)** Fibrosis of the myocardium was analyzed by Sirius Red staining in cMy-mOVA and cMy-mOVA+OT-I mice after sham and TAC surgery. The bars indicate 100 μm. **(C)** The areas containing collagen were determined on complete left ventricular cross sections of cMy-mOVA (sham $n = 14$, TAC $n = 10$) and cMy-mOVA+OT-I mice (sham $n = 11$, TAC $n = 9$). Means plus SEM are shown in **(A,C)**. The *P*-value of a Kruskal-Wallis test comparing all groups is indicated. Differences between two groups were analyzed by *U*-tests and significant *P*-values are given in the panels ($^{*}P < 0.05$, $^{**}P < 0.01$, $^{***}P < 0.001$). The Bonferroni-Holm correction was used to adjust for multiple testing in the two group comparisons.

protein 4 (CTLA4)-Ig fusion protein, delays progression of TAC-induced heart failure (24, 25). The question which type of T cells is involved in pressure overload-induced heart failure has also been addressed by some studies. Specifically CD4^{+}-T cells appeared to be important since mice deficient for MHC class II molecules, which lack CD4^{+}-T cells were protected from progression into heart failure after TAC similarly to RAG2-deficient mice lacking all T cells and in contrast to CD8-deficient mice lacking CD8^{+}-T cells (22). We have recently demonstrated that possessing high numbers CD4^{+}-T cells with specificity for an antigen in cardiomyocytes can accelerate progression into heart failure after TAC (12). This effect was independent of autoantibodies suggesting that T helper cells can have a direct effect on maladaptive cardiac remodeling.

In the present study, we investigated the role of CD8^{+}-T cells with specificity for an antigen in cardiomyocytes during the progression of heart failure in response to pressure overload. We show that CTL with specificity for OVA can become activated after TAC in cMy-mOVA mice expressing OVA in cardiomyocytes. The cytotoxic activity was detected after OVA-specific restimulation of CTL *in vitro*. The CTL activity was on average low, suggesting that its induction is an inefficient process. Moreover, it appeared to be unlikely that such a low-grade CTL activity has a major impact on heart function. This is in agreement with the finding by Laroumanie and colleagues that mice lacking CD8^{+}-T cells were not protected from TAC-induced heart failure (22). However, mice possessing higher numbers of CD8^{+}-T cells with specificity for antigens in cardiomyocytes might carry a substantially higher risk that such CTL become activated due to pressure overload and subsequently contribute to the deterioration of heart function. To elevate the number of CD8^{+}-T cells with specificity for an antigen in cardiomyocytes, we adoptively transferred CD8^{+}-T cells with that specificity from OT-I into cMy-mOVA mice before TAC. It has been previously shown that the adoptive transfer of naïve OVA-specific CD8^{+}-T cells from OT-I mice into cMy-mOVA mice does not cause myocarditis unless the mice are either immunized with OVA plus a strong adjuvant or are infected with an OVA-expressing virus (13, 26). In agreement with these observations, sham-operated mice that had received OT-I-derived CD8^{+}-T cells did not develop any signs of disease in our study. After TAC, these cMy-mOVA+OT-I mice developed a cardiac hypertrophy and progressed into heart failure similarly to cMy-mOVA control mice. Functionally, only the left ventricular dilation was significantly more pronounced in the cMy-mOVA+OT-I than cMy-mOVA mice. Although more T cells infiltrated the myocardium of cMy-mOVA+OT-I than cMy-mOVA mice, the cardiac fibrosis was similar. Systemically, an OVA-specific CTL activity was detectable also in these mice only after *in vitro* restimulation of splenocytes with the antigen. Even though this activity in the cMy-mOVA+OT-I mice was significantly higher after TAC than after sham operation, presumably only very few OVA-specific CTL became activated in response to TAC. This suggests that pressure overload does not provide sufficient danger signals or other adjuvant-like signals to break tolerance and to activate CTL robustly. Although they could exert a higher cytotoxic activity upon antigen-specific

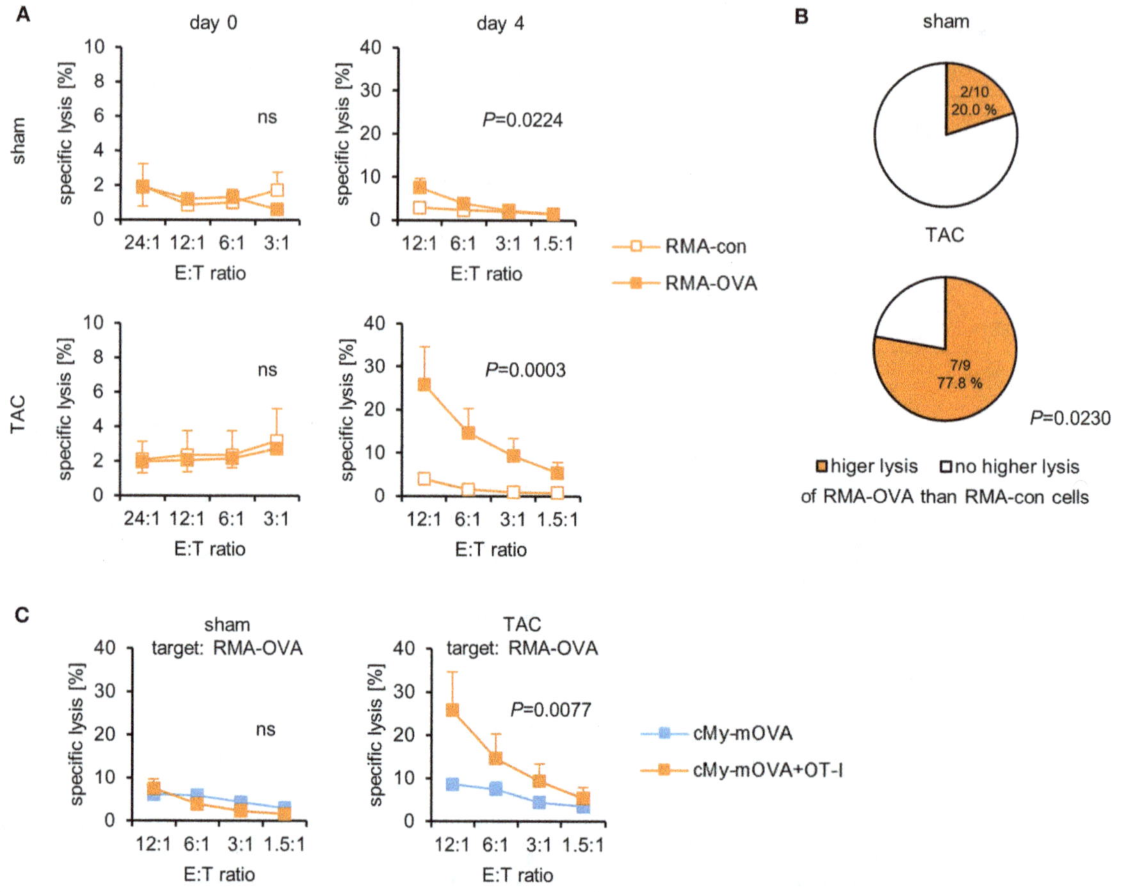

FIGURE 5 | OVA-specific CTL become activated in cMy-mOVA+OT-I mice after TAC and have a higher cytotoxic activity than OVA-specific CTL in cMy-mOVA mice. **(A)** The cytotoxic activity of splenocytes against RMA-OVA and RMA-con target cells was determined by ^{51}Cr-release assays at several CD3$^+$CD8$^+$ E:T ratios 10 weeks after sham ($n = 10$) or TAC ($n = 9$) surgery either directly after autopsy (day 0) or after restimulation *in vitro* with 1 µM OVA (day 4). Means and SEM are displayed. Differences between sham and TAC-operated mice were analyzed by 2-way ANOVA adjusted for the E:T ratios and the respective *P*-values are indicated (ns, non-significant). **(B)** The proportion of mice exerting a higher cytotoxic activity against RMA-OVA than RMA-con cells is displayed. The difference between sham and TAC-operated mice has been analyzed by Fisher's exact test and the *P*-value is displayed. **(C)** The OVA-specific cytotoxicity against RMA-OVA target cells of CTL from cMy-mOVA and cMy-mOVA+OT-I mice after sham ($n = 9$) or TAC ($n = 9$) surgery is compared by 2-way ANOVA adjusted for the E:T ratios and the respective *P*-value is indicated.

restimulation than non TCR-transgenic CTL with that specificity in cMy-mOVA mice, they did not significantly impair cardiac function.

At day 3 after the intervention, transferred OT-I-derived T cells were found in the blood and at one week also in the spleen of TAC and sham-operated mice. At these time points, they constituted 2 to 3% of the peripheral lymphocytes. At the end of the experiment, 10 weeks after the intervention, we did not detect the transferred cells in the spleen by flow cytometry anymore, suggesting that most OT-I-derived OVA-specific T cells were present in other compartments or got lost over time due to absence of an antigenic stimulation. However, the increased OVA-specific cellular cytotoxicity in the spleen and the higher numbers of T cells in heart of cMy-mOVA+OT-I mice indicate that at least some of the transferred T cells got activated after TAC and survived. It should be mentioned that the adoptive transfer even of high numbers of OT-I-derived CD8$^+$-T cells (10^7 in our experiment) into the cMy-mOVA+OT-I mice did not increase the OVA-specific CD8$^+$-T cells to similar numbers as reached for OVA-specific CD4$^+$-T cells in the double-transgenic cMy-mOVA-OT-II mice, in which stably most CD4$^+$-T cells are OVA-specific (12). A constant presence of similar numbers of OVA-specific CD8$^+$-T cells could potentially increase the risk to elicit a functionally relevant auto-reactivity also of CTL in cMy-mOVA mice after TAC. Unfortunately, due to the early death of the double-transgenic cMy-mOVA-OT-I mice, this has been impossible to achieve in our experiments. Moreover, it needs to be mentioned that the cMy-mOVA+OT-I displayed a more severe left ventricular dilation 8 weeks after TAC than cMy-mOVA mice. Hence, we cannot exclude that CD8$^+$-T cells with specificity for an antigen in cardiomyocytes would impair the cardiac function at later time points beyond the observation period of our study. Transferring OVA-specific CD4$^+$-T cells together with OVA-specific CD8$^+$-T cells before TAC could potentially support the survival of the OVA-specific CTL and might augment their effects in cMy-mOVA mice.

In comparison to $CD4^+$-T cells (12), $CD8^+$-T cells with specificity for a model antigen in cardiomyocytes have little impact on the progression of pressure overload-induced heart failure. This observation might be understandable in view of reports that cardiomyocytes largely lack MHC class I molecules under non-inflammatory conditions (18, 27) even though they are inducible by pro-inflammatory cytokines (18) and CTL-mediated killing of cardiomyocytes clearly occurs during viral myocarditis (13). A low expression level of MHC class I molecules on cardiomyocytes could explain why the OVA-specific $CD8^+$-T cells had little impact in the cMy-mOVA+OT-I mice after TAC although they reached the OVA-expressing tissue as suggested by the presence of higher numbers of $CD3^+$-T cells in the myocardium of these mice. In contrast, in cMy-mOVA-OT-II mice, OVA released from dying cells is expected to be taken-up by professional antigen specific cells, which then stimulate OVA-specific T helper cells to release cytokines involved in cardiac remodeling (12). Therefore, CTL with specificity for antigens in other myocardial cells than cardiomyocytes, e.g., cardiac fibroblasts, might have different consequences for heart function.

CONCLUSIONS

In this study, we have shown that CTL with specificity for a model antigen in cardiomyocytes, i.e., OVA in cardiomyocytes of cMy-mOVA mice, can become activated after TAC. Yet, this apparently is an inefficient process leading only to low-grade cytotoxicity. Adoptive transfer of OVA-specific $CD8^+$-T cells from TCR-transgenic OT-I mice does not substantially increase the risk to elicit a cytotoxic activity against OVA after TAC. In agreement with this finding, the progression from cardiac hypertrophy to heart failure was not significantly accelerated in these cMy-mOVA+OT-I mice. Thus, $CD8^+$-T cells with specificity for an antigen in cardiomyocytes, in contrast to $CD4^+$-T cells (12), apparently do not have a major impact on progression and mortality of pressure overload-induced heart failure.

AUTHOR CONTRIBUTIONS

RD designed the study. CG, AS, SM, CR, LE, and RD performed experiments and analyzed data. MD and W-HZ supervised echocardiography and the analysis of echocardiography data. VR helped with the adoptive transfers of CTL. GB contributed to the quantitative evaluation of histological data. AL provided the cMy-mOVA mice. KT and GH supervised the mouse surgery. RD wrote the manuscript, which all authors revised. All authors approved the final version of the manuscript.

FUNDING

The Deutsche Forschungsgemeinschaft (DFG) through the collaborative research center SFB 1002 (TPs B4 to KT and GH, C04 to W-HZ, C05 to RD, and S1 to W-HZ.) has supported this study. The authors received support from the German Center for Cardiovascular Research (DZHK). We acknowledge support by the Open Access Publication Funds of the Göttingen University.

ACKNOWLEDGMENTS

We are thankful for the excellent technical assistance of R. Blume, B. Knocke, S. Wollborn, S. Zafar, and M. Zoremba of the Service Project S1 of the SFB1002.

REFERENCES

1. Van Linthout S, Tschöpe C. Inflammation - cause or consequence of heart failure or both? *Curr Heart Fail Rep.* (2017) 14:251–65. doi: 10.1007/s11897-017-0337-9
2. Stephenson E, Savvatis K, Mohiddin SA, Marelli-Berg FM. T-cell immunity in myocardial inflammation: pathogenic role and therapeutic manipulation. *Br J Pharmacol.* (2016) 174:3914–25. doi: 10.1111/bph.13613
3. Torre-Amione G, Kapadia S, Benedict C, Oral H, Young JB, Mann DL. Proinflammatory cytokine levels in patients with depressed left ventricular ejection fraction: a report from the Studies of Left Ventricular Dysfunction (SOLVD). *J Am Coll Cardiol.* (1996) 27:1201–6. doi: 10.1016/0735-1097(95)00589-7
4. Mann DL. Innate immunity and the failing heart: the cytokine hypothesis revisited. *Circ Res.* (2015) 116:1254–68. doi: 10.1161/CIRCRESAHA.116.302317
5. Chung ES, Packer M, Lo KH, Fasanmade AA, Willerson JT, Anti-TNF Therapy against Congestive Heart Failure Investigators. Randomized, double-blind, placebo-controlled, pilot trial of infliximab, a chimeric monoclonal antibody to tumor necrosis factor-alpha, in patients with moderate-to-severe heart failure: results of the anti-TNF Therapy Against Congestive Heart Failure (ATTACH) trial. *Circulation* (2003) 107:3133–40. doi: 10.1161/01.CIR.0000077913.60364.D2
6. Mann DL, Mcmurray JJ, Packer M, Swedberg K, Borer JS, Colucci WS, et al. Targeted anticytokine therapy in patients with chronic heart failure: results of the Randomized Etanercept Worldwide Evaluation (RENEWAL). *Circulation* (2004) 109:1594–602. doi: 10.1161/01.CIR.0000124490.27666.B2
7. Liu HR, Zhao RR, Jiao XY, Wang YY, Fu M. Relationship of myocardial remodeling to the genesis of serum autoantibodies to cardiac beta(1)-adrenoceptors and muscarinic type 2 acetylcholine receptors in rats. *J Am Coll Cardiol.* (2002) 39:1866–73. doi: 10.1016/S0735-1097(02)01865-X
8. Jahns R, Boivin V, Hein L, Triebel S, Angermann CE, Ertl G, et al. Direct evidence for a beta 1-adrenergic receptor-directed autoimmune attack as a cause of idiopathic dilated cardiomyopathy. *J Clin Invest.* (2004) 113:1419–29. doi: 10.1172/JCI20149
9. Wallukat G, Schimke I. Agonistic autoantibodies directed against G-protein-coupled receptors and their relationship to cardiovascular diseases. *Semin Immunopathol.* (2014) 36:351–63. doi: 10.1007/s00281-014-0425-9
10. Deubner N, Berliner D, Schlipp A, Gelbrich G, Caforio AL, Felix SB, et al. Cardiac beta1-adrenoceptor autoantibodies in human heart disease: rationale and design of the Etiology, Titre-Course, and Survival (ETiCS) Study. *Eur J Heart Fail.* (2010) 12:753–62. doi: 10.1093/eurjhf/hfq072
11. Felix SB, Beug D, Dorr M. Immunoadsorption therapy in dilated cardiomyopathy. *Expert Rev Cardiovasc Ther.* (2015) 13:145–52. doi: 10.1586/14779072.2015.990385
12. Gröschel C, Sasse A, Röhrborn C, Monecke S, Didié M, Elsner L, et al. T helper cells with specificity for an antigen in cardiomyocytes promote pressure overload-induced progression from hypertrophy to heart failure. *Sci Rep.* (2017) 7:15998. doi: 10.1038/s41598-017-16147-1
13. Grabie N, Delfs MW, Westrich JR, Love VA, Stavrakis G, Ahmad F, et al. IL-12 is required for differentiation of pathogenic CD8+ T cell effectors that cause myocarditis. *J Clin Invest.* (2003) 111:671–80. doi: 10.1172/JC I16867
14. Barnden MJ, Allison J, Heath WR, Carbone FR. Defective TCR expression in

transgenic mice constructed using cDNA-based alpha- and beta-chain genes under the control of heterologous regulatory elements. *Immunol Cell Biol.* (1998) 76:34–40. doi: 10.1046/j.1440-1711.1998.00709.x

15. Hogquist KA, Jameson SC, Heath WR, Howard JL, Bevan MJ, Carbone FR. T cell receptor antagonist peptides induce positive selection. *Cell* (1994) 76:17–27.
16. Toischer K, Rokita AG, Unsöld B, Zhu W, Kararigas G, Sossalla S, et al. Differential cardiac remodeling in preload versus afterload. *Circulation* (2010) 122:993–1003. doi: 10.1161/CIRCULATIONAHA.110.943431
17. Montes-Cobos E, Li X, Fischer HJ, Sasse A, Kugler S, Didié M, et al. Inducible knock-down of the mineralocorticoid receptor in mice disturbs regulation of the renin-angiotensin-aldosterone system and attenuates heart failure induced by pressure overload. *PLoS ONE* (2015) 10:e0143954. doi: 10.1371/journal.pone.0143954
18. Didié M, Galla S, Muppalla V, Dressel R, Zimmermann WH. Immunological properties of murine parthenogenetic stem cell derived cardiomyocytes and engineered heart muscle. *Front Immunol.* (2017) 8:955. doi: 10.3389/fimmu.2017.00955
19. Isernhagen A, Malzahn D, Viktorova E, Elsner L, Monecke S, von Bonin F, et al. The MICA-129 dimorphism affects NKG2D signaling and outcome of hematopoietic stem cell transplantation. *EMBO Mol Med.* (2015) 7:1480–502. doi: 10.15252/emmm.201505246
20. Dressel R, Nolte J, Elsner L, Novota P, Guan K, Streckfuss-Bömeke K, et al. Pluripotent stem cells are highly susceptible targets for syngeneic, allogeneic, and xenogeneic natural killer cells. *FASEB J.* (2010) 24:2164–77. doi: 10.1096/fj.09-134957
21. Gröschel C, Hübscher D, Nolte J, Monecke S, Sasse A, Elsner L, et al. Efficient killing of murine pluripotent stem cells by natural killer (NK) cells requires activation by cytokines and partly depends on the activating NK receptor NKG2D. *Front Immunol.* (2017) 8:870. doi: 10.3389/fimmu.2017.00870
22. Laroumanie F, Douin-Echinard V, Pozzo J, Lairez O, Tortosa F, Vinel C, et al. CD4+ T cells promote the transition from hypertrophy to heart failure during chronic pressure overload. *Circulation* (2014) 129:2111–24. doi: 10.1161/CIRCULATIONAHA.113.007101
23. Nevers T, Salvador AM, Grodecki-Pena A, Knapp A, Velazquez F, Aronovitz M, et al. Left ventricular T-cell recruitment contributes to the pathogenesis of heart failure. *Circ Heart Fail.* (2015) 8:776–87. doi: 10.1161/CIRCHEARTFAILURE.115.002225
24. Wang H, Kwak D, Fassett J, Hou L, Xu X, Burbach BJ, et al. CD28/B7 deficiency attenuates systolic overload-induced congestive heart failure, myocardial and pulmonary inflammation, and activated T cell accumulation in the heart and lungs. *Hypertension* (2016) 68:688–96. doi: 10.1161/HYPERTENSIONAHA.116.07579
25. Kallikourdis M, Martini E, Carullo P, Sardi C, Roselli G, Greco CM, et al. T cell costimulation blockade blunts pressure overload-induced heart failure. *Nat Commun.* (2017) 8:14680. doi: 10.1038/ncomms14680
26. Tarrio ML, Grabie N, Bu DX, Sharpe AH, Lichtman AH. PD-1 protects against inflammation and myocyte damage in T cell-mediated myocarditis. *J Immunol.* (2012) 188:4876–84. doi: 10.4049/jimmunol.1200389
27. Seko Y, Tsuchimochi H, Nakamura T, Okumura K, Naito S, Imataka K, et al. Expression of major histocompatibility complex class I antigen in murine ventricular myocytes infected with Coxsackievirus B3. *Circ Res.* (1990) 67:360–7.

Permissions

All chapters in this book were first published in CIICD, by Frontiers; hereby published with permission under the Creative Commons Attribution License or equivalent. Every chapter published in this book has been scrutinized by our experts. Their significance has been extensively debated. The topics covered herein carry significant findings which will fuel the growth of the discipline. They may even be implemented as practical applications or may be referred to as a beginning point for another development.

The contributors of this book come from diverse backgrounds, making this book a truly international effort. This book will bring forth new frontiers with its revolutionizing research information and detailed analysis of the nascent developments around the world.

We would like to thank all the contributing authors for lending their expertise to make the book truly unique.

They have played a crucial role in the development of this book. Without their invaluable contributions this book wouldn't have been possible. They have made vital efforts to compile up to date information on the varied aspects of this subject to make this book a valuable addition to the collection of many professionals and students.

This book was conceptualized with the vision of imparting up-to-date information and advanced data in this field. To ensure the same, a matchless editorial board was set up. Every individual on the board went through rigorous rounds of assessment to prove their worth. After which they invested a large part of their time researching and compiling the most relevant data for our readers.

The editorial board has been involved in producing this book since its inception. They have spent rigorous hours researching and exploring the diverse topics which have resulted in the successful publishing of this book. They have passed on their knowledge of decades through this book. To expedite this challenging task, the publisher supported the team at every step. A small team of assistant editors was also appointed to further simplify the editing procedure and attain best results for the readers.

Apart from the editorial board, the designing team has also invested a significant amount of their time in

understanding the subject and creating the most relevant covers. They scrutinized every image to scout for the most suitable representation of the subject and create an appropriate cover for the book.

The publishing team has been an ardent support to the editorial, designing and production team. Their endless efforts to recruit the best for this project, has resulted in the accomplishment of this book. They are a veteran in the field of academics and their pool of knowledge is as vast as their experience in printing. Their expertise and guidance has proved useful at every step. Their uncompromising quality standards have made this book an exceptional effort. Their encouragement from time to time has been an inspiration for everyone.

The publisher and the editorial board hope that this book will prove to be a valuable piece of knowledge for

researchers, students, practitioners and scholars across the globe.

List of Contributors

Rui Zhang, Qi Luo and Chengwu Shen
Department of Pharmacy, Shandong Provincial Hospital Affiliated to Shandong University, Jinan, China

Lin Xu
Department of Thoracic Surgery, Shandong Provincial Hospital Affiliated to Shandong University, Jinan, China

Dong Zhang
Department of Urology, Shandong Provincial Hospital Affiliated to Shandong University, Jinan, China

Bo Hu
Minimally Invasive Urology Center, Shandong Provincial Hospital Affiliated to Shandong University, Jinan, China

Dan Han
Department of Pharmacy, Nanjing Drum Tower Hospital, The Affiliated Hospital of Nanjing University Medical School, Nanjing, China

Jiangbing Li
Department of Cardiology, Shandong Provincial Hospital Affiliated to Shandong University, Jinan, China

Jessie van Wezenbeek, Justin M. Canada, Krishna Ravindra, Salvatore Carbone, Cory R. Trankle, Dinesh Kadariya, Leo F. Buckley, Marco Del Buono, Hayley Billingsley, Michele Viscusi and Antonio Abbate
VCU Pauley Heart Center, Virginia Commonwealth University, Richmond, VA, United States

George F. Wohlford and Benjamin Van Tassell
Department of Pharmacotherapy and Outcome Sciences, Virginia Commonwealth University, Richmond, VA, United States

Ross Arena
Department of Physical Therapy, College of Applied Health Sciences, University of Illinois, Chicago, IL, United States

Kazuko Tajiri and Masaki Ieda
Department of Cardiology, Faculty of Medicine, University of Tsukuba, Tsukuba, Japan

Micaela Fredi, Laura Andreoli, Franco Franceschini and Angela Tincani
Rheumatology and Clinical Immunology Unit, Department of Clinical and Experimental Science, ASST Spedali Civili, University of Brescia, Brescia, Italy

Beatrice Bacco and Tiziana Bertero
S.S.d.D.U. Immunologia, Allergologia, A.O. Ordine Maurziano di Torino, Torino, Italy

Alessandra Bortoluzzi, Marcello Govoni and Melissa Padovan
UO e Sezione di Reumatologia, Dipartimento di Scienze Mediche, Universita' degli Studi di Ferrara, Cona, Italy

Silvia Breda
Struttura Complessa Medicina Interna, ASST Papa Giovanni XXIII, Bergamo, Italy

Veronica Cappa and Stefano Calza
Unit of Biostatistics, Biomathematics, and Bioinformatics, Department of Molecular and Translational Medicine, University of Brescia, Brescia, Italy

Fulvia Ceccarelli, Antonina Minniti and Roberta Priori
UO Complessa Reumatologia, Policlinico Umberto I-University La Sapienza, Rome, Italy

Rolando Cimaz
Anna Meyer Children's Hospital, University of Firenze, Firenze, Italy

Salvatore De Vita and Emma Di Poi
Clinica di Reumatologia, Azienda Sanitaria Universitaria Integrata di Udine, Udine, Italy

Elena Elefante, Marta Mosca and Chiara Tani
UO Reumatologia, Dipartimento di Medicina Clinica e Sperimentale, Universita' di Pisa, Pisa, Italy

Maria Gerosa
Istituto Ortopedico Gaetano Pini, University of Milan, Milan, Italy

Ariela Hoxha, Amelia Ruffatti and Marta Tonello
Unità di Reumatologia, Dipartimento di Medicina, Università di Padova, Padova, Italy

Andrea Lojacono and Sonia Zatti
Department of Obstetrics and Gynecology, ASST Spedali Civili and University, Brescia, Italy

Luca Marozio
Ginecologia e Ostetricia 1, Dipartimento di Scienze Chirurgiche, Università di Torino, Turin, Italy

Alessandro Mathieu and Matteo Piga
Cattedra e Struttura Complessa di Reumatologia, Universita' degli Studi e AOU di Cagliari, Cagliari, Italy

Pier Luigi Meroni
Immunorheumatology Research Laboratory, Istituto Auxologico Italiano, Milan, Italy

Marina Muscarà
UO Reumatologia, ASST Ospedale Niguarda, Milan, Italy

Véronique Ramoni
Rheumatology, IRCCS Policlinico San Matteo Foundation, University of Pavia, Padova, Italy

Laura Trespidi
Dipartimento per la Salute della Donna, Bambino e Neonato, Fondazione Ospedale Maggiore, Milan, Italy

Antonio Brucato
Struttura Complessa Medicina Interna, ASST Papa Giovanni XXIII, Bergamo, Italy
Dipartimento di Scienze Biomediche e Cliniche "Sacco", Università degli Studi di Milano, Milan, Italy

Elena Bartoloni, Alessia Alunno, Valentina Valentini, Filippo Luccioli, Eleonora Valentini, Giuliana Maria Concetta La Paglia, Maria Comasia Leone, Giacomo Cafaro, Elisa Marcucci and Roberto Gerli
Rheumatology Unit, Department of Perugia, University of Perugia, Perugia, Italy

William Bracamonte-Baran, Guobao Chen, Monica V. Talor, Hee Sun Choi and David Nauen
Department of Pathology, School of Medicine, Johns Hopkins University, Baltimore, MD, United States

Xuezhou Hou
W. Harry Feinstone Department of Molecular Microbiology and Immunology, Bloomberg School of Public Health, Johns Hopkins University, Baltimore, MD, United States

Giovanni Davogustto and Heinrich Taegtmeyer
Division of Cardiology, Department of Internal Medicine, University of Texas Medical School at Houston, Houston, TX, United States

Jungeun Sung
School of Medicine, Institute of Genetic Medicine, Johns Hopkins University, Baltimore, MD, United States

David Joel Hackam
Division of General Pediatric Surgery, Johns Hopkins University and Bloomberg Children's Center, Johns Hopkins Hospital, Baltimore, MD, United States

Jana Petrkova
Department of Pathological Physiology, Faculty of Medicine Dentistry, Palacky University, Olomouc, Czechia

Daniela Čiháková
Department of Pathology, School of Medicine, Johns Hopkins University, Baltimore, MD, United States
W. Harry Feinstone Department of Molecular Microbiology and Immunology, Bloomberg School of Public Health, Johns Hopkins University, Baltimore, MD, United States

Yongxia Sarah Qu
Department of Cardiology, New York Presbyterian Brooklyn Methodist Hospital, Brooklyn, NY, United States
VA New York Harbor Healthcare System and State University of New York Downstate Medical Center, Brooklyn, NY, United States

Pietro Enea Lazzerini, Pier Leopoldo Capecchi and Franco Laghi-Pasini
Department of Medical Sciences, Surgery and Neurosciences, University of Siena, Siena, Italy

Nabil El Sherif
VA New York Harbor Healthcare System and State University of New York Downstate Medical Center, Brooklyn, NY, United States

Mohamed Boutjdir
VA New York Harbor Healthcare System and State University of New York Downstate Medical Center, Brooklyn, NY, United States
NYU School of Medicine, New York, NY, United States

Jianqiang Zhang and Qiuyue Chen
Department of Immunology, School of Medicine, Yangtze University, Jingzhou, China

Jixin Zhong
Cardiovascular Research Institute, Case Western Reserve University, Cleveland, OH, United States

Chaohong Liu
Department of Microbiology, School of Basic Medicine, Tongji Medical College, Huazhong University of Science & Technology, Wuhan, China

Bing Zheng and Quan Gong
Department of Immunology, School of Medicine, Yangtze University, Jingzhou, China
Clinical Molecular Immunology Center, School of Medicine, Yangtze University, Jingzhou, China
Internal Medicine I - Cardiology, Palacky University and University Hospital, Olomouc, Czechia

Jaroslav Michalek
Department of Clinical and Molecular Pathology, Faculty of Medicine and Dentistry, Palacky University, Olomouc, Czechia

Jana Borucka
Department of Pathological Physiology, Faculty of Medicine Dentistry, Palacky University, Olomouc, Czechia
Faculty of Medicine and Dentistry, Institute of Molecular and Translational Medicine, Palacky University, Olomouc, Czechia

Martin Kalab
Department of Cardiac Surgery, Palacky University and University Hospital, Olomouc, Czechia

Petra Klevcova
Department of Pathological Physiology, Faculty of Medicine Dentistry, Palacky University, Olomouc, Czechia

Milos Taborsky
Internal Medicine I - Cardiology, Palacky University and University Hospital, Olomouc, Czechia

Martin Petrek
Department of Pathological Physiology, Faculty of Medicine Dentistry, Palacky University, Olomouc, Czechia
Faculty of Medicine and Dentistry, Institute of Molecular and Translational Medicine, Palacky University, Olomouc, Czechia
Laboratory of Cardiogenomics, University Hospital Olomouc, Olomouc, Czechia

Juan C. Sáez
Departamento de Fisiología, Pontificia Universidad Católica de Chile, Santiago de Chile, Chile
Instituto de Neurociencias, Centro Interdisciplinario de Neurociencias de Valparaíso, Universidad de Valparaíso, Valparaíso, Chile

Susana Contreras-Duarte
Departamento de Fisiología, Pontificia Universidad Católica de Chile, Santiago de Chile, Chile
Departamento de Ginecología y Obstetricia, Escuela de Medicina, Facultad de Medicina, Pontificia Universidad Católica de Chile, Santiago, Chile

Gonzalo I. Gómez, Valeria C. Labra, Cristian A. Santibañez, Rosario Gajardo-Gómez, Beatriz C. Avendaño, Esteban F. Díaz, Trinidad D. Montero and Juan A. Orellana
Departamento de Neurología, Escuela de Medicina and Centro Interdisciplinario de Neurociencias, Facultad de Medicina, Pontificia Universidad Católica de Chile, Santiago, Chile

Victoria Velarde
Departamento de Fisiología, Pontificia Universidad Católica de Chile, Santiago de Chile, Chile

Stephanie A. Legere and Ian D. Haidl
Departments of Microbiology and Immunology, Dalhousie University, Halifax, NS, Canada

Jean-François Légaré
Department of Pathology, Dalhousie University, Halifax, NS, Canada
Department of Surgery, Dalhousie Medicine New Brunswick, Saint John, NB, Canada

Jean S. Marshall
Departments of Microbiology and Immunology, Dalhousie University, Halifax, NS, Canada
Department of Pathology, Dalhousie University, Halifax, NS, Canada

Jing Chen, Jinsheng Lai, Mengying He, Guoran Ruan, Zhongwei Yin, Jin Wang , Chen Chen and Dao Wen Wang
Division of Cardiology, Department of Internal Medicine, Tongji Hospital, Tongji Medical College, Huazhong University of Science and Technology, Wuhan, China
Hubei Key Laboratory of Genetics and Molecular Mechanisms of Cardiological Disorders, Wuhan, China

Bei Wang
Division of Cardiology, Department of Internal Medicine, Tongji Hospital, Tongji Medical College, Huazhong University of Science and Technology, Wuhan, China
Hubei Key Laboratory of Genetics and Molecular Mechanisms of Cardiological Disorders, Wuhan, China
Department of Rheumatology and Immunology, Tongji Hospital, Tongji Medical College, Huazhong University of Science and Technology, Wuhan, China

Zachary Braunstein
Department of Internal Medicine, The Ohio State University, Columbus, OH, United States

Katherine Cianflone
Centre de Recherche de l'Institut Universitaire de Cardiologie & Pneumologie de Québec, Université Laval, Québec, QC, Canada

Qin Ning
Department of Infectious Disease, Institute of Infectious Disease, Tongji Hospital, Tongji Medical College, Huazhong University of Science and Technology, Wuhan, China

Appakkudal R. Anand
L&T Microbiology Research Centre, Vision Research Foundation, Sankara Nethralaya, Chennai, India
Department of HIV/AIDS, National Institute for Research in Tuberculosis, Chennai, India

Bernhard Maisch
Faculty of Medicine, and Heart and Vessel Center, Philipps-University, Marburg, Germany

Gladys Rachel
Department of HIV/AIDS, National Institute for Research in Tuberculosis, Chennai, India

Durgadevi Parthasarathy
L&T Microbiology Research Centre, Vision Research Foundation, Sankara Nethralaya, Chennai, India

Jun-Yan Xu, Yu-Yan Xiong and Yue-Jin Yang
State Key Laboratory of Cardiovascular Disease, Department of Cardiology, Fuwai Hospital, National Center for Cardiovascular Diseases, Chinese Academy of Medical Science and Peking Union Medical College, Beijing, China

Xiao-Tong Lu
National Cancer Center/National Clinical Research Center for Cancer/Cancer Hospital, Chinese Academy of Medical Sciences and Peking Union Medical College, Beijing, China

Di Wang
Engineering Research Center of Chinese Ministry of Education for Edible and Medicinal Fungi, Jilin Agricultural University, Changchun, China
School of Life Sciences, Jilin University, Changchun, China

Xue Jiang, Shanshan Teng and Yaqin Zhang
School of Life Sciences, Jilin University, Changchun, China

Yang Liu, Xiao Li and Yu Li
Engineering Research Center of Chinese Ministry of Education for Edible and Medicinal Fungi, Jilin Agricultural University, Changchun, China

Hui Jiang, Zhiqiang Li and Xian-Cheng Jiang
Department of Cell Biology, State University of New York Downstate Medical Center, Brooklyn, NY, United States
Molecular and Cellular Cardiology Program, VA New York Harbor Healthcare System, Brooklyn, NY, United States

Chongmin Huan
Department of Cell Biology, State University of New York Downstate Medical Center, Brooklyn, NY, United States
Molecular and Cellular Cardiology Program, VA New York Harbor Healthcare System, Brooklyn, NY, United States
Department of Surgery, State University of New York Downstate Medical Center, Brooklyn, NY, United States

Seung E. Baek, So Y. Park, Sun S. Bae and Chi D. Kim
Department of Pharmacology, School of Medicine, Pusan National University, Yangsan, South Korea
Gene and Cell Therapy Research Center for Vessel-Associated Diseases, Pusan National University, Yangsan, South Korea

Koanhoi Kim and Won S. Lee
Department of Pharmacology, School of Medicine, Pusan National University, Yangsan, South Korea

Carina Gröschel, Sebastian Monecke and Ralf Dressel
Institute of Cellular and Molecular Immunology, University Medical Center Göttingen, Göttingen, Germany
DZHK (German Center for Cardiovascular Research), Partner Site Göttingen, Göttingen, Germany

André Sasse, Charlotte Röhrborn and Leslie Elsner
Institute of Cellular and Molecular Immunology, University Medical Center Göttingen, Göttingen, Germany

Michael Didié
DZHK (German Center for Cardiovascular Research), Partner Site Göttingen, Göttingen, Germany
Institute of Pharmacology and Toxicology, University Medical Center Göttingen, Göttingen, Germany
Department of Cardiology and Pneumology, University Medical Center Göttingen, Göttingen, Germany

Verena Reupke
Central Animal Facility, University Medical Center Göttingen, Göttingen, Germany

Gertrude Bunt
Clinical Optical Microscopy, Department of Neuropathology, University Medical Center Göttingen, Göttingen, Germany

Andrew H. Lichtman
Department of Pathology, Brigham and Women's Hospital, Harvard Medical School, Boston, MA, United States

Karl Toischer and Gerd Hasenfuß
DZHK (German Center for Cardiovascular Research), Partner Site Göttingen, Göttingen, Germany
Department of Cardiology and Pneumology, University Medical Center Göttingen, Göttingen, Germany

Wolfram-Hubertus Zimmermann
DZHK (German Center for Cardiovascular Research), Partner Site Göttingen, Göttingen, Germany
Institute of Pharmacology and Toxicology, University Medical Center Göttingen, Göttingen, Germany

Index

www.ingramcontent.com/pod-product-compliance
Lightning Source LLC
LaVergne TN
LVHW081037210926
848485LV00004B/1043